Nursing Assistant
A Nursing Process Approach

BASICS

Barbara R. Hegner, MSN, RN
(deceased)

Barbara Acello, MS, RN
Independent nurse consultant
and educator

Esther Caldwell, MA, PhD
Consultant in Vocational
Education

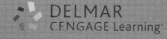

DELMAR
CENGAGE Learning

Australia • Brazil • Japan • Korea • Mexico • Singapore • Spain • United Kingdom • United States

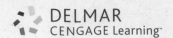

Nursing Assistant: A Nursing Process Approach—BASICS
by Barbara R. Hegner, Barbara Acello, and Esther Caldwell

Vice President, Career and Professional Editorial: Dave Garza

Director of Learning Solutions: Matthew Kane

Senior Acquisitions Editor: Maureen Rosener

Managing Editor: Marah Bellegarde

Product Manager: Jadin Babin-Kavanaugh

Editorial Assistant: Chiara Astriab

Vice President, Career and Professional Marketing: Jennifer McAvey

Executive Marketing Manager: Michele McTighe

Marketing Coordinator: Scott Chrysler

Production Director: Carolyn Miller

Production Manager: Andrew Crouth

Senior Content Project Manager: Kenneth McGrath

Senior Art Director: Jack Pendleton

Technology Project Manager: Benjamin Knapp

Technology Project Manager: Chris Catalina

For product information and technology assistance, contact us at
Cengage Learning Customer & Sales Support, 1-800-354-9706
For permission to use material from this text or product, submit all requests online at **www.cengage.com/permissions**
Further permissions questions can be e-mailed to
permissionrequest@cengage.com

Library of Congress Control Number: 2009923449

ISBN-13: 978-1-4283-1746-8

ISBN-10: 1-4283-1746-5

Delmar
5 Maxwell Drive
Clifton Park, NY 12065-2919
USA

Cengage Learning is a leading provider of customized learning solutions with office locations around the globe, including Singapore, the United Kingdom, Australia, Mexico, Brazil, and Japan. Locate your local office at: **international.cengage.com/region**

Cengage Learning products are represented in Canada by Nelson Education, Ltd.

To learn more about Delmar, visit **www.cengage.com/delmar**

Purchase any of our products at your local college store or at our preferred online store **www.ichapters.com**

Notice to the Reader

Publisher does not warrant or guarantee any of the products described herein or perform any independent analysis in connection with any of the product information contained herein. Publisher does not assume, and expressly disclaims, any obligation to obtain and include information other than that provided to it by the manufacturer. The reader is expressly warned to consider and adopt all safety precautions that might be indicated by the activities described herein and to avoid all potential hazards. By following the instructions contained herein, the reader willingly assumes all risks in connection with such instructions. The publisher makes no representations or warranties of any kind, including but not limited to, the warranties of fitness for particular purpose or merchantability, nor are any such representations implied with respect to the material set forth herein, and the publisher takes no responsibility with respect to such material. The publisher shall not be liable for any special, consequential, or exemplary damages resulting, in whole or part, from the readers' use of, or reliance upon, this material.

Printed in China
3 4 5 6 7 17 16 15 14

brief TABLE OF CONTENTS

CONTENTS

SECTION 1

INTRODUCTION TO NURSING ASSISTING   1

SECTION 2

SCIENTIFIC PRINCIPLES   39

SECTION 3

SECTION 4

SECTION 5

SECTION 6

SECTION 7

SECTION 10

SECTION 11

SECTION 12

SECTION 13

LIST *of* PROCEDURES

Icon Key: **OBRA** = OBRA   ✋ = PPE   **DVD** = DVD icon   **WWW.** = online

BARBARA R. HEGNER

Barbara Robinson Hegner, RN, MSN, was a graduate of a three-year diploma nursing program where direct and total care was the focus. She earned a BSN at Boston College and an MS in nursing from Boston University, with a minor in biologic sciences. She was Professor Emerita of Nursing and Life Sciences at Long Beach City College, Long Beach (CA).

Throughout her professional career, she had a deep interest in both hospital-based and long-term care nursing.

It was Ms. Hegner's belief that ensuring the rights and well-being of all patients and residents requires the care of competent, caring nursing assistants under the supervision of professional nurses. The nursing assistants who provide this care should be thoroughly trained and consistently encouraged, evaluated, and given the opportunity for continued learning. Providing the tools to prepare these health care providers in the most effective and efficient way is the goal of *Nursing Assistant, A Nursing Process Approach—BASICS.*

BARBARA ACELLO

Barbara Acello, MS, RN, is an independent nurse consultant and educator in Denton, Texas. She is a member of the Texas Nurses' Association, NANDA International, and American College of Healthcare Administrators (ACHCA). She is the recipient of the 2006 ACHCA education award and 2008 ACHCA journalism award. Mrs. Acello is a proponent and supporter of CNAs. She has written many textbooks, journal articles, and other materials related to nursing assistant education. She believes the nursing assistant is the most important caregiver in the health care facility.

INTRODUCTION

The passage of the Omnibus Budget Reconciliation Act (OBRA) of 1987, which included the Nursing Home Reform Act, was the first federal legislation to address standards for certification of nursing assistants as health care providers in long-term care. This legislation has influenced both the education and practice of all nursing assistants.

Following the enactment of OBRA, the National Council of State Boards of Nursing, Inc., developed the Nurse Aide Competency Evaluation Program as the guideline for evaluating nursing assistant education to meet the specific needs of health care consumers. Individual states have developed training programs that meet and, in many cases, exceed the minimum requirements of the federal government.

Nursing assistants are important members of the nursing team (one part of the interdisciplinary health care team that plans and provides care to patients). Nursing assistants make valuable contributions to the nursing process that the professional nurse follows in assessing the patients' needs, planning interventions, implementing care, and evaluating outcomes. Nursing assistants must be helped to see the vital role their accurate observations, reporting skills, and careful attention to instructions play in the overall success of the nursing care plan. Only then can they recognize their full value as part of the nursing team.

This text is designed for nursing assistant programs that are 75 to 150 hours in length. Basic "need to know" information is provided. The goal of this text and supplement package is to provide the tools that instructors can use to teach nursing assistants to meet high standards of care. This will enable them to help patients achieve a desirable level of comfort, restoration, and wellness while protecting and respecting patients' rights as health care consumers.

THE FUTURE

The ways in which health care is provided in the United States continue to change. Emphasis continues to be placed on maintaining wellness, limiting length of stay in acute care facilities, controlling costs through managed care, providing short- and long-term rehabilitation and restorative care in more cost-effective settings, and increasing home care services. In addition, the population of the United States is aging, with the greatest increase in the number of people over 65 years of age. As a result, restorative care and home care services will be major components in health care. Nursing assistants will provide much of this care. It is essential that nursing assistants be prepared to assume these vital responsibilities.

EXTENSIVE TEACHING AND LEARNING PACKAGE

Delmar Cengage Learning has provided a complete learning package to accompany *Nursing Assistant: A Nursing Process Approach—Basics.*

Student and Instructor Resources

The following resources were developed to help students learn and practice the information essential to becoming certified as a skilled nursing assistant:

StudyWare CD-ROM

The CD-ROM included in the back of this text features quizzes, games, and case studies. Students can take the quizzes in Practice Mode to improve mastery of the material; instant feedback tells whether an answer is right or wrong, and explains why. Quiz Mode allows students to test themselves and keep a record of their scores. Study-Ware games, flashcards, and image labeling exercises reinforce unit content, and the unique critical thinking case studies help synthesize and apply unit topics to real-world scenarios. Video clips from Delmar's Basic Core Skills for Nursing Assistants DVD series are also included.

Student Workbook

ISBN 1428317473

The student workbook directly correlates to the textbook. This competency-based supplement includes critical thinking questions, multiple-choice questions similar to those seen in the state certification examination, and challenging items such as word games, puzzles, and exercises to help students understand essential content and master spelling and definitions of key terms. A section on studying for the state written and competency examination will help prepare students who will be taking a state certification exam.

Student Resources at the Online Companion

The Online Companion features additional resources to supplement the book content, plus up-to-date information on ever-changing practices and standards in nursing assisting, as well as additional unit content. To access, go to www.delmarlearning.com/companions, click on 'Nursing' from the left navigation menu. Scroll down to select *Nursing Assistant: a Nursing Process Approach-BASICS*, then click on 'Student Resources.'

Instructor Resources

The following resources were developed to aid instructors in teach the content found in Nursing Assistant: A Nursing Process Approach—BASICS.

Instructor Resource CD-ROM
ISBN 1428317481

The Instructor Resource CD-ROM contains everything you need to teach Nursing Assistant: A Nursing Process Approach—BASICS. The following are included on the CD-ROM:

- **Instructor's Manual**—this contains the answer keys to all textbook and student workbook exercises, in addition to lesson plans, instructor resources, quizzes, testing materials, procedure checklists, and transparency images. The instructor's manual is available electronically on this CD-ROM and at the Online Companion.
- **Computerized Test Bank** with more than 1900 questions written in *ExamView*® Pro test-generating software.
- **Presentations written in PowerPoint™** featuring over 900 slides with illustrations from the textbook.

Instructor Resources at the Online Companion

For your convenience, this online resource features the same great supplements found on the Instructor Resource CD-ROM, including the Instructor's Manual, Computerized Test Bank, and Presentations written in PowerPoint. All instructor resources at the Online Companion are password-protected. Go to www.delmarlearning.com/companions, click on 'Nursing' from the left navigation menu. Scroll down to select *Nursing Assistant: a Nursing Process Approach-BASICS*. Please contact your sales rep for the user id and password log-in combination, or see the Instructor's Manual.

WebTutor Advantage on WebCT and Blackboard
WebCT: 142831749X   Blackboard: 1428317503

This course cartridge for Blackboard and WebCT can be used to supplement on-campus course delivery or as the course management platform for an online course. Web-Tutor™ provides communication tools to instructors and students, including a course calendar, chat, e-mail, and threaded discussions. Each unit contains the following items:

- Advance Preparation—details what a student should do before starting each online unit
- Unit Objectives—alert the student to what is expected as outcomes for each unit
- Class Notes—helpful tips that provide further clarification and expansion of text content
- Frequently Asked Questions (FAQs)—provide answers to questions that students commonly ask
- Glossary of terms—specific to the unit; this material is also rolled into a comprehensive glossary for the course
- Discussion Topics—provide interactive classroom discussion by means of a threaded bulletin board
- Learning Links—require students to search the Web for information to reinforce and expand learning; students report their findings to instructors through e-mail

- Online Exercises—provide further reinforcement of learning with immediate feedback WebTutor™ also includes a midterm test and a final test.

WebTutor™
WebCT 142831749X,   BlackBoard 1428317503

This course cartridge for Blackboard and WebCT can be used to supplement on-campus course delivery or as the course management platform for an online course. WebTutor™ provides communication tools to instructors and students, including a course calendar, chat, e-mail, and threaded discussions. Each unit contains the following items:

- Advance Preparation—details what a student should do before starting each online unit
- Unit Objectives—alert the student to what is expected as outcomes for each unit
- Class Notes—helpful tips that provide further clarification and expansion of text content
- Frequently Asked Questions (FAQs)—provide answers to questions that students commonly ask
- Glossary of terms—specific to the unit; this material is also rolled into a comprehensive glossary for the course
- Discussion Topics—provide interactive classroom discussion by means of a threaded bulletin board

Basic Core Skills for Nursing Assistants DVD Series
ISBN 1418029599

Skills-based videos to accompany many of the procedures in the text! Each of the 76 core procedures is presented step-by-step for maximum effectiveness. In addition to the procedures, general guidelines are included for lifting and moving, ambulation, handling clean or soiled linen, and observation and reporting. These videos are great for in-class demonstration to help prepare students for exams or for clinical rotations. This series includes the following modules:

Module 1	Obstructed Airway, Handwashing, Beginning and Completion Procedure Actions, Communication Skills
Module 2	Personal Protective Equipment, Standard Precautions, and Transmission Based Precautions
Module 3	Positioning, Transfers, and Ambulation
Module 4	Bedmaking and Bathing
Module 5	Bladder, Bowel, and Perineal Care
Module 6	Personal Care
Module 7	Dressing, Meal Care, and Restraints
Module 8	Vital Signs, Height, and Weight
Module 9	Observation/Reporting Guidelines and Postmortem Care
Module 10	Range of Motion and Mechanical Lift

For your convenience, a DVD icon appears in the text on every procedure that has a corresponding video clip.

SUPPLEMENT	WHAT'S ON IT
StudyWare Software CD-ROM	This is the CD-ROM found in the back of this textbook. It features quizzes and games for each unit, plus case studies and video clips from Delmar's *Basic Core Skills for Nursing Assistants* DVD Series.
Student Workbook	This competency-based supplement follows the textbook and includes critical thinking questions, multiple-choice questions similar to those seen in state certification exams, and challenging items such as word games, puzzles, and exercises to help students understand essential content.
Instructor Resources	Includes the **Instructor's Manual** with answer keys to book and workbook, plus over 1900-question test bank, and a 900-slide presentation written in PowerPoint™.
Student Resources at the Online Companion	**Student Resources** include additional unit content, procedures, and information on the ever-changing practices and standards in Nursing Assisting.
Instructor Resources at the Online Companion	**Instructor Resources** are password-protected and include the test bank, presentations in PowerPoint™, and Instructor's Manual.
WebTutor™ Advantage	Available on WebCT or Blackboard, the WebTutor™ provides the foundation for an online course to extend learning beyond the classroom. Features include: • Objectives • Study Tips • Class Notes (with PowerPoint) • Discussion questions • Email, chat capability • Chapter Quizzes with immediate feedback • Preloaded test bank for instructors • Web links
Basic Core Skills for Nursing Assistants DVD-ROM	Skills-based videos available for separate purchase, featuring 76 core procedures presented in step-by-step format.

ACKNOWLEDGMENTS

Each book provides an opportunity to acknowledge the contributions of a number of individuals.

First, my husband, Francis; son Jon; and granddaughter Brooklyn have given greatly of themselves while I worked on this manuscript. I appreciate their love and support.

A book of this size represents an enormous investment of time and talent by many dedicated individuals. I sincerely appreciate the support and assistance of the following individuals at Delmar Learning: Jadin Babin-Kavanaugh, product manager, whose support was invaluable in manuscript construction and development; and Matthew Seeley, acquisitions editor, whose vision and tolerance of my idiosyncrasies is sincerely appreciated. I am always delighted when Brooke Graves lends her many copyediting talents to my projects.

Reviewers

The revision was aided by a dedicated group of instructors who reviewed content at different stages of the revision process. For their valuable suggestions and insights, the publisher and author would like to thank the following:

Lois Stotter, MSN, RN
Dorsey Schools
Madison Heights, MI

Deb McClain, RN, BSN, CRRN
Hagerstown Community College
Hagerstown, MD

Betty Earp, BSN, RN
Maricopa Community Colleges
Mesa Community College
Mesa, AZ

Jean Lashbrook, RN
Texas State Technical College
Harlingen, TX

Marty Bachman, PhD, RN
Front Range Community College
Fort Collins, CO

HOW TO USE *this* BOOK

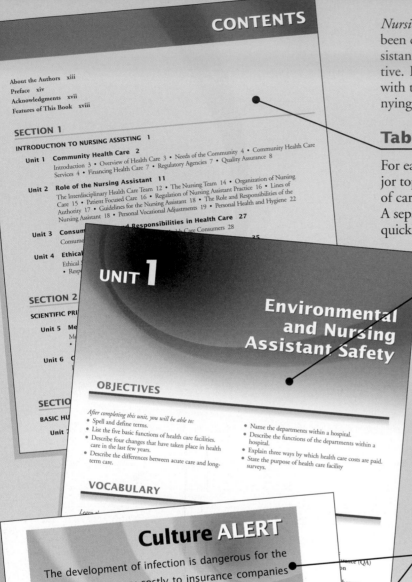

UNIT 1

Environmental and Nursing Assistant Safety

OBJECTIVES

After completing this unit, you will be able to:
• Spell and define terms.
• List the five basic functions of health care facilities.
• Describe four changes that have taken place in health care in the last few years.
• Describe the differences between acute care and long-term care.

• Name the departments within a hospital.
• Describe the functions of the departments within a hospital.
• Explain three ways by which health care costs are paid.
• State the purpose of health care facility surveys.

VOCABULARY

Learn t...

Nursing Assistant: A Nursing Process Approach—Basics has been carefully designed to make the mastery of nursing assistant tasks and responsibilities easier and more productive. For best results, you may want to become familiar with the features incorporated into this text and accompanying learning tools.

Table of Contents

For each unit, the table of contents lists the unit title, major topic headings, and general guidelines for specific areas of care and topics of importance to the nursing assistant. A separate listing helps you locate patient care procedures quickly and easily.

Unit Opening Page

Each unit opening page contains objectives and vocabulary terms.

The **objectives** help you know what is expected of you as you read the text. Your success in mastering each objective is measured by the review questions at the end of each unit.

The **vocabulary** list alerts you to new terms presented in the unit. When each term is first used in the unit, it is highlighted in boldface and color. Each term is defined at this point in the unit. Read the definition of the term and note the context in which it is used so that you will feel comfortable in using the term. Note that the glossary at the back of the book also defines these highlighted terms.

Text Alerts

The alerts provide important content on infection control, OSHA, communication, age-appropriate care, legal implications, safety, difficult situations, and clinical information related to patient care. These alerts make the learner aware of best practices in patient care, include practical tips based on experience, and highlight critical infection control, safety, and other OSHA workplace guidelines.

Culture ALERT

The development of infection is dangerous for the patient and is very costly to insurance companies and the hospital. Prevention of infection is a major nursing assistant function. Prevention of infection is a major nursing assistant function. Prevention of infection is a...

Critical Information ALERT

Know the location of the know the location of the tube at all times and avoid pulling on it. Avoid pulling on the tube when moving and transferring the patient. Serious com... feeding tube is dislodg... feeding tube must be k... times the skin around a... ered with gauze. After t...nent. dressing is necessary. If t...spital tric tube, it may be clippe... to prevent pulling. ■

Safety ALERT

Know the location of the know the location of the tube at all times and avoid pulling on it. Avoid pulling on the tube when moving and transferring the patient. Serious complications can result if a feeding tube is dislodged. The skin around the feeding tube must be kept clean and dry. Sometimes the skin around a gastrostomy tube is covered with gauze. After the incision has healed, no dressing is necessary. If the patient has a nasogastric tube, it may be clipped to the gown or clothing to prevent pulling. ■

Patients may b...
within a hospit...
will go from the...
to the surgical r...

safety data sheets,
An OSHA survey
a tour of all areas o...

Inspector C T...
health and safety
recommendations...

...ll cleaning
...ent.
...billing,
...rns.
...catalogs all

FINANCI...

Health care is p...
• Insurance. E...
or persons m...
• **Medicare** is a...
portion of he...
over and for y...
abled and wh...

OSHA Surveys

The **Occupational Safety** ...ls for the
(OSHA) also surveys health c...
...ernmental agency that prot...us and
...d perform
...nning the
...OSHA inspectors...

Photographs and Illustrations

Numerous color illustrations and photos help to clarify and reinforce the unit content. Many figures are used in the procedures to help you visualize critical step-by-step information. Full-color anatomy drawings help you to locate body components and understand body organization.

Guidelines

"Guidelines for . . ." boxes highlight important points that you need to remember for specific situations or types of care. They are presented in an easy-to-use format that you can refer to repeatedly until you know the actions you must take when confronted with the situation.

Procedures

The textbook contains 114 clinical procedures in a step-by-step format. Each procedure reminds you to perform both beginning and ending actions. Any notes or cautions about performing the procedure are given. The steps take you carefully through the procedure, emphasizing at all times the need to work safely and to protect the patient's privacy. Icons accompanying each procedure help you easily identify procedures that contain key OBRA and PPE standards, as well as procedures for which a corresponding video is available on *Delmar's Basic Core Skills for Nursing Assistants* video series. Additional state- and facility-specific procedures are located in the Online Companion to this book.

Unit Reviews and Testing Material

A variety of review questions at the end of each unit test your understanding of the unit content. Each review contains a Nursing Assistant Challenge that presents a typical clinical situation and asks questions about your response to the situation. These questions help you master critical thinking skills and require you to integrate what you have learned to arrive at an appropriate solution or set of actions.

FIGURE 5-18 The central nervous system

Lateral ventricles (2)
- Skull
- Frontal lobe
- Temporal lobe
- Pituitary gland
- Midbrain
- Pons
- Medulla oblongata
- Spinal cord
- Parietal lobe
- Convolutions (gyri)
- Sulci
- Dura mater
- Arachnoid
- Pia mater — Meninges
- Third ventricle
- Cerebral
- Fourth ventricle
- Cerebellum

GUIDELINES for
Charting

- Check for: right patient, right chart, right form, right room
- Fill out new headings completely
- Use correct color of ink
- Date and time each entry
- Chart entries in co
- Make entries brief
- Print or write clea
- Spell each word
- Leave no blank
- Do not use the
- Do not use dif
- Sign each ent and job title
- Make correc entry; then your initials

PROCEDURE

26
MEASURING A RECTAL TEMPERATURE

Note: The guidelines for this procedure vary slightly from state to state, and from one facility to the next. Your instructor will inform you if the sequence in your state or facility differs from the procedure listed here. Know and follow the required sequence for your facility and state.

1. Carry out initial procedure actions.
2. Assemble equipment on a tray:
   - Gloves
   - Glass or digital thermometer or electronic thermometer with rectal (red) probe
   - Probe cover or plastic sheath
   - Lubricant
3. If using a glass thermometer, rinse the disinfectant off and dry the thermometer. Shake the glass thermometer down to 96°F. Cover the thermometer or probe with a plastic sheath or probe cover.

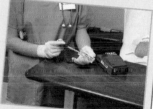

FIGURE 18-9 Apply a small amount of lubricant to the tip of the sheath. (© Delmar/Cengage Learning)

alarm sounds on the electronic or digital thermometer. Discard the cover.
8. Hold the glass thermometer at eye level and

REVIEW

A. Multiple Choice
Select the one best answer for each of the following.

1. Successful communication is essential for
   a. body language to be meaningful.
   b. patients only.
   c. staff only.
   d. safe care.
2. Verbal communication includes
   a. talking and listening.
   b. facial expressions.
   c. reading reports.
   d. using a fax machine.
3. For successful communication to occur, all of the following elements must be present except
   a. receiver.
   b. hearing.
   c. feedback.
   d. sender.
4. Examples of nonverbal communication include
   a. reading and using the patient's care plan.
   b. answering the telephone.
   c. listening to the shift report.
   d. conversing with patients.
5. Demonstrating your understanding of a message by stating the message in your own words is
   a. channeling.
   b. rephrasing and restating.
   c. paraphrasing.
   d. reorganizing.

6. The portion of communication that influence on the receiver's interpreta message is the
   a. body language.
   b. tone of voice.
   c. pitch of voice.
   d. eye contact.
7. The document that shows the line of communication is the
   a. staff development chart.
   b. employee personnel handbook.
   c. policy and procedure manual.
   d. organizational chart.
8. Examples of manuals that are found include
   a. computer manual, administrative quality assurance manual.
   b. procedure manual, infection cont disaster manual.
   c. employee assistance program man manual, benefits manual.
   d. isolation manual, X-ray manual, manual.
9. The patient's care plan provides infor
   a. nursing assistant assignments.
   b. employee benefits.
   c. fire drill procedures.
   d. licensed personnel only.
10. The patient's medical record or chart
    a. used only by the physician.

Dedication

This text is dedicated to the memory of Barbara R. Hegner. Barbara was a visionary who saw the need for formalized instructional materials to help educate and develop skilled nursing assistants. She was committed to this unique and important group of health care professionals.

SECTION 1

Introduction to Nursing Assisting

UNIT 1

Community Health Care

OBJECTIVES

After completing this unit, you will be able to:
- Spell and define terms.
- List the five basic functions of health care facilities.
- Describe the differences between acute care and long-term care.
- Name at least five departments within a hospital and state their functions.
- Describe patient-focused care.
- State the purpose of health care facility surveys.

VOCABULARY

Learn the meaning and the correct spelling of the following words and phrases:

acute illness	hospital	Occupational Safety and	prenatal
chronic illness	Joint Commission	Health Administration	psychiatric
citation	long-term acute care	(OSHA)	quality assurance (QA)
client	hospital (LTACH)	patient	resident
community	Magnet Program for	patient-focused care	skilled care facility
cross-training	Excellence in Nursing	pediatric	survey
facility	Services	post-anesthesia recovery	surveyor
health care consumer	managed care	(PAR)	
hospice	obstetric	postpartum	

INTRODUCTION

Nursing assistants play an important role in the care of people who are ill or injured. You will care for patients under the direction and supervision of licensed, professional health care workers, such as physicians (doctors) and nurses. The place where care is given is called a health care **facility**. A **hospital** provides a full range of health care services. Highly technical services are available there. Some hospitals provide general care for patients with many conditions. Others provide only specialized services, such as care for patients with cancer. A **skilled care facility** provides care to persons whose conditions are stable but who need monitoring, nursing care, and treatments. All health care facilities have five basic functions:

1. Providing services for the ill and injured (Figure 1-1).
2. Preventing disease.
3. Promoting individual and community health.
4. Educating health care workers (Figure 1-2).
5. Promoting research in medicine and nursing.

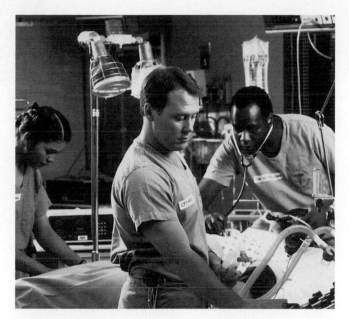

FIGURE 1-1 Health care facilities provide routine, emergency, and surgical services to many different types of patients. *("Be All You Can Be," Courtesy United States Government, as represented by the Secretary of the Army)*

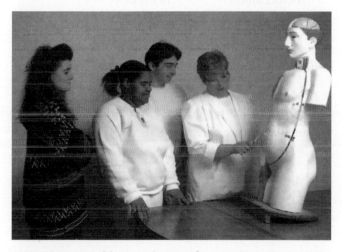

FIGURE 1-2 Health care changes frequently, and education is an important objective for personnel. *(© Delmar/ Cengage Learning)*

OVERVIEW OF HEALTH CARE

Health care workers today give **patient-focused care**. This type of care focuses on the unique individual needs of each person. Physical, mental, and emotional needs are all considered.

People are living longer, so quality of life is an important concern. Quality-of-life policies focus on providing care in an environment that humanizes and individualizes each patient. Some health care decisions are made with the patient's future quality of life in mind. Preserving the quality of life is sometimes more important than increasing the length of life.

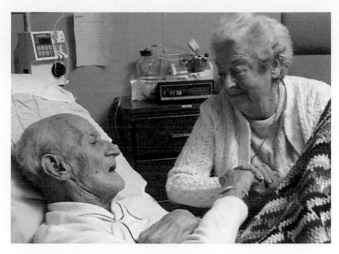

FIGURE 1-3 An aging population needs more health care services to manage illness and disability. *(© Delmar/Cengage Learning)*

Many changes have occurred in health care within the past few decades because:

- People are living longer. Their need for health care increases with age (Figure 1-3).
- Advances in technology mean that more lives are saved. However, some of these individuals need continuing care.
- The cost of health care has increased because of the demand for services and use of expensive technology.
- Science has created many ethical (moral) questions that must be answered.

Patients are discharged earlier from hospitals to reduce costs. These patients may still require health care. This care can be given more economically in other settings. Diagnostic tests and procedures are provided in outpatient facilities. Most health care is paid for with insurance. Insurance companies use **managed care** to provide efficient services at the lowest cost. Briefly, this means that the insurance company will:

- Preapprove some procedures and tests.
- Negotiate with some facilities and professionals to provide care at a lower cost to the company's members.
- Approve a certain number of days of hospitalization for specific diagnoses. If the patient must stay longer, the hospital must get approval from the insurer, or payment may be denied.
- Require that some procedures be done on an outpatient basis.

Infection Control ALERT

The development of infection is dangerous for the patient and is very costly to insurance companies and the hospital. Prevention of infection is a major nursing assistant function. ∎

NEEDS OF THE COMMUNITY

People who live in a common area and share common health needs form a **community**. The community may provide waste disposal, safe drinking water, services to ensure that food in stores and restaurants is wholesome, and some health services.

Public health laws regulate these services and are enforced by government agencies.

Health care is needed throughout life. The care may be short-term or long-term and includes:

- Preventive care to maintain good health.
- **Prenatal** care (care of the mother during pregnancy).
- Health education.
- Emergency care for sudden illness or injury.
- Surgery to repair an injured body part or remove a diseased organ.
- Rehabilitation to help a person regain abilities lost due to illness or injury.
- Long-term care for persons with chronic conditions.
- **Hospice** care for patients who are dying and their families.

Persons receiving health care are called **health care consumers**. They are also identified by the type of care they need:

- **Patient** is a person who receives care in a hospital.
- **Client** is a person who is cared for at home.
- **Resident** is the recipient of care in a long-term care facility.

HEALTH CARE SERVICES

There are two main types of health care facilities: those that provide short-term care and those that provide long-term care (Table 1-1). Short-term (acute) care is given to persons with minor problems, and those who need surgery or care for acute illnesses or injuries. An **acute illness** comes on suddenly and requires immediate treatment. Heart attacks, severe burns, strokes, and uncontrolled diabetes are examples of acute conditions.

Long-term care is given to persons who have chronic conditions. A **chronic illness** is one that is treatable but not curable and is expected to require lifelong care.

Hospitals

Most hospitals care for patients of all ages and patients with a variety of problems. Some take care of patients with special conditions or care for specific age groups:

- **Pediatric** hospitals care only for children from birth to age 18.
- **Psychiatric** hospitals provide care for persons with mental illness.

TABLE 1-1 TYPES OF HEALTH CARE FACILITIES

Short-Term Care	Long-Term Care
Hospitals	Long-term acute care hospitals Subacute and transitional care facilities Skilled care facilities (SNF) and nursing facilities (NF)
Urgent care facilities	Adult day care
Surgicenters	Assisted living facilities Rehabilitation centers
Outpatient clinics	Respite care (temporary care)
Psychiatric hospitals	Group homes, homes for persons with mental retardation, and psychiatric hospitals
Physician's offices	Home care

- **Rehabilitation** hospitals help individuals regain skills and abilities that were lost as a result of illness or injury. If complete restoration is not possible, the patient is restored to his or her highest level of function.
- **Long-term acute care hospitals (LTACH)** are licensed hospitals that care for patients who are expected to have a lengthy stay. To be accepted, the patient must have a medically complex condition, need acute care services, and have a good chance of improvement. The level of care is higher than in long-term care facilities and other chronic care settings.

Hospital Organization

Hospitals are set up to provide the most efficient delivery of care. Many departments meet the needs of patients 24 hours a day, 7 days a week (Figure 1-4).

- Medical department: cares for patients with medical conditions such as pneumonia or heart disease.
- Surgical department: cares for patients before, during, and after surgery. The **post-anesthesia recovery (PAR)** area is where patients are monitored until they are stable enough to leave the surgical department.
- Pediatric department: cares for sick or injured children.
- **Obstetric** department: cares for newborns and their mothers. This department includes the labor and delivery unit, the **postpartum** unit (for mothers who have given birth), and the nursery for care of newborns (Figure 1-5).

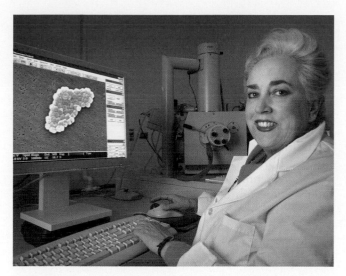

FIGURE 1-4 Many departments meet the needs of patients. Some require special equipment and are highly technical. This microbiologist is studying an electronic image of bacteria that cannot be seen with the eye. *(Courtesy of Centers for Disease Control and Prevention)*

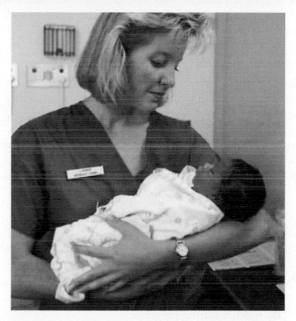

FIGURE 1-5 The obstetric department cares for mothers and newborn infants. *(© Delmar/Cengage Learning)*

- Emergency departments: care for persons with serious illness or injury.
- Critical care department: cares for critically ill patients who require constant monitoring and care.

Patients may be transferred from one unit to another within a hospital. For example, a patient having surgery will go from the operating room to the PAR room and then to the surgical nursing unit.

Cost containment is a priority, which means that the maximum benefit must be achieved for every dollar spent. Each worker must do everything possible to avoid waste and keep expenditures down.

PATIENT-FOCUSED CARE

The trend in health care has moved toward the patient-focused method of care delivery. This model of care emphasizes the needs of the patients rather than the workers. Team members make decisions jointly, and plan and deliver care to meet patient needs. This is faster and involves fewer individuals than other methods of care involving many departments. Thus, the patient is the focus of the service, and is a fully functional member of the team. The goals of patient-focused care are to:

- Limit the number of people involved in patient care.
- Contain costs.
- Meet patients' needs efficiently.

Staff members may be prepared as multiskilled workers by **cross-training** them to perform special skills. Multiskilled team members carry out treatments and provide services formerly given by other departments. For example, when a multiskilled nursing assistant has been **cross-trained** to draw blood, it is not necessary to call a technician from another department or move the patient out of the unit.

REGULATORY AGENCIES

Many external agencies regulate health care facilities. Some are branches of the state and federal government, but several are voluntary, private organizations.

Health care facilities must meet certain quality standards to operate. Various agencies inspect the facility to ensure that it meets health and safety rules. A **survey** is a review and evaluation to ensure that a facility is maintaining acceptable standards of practice. Many different agencies establish standards for health care facilities. Different types of facilities must meet different quality standards.

During a survey, a number of surveyors inspect conditions in the facility. **Surveyors** are representatives of the agency that reviews the facility.

The Joint Commission

The **Joint Commission** inspects and accredits health care providers. Participation in the accreditation process is voluntary. However, hospitals are not eligible to receive some types of payment unless they are accredited. Joint Commission sets very high standards for accreditation. Joint Commission surveyors visit periodically to ensure that the facility meets these standards.

OSHA Surveys

The **Occupational Safety and Health Administration (OSHA)** also surveys health care facilities. OSHA is a government agency that protects the health and safety of employees. OSHA inspectors review infection control, employee tuberculin testing, and other policies and practices. If the surveyor notes dangerous or unsafe conditions that could affect employee well-being, the facility may receive a **citation** or fine. A citation is a written notice that informs the facility of the violation of agency rules.

Magnet Hospitals

According to the American Hospital Association (AHA), 95% of all hospital care is given by nursing personnel. The quality of nursing services has a significant effect on patient outcomes. The **Magnet Program for Excellence in Nursing Services** recognizes hospitals for nursing excellence. This program is based on quality standards of nursing

practice. Attaining magnet designation is not easy. Hospitals that have achieved magnet status are usually very desirable places to work. Nurses and others like to work in an environment that recognizes their status and contributions.

QUALITY ASSURANCE

All health care facilities have a program called **quality assurance (QA)**. A quality assurance committee conducts reviews to identify problems. Restraint use, pressure ulcers, and infection control are some of the areas reviewed. Committee members make recommendations to improve care. Care and services should be adjusted regularly to meet patient needs. This prevents problems with regulatory agencies and improves the quality of care.

REVIEW

A. Multiple Choice

Select the one best answer for each of the following.

1. The general term for a person who needs health care is
   a. patient.
   b. resident.
   c. health care consumer.
   d. health care provider.

2. Psychiatric hospitals provide care only to
   a. children.
   b. persons with mental illness.
   c. persons with contagious diseases.
   d. dying persons.

3. Health care facilities
   a. treat most patients on an outpatient basis.
   b. must get the insurer's approval before providing emergency care.
   c. provide a variety of services to ill and injured persons.
   d. allow patients to stay as long as they want.

4. Health care has changed because
   a. there is less demand for services.
   b. people are living longer.
   c. the death rate is increasing.
   d. it is too expensive for most people.

5. Hospice care is provided to people who
   a. are dying.
   b. need rehabilitation.

   c. need surgery.
   d. are pregnant.

6. The emphasis of patient-focused care is
   a. the needs of the workers.
   b. each patient's individual needs.
   c. having workers from all departments provide care.
   d. involving family members in care.

7. Magnet hospitals
   a. have high-technology equipment.
   b. use the best doctors in their fields.
   c. are known for nursing excellence.
   d. hire only licensed professionals.

8. Prenatal care involves care of the
   a. mother during labor and delivery.
   b. mother during pregnancy.
   c. high-risk infant.
   d. infant immediately after birth.

9. The organization that accredits most health care facilities is
   a. OSHA.
   b. Medicare.
   c. Joint Commission.
   d. the quality assurance committee.

10. The purpose of quality assurance is to
    a. guarantee quality to the government.
    b. identify and correct problems.
    c. ensure that the facility gets paid.
    d. pass the accreditation inspection.

B. Nursing Assistant Challenge

Susanna Hernandez is a 34-year-old patient who was in an accident in which she fractured her pelvis, left femur (thigh bone), and right forearm. She formerly lived alone in an apartment and looked in on her elderly mother at the assisted living facility daily. After a long hospitalization, the doctor plans to discharge Susanna. She cannot ambulate (walk) and has difficulty feeding herself with her left hand. Consider how Ms. Hernandez will move through the health care system to regain her self-care ability.

11. Ms. Hernandez cannot feed herself or ambulate. What kind of assistance will she need after discharge?

12. Can she be discharged to her apartment, living alone? Explain your answer.

13. List the locations in which her continuing care could be provided.

UNIT 2

On the Job: Being a Nursing Assistant

OBJECTIVES

After completing this unit, you will be able to:
- Spell and define terms.
- Identify the members of the interdisciplinary health care team.
- Identify the members of the nursing team.
- Understand the legal limits of nursing assistant practice.
- List the job responsibilities of the nursing assistant.
- State the purpose of evidence-based practice.

- Make a chart showing your facility's lines of authority.
- Discuss the potential for career growth and advancement.
- Describe the importance of good human relationships and list ways of building productive relationships with patients, families, and staff.
- List the rules of personal hygiene and explain the importance of a healthy mental attitude.
- Describe the appropriate dress for the job.

VOCABULARY

Learn the meaning and the correct spelling of the following words and phrases:

assessment	hand-off communication	Nurse Aide Training	Omnibus Budget
assignment	interdisciplinary health	and Competency	Reconciliation Act
attitude	care team	Evaluation Program	(OBRA)
burnout	interpersonal	(NATCEP)	registered nurse (RN)
delegation	relationship	nurse practice act	scope of practice
empathy	licensed practical nurse	nursing assistant	shift report
evidence-based practice	licensed vocational nurse	nursing team	
(EBP)			

THE INTERDISCIPLINARY HEALTH CARE TEAM

The nursing assistant is an important member of the **interdisciplinary health care team** (Figure 2-1). In some facilities, this is called the *personal support team.* This team includes the patient, the physician, the nursing team, and others who provide services to patients (Figure 2-2). Members of the patient's family are also included, with the patient's permission.

The physician names the condition or illness (makes a diagnosis) and prescribes treatment. Physicians may specialize in one area of medical practice. Table 2-1 lists common medical specialties, and a description of the care provided by each.

The **nursing team** provides skilled nursing care. The team consists of registered nurses, licensed practical (or vocational) nurses, and nursing assistants. Registered nurses plan and direct the nursing care. All members of the team provide direct patient care.

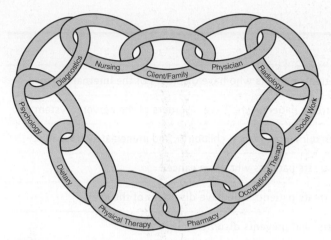

FIGURE 2-1 The interdisciplinary team members are like the links in a chain; they work together in providing services to patients. *(© Delmar/Cengage Learning)*

Specialists who may also be part of the team include dietitians, physical therapists, occupational therapists, speech therapists, respiratory therapists, and pharmacists. Table 2-2 provides an overview of the members of the health care team.

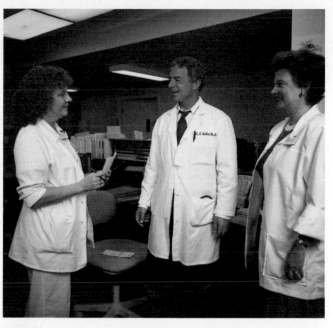

FIGURE 2-2 Each member of the health care team makes important contributions to the overall operation of the facility and well-being of patients. *(© Delmar/Cengage Learning)*

TABLE 2-1 MEDICAL SPECIALTIES

Specialty	Physician	Type of Care
Allergy	Allergist	Diagnoses and treats patients who have abnormal immune responses to foreign agents, such as substances or drugs.
Cardiovascular diseases	Cardiologist	Diagnoses and treats patients who have disorders of the heart and blood vessels.
Critical care	Intensivist	Specializes in intensive care and treats critically ill and injured patients.
Dermatology	Dermatologist	Diagnoses and treats patients who have disorders of the skin.
Endocrinology	Endocrinologist	Specializes in diabetes; diagnoses and treats conditions of the endocrine system.
Gastroenterology	Gastroenterologist	Diagnoses and treats patients who have disorders of the digestive system.
Gerontology	Gerontologist	Diagnoses and treats disorders of the aging person.
Gynecology	Gynecologist	Diagnoses and treats female reproductive disorders.
Hematology	Hematologist	Diagnoses and treats patients who have disorders of the blood and blood-forming organs.
Hospital care	Hospitalist	Has his or her primary practice in the hospital, rather than in an office. Admits patients, manages care, and reports to the patient's primary physician about the hospital course of treatment.

continues

TABLE 2-1 continued

Specialty	Physician	Type of Care
Internal medicine	Internist	Diagnoses and treats patients who have disorders of the internal organs.
Neurology	Neurologist	Diagnoses and treats patients who have disorders of the nervous system.
Obstetrics	Obstetrician	Cares for women during pregnancy, childbirth, and immediately thereafter.
Oncology	Oncologist	Diagnoses and treats patients who have cancer.
Ophthalmology	Ophthalmologist	Diagnoses and treats patients who have disorders of the eyes.
Pediatrics	Pediatrician	Diagnoses, treats, and prevents disorders in children.
Physical medicine	Physiatrist	Restores physical function for persons who have been injured or are disabled.
Psychiatry	Psychiatrist	Diagnoses and treats disorders of the mind.
Radiology	Radiologist	Diagnoses and treats disorders with X-rays and other forms of imaging technology.
Urology	Urologist	Diagnoses and treats disorders of the urinary tract and male reproductive tract.

TABLE 2-2 INTERDISCIPLINARY HEALTH CARE TEAM MEMBERS

Each discipline requires a specified course of study. Most require state licensing or certification from a professional association. Requirements vary from state to state for some disciplines.

Patient	The most important member of the team. The patient has input into the planning and implementation of care. The family may participate if the patient gives permission or if the patient is unable to participate.
Physician	Licensed to diagnose and treat disease and prescribe medications. Many specialty areas require additional education.
Clinical Nurse Specialist (CNS)	An advanced-practice registered nurse whose care focuses on a very specific patient population (e.g., medical, surgical, diabetic, geriatric, etc.).
Nurse Practitioner (NP)	A registered nurse with advanced education and experience that enables the NP to diagnose and manage common illnesses, either independently or as part of a team. A nurse practitioner can prescribe medications in most states.
Physician Assistant (PA)	A professional who is licensed to practice medicine only with physician supervision. PAs conduct physical exams, order and interpret tests, assist in surgery, and can write prescriptions in most states. PAs are educated in the medical model and their activities are designed to complement physician practice.
Registered Nurse (RN)	Licensed to make assessments and plan, implement, and evaluate nursing care. Supervises other nursing staff. Many specialty areas within nursing require additional education.
Licensed Practical Nurse (LPN or LVN)	Licensed to provide direct patient care under the supervision of a registered nurse. Called *licensed vocational nurse* in Texas and California.
Nursing Assistant	Has completed a state-approved course, has passed a competency examination, and is certified to provide direct patient care under the supervision of a licensed nurse.

TABLE 2-2 continued

Nutrition Assistant (Feeding Assistant)	After completing an approved class, may assist stable, long-term care facility residents with intake of food and fluids, under the direction of a licensed nurse.
Medication Aide (MA)	A certified nursing assistant who has taken additional classes in medication administration and passed a state examination. Allowed to give medications under the supervision of a licensed nurse. About 30 states permit medication aides to practice in various health care settings.
Restorative Assistant (RNA)	A certified nursing assistant who has additional education in restorative nursing care. Assists patients to attain and maintain their highest level of function, and prevents physical deformities.
Specialty Services	
Chaplain	Meets religious and spiritual needs of patients and provides emotional support.
Dietitian	Licensed to assess nutritional needs; plans menus and therapeutic diets and oversees food services.
Occupational Therapist (OT)	Assists patients to relearn activities of daily living, improve fine motor skills, and prevent deformities. OT assistants and aides work under therapist supervision.
Orthotist	Designs and fits braces and splints.
Physical Therapist (PT)	Assists patients to relearn mobility and ambulation skills, improve gross motor skills, and prevents deformities. PT assistants and aides work under therapist supervision.
Respiratory Therapist (also called respiratory care practitioner or RCP)	Evaluates and treats diseases and problems associated with breathing and the respiratory tract. Cares for persons who have sleep apnea.
Social Worker	Assesses and provides services to meet the nonmedical, psychosocial needs of patients.
Speech Therapist (also called speech-language pathologist; SLP)	Provides services to persons who have speech and swallowing disorders caused by illness or trauma.
Ancillary Clinical	
Pharmacist	Fills prescriptions for medications and acts as an information resource for maintaining safe drug therapy.
Phlebotomist	Uses needles to puncture veins for the purpose of drawing blood.
Laboratory Technician	Prepares specimens, operates automated analyzers, and performs manual tests.
Laboratory Technologist	Performs complex laboratory tests and examines blood, tissue, and other body substances.

In addition to these members of the interdisciplinary health care team, other employees in the health care facility provide services that benefit patients:

Administrator	Provides general administration and supervision of a department or facility.
Environmental Services	Maintain a clean and comfortable environment.
Volunteers	Provide personal services such as delivering mail, doing errands, and providing reading materials.

THE NURSING TEAM

The Registered Nurse

The **registered nurse (RN)** has completed a two-, three-, or four-year nursing program and passed a licensure examination given by the state. Registered nurses assess, plan for, evaluate, and coordinate the many aspects of patient care. They teach patients and their families about health practices, provide nursing care, delegate tasks, and supervise the persons to whom they delegate duties.

The Licensed Practical/ Vocational Nurse

The **licensed practical nurse** or **licensed vocational nurse** has completed a 1-year to 18-month training program and passed a licensure examination administered by the state. She or he is identified by the initials LPN or LVN. This nurse works under the supervision of a registered nurse.

The Nursing Assistant

The **nursing assistant** gives personal care to patients under the supervision of a licensed nurse (Figure 2-3). In the health care facility, the assistant is called by one of the following names:

- Patient care attendant
- Nurse's aide, nurse assistant, state-tested nursing assistant, nursing assistant, or certified nursing assistant
- Clinical support associate
- Nurse extender
- Health care assistant
- Personal care assistant
- Patient care technician

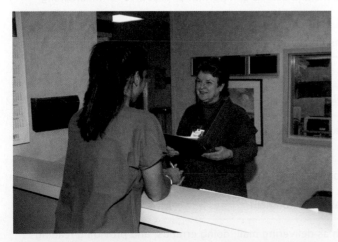

FIGURE 2-3 A professional nurse heads the nursing team and supervises nursing assistants and other team members. (© Delmar/Cengage Learning)

- Unlicensed assistive personnel (UAP)
- _____ care technician (the first part of the title designates the unit on which the assistant works, such as *critical* care technician, *surgical* care technician, and so forth)

REGULATION OF NURSING ASSISTANT PRACTICE

Nursing assistants must know the scope of their duties and the laws governing their practice. Each state identifies the duties and responsibilities of the assistant, and defines the education and level of competency required for safe practice.

In 1987, Congress passed a federal law that regulates the education and certification of nursing assistants. That law is called the **Omnibus Budget Reconciliation Act (OBRA)**. OBRA established the minimum requirements for nursing assistant programs. All persons working as nursing assistants must complete a competency evaluation program or approved course. The education of nursing assistants is under the jurisdiction of each state, guided by federal regulations.

The National Council of State Boards of Nursing, Inc., developed the **Nurse Aide Training and Competency Evaluation Program (NATCEP)**. NATCEP meets the requirements of OBRA, and serves as a guide for registering and awarding credentials to nursing assistants. NATCEP lists the skills to be achieved. Programs may exceed these minimums.

The nursing assistant class must include a minimum of 75 hours of theory and practice. Some states require 80 to 175 program hours in written or oral and clinical skills in several areas:

- Basic nursing skills, including infection control
- Basic restorative services
- Mental health and social service needs
- Personal care skills
- Resident rights and good communication
- Safety and emergency care

Other rules that affect nursing assistant practice require:

- Successful completion of a competency evaluation program. Assistants who have completed the program have at least three opportunities to pass the state test.
- Completion of a new program or retesting by nursing assistants who have not given nursing care for pay for a continuous 24-month period.
- Continuing education (12 to 24 hours per year, in some states).

Become familiar with the rules for nursing assistant practice in your state and facility and be sure you meet the requirements. In some states and facilities, you may be required to take special classes before being allowed to work on the nursing unit. For example, your facility may require you to complete a cardiopulmonary resuscitation (CPR) class. Some states require additional classes to learn about abuse of elderly and disabled persons.

THE ROLE AND RESPONSIBILITIES OF THE NURSING ASSISTANT

The nursing assistant gives physical care and emotional support to patients under the direction of the licensed nurse. You have an important role and can contribute much to the patient's comfort and safety. You will make observations during care, report them to the nurse, and record them on the patient's chart. Nursing assistant responsibilities vary from one facility to the next. An overview of nursing assistant responsibilities is provided in Table 2-3.

TABLE 2-3 TYPICAL JOB DESCRIPTION FOR A NURSING ASSISTANT

Nursing assistants commonly participate in the nursing process by carrying out the activities listed here.

1. Assist with patient assessment and care planning.

   a. Check and record vital signs

   b. Measure height and weight

   c. Measure intake and output

   d. Collect specimens

   e. Test urine and feces

   f. Observe patient response to care

   g. Report and record observations of patients' conditions

2. Assist patients in meeting nutrition and elimination needs.

   a. Check food trays

   b. Pass food trays

   c. Feed patients

   d. Provide fresh drinking water and nourishments

   e. Assist with bedpans, urinals, and commodes

   f. Empty urine collection bags

   g. Assist with colostomy care

   h. Give enemas

   i. Observe feces and urine

   j. Monitor intake and output

3. Assist patients with mobility.

   a. Turn and position patients

   b. Provide range-of-motion exercises

   c. Transfer patients to wheelchair or stretcher

   d. Assist with ambulation

4. Assist patients with personal hygiene and grooming.

   a. Bathe patients

   b. Provide nail and hair care

   c. Give oral hygiene

   d. Provide denture care

   e. Shave patients

   f. Assist with dressing and undressing

5. Assist with patient comfort and anxiety relief.

   a. Protect patient privacy and maintain confidentiality

   b. Keep call signal within patient's reach

   c. Answer call signal promptly

   d. Provide orientation to the room or unit and to other patients and visitors

   e. Assist patients with communications

   f. Protect personal possessions

   g. Provide diversional activities

   h. Give backrubs

   i. Prepare hot and cold applications

6. Assist in promoting patient safety and environmental cleanliness.

   a. Use side rails and restraints appropriately

   b. Keep patient unit clean and free of clutter

   c. Make beds

   d. Clean and care for equipment

   e. Carry out isolation precautions

continues

TABLE 2-3 continued

f. Practice medical asepsis and infection control
g. Practice standard precautions
h. Observe oxygen precautions
i. Assist in keeping recreational and nonpatient areas clean and free of hazards
j. Participate in fire drills and patient evacuation procedures
7. Assist with unit management and efficiency.
a. Admit, transfer, and discharge patients
b. Transport patients
c. Take specimens to lab
d. Assist with special procedures
e. Do errands as required
f. Assist with cost-containment measures
g. Answer the telephone
h. Document care provided and assist with unit recordkeeping

Not everyone can be a nursing assistant. Nursing assistants are special people: they are interested in others, they take pride in themselves, and they are willing to learn the skills necessary to care for those who are ill.

Your interest and caring are valuable assets to the nursing team. You are the person the patient sees most often. You may observe and hear things that others will not. This provides insight into the patient's illness and attitude. For example, the patient is far more likely to tell you of "minor complaints" that may not be minor at all. Inform the nurse of these things; he or she will pass the information on to others, if appropriate. Competent, caring nursing assistants make a valuable contribution to patient comfort and safety.

Nurse Practice Act

Nursing practice is regulated by a board of nursing, or other governing body, in each state. This agency governs nursing practice by establishing a **nurse practice act**. The nurse practice act describes the nursing scope of practice in your state. This may vary slightly from one state to the next. The act is used as a guide when agencies develop job descriptions, and such laws determine which skills and tasks you can perform.

Scope of Practice

Scope of practice means the skills the nursing assistant is legally permitted to perform by state regulations and facility policies. If someone asks you to perform a task that is clearly out of your scope of practice, such as giving medications, explain in a courteous manner that you are not technically or legally prepared to do the task. Report the incident to the nurse.

Be willing to learn new skills. For example, suppose that your unit has purchased new lifting equipment. Listen and watch carefully as instructions for operating the lift are given. Seek supervision as you practice until both you and your supervisor feel that you use the lift safely. Health care is an ever-changing profession. Nursing assistant practice will continue to change and evolve over time as a result of changes in reimbursement, evidence-based practice, and patient-focused care.

Expanded Scope of Practice

In many states and facilities, experienced nursing assistants can expand their scope of practice by taking classes to gain information and learn new skills. These programs provide the opportunity for career advancement. Successfully completing a class of this type will enable the assistant to practice advanced skills.

There are many opportunities for qualified health care workers. Many facilities have special programs, such as career ladders for career advancement. You will find that you have chosen a career with unlimited opportunities for personal growth and satisfaction.

EVIDENCE-BASED PRACTICE

For many years, health care workers based their practice on "whatever worked," including intuition, education, and past experience. Scientific evidence and research were largely nonexistent. The lack of research led to home remedies, unqualified caregivers, treatments and cures that were not always effective, and treatments that were harmful in some cases. Over time, the nursing community realized that professional practice must be validated and confirmed by scientific evidence.

Evidence-based practice (EBP) is an approach that guides decision-making by identifying evidence for a treatment or particular way of doing things, then rating that practice according to the strength of the evidence. This approach opposes the use of tradition and rules of thumb. With EBP, workers consider individual patient variables when selecting approaches to patient care. The goal of EBP is to improve patient outcomes by eliminating scientifically unsound, unsafe, and risky practices. Research must be done and solid evidence of effectiveness must be present for a method to be included in EBP. The EBP approach encourages professionals to use the strongest and best evidence possible when making clinical decisions. EBP involves developing guidelines for best practices based on the strength of the evidence instead of tradition, gut feelings, or rules of thumb (estimation). Professionals also use EBP for developing procedures, practices, and guidelines, and for educating health care workers. This results in safe, cost-effective patient care. The information and procedures you are learning in your nursing assistant class have been proven valid and effective, based on the strength of the available evidence.

ASSESSMENT

A nursing **assessment** is a complete nursing evaluation of the patient, followed by an analysis and synthesis of the information collected. By law, only an RN can assess patients. Assessment cannot be delegated. However, it is within the scope of nursing assistant practice to collect data for the complete assessment. For example, taking vital signs, height, and weight is part of some assessments. The nursing assistant can obtain these data. Making observations and reporting them to the nurse are also contributions to the overall assessment, and are well within the scope of nursing assistant practice. The RN uses all the data collected to define the big picture, and uses the information to develop the plan of nursing care that guides all staff in the care of the patient. You will learn more about assessment in Unit 8.

LINES OF AUTHORITY

Nursing assistants receive their **assignments** from the team leader or charge nurse, and report completion of the assignment to the same person. This is the assistant's immediate line of authority and communication.

The assistant works with a team whose leader is a licensed nurse. When you work as part of a team, your immediate superior is the team leader. The team leaders receive their instructions from the charge nurse. The charge nurse is responsible for the total care of a certain number of patients. Sometimes this includes all the patients on a wing, a unit, or a floor of the facility. Supervisors are responsible for several charge-nurse units. They receive direction from the director of nursing. The complexity of staffing varies with each health care facility. You must learn the lines of authority in your facility, as shown in Figure 2-4. As a student, your immediate authority is your instructor.

The physician directs the patient's medical care. The registered nurse carries out the physician's orders and plans and evaluates the nursing care. When you accept the responsibility for an assignment, you must understand what is expected and be able to handle it. *If you have any doubts, discuss them with the supervising nurse* (Figure 2-5).

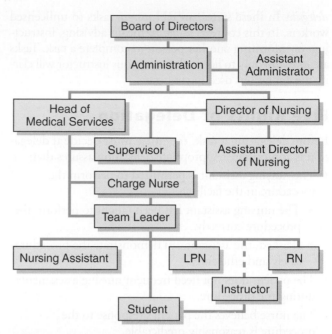

FIGURE 2-4 Typical model of nursing department lines of authority. The diagram may vary slightly from one facility to the next. *(© Delmar/Cengage Learning)*

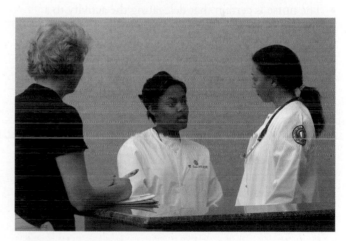

FIGURE 2-5 If you have a question, consult your supervisor. *(© Delmar/Cengage Learning)*

Delegation

Delegation is the transfer of responsibility for the performance of a nursing activity from a nurse to someone who does not already have that authority. Once the task has been delegated, only the person given the authority may perform the procedure. In other words, this person cannot delegate the assignment to someone else. The licensed nurse is accountable for the task and its outcome. He or she must be confident that the unlicensed person can complete the assignment correctly.

In some states, the nurse practice act describes how nurses assign or delegate duties. Some states have passed laws that specifically prohibit nursing assistants from performing certain activities. Some states further define the terms *assign* and *delegate*. In these states, an RN *assigns* tasks to unlicensed workers. In this context, *assigning* means advising, instructing, or informing another person to complete a task. Tasks are *delegated* only to licensed nurses. Your instructor will clarify the definitions used in your state.

Five Rights of Delegation

Before delegating a task, the nurse must decide if delegation is appropriate. Appropriate delegation assures that:

- The nursing assistant is permitted to perform the procedure in the facility.
  - The nursing assistant has been taught to perform the procedure correctly.
  - If asked, the assistant can demonstrate the procedure safely and efficiently.
- The patient does not need frequent nursing assessments during the procedure.
- The nurse believes the patient's response to the procedure is reasonably predictable.
  - In the nurse's opinion, the nursing assistant will obtain the same or similar results from performing the procedure as an RN would.
- The nurse is certain that delegating the activity to a nursing assistant is not against the law.

The National Council of State Boards of Nursing has developed a guide called the "Five Rights of Delegation." Nurses use this list to help them delegate correctly. Reading this list will help you learn if a delegation is appropriate. The rights are:

- *Right Task*—the task is one that can legally be done by a nursing assistant who has been taught the proper way to do the procedure. Further, your instructor or other licensed nurse must have checked your competency in the procedure and approved you to perform it on patients. You must be permitted to perform the procedure according to your state law and facility policy.
- *Right Circumstances*—the nursing assistant understands the purpose of the procedure, can perform it safely, and has the right supplies or equipment to perform the procedure safely.
- *Right Person*—the right person delegates the right task to the right nursing assistant, to be performed on the right patient.
- *Right Direction/Communication*—the nurse delegating the activity has given complete instructions, has described the procedure clearly, and has identified the limits (if any) and expected outcome(s) of the procedure. Always ask for directions if you do not understand your assignment.
- *Right Supervision*—the nurse delegating the activity has answered the nursing assistant's questions and is available to manage changes in the patient's condition. The nursing assistant reports completion of the task and the patient's response to the nurse who delegated the activity.

In some situations, delegating even simple activities is inappropriate. For example, the nursing assistant routinely takes the vital signs of stable patients. However, assigning a nursing assistant to take the vital signs of an unstable patient may be an inappropriate delegation. In this situation, the patient needs the assessment skills of a licensed nurse. Do not feel offended if the nurse takes the vital signs or performs other patient care duties in a situation like this.

Delegated Activities

As you can see, delegating activities is a serious matter for nurses. When you accept the responsibility for a delegated task, you are responsible for your own actions. If you think that performing a procedure is unsafe for the patient, discuss your feelings with the RN. Report your observations about the patient's condition, and be prepared to explain why you are uncomfortable about doing the procedure. Ask for help, if necessary.

You may refuse a delegation if you believe that a procedure is not within your legal scope of practice, if you have not been taught and approved to perform it, or if you believe that the activity will harm the patient. If you are unsure how to carry out a procedure, inform the nurse. Do not feel embarrassed. It is better to ask for help than to make an error and injure a patient. Likewise, if you do not understand the instructions, or do not have the proper supplies, you may also refuse until the problem has been addressed. However, you must explain the reason for your refusal to the RN. He or she can probably resolve your concerns, enabling you to safely complete the activity. Do not refuse because you do not have time, or because the procedure is unpleasant.

Good communication is the key to successful delegation and patient safety. Be honest, tactful, and sensitive. If honest communications are ineffective, you can use the chain of command to address the problem with the next person in line. If you are assigned to a task, your supervisor assumes that you will do it. Never ignore an assignment. If you cannot complete the activity, discuss the situation with your supervisor.

YOUR WORKDAY: MANAGING AN ASSIGNMENT

Your work day will begin with communication, in the form of a **shift report**. This is described in greater detail in Unit 8. Oral reports are used frequently to communicate information about patients. The nurse who worked the previous shift will report to oncoming staff. In some facilities, the shift report is tape-recorded. Listen carefully to the report, because it will help you plan your **assignment** (Figure 2-6). Your assignment tells you:

- Which patients you will care for during your shift
- The procedures you will need to do for these patients

	CNA ASSIGNMENT SHEET								**DATE** 4-18-XX	
Rm.	Resident	Bath	Pos. Sched.	ROM	V.S.	WT.	B+B	ADL Prog.	Transfer	Safety
101A	J. Damski	X	X	X			X	X	2+TB	X
101B	G. Jones		X	X	X	X			Mech Lift	
102A	C. Hernandez	X				X			Indep.	
102B	R. Lattini	X	X	X			X		2+TB	X
103	N. Goldberg	X			X	X	X		SBA	
104A	M. Welch		X	X					Mech Lift	
104B	L. Ordoni		X	X			X	X	1+TB	X
105	B. Brinzoski	X			X		X		Indep.	
106A	A. Feinstein	X				X		X	1+TB	
106B	D. Farmell		X	X	X		X	X	2+TB	
107	T. Green	X	X	X		X	X		2+TB	
108A	H. Johnson	X	X	X	X			X	2+TB	
108B	B. Miller		X	X		X			1+TB	X

FIGURE 2-6 The assignment sheet provides an overview of patient needs and activities. (© Delmar/Cengage Learning)

Your supervising nurse will give you additional information about your assignment based on the shift report. This information will include orders, procedures, care, and observations to make for specific patients. Unit 8 gives additional information about oral reports.

Report the completion of your assignment, and the patient's response, to the nurse. You may be tempted to skip reporting if you will be documenting the activity. Do not give in: Reporting even simple things may be important.

ORGANIZING YOUR TIME

Successful time management is a key to nursing assistant success. You cannot master time management skills in the classroom. However, you can practice and use good organizational skills in the skills lab and clinical portions of your class until they become automatic. This will translate to good organization on the nursing unit. Mastering good organization and time management skills helps you work more efficiently, and reduces stress. Once mastered, organizational skills become a part of you, and you will not have to think about them. A bonus is that these skills are also very useful at home and in your personal life.

Time is a borrowed commodity. Once used, it is gone and cannot be replaced or reclaimed. You can only manage yourself in relation to time. Each day begins with 86,400 seconds, 1440 minutes, or 24 hours. This equals 168 hours each week. If you work an 8-hour shift, you have:

- 28,800 seconds or 480 minutes in which to get your work done each day.

If you work a 12-hour shift, you have:

- 43,200 seconds or 600 minutes in which to get your work done each day.

The total time available for getting your work done is set by your employer. You can only control how you use that time. Cutting corners, skipping breaks, and working longer hours are not good techniques for managing time, and may cause ethical and legal problems for you. At best, managing time in this manner is stressful. At worst, it is dangerous. You manage the time available. It does not manage you. Do this by *working smarter, not harder*.

Developing and Perfecting Time Management Skills

Lack of good organizational skills plagues health care workers at all levels. Avoid becoming so focused on *tasks* that you fail to see the larger picture of things for which you are responsible, such as:

- Making important or significant observations as you circulate around the unit.

- Overseeing your patients; noticing if certain patients are becoming sick, having behavior problems, or developing other abnormalities.
- Informing the nurse of patients' problems, complaints, and changes in condition.

Making Rounds

If you do not manage your time, others will do it for you. This can be both difficult and stressful. Making rounds is an important part of your time management strategy. Making regular rounds will save you many trips up and down the hallway, and give you a more complete picture of patient needs. Patients and their families will feel confident and secure in your ability. Setting priorities and focusing on efficiency are key assets in developing good time management skills. Avoid losing your focus. Ensuring quality care and patient safety are your top priorities. Perfecting good organization and time management skills will make a difference in your personal life and the care you give.

- Establish and develop a systematic daily routine for things.
  - Make rounds as soon as possible after report to identify patient needs and problems. Meet immediate needs during this round, such as assisting with toileting.
  - Develop your plan for each patient while making rounds.
- Practice good communication skills with patients and families while making rounds; this will save you time and prevent them from calling you to the room later. Let them know you are on top of things. Ask questions and obtain patient input on the plan you are mentally formulating.
  - Stop to visit briefly with concerned family members. Do not wait for them to seek you out. This may seem like a time waster, but it promotes satisfaction, gains support, and may end up saving you time. Offer simple information to families. For example, "Your mother ate a good breakfast today," "The night nurse said your father had a restful night," or "Your auntie really enjoyed her visit from the church members yesterday."
  - Families usually know the patient well. They may offer important information about the patient. Do not be timid about asking for their opinion. For example, "Does he seem stronger to you?"
  - Avoid becoming defensive if family members express concerns about patient conditions. Report concerns, observations, and needs to the nurse after you have made rounds on all your patients. Listen to what patients have to say. Tell them what you will do about their concern, and give them a follow-up time if needed, such as, "I will let you know tomorrow." Thank them for sharing their concerns. Keep the nurse informed.
- Determine which patients need frequent monitoring.
  - *Monitoring* is simple oversight, such as looking in on or speaking with a patient, taking or reviewing vital signs, watching for new problems and changes in condition, and addressing known problems.

Develop a personal plan for organizing your time by following these suggestions:

- Plan and organize your work. Be sure the plan is realistic.
  - Write down your plan; make a new "to do" list every day. Putting the plan in writing is important.
- List your main goals for the day. Your goals will help ensure that the most important tasks are done. Review each item on your list and ask yourself it makes the best use of your time.
  - Goals without deadlines are dreams. Set realistic and achievable deadlines.
  - Everything designated as a top priority must be completed immediately.
  - Next-level priorities must be done a few minutes after top priorities are finished.
- Schedule your breaks into the plan. Take breaks at the assigned times. These are important to reduce stress and prevent injury. Avoid overloading yourself. Avoid taking work with you on your breaks.
- Be flexible. Expect the unexpected. Accept that you may have to change your plan if conditions and patient needs change.
  - Accept that your priorities may change.
  - Identify "no options" activities. These are things that *must* be done during your shift, without exception.
- Identify events that must be done by specific times, and distinguish them from things you can take care of later.
- Identify the what, where, when, why, who, and how of your priorities; this will help you devise a strategy and plan for completing your priority items.
- *You control* the timing of events for which you are responsible.
- Emergencies, new admissions, and patient or family demands are imposed on you by others, and you cannot control them. Accept this as a fact, and learn to remain calm when things change suddenly. On most days, these things will not be a burden if you do a good job organizing and managing your time regarding events you can control.
- Focus on the patients' *needs* instead of *tasks* that must be done; by focusing on needs, you will complete the necessary tasks with far less stress.
- Avoid repetition. Plan to do like jobs at the same time. Do them right the first time to avoid having to redo them.
- Plan to do things simultaneously. For example, you must remain in the patient's room while she washes at the sink. Use that time productively! Make the bed or do another task instead of waiting impatiently.
- When you have a task to complete, set a time limit for yourself. Be reasonable.
  - Avoid becoming distracted. Focus on the task at hand.

- Break tasks and responsibilities into smaller, more manageable pieces, if possible.
- Constantly evaluate your efficiency and time management skills and work on improving them.

Try to break your own record on time-consuming tasks. If a job takes 30 minutes today, try to get it done in 29 minutes tomorrow. Save a few seconds to a minute a day until you have streamlined the task as much as possible. One caveat, however: Avoid cutting corners for the sake of saving time. The time you save is not worth the price you will pay for harming a patient or making a major error. If cutting corners is the only way you feel you can save time, try a different routine.

Before beginning a task, organize what you will need:

- When beginning a project, gather and organize your supplies in advance.
- Take everything you will need into the patient's room at once so you do not waste time and energy making trips up and down the hall to retrieve forgotten items.
- Communicate with peers, colleagues, and others throughout your shift. Good communication helps ensure success.
  - Be tactful and polite in all communications.
  - Treat others with dignity, respect, and integrity.
- Be assertive.
  - Help others when you can. Do not be afraid to ask for help when you need it.
- Avoid wasting time; remain organized so you make good use of your time.
- Note whether patients are sick, unstable, or displaying behavior problems; develop a plan for nursing assistant action. Keep the nurse informed.
  - Take the blinders off! Continue to make important observations as you circulate around the unit.

HAND-OFF COMMUNICATION

Hand-off communication is essential communication that must occur when patient care is transferred from one worker or department to another worker or department. It is similar to your shift report, but is usually about only one patient. In hand-off communication, one worker communicates directly with the next person who will be responsible for the patient's care. Transfer of care is a very vulnerable time for the patient and is one of the times when errors are most likely to occur. Information in a hand-off communication includes:

- The patient's situation and background.
- Relevant observations and findings, especially changes and abnormalities.
- Recommendations and special orders or information for continuity of ongoing care.

Hand-off communication must be accurate, clear, and complete. It should also include an opportunity to ask questions. As a nursing assistant, you will be giving and receiving hand-off information. Write down information about patients, if necessary, and refer to your notes as needed.

Teamwork

Various models of patient care are successful because they promote cooperation and teamwork. Learning to work with others as a member of a team is one of the most important skills to master during your nursing assistant education. Team members work together to: perform job duties and provide patient care; coordinate work assignments; cooperate with others; and share resources and information. You can be an effective team member by:

- Recognizing that all team members are important and appreciating their contributions.
- Contributing to care plans by sharing your observations and ideas.
- Cooperating with others to provide patient-focused care.

PERSONAL VOCATIONAL ADJUSTMENTS

You will have to make some personal adjustments to your new work situation. You must obey facility rules and orders from supervisors even if you do not agree with them. Rules are created to protect the welfare of both patients and employees. You must also learn to accept constructive criticism and profit from it. You show your maturity in many ways. You demonstrate:

- Dependability and accuracy by reporting for duty on time (Figure 2-7) and completing your assignments carefully.
- Respect for your coworkers and the value of teamwork when you are ready to help.
- Understanding of human relationships by being empathetic, patient, and tactful with others.

Interpersonal Relationships

An **interpersonal relationship** is a connection between people. You develop interpersonal relationships with everyone you know. Some are deep and lasting, while others are only casual. To some degree, you react to others and they react to you. Friendship is a good example of an interpersonal relationship that is satisfactory to both parties.

Much of the satisfaction that a nursing assistant gets from work comes from the quality of the relationships with staff and patients. Good relationships begin with your own personality and attitude. If you are a warm and accepting person with a positive attitude, others will respond in the same way. If you walk down the street and someone smiles at you, you will probably smile back. Most human relationships

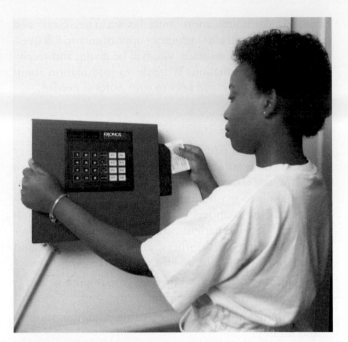

FIGURE 2-7 Reporting for work on time is a sign of responsibility and demonstrates dependability. *(© Delmar/Cengage Learning)*

are like this. It is not necessary for you to like someone else to be pleasant and cooperative with him or her as you carry out your duties (Figure 2-8).

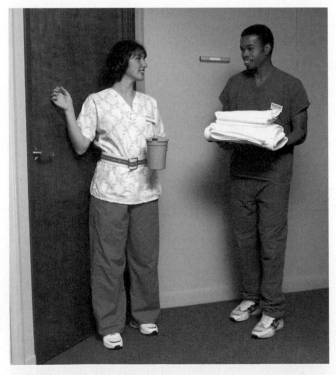

FIGURE 2-8 A positive attitude and spirit of cooperation are employee attributes that make the workplace pleasant. *(© Delmar/Cengage Learning)*

Staff Relationships

You are part of the staff of a health care facility. All workers share a single goal: to help the patients. This single purpose bonds you into a unit that must work together. Good interpersonal relationships will make your working hours satisfying and productive. Good relationships can be formed if you:

- Remember that each of you has a specific role to fulfill and jobs to carry out.
- Do not overstep your authority or criticize others.
- Listen to instructions carefully. Phrase questions in such a way that your supervisor knows you are looking for clarification, not challenging authority.
- Remember that your tone of voice and body language can change your message.
- Carry out your assignment and inform the nurse in advance if you cannot complete your work.
- Offer help to others and accept help when you need it. Coworkers must help one another when a task is difficult or physically taxing (for example, lifting a heavy patient or moving equipment). Simply being available when another team member gets behind in his or her work is a great help.
- Have a cheerful, positive attitude. This is as important for relationships with other workers as it is in establishing rapport (mutual trust and understanding) with patients.
- Extend the same courtesy to staff members that you would to patients.
- Always keep your common goal in mind. Recognize coworkers as important members of the total team.

Attitude

The most important characteristic that you bring to your job is your **attitude**. Your attitude develops throughout your lifetime, and is shaped by your experiences. Some people think "having an attitude" means being negative, but all people show attitude through their behavior. Sometimes the attitude is good and sometimes it is poor.

All the other characteristics described are an outer reflection of your inner feelings—of your view of yourself and others. Your attitude should reflect:

- Caring
- Courtesy
- Cooperation
- Emotional control
- Empathy (understanding)
- Tact
- Patience

Patients have the right and need to be cared for in a calm, unhurried atmosphere by people with a caring attitude.

Patient Relationships

Patients come in all sizes, shapes, and ages. Some have major, complicated illnesses. Others have physical problems. Some are in the facility to begin their lives. Others will end their lives there. A good nursing assistant shows **empathy** (understanding) for patients by being eager to serve and by using a gentle touch.

Every patient presents a unique set of problems and concerns. Never forget that, to the patient, her or his own problems are the most important.

Meeting the Patient's Needs

Patients' personalities are also shaped by their life experiences, which are now complicated by illness. Their social, spiritual, and physical needs must be met despite their admission to a health care facility. Illness limits their ability to satisfy these needs. This is frustrating and strains the patient's ability to establish and maintain relationships.

Some patients become irritable, complaining, and uncooperative because of:

- Fears about their diagnosis, disfigurement, disability, and death
- Pain
- Unrealistic or mistaken perceptions of activities around them
- Uncertainties about the future
- Worries about family
- The loss or lack of social support systems
- Dependence on others
- Financial concerns

Offer emotional support (Figure 2-9), listen carefully, and report the patient's concerns to the nurse.

Meeting the Family's Needs

Families and friends are very concerned when a loved one is in a health care facility, especially if that person has a life-threatening illness. This causes them to feel stressed, and they need to be reassured. Their anxiety may make them demanding and uncooperative.

The nursing assistant who understands human behavior makes allowances for these stresses and realizes that ill people, coworkers, and families under stress may be touchy. This is why sensitivity and awareness of the needs of others are so important (Figure 2-10). Having patience and tact is important. Sometimes listening quietly or rephrasing your sentences can change an entire interaction. Try to be aware of both your words and your body language. Clues such as tone of voice or a hand movement may reveal much about the inner feelings of others. People are three-dimensional. They are physical, emotional, and social beings. You will learn additional techniques for effective communication in Unit 7.

Personal Health and Hygiene

Good personal grooming is essential, because the nursing assistant is in close contact with patients (Figure 2-11). The work can be physically challenging, so body odors must be controlled. The assistant may be the last to know that he or she has bad breath or body odor. A daily shower or bath and the use of an antiperspirant/deodorant are essential. Keep the mouth and teeth clean. Recognize that strong perfumes, aftershave lotions, and cigarette odors are often offensive to patients.

Keep your hair clean and short or tied back in a controlled style. Keep your fingernails short and clean. Avoid wearing nail polish.

Jewelry is a ready medium for bacterial growth. It may also injure the patient or the assistant. Long, dangling earrings can be caught in linen or pulled out by a patient.

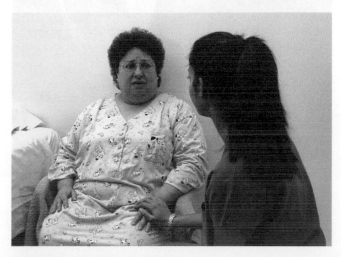

FIGURE 2-9 A worried patient is reassured by gentle touch. *(© Delmar/Cengage Learning)*

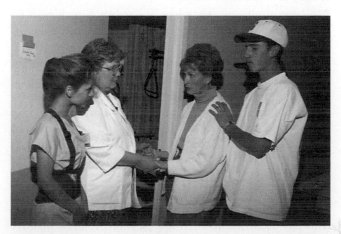

FIGURE 2-10 Concerned family members also need support from staff. *(© Delmar/Cengage Learning)*

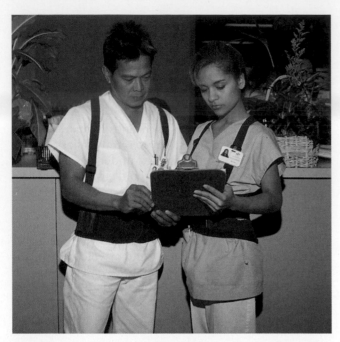

FIGURE 2-11 Well-groomed caregivers instill confidence in patients. *(© Delmar/Cengage Learning)*

Most facilities permit staff to wear wedding rings and small earrings. A watch with second hand is needed to measure vital signs.

Uniforms

Many facilities allow workers to select the type and style of their uniforms. Traditionally, patients could identify workers' job positions by their uniforms, which included caps. Today, it is difficult to distinguish one worker from another. It is no wonder that patients may be confused. Because of this, some facilities require personnel to wear a name badge or photo identification tag while on the job. The name badge may state only your first name and title. Some facilities do not list workers' last names on name badges, as a security measure.

Wear your uniform only when you are on duty. If your facility provides an area for changing your uniform, take advantage of it. If not, wear a cover-up as you travel to and from work so you will not spread germs. When you get home, remove your uniform, fold it inside out, and put it in the laundry. This keeps the dirtiest part of your uniform away from other clothes. Wear a fresh uniform that is clean and in good repair each day. Stockings and socks should be freshly laundered. Clean shoes and shoelaces daily. You will be less fatigued if your shoes give proper support to the feet and fit well.

Remember that your appearance reflects your pride in yourself and your work. Well-groomed nursing assistants who pay attention to their appearance project a positive image and send a nonverbal message that says they have the same pride and caring attitude toward their work. If you are well groomed and have good personal habits, patients will feel more secure, and other staff will regard you as mature and reliable.

Reducing Stress

Your work is physically and emotionally demanding because you must give so much of yourself to those in your care. To stay healthy and do your best, you will need:

- Sufficient rest
- Good nutrition
- Satisfying leisure activities (Figure 2-12)
- Ways of reducing stress

Burnout is total mental, emotional, and sometimes physical exhaustion. Burnout is common in health care workers. You can reduce stress by balancing your work with rest and recreation.

Some facilities offer programs to help employees reduce stress. Group discussions, exercise programs, and special counseling are available for stress management and to meet special circumstances, such as when a patient dies or when conflicts arise. Death is always a possibility, but staff members usually focus on improvement and recovery. The loss of a patient, especially a child, can be very stressful. Caring for an abuse victim also takes a great toll on the staff.

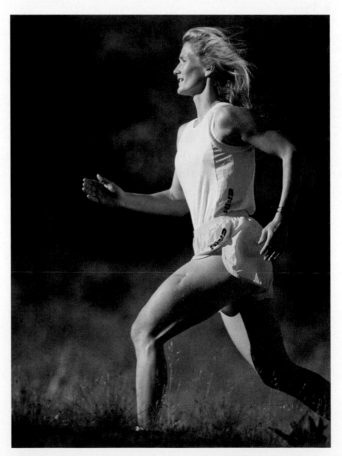

FIGURE 2-12 Strive to balance your life between work, recreational activities, and family responsibilities. *(Courtesy of PhotoDisc)*

Change

Change is ongoing in the health care industry. Learn to accept this as a fact from the outset of your health care career. New competitors build facilities and take away established customers (patients); technology changes; new research reveals different methods of patient care; changes in laws alter the way services are given; patients have high expectations. Change is never really finished. It can be very disruptive, unpredictable, and difficult for everyone. Venturing into unknown territory can be threatening. Workers faced with change may feel stressed and insecure, believing that change will expose their shortcomings. When workers resist change, negative attitudes cause turmoil for others.

The ability to cope with change is an asset that all workers must master. Try these strategies:

- Learn all you can about the change and your responsibilities.
- Try to understand the need for and value of the change.
- Find ways of adapting to the change.
- Be open-minded and flexible.
- Cooperate with others and be a team player.
- Adjust your attitude. View change as an opportunity for new challenges, growth, and accomplishment.
- Keep your sense of humor. Make change fun. Try to have a good time despite the discomfort you feel.
- Compensate for the stress by making time for activities you enjoy.

Remember the old adage: "Change is inevitable, but growth is optional." Viewing each change as an opportunity for growth will do more than help you survive. Having a positive attitude and using change as an opportunity for growth will help you thrive in the ever-changing workplace.

Personal Stress Reduction

Some people use food, alcohol, or other drugs to reduce stress. These substances can cause serious health problems. Chemicals and drugs alter the body's chemistry, causing thought and behavior problems. Drug use can become addictive and may cause death. To reduce stress:

- Talk to your supervisor; a team conference may help.
- Try sitting for a few moments with your feet up.
- Shut your eyes and take some deep breaths.
- With your eyes shut, picture a special place you like and, in your mind, take yourself there.
- Take a warm, relaxing bath.
- Listen to some quiet music.
- Carry out a relaxation exercise.
- Make yourself a cup of herbal tea and drink it slowly.
- Exercise.
- Devote time to hobbies such as sewing, painting, or playing a musical instrument.
- Go for a walk.
- Take advantage of available stress-reduction programs.
- Sing! Singing is a good stress reducer.
- Read a book.
- Meditate.
- Treat yourself to an activity you enjoy.

Professional and personal adjustments are easier if the nursing assistant:

- Understands and follows facility policies and procedures.
- Treats patients, coworkers, and visitors with respect.
- Practices proper hygiene and grooming, good nutrition, and stress reduction.

REVIEW

A. Multiple Choice

Select the one best answer for each of the following.

1. The team member who writes the medical orders for patient care is the
   a. registered nurse.
   b. social worker.
   c. physician. ✓
   d. dietitian.

2. A nursing assistant who has a question regarding an assignment should ask the
   a. physician.
   b. charge nurse.

   c. physiotherapist.
   d. administrator.

3. A patient tells you that he has difficulty making a fist because his hand feels weak. He did not mention this fact to the nurse. You must
   a. ignore it. The patient should have told the nurse.
   b. tell another assistant.
   c. tell the nurse.
   d. tell the physician.

4. You demonstrate maturity by
   a. rushing assignments.
   b. being disrespectful to coworkers.

   c. "bending" the rules.

   d. reporting for duty on time. ✓

5. The OBRA laws of 1987 govern

   a. hospital accreditation.

   b. infection control issues.

   c. nursing assistant education. ✓

   d. employee health.

6. Nursing care is

   a. occupationally oriented.

   b. patient-focused.

   c. cross-trained.

   d. physician directed.

7. Nursing care is planned and directed by the

   a. registered nurse.

   b. physician.

   c. licensed practical nurse.

   d. administrator.

8. The most important member of the interdisciplinary team is the

   a. registered nurse.

   b. physician.

   c. nursing assistant.

   d. patient. ✓

9. A patient's family may participate in care conference

   a. if they want to attend.

   b. with a physician's order.

   c. with the patient's permission ✓

   d. if they are available.

10. Burnout is

   a. disagreement with a coworker.

   b. feeling overwhelming stress. ✓

   c. a mental health condition.

   d. usually a result of change.

B. Nursing Assistant Challenge

Read each clinical situation and answer the questions.

11. Enrique is given his assignment and has questions.

   a. He must check his assignment with _____.

   b. One of his assignments is to bathe patients. Is this appropriate? _____

   c. One of his assignments is to give medications. Is this appropriate? _____

12. Felicia once worked as a part-time assistant to an elderly woman, but was never certified as a nursing assistant. What can you tell her about the requirements?

   a. Is a competency evaluation program required? _____

   b. How many opportunities are there to meet requirements? _____

   c. How much continuing education is required once certification is granted? _____

13. Peggy reported for duty wearing bracelets, long earrings, and pale pink nail polish. Her uniform was clean and crisp, but the hem was hanging down on one side. Her shoes were dirty. List ways in which her appearance can be improved.

UNIT 3

Consumer Rights and Responsibilities in Health Care

OBJECTIVES

After completing this unit, you will be able to:
- Spell and define terms.
- Explain the purpose of health care consumer rights.

- Describe four items that are common to Residents' Rights, the Patients' Bill of Rights, and the Clients' Rights in Home Care.
- List five responsibilities of health care consumers.

VOCABULARY

Learn the meaning and the correct spelling of the following words and phrases:

advance directives	corporal punishment	informed consent	Patients' Bill of Rights
Clients' Rights	grievance	involuntary seclusion	Residents' Rights

CONSUMER RIGHTS

All citizens in the United States have certain rights that are guaranteed by law. These rights are granted to ensure that health care consumers will receive quality care. There are different documents setting out rights, and the one that applies depends on where care is given. Staff must be familiar with and protect each patient's rights. A copy of the **Residents' Rights** is given to each person upon admission to a long-term care facility (Figure 3-1). The **Patients' Bill of Rights** is given to patients upon admission to a hospital. Persons receiving care in their homes are given a copy of the **Clients' Rights**. Each of these documents is similar and emphasizes the right of the patient, resident, or client to:

- Be treated with respect and dignity; this includes the right to privacy and confidentiality.

- Open and honest communication with caregivers.
- Make health care decisions and participate in care planning. **Informed consent** means that the person gives permission for care only after full disclosure of the purpose of the procedure, the benefits, and risks involved (Figure 3-2).
- Be informed of their rights concerning **advance directives** (documents that describe the person's wishes for treatment at the end of life [see Unit 33]).
- Receive continuity of care.
- Be informed of resources for resolving conflicts or grievances. A **grievance** is a situation in which the consumer feels there are grounds for complaint.

Figures 3-3, 3-4, and 3-5 reproduce each of these rights documents.

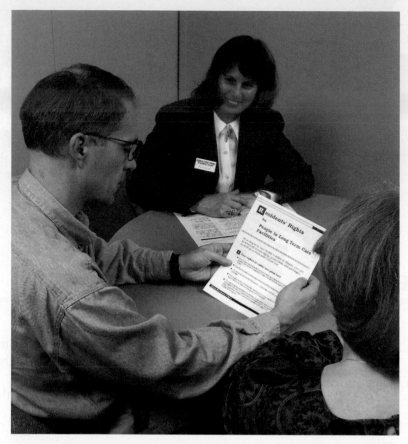

FIGURE 3-1 The Residents' Bill of Rights is presented to each resident (or the resident's legally responsible party) when the resident is admitted to a long-term care facility. (© Delmar/Cengage Learning)

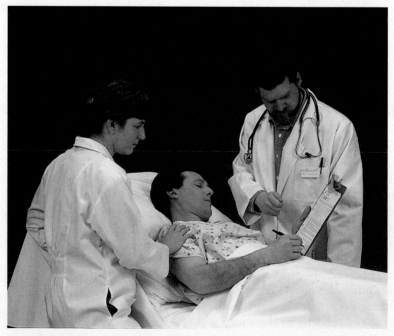

FIGURE 3-2 Informed consent is necessary for some procedures. (© Delmar/Cengage Learning)

Residents' Rights

This is an abbreviated version of the Residents' Rights as set forth in the Omnibus Budget Reconciliation Act. This document must be given to all residents and/or their families prior to admission to a long-term care facility.

1. The resident has the right to free choice, including the right to:
   - choose an attending physician
   - full advance information about changes in care or treatment
   - participate in the assessment and care planning process
   - self-administer medications if the resident is able to safely do so
   - consent to participate in experimental research
2. The resident has the right to freedom from abuse and restraints, including freedom from:
   - physical, sexual, mental abuse
   - **corporal punishment** (the use of physical force) and **involuntary seclusion** (isolating a resident without a medical reason)
   - physical and chemical restraints
3. The resident has the right to privacy, including privacy for:
   - treatment and nursing care
   - receiving/sending mail
   - telephone calls
   - visitors
4. The resident has the right to confidentiality of personal and clinical records.
5. The resident has the right to accommodation of needs, including:
   - choices about life
   - receiving assistance in maintaining independence

6. The resident has the right to voice grievances.
7. The resident has the right to organize and participate in family and resident groups.
8. The resident has the right to participate in social, religious, and community activities, including the right to:
   - vote
   - keep religious items in the room
   - attend religious services
9. The resident has the right to examine survey results and correction plans.
10. The resident has the right to manage personal funds.
11. The resident has the right to information about eligibility for Medicare/Medicaid funds.
12. The resident has the right to file complaints about abuse, neglect, or misappropriation of property.
13. The resident has the right to information about advocacy groups.
14. The resident has the right to immediate and unlimited access to family or relatives.
15. The resident has the right to share a room with the spouse if they are both residents in the same facility.
16. The resident has the right to perform or not perform work for the facility if it is medically appropriate for the resident to work.
17. The resident has the right to remain in the facility except in certain circumstances.
18. The resident has the right to use personal possessions.
19. The resident has the right to notification of change in condition.

FIGURE 3-3 Residents' Bill of Rights. (© Delmar/Cengage Learning)

The Patients' Bill of Rights

Introduction

Effective health care requires collaboration between patients and physicians and other health care professionals. Open and honest communication, respect for personal and professional values, and sensitivity to differences are integral to optimal patient care. As the setting for the provision of health services, hospitals must provide a foundation for understanding and respecting the rights and responsibilities of patients, their families, physicians, and other caregivers. Hospitals must ensure a health care ethic that respects the role of patients in decision making about treatment choices and other aspects of their care. Hospitals must be sensitive to cultural, racial, linguistic, religious, age, gender, and other differences as well as the needs of persons with disabilities.

The American Hospital Association presents *The Patients' Bill of Rights* with the expectation that it will contribute to more effective patient care and be supported by the hospital on behalf of the institution, its medical staff, employees, and patients. The American Hospital Association encourages health care institutions to tailor this bill of rights to their patient community by translating and/or simplifying the language of this bill of rights as may be necessary to ensure that the patients and their families understand their rights and responsibilities.

Bill of Rights*

1. The patient has the right to considerate and respectful care.

2. The patient has the right to and is encouraged to obtain from physicians and other direct caregivers relevant, current, and understandable information concerning diagnosis, treatment, and prognosis.

   Except in emergencies when the patient lacks decision-making capacity and the need for treatment is urgent, the patient is entitled to the opportunity to discuss and request information related to the specific procedures and/or treatments, the risks involved, the possible length of recuperation, and the medically reasonable alternatives and their accompanying risks and benefits.

   Patients have the right to know the identity of physicians, nurses, and others involved in their care, as well as when those involved are students, residents, or other trainees. The patient also has the right to know the immediate and long-term financial implications of treatment choices, insofar as they are known.

3. The patient has the right to make decisions about the plan of care prior to and during the course of treatment and to refuse a recommended treatment or plan of care to the extent permitted by law and hospital policy and to be informed of the medical consequences of this action. In case of such refusal, the patient

is entitled to other appropriate care and services that the hospital provides or transfer to another hospital. The hospital should notify patients of any policy that might affect patient choice within the institution.

4. The patient has the right to have an advance directive (such as a living will, health care proxy, or durable power of attorney for health care) concerning treatment or designating a surrogate decision maker with the expectation that the hospital will honor the intent of that directive to the extent permitted by law and hospital policy.

   Health care institutions must advise patients of their rights under state law and hospital policy to make informed medical choices, ask if the patient has an advance directive, and include that information in patient records. The patient has the right to timely information about hospital policy that may limit its ability to implement fully a legally valid advance directive.

5. The patient has the right to every consideration of privacy. Case discussion, consultation, examination, and treatment should be conducted so as to protect each patient's privacy.

These rights can be exercised on the patient's behalf by a designated surrogate or proxy decision maker if the patient lacks decision-making capacity, is legally incompetent, or is a minor.

The Patients' Bill of Rights was first adopted by the American Hospital Association in 1973. This revision was approved by the AHA Board of Trustees on October 21, 1992.

AHA

FIGURE 3-4 Patients' Bill of Rights. *(© Delmar/Cengage Learning)*

continues

6. The patient has the right to expect that all communications and records pertaining to his/her care will be treated as confidential by the hospital, except in cases such as suspected abuse and public health hazards when reporting is permitted or required by law. The patient has the right to expect that the hospital will emphasize the confidentiality of this information when it releases it to any other parties entitled to review information in these records.

7. The patient has the right to review the records pertaining to his/her medical care and to have the information explained or interpreted as necessary, except when restricted by law.

8. The patient has the right to expect that, within its capacity and policies, a hospital will make reasonable response to the request of a patient for appropriate and medically indicated care and services. The hospital must provide evaluation, service, and/or referral as indicated by the urgency of the case. When medically appropriate and legally permissible, or when a patient has so requested, a patient may be transferred to another facility. The institution to which the patient is to be transferred must first have accepted the patient for transfer. The patient must also have the benefit of complete information and explanation concerning the need for, risks, benefits, and alternatives to such a transfer.

9. The patient has the right to ask and be informed of the existence of business relationships among the hospital, educational institutions, other health care providers, or payers that may influence the patient's treatment and care.

10. The patient has the right to consent to or decline to participate in proposed research studies or human experimentation affecting care and treatment or requiring direct patient involvement, and to have those studies fully explained prior to consent. A patient who declines to participate in research or experimentation is entitled to the most effective care that the hospital can otherwise provide.

11. The patient has the right to expect reasonable continuity of care when appropriate and to be informed by physicians and other caregivers of available and realistic patient care options when hospital care is no longer appropriate.

12. The patient has the right to be informed of hospital policies and practices that relate to patient care, treatment, and responsibilities. The patient has the right to be informed of available resources for resolving disputes, grievances, and conflicts, such as ethics committees, patient representatives, or other mechanisms available in the institution. The patient has the right to be informed of the hospital's charges for services and available payment methods.

The collaborative nature of health care requires that the patients, or their families/surrogates, participate in their care. The effectiveness of care and patient satisfaction with the course of treatment depend, in part, on the patient fulfilling certain responsibilities. Patients are responsible for providing information about past illnesses, hospitalizations, medications, and other matters related to health status. To participate effectively in decision making, patients must be encouraged to take responsibility for requesting additional information or clarification about their health status or treatment when they do not fully understand information and instructions. Patients are also responsible for ensuring that the health care institution has a copy of their written advance directive if they have one. Patients are responsible for informing their physicians and other caregivers if they anticipate problems in following prescribed treatment.

Patients should also be aware of the hospital's obligation to be reasonably efficient and equitable in providing care to other patients and the community. The hospital's rules and regulations are designed to help the hospital meet this obligation. Patients and their families are responsible for making reasonable accommodations to the needs of the hospital, other patients, medical staff, and hospital employees. Patients are responsible for providing necessary information for insurance claims and for working with the hospital to make payment arrangements, when necessary.

A person's health depends on much more than health care services. Patients are responsible for recognizing the impact of their life style on their personal health.

Conclusion

Hospitals have many functions to perform, including the enhancement of health status, health promotion, and the prevention and treatment of injury and disease; the immediate and ongoing care and rehabilitation of patients; the education of health professionals, patients, and the community; and research. All these activities must be conducted with an overriding concern for the values and dignity of patients.

Clients' Rights in Home Care

The persons receiving home health care services or their families possess basic rights and responsibilities. As the client, you have:

The right to:
1. be treated with dignity, consideration, and respect
2. have your property treated with respect
3. receive a timely response from the agency to requests for service
4. be fully informed on admission of the care and treatment that will be provided, how much it will cost, and how payment will be handled
5. know in advance if you will be responsible for any payment
6. be informed in advance of any changes in your care
7. receive care from professionally trained personnel, and to know their names and responsibilities
8. participate in planning care
9. refuse treatment and be told the consequences of your action
10. expect confidentiality of all information
11. be informed of anticipated termination of service
12. be referred elsewhere if you are denied services solely based on your inability to pay
13. know how to make a complaint or recommend a change in agency policies and services

The responsibility to:
1. remain under a doctor's care while receiving services
2. provide the agency with a complete health history
3. provide the agency all requested insurance and financial information
4. sign the required consents and releases for insurance billing
5. participate in your care by asking questions, expressing concerns, and stating if you do not understand
6. provide a safe home environment in which care can be given
7. cooperate with your doctor, the staff, and other caregivers
8. accept responsibility for any refusal of treatment
9. abide by agency policies that restrict the duties our staff may perform
10. advise agency administration of any dissatisfaction or problems with your care

FIGURE 3-5 Clients' Rights in Home Care. (© Delmar/Cengage Learning)

RESPONSIBILITIES OF HEALTH CARE CONSUMERS

Consumers also have certain responsibilities. These responsibilities include:

- Maintaining personal health care records.
- Communicating openly and honestly with the physician and other caregivers.
- Learning how to manage their own health (Figure 3-6).
- Asking questions if they do not understand instructions or explanations.
- Accepting financial responsibility for payment.

The rights of health care consumers have both a legal and an ethical basis. Legal and ethical aspects are discussed in Unit 4.

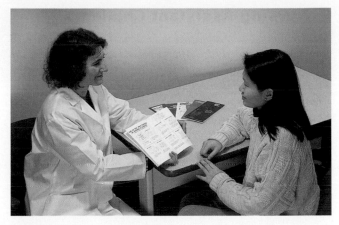

FIGURE 3-6 The RN develops a plan to teach the patient how to manage her own health. *(© Delmar/Cengage Learning)*

REVIEW

A. Multiple Choice

Select the one best answer for each of the following.

1. The Residents' Rights document is given to persons before they are admitted to
   a. home care.
   b. a long-term care facility. ✔
   c. the hospital.
   d. hospice services.

2. All types of consumer rights documents state that the consumer has the right to
   a. be treated in a respectful, dignified manner. ✔
   b. select the individuals who will be assigned to provide health care.
   c. private-duty nursing care, if desired by the patient or family.
   d. withhold personal information about his or her medical condition.

3. The purpose of advance directives is to
   a. give instructions for end-of-life care. ✔
   b. enable patients to choose their caregivers.
   c. provide a resource for resolving conflicts.
   d. permit the physician to prescribe treatment.

4. Health care consumers must
   a. leave their bad habits at home.
   b. study medical books.

   c. keep their own medical records.
   d. communicate honestly with caregivers. ✔

5. What is your best response when a patient complains about the care?
   a. Call the patient's family and ask them to transfer the patient.
   b. Listen carefully and report the complaint to the ✔ nurse.
   c. Help the patient write a letter of complaint to the state.
   d. Tell the patient that conditions cannot be changed.

6. When a patient feels that his or her rights have been violated, he or she has the right to
   a. leave the facility without paying for the care.
   b. remain in the facility without paying the bill.
   c. call the police or sheriff.
   d. file a grievance.

7. Patients' possessions, such as photographs and letters, should be:
   a. placed in the facility's safe.
   b. sent home with family members.
   c. handled with respect and care.
   d. put away where no one can see them. ✗

B. Nursing Assistant Challenge

Mr. Delmonico was admitted to General Hospital for surgery to repair a fractured hip. After a few days in the hospital, he will be transferred to Memorial Nursing Center, a skilled care facility, for additional rehabilitation. After discharge from Memorial, it is expected that he will need home care for four to six weeks. Briefly explain how the different rights set out in each document will affect Mr. Delmonico's care.

8. Consider Mr. Delmonico's diagnosis and the services he will need for recovery. Which aspects of the Patients' Bill of Rights pertain to his hospital care?

9. Discuss the statements in the Residents' Rights document that pertain specifically to rehabilitation and independence.

10. For which items in the Clients' Rights document would the nursing assistant be responsible?

UNIT **4**

Ethical and Legal Issues Affecting the Nursing Assistant

OBJECTIVES

After completing this unit, you will be able to:

- Spell and define terms.
- Describe the legal responsibilities of a nursing assistant.
- Describe how to protect the patients' right to privacy.
- Define abuse and neglect, and give examples of each.
- Define sexual harassment and give examples of activities that may be perceived as being sexually harassing.

VOCABULARY

Learn the meaning and the correct spelling of the following words and phrases:

abuse	ethical standards	libel	sexual harassment
aiding and abetting	false imprisonment	malpractice	slander
assault	informed consent	mental abuse	theft
battery	invasion of privacy	neglect	verbal abuse
coercion	involuntary seclusion	negligence	
confidential	legal standards	physical abuse	
defamation	liable	sexual abuse	

LEGAL AND ETHICAL STANDARDS

You will be faced with decisions about your actions at work each day. Some of these decisions involve being morally right or wrong. Others involve the legality of your behavior. Two sets of rules help govern the moral and legal actions you will take.

1. **Ethical standards** are guides to moral behavior. You must follow these rules if you are to give safe, correct care.

2. **Legal standards** are guides to lawful behavior. Workers who break the law may be prosecuted and found **liable**

(held responsible) for injury or damage. Legal guilt can result in the payment of fines or imprisonment.

The legal and ethical standards ensure that only safe, quality care is given. Following them also protects the caregiver. Some rules governing moral and legal actions cover the same areas.

ETHICS QUESTIONS

Probably at no other time in history have the questions of medical ethics been under such scrutiny. As a nursing assistant, you will take directions from and be ruled by the legal and ethical guidelines established by your facility.

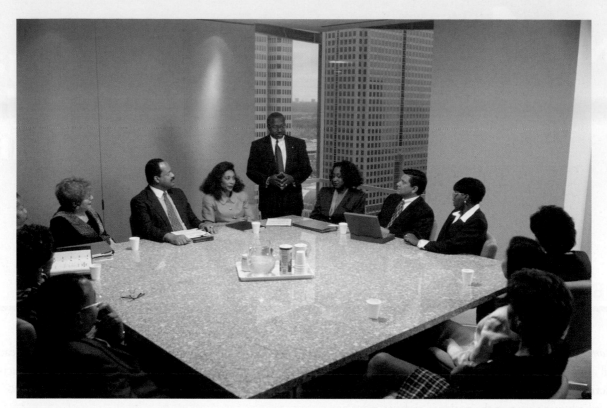

FIGURE 4-1 The ethics committee often discusses complex patient situations and sometimes must make difficult decisions. *(Courtesy of Photodisc)*

Most facilities have ethics committees (Figure 4-1) that advise the staff on ethical matters. Committee members review any problems and make recommendations to the staff, patients, and patients' families. Sometimes the choices are difficult, such as when doctors recommend removing life support and the patient's family disagrees with the decision. In situations like this, the family has the option of moving the patient to another facility within a given time frame, such as 10 days. However, finding a new placement is often difficult and time-consuming. Care for such patients is usually highly technical and very expensive. A facility that is qualified and willing to accept the patient may be hundreds of miles away.

Respect for Life

One of the most basic rules of ethics is that life is precious. The promotion of health and the quality of life are primary goals of health care facilities (Figure 4-2). Death is a natural progression of life. When death is certain, the goal is to keep the dying person comfortable. Health care workers are expected to maintain quality of life and make terminally ill patients comfortable.

Respect for the Individual

Respect for each patient as a unique individual is another basic ethical principle.

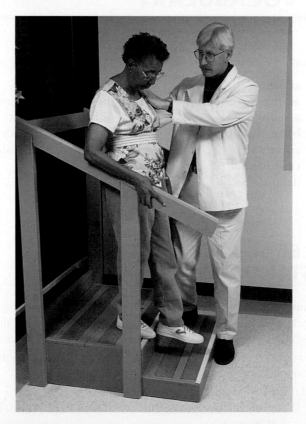

FIGURE 4-2 Promoting good health and the highest possible quality of life are primary goals. *(© Delmar/Cengage Learning)*

You may find the differences that make the patient so special also make dealing with the patient challenging or difficult. If you respect each patient as a valuable person, you can learn to accept and work with each one in the best possible way.

PATIENT INFORMATION

Information about patients is privileged and must not be shared with others (Figure 4-3).

Confidentiality concerns fall into three main categories:

1. Discuss patient information only in private areas.
   a. Avoid discussing a patient's condition while in the patient's room.
   b. Never discuss patients with your family or others.
   c. Avoid discussing patients during breaks, or in public areas of the facility.
2. Discuss information only with the proper people.
   a. Other people may ask for information about patients; you must know who is entitled to what information.
   b. Discuss patients only with your supervisor in a private area.
   c. Learn to evade inquiries tactfully by referring the questioner to the nurse.
3. Respect patients' personal religious beliefs or absence of beliefs.
   a. Treat religious articles with respect.
   b. Do not impose your own beliefs on patients.

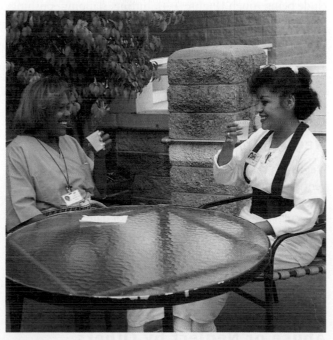

FIGURE 4-3 Patient information is always confidential and must never be discussed casually. *(© Delmar/Cengage Learning)*

c. Assist patients to practice their beliefs, if requested to do so.
d. Provide privacy during clergy visits.

TIPPING

Patients are charged for the services they receive. Your salary is included in that charge. If patients offer you money, firmly and courteously refuse.

As you can see, the ethical code ensures that each patient is treated with dignity and respect in ways that always promote safe care.

LEGAL ISSUES

Laws are passed by governments and must be obeyed by citizens. Persons who break the law may be liable (responsible) for fines or subject to imprisonment. You need not fear breaking laws if you:

- Stay within your scope of practice and do not overstep your authority. In this situation, the scope of practice is what a reasonable nursing assistant would do in a similar situation. Your job description, textbook, and facility policies and procedures are guides to the scope of nursing assistant practice. Your instructor is also an excellent source of information.
- Carry out procedures carefully and as you were taught.
- Request guidance from the nurse before taking action in a questionable situation.
- Keep patient safety and well-being foremost in your mind.
- Make sure you understand the directions before giving care.
- Do your job according to facility policy and your job description.
- Respect the patient's belongings (property).

Negligence

Negligence is failure to exercise the degree of care considered reasonable under the circumstances. Negligence is carelessness. It may be accidental or deliberate. It may result from an action or an omission (failure to act). For example, not feeding a confused patient because she is a slow eater and you are short on time is negligent. Forgetting to give a tray to a confused patient who feeds himself is also a negligent act. Either way, the patient is not given the expected level of care.

Malpractice is improper or negligent conduct that results in harm to a patient. For example, the care plan notes that the patient needs a two-person transfer. You transfer the patient alone, and he falls and is injured.

Theft

Taking anything that does not belong to you is **theft**. The patients' rights document refers to this action as the "misappropriation of property." You are guilty of **aiding and abetting** if you see someone committing a crime and do not report it.

Defamation

Harming another person by making false statements is called **defamation**. You commit defamation if you make the statement verbally (**slander**) or in writing (**libel**).

False Imprisonment

Restraining a person's movement without proper authorization is **false imprisonment**. For example, patients have the right to leave the hospital *with or without* the doctor's permission. If you interfere with this right, you are guilty of false imprisonment.

Assault and Battery

Assault means trying or threatening to touch a person's body without permission, causing the person to fear harm. **Battery** is touching a person without permission.

Care is always given with the patient's permission or **informed consent**. The patient must know about and agree to the care before you begin. Consent may be withdrawn at any time. You can avoid legal pitfalls by:

- Carefully explaining what you plan to do.
- Making sure the patient understands what you plan to do, when you plan to do it, how you plan to do it, and what the expected outcome will be.
- Giving the patient an opportunity to ask questions or refuse.
- Never performing care against a patient's wishes, and reporting refusals of care to the nurse.

Coercion means forcing a patient to do something against his or her wishes. Refusal of treatment creates a dilemma for the nursing assistant when the person is confused. A family member or other responsible person consents to facility admission and treatment for patients who are confused. We presume that the patient would agree to the care if he or she were mentally able to do so. The patient may refuse a procedure, such as a bath, but a legally responsible person has already consented to routine facility care, so you may perform it. However, it is always best to gain the patient's cooperation. Return later and try again. Try to avoid forcing the patient. Consult the nurse if in doubt about how to handle refusals of care.

Abuse

Abuse is any deliberate action that causes harm to a patient. Abuse is a criminal action. It may be verbal, sexual, physical, or mental.

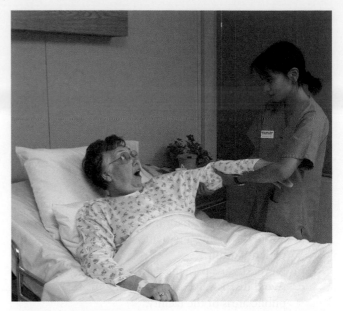

FIGURE 4-4 Handling a patient roughly is physical abuse. *(© Delmar/Cengage Learning)*

Verbal abuse may be directed toward the patient or expressed about the patient. You are guilty of verbal abuse if you swear at a patient, call the patient names, or tease or embarrass the patient. (Teasing and embarrassing may also constitute mental abuse, depending on the situation.)

Sexual abuse is inappropriate touching, forcing a person to perform sexual acts, or behavior that is seductive, harassing, or reasonably interpreted as sexual by the patient.

Physical abuse is a deliberate action that physically harms the patient or causes pain. Examples of physical abuse include being rough (Figure 4-4), hitting, slapping, pushing, kicking, or pinching a patient.

Mental abuse includes causing the patient to feel afraid, threatening to withhold care or cause harm, or making fun of the person (Figure 4-5). Calling the patient by names such as "honey" and "grandma" is another way of belittling the patient.

Neglect

Neglect is the failure to provide the care necessary to prevent discomfort, avoid physical harm, or avoid mental anguish. It includes accidentally or deliberately withholding care, such as assistance with activities of daily living, or failure to provide food or fluids. Simply put, it is not doing what you are supposed to do in the care of a patient.

Involuntary seclusion is the separation of a patient from others against the person's will. Separation may be permitted in some situations as part of a therapeutic plan of care.

Abuse or Neglect by Others

Inform the nurse if you suspect that a patient is being abused or neglected. Anyone may be abused, but the old

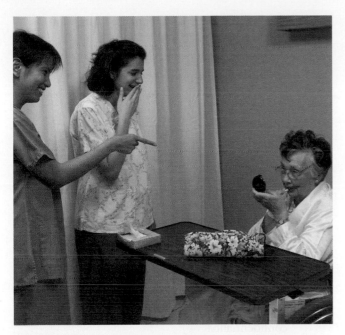

FIGURE 4-5 Making fun of a patient is psychological abuse. (© Delmar/Cengage Learning)

and the young are the most vulnerable. Usually, the caregiver or a family member is the abuser.

You are not responsible for determining whether a patient has been abused or neglected. You *are* responsible for reporting signs or symptoms that might be the result of abuse or neglect. These include:

- Statements by the patient that reflect or suggest neglect or abuse
- Unexplained bruises or injuries
- Signs of neglect, such as poor personal hygiene
- A change in personality

These are not conclusive signs of abuse, but they do demand further investigation by the nurse.

Review the stress management techniques in Unit 2 if you feel that your own tolerance or patience are being tested or you need to find ways of relieving stress. It is never acceptable to take out your frustrations on patients!

Invasion of Privacy

Personal information about patients must be kept **confidential**. To do otherwise is an **invasion of privacy**. Invading the privacy of another is against the law.

You can protect the patient's privacy by:

- Protecting the patient's body from exposure.
- Knocking and pausing before entering a room.
- Drawing curtains when providing care.
- Speaking quietly so that others do not hear sensitive or private conversations with the patient or other workers.
- Leaving when visitors come to see the patient, and staying away while they are present.
- Abiding by the rules of confidentiality.

SEXUAL HARASSMENT

Some people are unaware that their words or behavior constitute **sexual harassment**. A simple definition of *sexual harassment* is unwelcome sexual advances, requests for sexual favors, and other verbal or physical conduct of a sexual nature. The other party may be a patient or coworker, of the same gender or the opposite gender. Sexual harassment is illegal. The facility has a duty to protect both patients and staff from sexual harassment, and to avoid repeated incidents once harassment has been reported. Your facility will have policies and procedures regarding actions to take and possible penalties if harassment occurs.

REVIEW

A. Multiple Choice

Select the one best answer for each of the following.

1. You overhear another assistant yelling at Mrs. Ryan. The assistant is guilty of
   a. negligence.
   b. slander.
   c. abuse. ✓
   d. invasion of privacy.

2. Mr. Deonne offers you two dollars for picking up a newspaper from a machine in the lobby for him. You will

   a. ignore the money and pretend not to see it.
   b. take the money—you earned it.
   c. report the matter to the supervisor.
   d. politely refuse, because tipping is not allowed. ✓

3. You see another nursing assistant hitting a confused patient. What is your best response?
   a. Call the patient's family immediately.
   b. Report this to your supervisor. ✓
   c. Make the assistant promise not to do this again.
   d. Do nothing, because it is not your responsibility.

4. Mr. Chan's daughter asks what her father's blood pressure reading is. You will
   a. tell her.
   b. say you don't know.
   c. refer her to the nurse. ✓
   d. refer her to the physician.

5. You observe another worker slipping a patient's rosary into her pocket. You will
   a. do nothing.
   b. inform the nurse. ✓
   c. tell the patient.
   d. call the police.

6. You hear a housekeeper cursing at a patient. You should
   a. pretend that you did not hear.
   b. ask the other nursing assistants for advice.
   c. report this information to your supervisor. ✓
   d. report this information to the housekeeper's supervisor.

7. A nursing assistant listens when a patient makes phone calls. The assistant is guilty of
   a. invasion of privacy. ✓
   b. defamation.
   c. negligence.
   d. libel.

8. An assistant forgets to care for a confused patient. This is an example of
   a. abuse.
   b. libel.
   c. slander.
   d. neglect. ✓

9. Mrs. Rosario has very fragile skin that tears and bruises easily. The nurse instructed the nursing assistants to handle this patient gently. Tony is in a hurry and bumps Mrs. Rosario's leg against the side rail, causing a large skin tear. This is an example of
   a. slander.
   b. abuse.
   c. libel.
   d. negligence. ✓

10. Mr. McNally says he is tired and does not want his bath right now. You should
    a. tell him you will not have time to bathe him later.
    b. ask him when he would like you to return.
    c. advise him that the doctor insists that he bathe.
    d. skip the bath for today.

11. Mr. Strong, a confused patient, has a visitor. After the visitor leaves, you discover a large bruise on the patient's arm that was not there previously. You should
    a. notify the nurse.
    b. call the police.
    c. do nothing.
    d. cover the bruise with clothing.

12. A patient tells you that she no longer wants to live. She confides that she is collecting her medicine so she can take an overdose and die. You should
    a. tell no one, out of respect for the patient's right to confidentiality.
    b. notify the patient's husband when he visits.
    c. inform the nurse immediately. ✓
    d. notify the doctor when she makes rounds.

13. Which of the following is an example of a violation of the patient's right to confidentiality?
    a. Discussing the patient's condition during a care conference
    b. Reporting an observation to the nurse
    c. Discussing the patient's condition in a crowded elevator ✓
    d. Writing the patient's vital signs on a scrap of paper

B. Nursing Assistant Challenge

Describe the correct nursing assistant action in each of the following situations.

14. Ms. Harvey is dying. Her doctors believe that she will live only a few days. What is your responsibility to this patient? _____

15. Mrs. Wybok insists on saying her prayers every morning just as breakfast is ready. _____

16. Mr. Bishop's daughter asks you what medicine the doctor ordered for her father's heart condition. _____

SECTION 2

Scientific Principles

UNIT 5

Medical Terminology and Body Organization

OBJECTIVES

After completing this unit, you will be able to:

- Spell and define terms.
- Write the abbreviations commonly used in health care facilities.
- Describe the organization of the body, from simple to complex.
- Name four types of tissues and their characteristics.
- Name and locate major organs as parts of body systems, using proper anatomic terms.
- State the location and functions of each body system.

VOCABULARY

Learn the meaning and the correct spelling of the following words and phrases:

abbreviation	clitoris	genitalia	medial
abduction	cochlea	glucagon	medulla
adduction	combining form	gonads	meninges
adrenal glands	conjunctiva	health	myocardium
alveoli	cornea	hormones	nephrons
anatomic position	cortex	inferior	nerves
anatomy	Cowper's glands	insertion	neurons
anterior	defecation	insulin	neurotransmitters
atrium	dendrites	integument	organs
axons	dermis	involuntary muscles	origin
brain stem	disease	iris	ossicles
bronchi	distal	islets of Langerhans	ovaries
bronchioles	dorsal	kidneys	ovulation
bursae	ejaculatory duct	labia majora	ovum
capillaries	endocrine glands	labia minora	oxygen (O_2)
carbon dioxide (CO_2)	epidermis	lacrimal glands	oxygenation
cardiac cycle	epididymis	larynx	pallor
cardiac muscle	erythrocytes	lateral	parathyroid glands
cell	eustachian tubes	leukocytes	pelvis
cerebellum	extension	ligaments	penis
cerebrospinal fluid (CSF)	fallopian tubes (oviducts)	lymph	pharynx
cerebrum	flexion	lymphatic vessels	physiology

pineal body	rubra	testosterone	urinary meatus
pituitary gland	semicircular canals	tetany	uterus
plasma	seminal vesicles	thrombocytes	vagina
pleura	sperm	thyroid gland	vas deferens
posterior	stimulus	tissues	ventilation
prefix	subcutaneous tissue	trachea	ventral
prostate gland	suffix	tympanic membrane	ventricle
proximal	superior	umbilicus	visceral muscles
pupil	synapse	ureters	vocal cords
quadrant	systems	urethra	voluntary muscles
retention	tendons	urinalysis	vulva
rotation	testes	urinary bladder	word root

MEDICAL TERMINOLOGY

Medical science and health care have a special language called *medical terminology*. In this language, the terms are formed by building on common word parts (Figure 5-1). Terms are developed by combining:

- **Word root**—the foundation of a medical term. A word root usually, but not always, refers to the part of the body or condition that is being treated, studied, or named by the term.
- **Combining form**—a vowel may be added to the end of the word root to make it easier to form medical words. This combination of the word root and vowel is called a *combining form*.
- **Prefix**—word part added to the beginning of a word to change or add to its meaning.
- **Suffix**—word part added to the end of a word to change or add to its meaning.
- **Abbreviation**—shortened form of a word (often letters). You already know the abbreviation RN (registered nurse). You will soon become familiar with additional abbreviations that are common to the world of medicine and health care.

Each facility has a listing of abbreviations that may and may not be used. Check your facility's list to determine which abbreviations have been approved for use.

Medical Word Parts

Word roots Familiarity with the important word parts comes from study and repeated usage. You will gain experience with the word parts as you practice reporting and charting, and by communicating with your coworkers.

Legal ALERT

Documentation is a means of communication (Figure 5-2). Abbreviations must be clear, and others must know their meanings, if you are to communicate effectively. ■

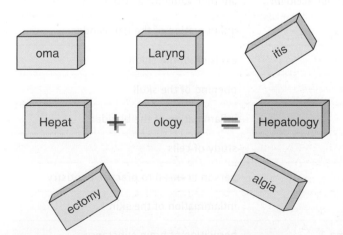

FIGURE 5-1 New words can be formed by combining different prefixes and suffixes. (© Delmar/Cengage Learning)

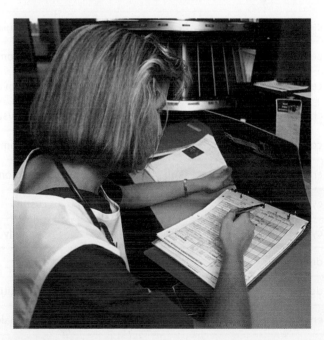

FIGURE 5-2 Documentation is a very important responsibility. (© Delmar/Cengage Learning)

A single medical word root may be used in different parts of a word, but it still has a specific meaning. For example, the root *cyte* means cell:

- *Cyt*ology—the study of cells
- Leuko*cyte*—a white blood cell
- Poly*cyt*osis—an illness in which there are too many blood cells

No matter where the form *cyte* occurs in a medical word, it refers to cells. It may be a prefix, a suffix, or a word root. Word roots are often derived from Greek or Latin. For example, the word root *nephro* is derived from the word for

kidney. This root may be used to form a variety of medical terms. For example:

- Nephroma—a tumor of the kidney
- Nephrectomy—surgical excision of the kidney
- Nephrolithiasis—presence of kidney stones

Give special attention to the exercises and activities in this unit. Learning the new words and parts of words in this unit will make it easier for you to determine the meanings of medical terms. Table 5-1 lists combining forms (word roots plus vowel).

TABLE 5-1 COMBINING FORMS

Combining Form	Meaning	Example	Meaning
abdomin (o)	abdomen	abdominal	portion of body between the thorax and pelvis
aden (o)	gland	adenoma	a glandular tumor
angi (o)	vessel	angioedema	recurrent large areas of subcutaneous edema of sudden onset (commonly an allergic reaction to foods or drugs)
arteri (o)	artery	arteriogram	X-ray of an artery after injection of contrast medium (dye)
arthr (o)	joint	arthritis	inflammation of a joint
bronch (i) (o)	bronchus	bronchiectasis	condition in which one of the larger passages conveying air to and within the lungs becomes abnormally enlarged
cardi (o)	heart	cardialgia	pain in the region of the heart
cephal (o)	head	cephaloma	soft or encephaloid tumor
cerebr (o)	brain	cerebrovascular accident	another name for a stroke
chol (e)	bile	cholecystitis	inflammation of the gallbladder
col (o)	colon, large intestine	colectomy	excision of the colon
crani (o)	skull	craniotomy	opening of the skull
cyst (o)	bladder, cyst	cystitis	inflammation of the bladder
cyt (o)	cell	cytology	study of cells
dent (i) (o)	tooth	dentist	person licensed to practice dentistry
dermat (o)	skin	dermatitis	inflammation of the skin
encephal (o)	brain	encephaloma	herniation of brain substance
enter (o)	small intestine	enteritis	inflammation of the intestines

TABLE 5-1 continued

Combining Form	Meaning	Example	Meaning
erythr (o)	red	erythroblastosis	presence of many red blood cells
fibr (o)	fiber	fibroadenoma	benign growth commonly occurring in breast tissue
gastr (o)	stomach	gastritis	inflammation of the lining of the stomach
geront (o)	elderly	gerontology	scientific study of process and problems related to aging
gloss (o)	tongue	glossodynia	burning or painful tongue
glyc (o)	sugar	glycosuria	excretion of sugar in the urine
gynec (o)	female	gynecomastia	excessive development of male mammary glands
hem (o)	blood	hematuria	discharge of blood in urine
hepat (o)	liver	hepatitis	inflammation of the liver
hydr (o)	water	hydrocephalus	enlargement of the cranium caused by abnormal accumulation of fluid
hyster (o)	uterus	hysterectomy	surgical removal of the uterus
lapar (o)	abdomen, flank, loin	laparoscopy	examination of the contents of the abdomen through an instrument (scope) passed through the abdominal wall
laryng (o)	larynx	laryngectomy	partial or total removal of the larynx by surgery
lith (o)	stone	lithiasis	formation of stones in any hollow structure of the body
mamm (o)	breast	mammography	imaging examination of the breasts
mast (o)	breast	mastitis	inflammation of the breast
men (o)	menstruation	menorrhagia	excessive menstrual flow
my (o)	muscle	myalgia	muscular pain
myel (o)	bone marrow, spinal cord	myelocele	protrusion of the spinal cord
nephr (o)	kidney	nephrolithiasis	presence of renal calculi (kidney stones)
neur (o)	nerve	neuropathy	any disease of the nervous system
ocul (o)	eye	oculodynia	pain in the eyeball
ophthalm (o)	eye	ophthalmoscope	instrument used to view the inside of the eye
oste (o)	bone	osteitis	inflammation of the bone

continues

TABLE 5-1 continued

Combining Form	Meaning	Example	Meaning
ot (o)	ear	otitis media	inflammation of the middle ear
ped (i) (o)	child	pedodontics	dental care of children
pharyng (o)	throat, pharynx	pharyngitis	inflammation of the pharynx
phleb (o)	vein	phlebitis	inflammation of a vein
pneum (o)	lung, air, gas	pneumonectomy	resection of lung tissue
proct (o)	rectum	proctoscopy	rectal exam with a proctoscope
psych (o)	mind	psychology	study of human behavior
pulm (o)	lung	pulmonary	pertaining to the lungs
py (o)	pus	pyogenic	producing pus
rect (o)	rectum	rectocele	hernial protrusion of part of the rectum into the vagina
rhin (o)	nose	rhinorrhea	discharge from nasal mucous membrane
splen (o)	spleen	splenoma	enlarged spleen
stern (o)	sternum	sternotomy	incision into or through the sternum
thorac (o)	chest	thoracotomy	opening of the chest
thromb (o)	clot	thrombocytopenia	abnormally small number of platelets in the circulating blood
tox (o)	poison	toxoplasmosis	disease produced by a parasite; can cause birth defects if acquired during pregnancy
trache (o)	trachea	tracheotomy	incision of the trachea for exploration
ur (o)	urine, urinary tract, urination	urinalysis	analysis of the urine
urethr (o)	urethra	urethralgia	pain in the urethra
urin (o)	urine	urinometer	an instrument for determining the specific gravity of urine
uter (i) (o)	uterus	uterotonic	drugs that give tone to uterine muscle
ven (o)	vein	venostat	any instrument used to suppress venous bleeding

Prefixes and Suffixes

Many medical words have common beginnings (prefixes) or common endings (suffixes). You can put together many new words by using prefixes and suffixes. Many common ones are listed in Tables 5-2 and 5-3.

TABLE 5-2 COMMON PREFIXES

Prefix	Meaning	Example	Meaning
a-	without	asepsis	without infection
brady-	slow	bradycardia	slow heart rate
dys-	pain or difficulty	dysuria	painful urination
hyper-	above, excessive	hypertension	high blood pressure
hypo-	low, deficient	hypotension	low blood pressure
pan-	all	pandemic	widespread epidemic
poly-	many	polyuria	excessive urine
post-	after	postoperative	after surgery
pre-	before	premenstrual	before the menses
retro-	behind, backward	retrograde	moving backward, degenerating
tachy-	fast	tachycardia	pulse rate above normal

TABLE 5-3 COMMON SUFFIXES

Suffix	Meaning	Example	Meaning
-algia	pain	arthralgia	pain in the joints
-ectomy	removal of	appendectomy	removal of the appendix
-emia	blood	anemia	lacking sufficient quality or quantity of blood
-gram	record	electrocardiogram	record of heart function produced by an electrocardiograph machine
-itis	inflammation	appendicitis	inflammation of the appendix
-logy	study of	hematology	study of blood
-oma	tumor	fibroma	a tumor containing fibrous tissue
-otomy	incision	tracheotomy	incision into the trachea
-plegia	paralysis	hemiplegia	paralysis of one side of the body
-pnea	breathing, respiration	apnea	temporary absence of respirations
-scope	examination instrument	otoscope	instrument for inspecting the ear
-scopy	examination using a scope	proctoscopy	rectal exam with a proctoscope

Common Abbreviations

Table 5-4 lists abbreviations and their meanings. They have been grouped according to most common usage for easier learning. Other abbreviations are presented in following units, within the context in which they are most often used.

TABLE 5-4 COMMON ABBREVIATIONS

Body Parts

ABCs	airway, breathing, circulation
abd	abdomen
ant	anterior
ax	axillary
BLE	both lower extremities
GI	gastrointestinal
GU	genitourinary

Patient Orders and Charting

ā	before
AAROM	active assistive (assisted) range of motion
ADL	activities of daily living
ad lib	as desired
adm	admission; administer; administrator
AEB	as evidenced by
AKA	also known as
AMA	against medical advice
amb	ambulate, ambulatory
AROM	active range of motion
ASAP	as soon as possible
assist	assistance
as tol	as tolerated
B, Ⓑ	bilateral, both
bilat	bilateral
BLE	both lower extremities
BM	bowel movement

BP, B/P	blood pressure
BPM	beats per minute
BR	bedrest; bathroom
BRP	bathroom privileges
BS	blood sugar
BSC	bedside commode
BUE	both upper extremities
c̄	with
cal	calorie
cath	catheterize, catheter
ck or ✓	check
ck freq ✓	check frequently
cl liq	clear liquid
c/o	complains of
CP	care plan; chest pain
CPM	continuous passive motion
CPR	cardiopulmonary resuscitation
DAT	diet as tolerated
DNR	do not resuscitate
Dr	doctor
DSD	dry sterile dressing
Dx	diagnosis
Et, et	and
ETOH	ethanol (used to refer to alcoholic beverages)
eval	evaluation
ex, ex	exercise, example
exam	examination
ext	extension; extremity; external
F	fair
FB	foreign body
FE	Fleet's enema
flex	flexion

TABLE 5-4 continued

FU, f/u	follow-up		mod	moderate
FUO	fever of unknown origin		N/A	not applicable
FWB	full weight bearing		N/C, no c/o	no complaints
G	good		neg, ⊖	negative
g/c, GC	geriatric chair		NG	nasogastric
GT, g/t	gastrostomy tube		NKA	no known allergies
H_2O	water		NPO	nothing by mouth
H_2O_2	hydrogen peroxide		N/S, NSS	normal saline solution
HOB	head of bed		N & V, N&V	nausea and vomiting
HOH	hard of hearing		NWB	no weight bearing
Ht	height		O_2	oxygen
Hx	history		OOB	out of bed
Ⓘ	independent		O, OS	oral; mouth
I&O	intake and output		P	poor, pulse
IM	intramuscular		per	by
IV	intravenous		po, PO	by mouth
JT	jejunostomy tube		postop	postoperative
K^+	potassium		preop	preoperative
Kcal, kcal	kilocalorie, calorie		prep	prepare
L	left, liter		PRN	whenever necessary, as needed
lat	lateral		PROM	passive range of motion
LBP	low back pain		PWB	partial weight bearing
lg, lge, L	large		Px	prognosis (prog)
liq	liquid		q̄	each, every
L/min, LPM	liters per minute		qs	sufficient quantity, enough
LOC	loss of consciousness, level of consciousness		R	rectal; respiration; right
max	maximum		re:	regarding
min	minimum		rehab	rehabilitation
meds	medications		rt, (R)	right
mmHg	millimeters of mercury		r/t	related to

continues

TABLE 5-4 continued

Patient Orders and Charting

RT	respiratory therapy
Rx	treatment; prescription
$\bar{s}$	without
s/s, S&S	signs and symptoms
S, sm	small
SOB	short(ness) of breath
SBA	standby assistance
SSE	soapsuds enema
stat	at once; immediately
T, temp	temperature
TIAN	toilet in advance of need
TKO	to keep open
TLC	tender loving care
TPN	total parenteral nutrition
TPR	temperature, pulse, respirations
trach	tracheostomy
TWE	tap water enema
Tx	treatment
VC	verbal cues
VS	vital signs
w/c, WC	wheelchair
WB	weight bearing
WBAT	weight bearing as tolerated
Wt	weight

Tests

BS	blood sugar
C&S	culture and sensitivity
CBC	complete blood count
CXR	chest X-ray
FBS	fasting blood sugar
FSBS	fingerstick blood sugar
H&H	hemoglobin and hematocrit
spec	specimen
UA, U/A	urinalysis

Time Abbreviations

$\bar{ac}$	before meals
AM	morning
BID	twice a day
D	day
H	hour
noc	night
OC, oc	on call
$\bar{p}$	after
$\bar{pc}$	after meals
PM	evening or afternoon
$\bar{q}$ h	every hour
$\bar{q}$ 4h	every four hours
QID	four times a day
TID	three times a day
WA, W/A	while awake
x, X	times
x2, x3	two times, three times, . . .

Common Numbers

1°	first; primary; first degree
2°	second; secondary to; second degree
3°	third; tertiary; third degree
1x	one time, one person
2x	two times, two people

TABLE 5-4 continued

Measurements and Volume	
amt	amount
gtt	drop
mL	milliliter
L	liter
oz	ounce

Weight/Height	
cm	centimeter
ft	feet
Ht, ht	height
kg	kilogram
lb	pound(s)
in	inch(es)
oz	ounce
wt	weight

Temperature	
°	degrees
ax	axillary
F	Fahrenheit
C	Celsius, centigrade
O	oral
R	rectal

Symbols	
♂	male
♀	female
↑	up, increase
↓	down, decrease
=	parallel
Δ	change to
∅	zero, none, nothing
*	important

BODY ORGANIZATION

Health is a state of well-being in which the body and mind are functioning properly. **Disease** is any change from the healthy state. Disease takes many forms. Medical science is the study of disease and its effects on the human body. These effects are easier to understand when you have a clear picture in your mind of a normal and properly functioning body. The first step is to understand the organization of the body.

Anatomic Terms

You will understand the **anatomy** (structure) and **physiology** (function) of the body most easily if you study them in an orderly manner. Medical language uses special terms to describe the relationship of one body part to another.

Whenever we describe the relationship of the body parts, we refer to the **anatomic position** (Figure 5-3), which is:

- Standing erect with feet together or slightly separated
- Facing the observer
- Arms at the sides with the palms forward

In our own minds, we should always position the body in this way before describing any body part or area. The patient's right side is opposite to your left and your left is opposite to the right of the patient.

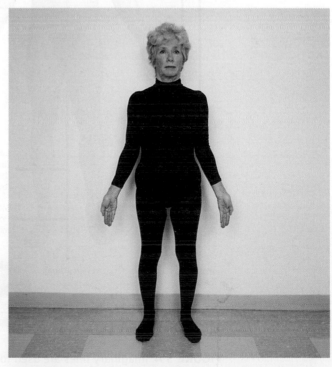

FIGURE 5-3 All references to body parts are made in relationship to the anatomic position. (© Delmar/Cengage Learning)

Descriptive Terms

Imaginary lines drawn through the body (Figure 5-4) provide us with other reference terms.

- A line drawn down the center of the body from head to foot (the *midline*) divides the body into equal sides. Note that the body has the same parts on either side. For example, there is an arm, a leg, an eye, and half of a nose on each side of the line.
- Parts close to this line are **medial** to the line.
- Parts farther away from the line are **lateral** to the line.

For example, in the anatomic position, the thumbs are more lateral to the line and the little fingers are more medial to the line.

Another line drawn parallel to the floor divides the body into upper and lower parts. This line can be drawn at any level on the body as long as the line is parallel to the floor.

- Parts located above this line are **superior** to the line.
- Parts located below this line are **inferior** to the line.

For example, if the line is drawn between the knees and ankles, the knees are superior to the ankles and the ankles are inferior to the knees.

A third line can be drawn to divide the body into front and back.

- Parts in front of this line are **anterior** or **ventral** to the line.
- Parts in back of this line are **posterior** or **dorsal** to the line.

Points of Attachment

The arms and legs are called the *extremities* of the body. The arms are attached to the body at the shoulders. The

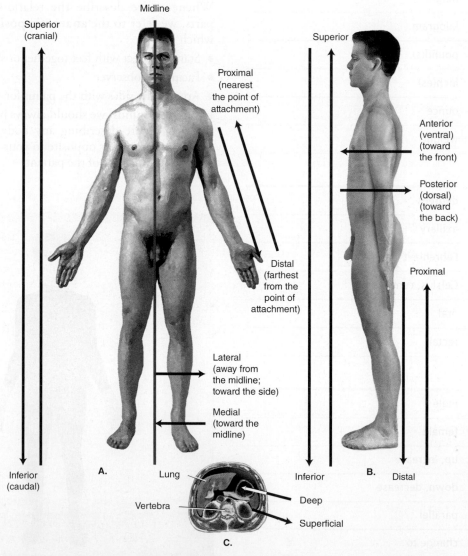

FIGURE 5-4 Imaginary lines are used to section the body to make it easier to locate parts. Directional terms relate to the anatomic position. (A) Anatomic position. (B) Lateral views of the body. (C) Directional terms *deep* and *superficial*. (© *Delmar/Cengage Learning*)

legs are attached to the body at the hips. Two terms are used to describe the relationship between the parts of the extremities and their points of attachment to the body.

● **Proximal** means closest to the point of attachment.
● **Distal** means farthest away from the point of attachment.

Because the upper arm is closest to the shoulder, where it is attached, this part is *proximal* when compared to the fingers, which are farthest away. The fingers are *distal* or farthest away from the point of attachment of the upper extremity.

Abdominal Regions

The abdomen is divided into four **quadrants**, with the **umbilicus** (navel) at the central point (Figure 5-5A). The abdomen can also be divided into nine regions (Figure 5-5B). Knowing these areas will be important as you report and document your observations.

ORGANIZATION OF THE BODY

All parts of the body are interdependent. The basic unit of the body is the **cell**. Groups of similar cells are organized into **tissues**. Different tissues form **organs**. The organs are organized into **systems** that perform the body functions.

Cells

Each cell performs the same basic functions that the total body performs, but on a smaller scale. These functions are breathing (respiration), reproduction, nutrition, and excretion (eliminating wastes).

● Epithelial cells, which are very close together, form protective coverings and sometimes produce body fluids.
● Nerve cells carry electrical messages to and from the different parts of the body, coordinating activities and making us aware of changes in the environment.
● Muscle cells can shorten or lengthen, changing their shape and the position of parts to which they are attached. They also surround and control the size of body openings, such as the mouth.
● Connective tissue cells are present throughout the body in many different types. They support and connect body parts.

Tissues

Groups of similar cells are organized into tissues.
● Epithelial tissue is specialized in its ability to absorb, secrete (produce) fluids, excrete (eliminate) waste products, and protect.
● Nervous tissue forms the brain and spinal cord and the nerves throughout the body. The activities of the rest of the body are directed through the nervous tissues.

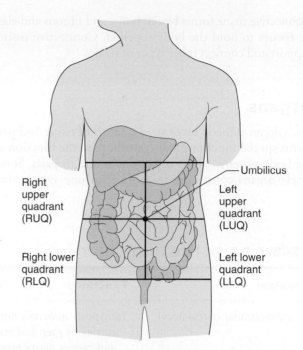

FIGURE 5-5A Division of the abdomen into four quadrants. *(© Delmar/Cengage Learning)*

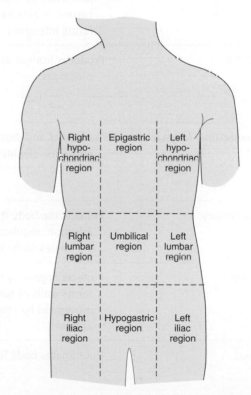

FIGURE 5-5B Nine regions of the thorax and abdomen. *(© Delmar/Cengage Learning)*

Three kinds of muscle tissue are found in the body:
● Skeletal (voluntary) muscle is attached to bones for movement.
● Cardiac muscle forms the heart wall.
● Smooth muscle (involuntary muscle) (visceral) forms the walls of body organs such as the stomach and intestines.

Connective tissue forms blood, bone, and fibrous and elastic tissues to hold the body together. Connective tissues support and connect other types of tissues.

Organs

Each organ is made up of several kinds of tissue and performs special functions that contribute to the function of the body systems. Some organs are found in pairs. Some single organs contribute to more than one system. For example, the pancreas contributes secretions to both the endocrine and digestive systems.

Systems

The body has 10 major body systems. Table 5-5 lists the organs that contribute to the function of each system. Notice that some organs are included with more than one system. For example, the ovaries contribute to the endocrine system by producing female hormones and to the reproductive system by producing the egg.

TABLE 5-5 SYSTEMS OF THE BODY

System	Function	Structures
Cardiovascular (circulatory)	Transports materials around the body; carries oxygen and nutrients to the cells and carries waste products away; part of the immune system that provides protective cells and chemicals to fight current infections and protect against future infections	Heart, arteries, capillaries, veins, spleen, lymph nodes, lymphatic vessels, blood, lymph
Endocrine	Produces hormones that regulate body processes	Pituitary gland, thyroid gland, parathyroid glands, thymus gland, adrenal glands, testes, ovaries, pineal body, islets of Langerhans in pancreas
Gastrointestinal (digestive)	Transports and digests food; absorbs nutrients; eliminates wastes	Mouth, esophagus, pharynx, stomach, small intestine, large intestine, salivary glands, teeth, tongue, liver, gallbladder, pancreas
Integumentary	Protects the body from injury and against infection, regulates body temperature, eliminates some wastes	Skin, hair, nails, sweat and oil glands
Muscular	Protects organs by forming body walls; forms walls of some organs; assists in movement by changing position of bones at joints	*Smooth* muscles—form walls of organs *Skeletal* muscles—attached to bones *Cardiac* muscles—form wall of heart
Nervous	Coordinates body functions	Brain, spinal cord, spinal nerves, cranial nerves, special sense organs such as eyes and ears
Reproductive	Reproduces the species; fulfills sexual needs; develops sexual identity	*Male:* Testes, epididymis, urethra, seminal vesicles, ejaculatory duct, prostate gland, bulbourethral glands, penis, spermatic cord *Female:* Breasts, ovaries, oviducts, uterus, vagina, Bartholin glands, vulva
Respiratory	Brings in oxygen and eliminates carbon dioxide	Sinuses, nose, pharynx, larynx, trachea, bronchi, lungs

TABLE 5-5 continued

Skeletal	Supports and protects body parts, produces blood cells, acts as lever in movement	Bones, joints
Urinary	Manages fluids and electrolytes of body, eliminates liquid wastes	Kidneys, ureters, urinary bladder, urethra
Sensory	Part of the nervous system, but often considered a system on its own	Eyes, ears; also senses of taste, touch, and smell

RESPIRATORY SYSTEM STRUCTURE AND FUNCTION

The respiratory system (Figure 5-6) is sometimes called the lifeline of the body. It extends from the nose to the tiny air sacs (**alveoli**) that make up the bulk of the lungs. Air is warmed, moistened, and filtered as it passes through the nasal cavities, which are separated by the nasal septum. The air passes through the **pharynx**, a passageway for both air and food, into the larynx and **trachea**. It then passes into the **bronchi** to join the upper respiratory tract to the lungs. Within the lungs, the bronchi branch into smaller and smaller divisions called **bronchioles**. The *alveoli* are tiny air sacs that extend from the bronchioles. The exchange of gases takes place in the alveoli (Figure 5-7).

The alveoli, bronchioles, and the important pulmonary blood vessels form the lungs. Figure 5-8 shows how oxygen and carbon dioxide are exchanged between the alveoli and the capillaries.

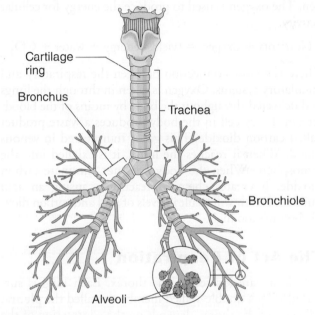

FIGURE 5-7 The lower respiratory tract. *(© Delmar/Cengage Learning)*

The purpose of this system is to bring **oxygen (O$_2$)** into the body to meet cellular needs and to expel **carbon dioxide (CO$_2$)**. Carbon dioxide is a gaseous metabolic waste produced by the cells.

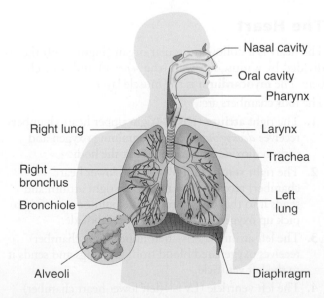

FIGURE 5-6 The respiratory system. *(© Delmar/Cengage Learning)*

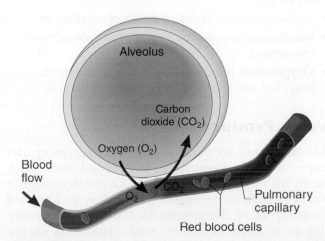

FIGURE 5-8 Oxygen and carbon dioxide are exchanged in the alveoli. *(© Delmar/Cengage Learning)*

Critical Information ALERT

The respiratory system is *very powerful*. The air released from an explosive cough moves at speeds up to 60 miles per hour (mph). A sneeze creates a force of air moving nearly 99 mph. It is impossible to sneeze with your eyes open. ∎

Each cell in the body must have a constant supply of oxygen. The oxygen is used to produce the energy for cellular activity:

Nutrients + oxygen = (yields) energy + water + CO_2

There is a close connection between the respiratory and circulatory systems. Oxygen is taken in through the lungs and delivered throughout the body by means of the bloodstream. Every cell in the body produces a waste product called carbon dioxide. This gas is transported in venous blood. When it reaches the lungs, it is exhaled into the atmosphere. When the body does not eliminate carbon dioxide, it creates chemical reactions causing an acid buildup. Death will result if levels of acid and carbon dioxide become too high.

The Act of Respiration

Two lungs are located in the thorax. Each lung is surrounded by a double-walled membrane called the **pleura**. The size of the thorax depends on the contraction of the diaphragm and intercostal muscles. When the diaphragm contracts, the thorax enlarges, expanding the lungs. Air carrying oxygen enters the lungs. When the muscles relax, the thorax becomes smaller. Air carrying carbon dioxide leaves the lungs and is breathed out.

- *Inspiration* (or inhalation) is the act of drawing air into the lungs.
- *Expiration* (or exhalation) is the act of expelling air.
- **Ventilation** (respiration) is the combination of these two actions.
- **Oxygenation** is the movement of oxygen from the lungs and into the blood to be carried to the cells.

Voice Production

The **larynx**, or voice box, is the part of the respiratory tract responsible for voice production. Two vocal cords stretch across the inside of the larynx. As air moves upward, it passes through an opening in the vocal cords. The vocal cords respond by changing the size of the opening, permitting air to reach the mouth, nasal cavities, and sinuses, where speech sounds are made when formed by the teeth, lips, and tongue.

CIRCULATORY SYSTEM STRUCTURE AND FUNCTION

The organs of the cardiovascular system include:

1. **Heart**—a central pumping station
2. **Blood vessels**
   a. Arteries—tubes that carry blood away from the heart.
   b. Veins—tubes that carry blood toward the heart.
   c. Capillaries—tubes that connect arteries and veins.
3. **Lymphatic vessels**—tubes that carry **lymph** (tissue fluid) to the bloodstream.
4. **Lymph nodes**—filter the lymph.
5. **Spleen**—organ that produces and stores some blood
6. **Blood**—a connective tissue made up of liquid (plasma) and cellular elements.

The Blood

The body contains 4 to 6 quarts (liters) of blood. Fifty-five percent of the blood is a watery solution called **plasma**, which contains antibodies (Unit 12) with which to fight infection; nutrients (Unit 26); gases such as oxygen and carbon dioxide; and waste products from the kidneys. Blood cells are produced mainly in the bone marrow and lymphatic tissues of the body:

- Red blood cells (RBCs or **erythrocytes**)—carry most of the oxygen and small amounts of carbon dioxide.
- White blood cells (WBCs or **leukocytes**)—fight infection.
- **Thrombocytes** (or platelets)—are parts of cells that initiate blood clotting.

The Heart

The heart is a hollow muscular organ (Figure 5-9) that is divided by a muscular wall (the *septum*) and four chambers. The **myocardium** is the muscle layer.

The four chambers are:

1. The right **atrium** (RA)—(right upper heart chamber) receives *deoxygenated blood* containing oxygen and carbon dioxide from throughout the body.
2. The right **ventricle** (RV)—(right lower heart chamber) receives blood from the right atrium and sends it to the lungs through the pulmonary artery to pick up oxygen and remove carbon dioxide.
3. The left atrium (LA)—(left upper heart chamber) receives oxygenated blood from the lungs and sends it to the left ventricle.
4. The left ventricle (LV)—(left lower heart chamber) receives blood from the left atrium and sends it out through the aorta to the entire body.

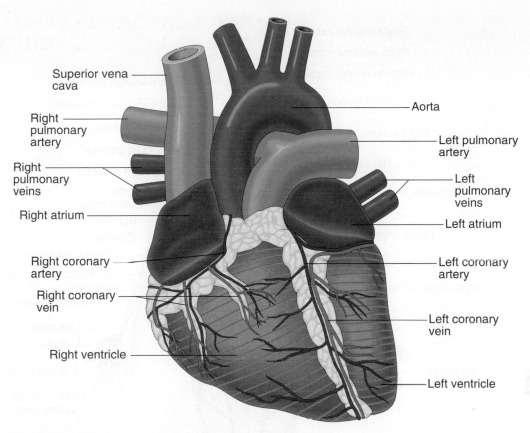

FIGURE 5-9 The heart. (© *Delmar/Cengage Learning*)

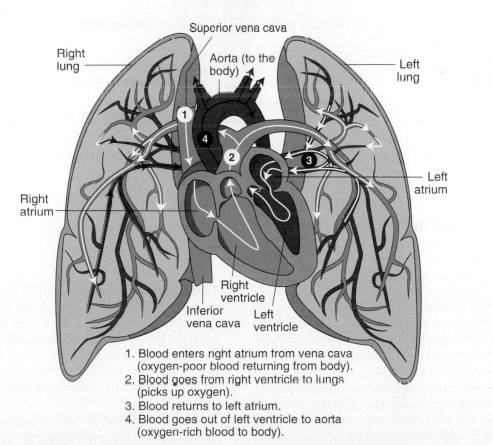

1. Blood enters right atrium from vena cava (oxygen-poor blood returning from body).
2. Blood goes from right ventricle to lungs (picks up oxygen).
3. Blood returns to left atrium.
4. Blood goes out of left ventricle to aorta (oxygen-rich blood to body).

FIGURE 5-10 Blood flows from the heart to the lungs, to the body, and back to the heart to begin the cycle again. (© *Delmar/Cengage Learning*)

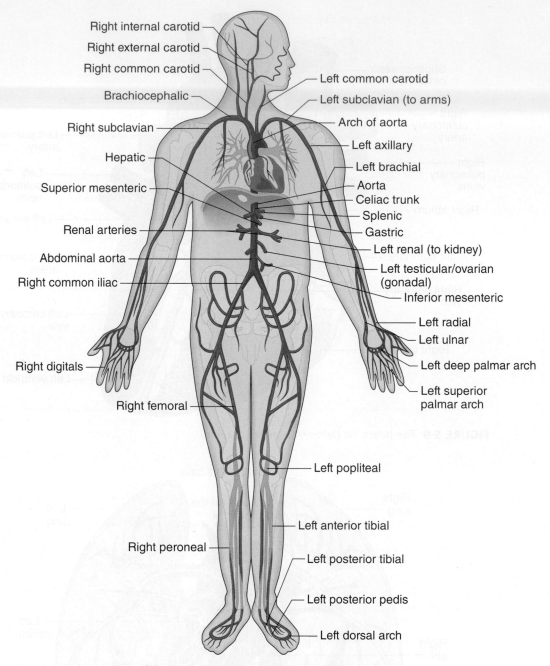

Right internal carotid

Right external carotid

Right common carotid

Brachiocephalic

Right subclavian

Hepatic

Superior mesenteric

Renal arteries

Abdominal aorta

Right common iliac

Right digitals

Right femoral

Right peroneal

Left common carotid

Left subclavian (to arms)

Arch of aorta

Left axillary

Left brachial

Aorta

Celiac trunk

Splenic

Gastric

Left renal (to kidney)

Left testicular/ovarian (gonadal)

Inferior mesenteric

Left radial

Left ulnar

Left deep palmar arch

Left superior palmar arch

Left popliteal

Left anterior tibial

Left posterior tibial

Left posterior pedis

Left dorsal arch

FIGURE 5-11 Arteries of the body. *(© Delmar/Cengage Learning)*

Valves separate the chambers of the heart. They also guard the exit of the pulmonary artery and aorta to prevent back-flow and maintain a constant forward motion of the blood. The pulmonary artery carries blood to the lungs. The aorta is the largest blood vessel in the body.

Nerve impulses make the heart contract regularly according to body needs. For example, when you run, your cells signal the brain that they need more oxygen. The brain sends a signal through the nerves telling the heart to supply more blood. The heart responds by beating faster, pumping oxygen-rich blood to the body.

The cardiac cycle The series of movements by which the heart pumps blood through the body is the **cardiac cycle** (Figure 5-10). First, *atria* relax and fill with blood while the lower chambers contract, forcing blood through the aorta and pulmonary arteries. Next, the lower chambers (*ventricles*) relax, and fill with blood from the contracting upper chambers. The cycle repeats about 70 to 80 times per minute.

The pulse you feel at the wrist corresponds with ventricular contraction. The sounds you hear when taking the apical pulse or measuring blood pressure are the sounds of valves closing during the cardiac cycle.

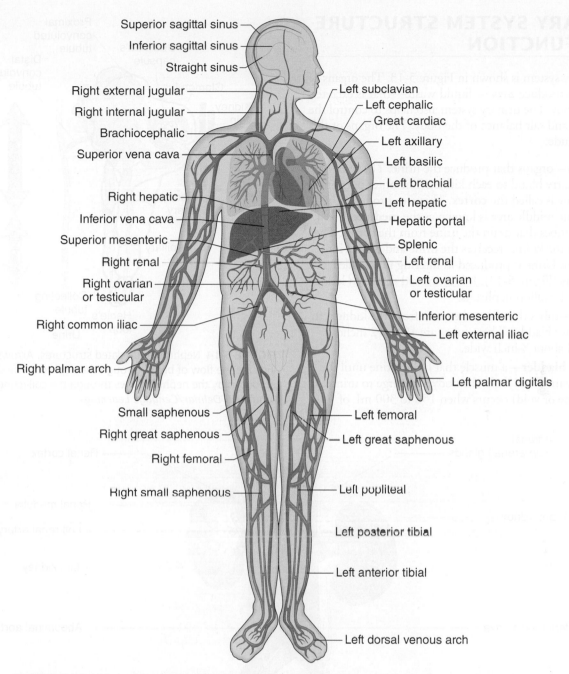

Superior sagittal sinus
Inferior sagittal sinus
Straight sinus
Right external jugular
Right internal jugular
Brachiocephalic
Superior vena cava
Right hepatic
Inferior vena cava
Superior mesenteric
Right renal
Right ovarian or testicular
Right common iliac
Right palmar arch
Small saphenous
Right great saphenous
Right femoral
Right small saphenous

Left subclavian
Left cephalic
Great cardiac
Left axillary
Left basilic
Left brachial
Left hepatic
Hepatic portal
Splenic
Left renal
Left ovarian or testicular
Inferior mesenteric
Left external iliac
Left palmar digitals
Left femoral
Left great saphenous
Left popliteal
Left posterior tibial
Left anterior tibial
Left dorsal venous arch

FIGURE 5-12 Veins of the body. (© *Delmar/Cengage Learning*)

The conduction system governs the rate and rhythm of the cardiac cycle. This system consists of neuromuscular tissue that sends out impulses. When the impulses reach the myocardial cells, those cells contract.

- The impulses begin at the SA node in the right atrium and spread across the atria.
- The atria contract.
- Impulses from the SA node reach the AV node in the right atrium.
- The messages spread through the bundle of His in the septum, then go through the Purkinje fibers to the walls of the ventricles.
- The ventricles contract, forcing the blood forward.

An electrocardiogram, called an ECG or an EKG, is a test that traces the electrical impulses of the heart. Heart disease may be detected with this test.

Blood Vessels

Many large arteries and veins take their names from the bones they are near or the part of the body they serve. For example, the femoral artery and vein run close to the femur (thigh bone). Figure 5-11 shows the arterial system that distributes blood from the heart. Figure 5-12 shows the venous system that returns blood to the heart.

URINARY SYSTEM STRUCTURE AND FUNCTION

The urinary system is shown in Figure 5-13. The organs of this system produce *urine*—liquid waste—that is excreted from the body. The urinary system also helps to control the vital water and salt balance of the body. The organs of this system include:

- **Kidneys**—organs that produce the urine. The renal arteries carry blood to each kidney. The outer portion of the kidney is called the **cortex**. This area produces the urine. The middle area is known as the **medulla**. It is a series of tubes that drain the urine from the cortex. The **pelvis** of the kidney receives the urine and directs it to the ureter. Urine is produced in filtering units called **nephrons** (Figure 5-14). It is estimated that each kidney contains 1 million nephrons.

- **Ureters**—tubes that carry the urine from the kidneys to the urinary bladder. These tubes are 10 to 12 inches long and about ¼-inch wide.

- **Urinary bladder**—a muscle that holds urine until the urine is eliminated from the body. The urge to urinate (micturate or void) occurs when 150 to 300 mL of

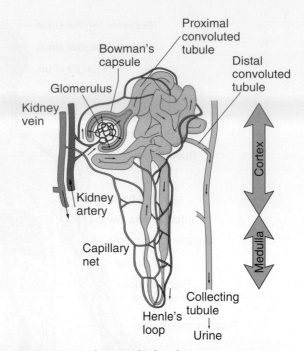

FIGURE 5-14 Nephron and related structures. Arrows indicate the flow of blood through the nephron. The urine produced by the nephron flows through the collecting tubule. (© *Delmar/Cengage Learning*)

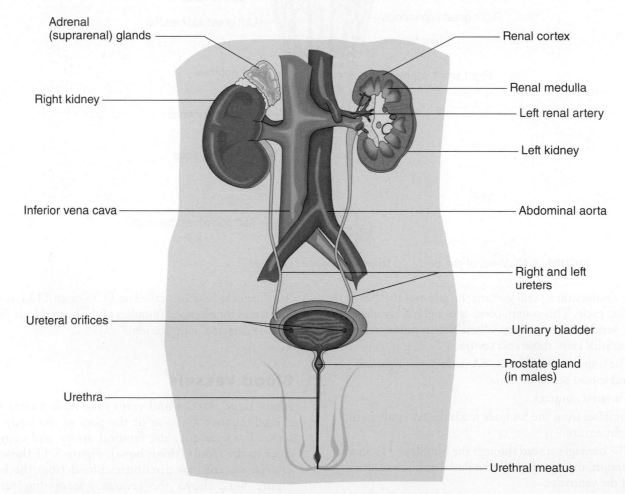

FIGURE 5-13 Structures of the urinary system. (© *Delmar/Cengage Learning*)

urine are in the bladder, although the bladder can hold more urine than this.

- **Urethra**—the tube that carries the urine to the outside. The female urethra is about 1 ½ to 2 inches long. The male urethra is about 6 to 8 inches long. The opening to the outside is called the external **urinary meatus**. The meatus is guarded by a round sphincter muscle that relaxes to release the urine.

Blood arriving at the kidneys carries waste products such as acids and salts that must be eliminated from the body. Urine is a liquid waste containing water and dissolved substances. These substances provide good information about the chemistry of the body and how well it is functioning. Tests are frequently performed on the urine (**urinalysis**). Urine samples must be obtained and preserved properly.

Inability to excrete urine that has been produced in the kidneys and is stored in the bladder is called **retention**.

ENDOCRINE SYSTEM STRUCTURE AND FUNCTION

The **endocrine glands** (Figure 5-15):

- Secrete **hormones** (chemical messengers that regulate the body's activities).
- Control body activities and growth.
- Are found as distinct glands or clusters of cells.
- Are subject to disease that can result in hyposecretion (underproduction) or hypersecretion (overproduction) of hormones.

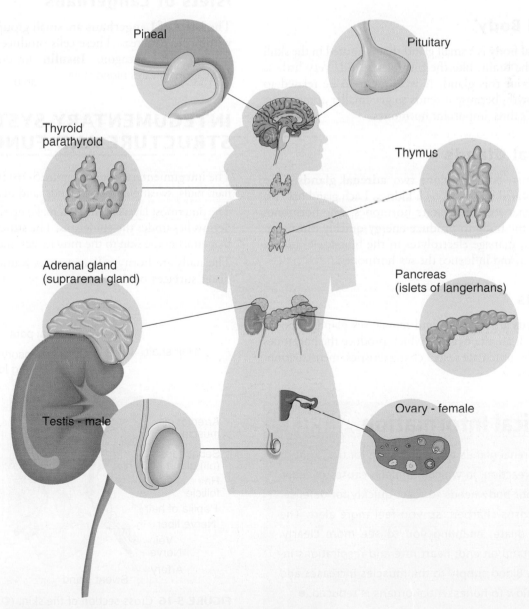

Pineal

Pituitary

Thyroid parathyroid

Thymus

Adrenal gland (suprarenal gland)

Pancreas (islets of langerhans)

Testis - male

Ovary - female

FIGURE 5-15 Endocrine system. (© *Delmar/Cengage Learning*)

Pituitary Gland

Because it controls most of the other glands, the **pituitary gland** is called the *master gland*. The pituitary gland secretes hormones that are responsible for many essential functions throughout the body.

Pineal Body

The **pineal body** is a small gland that is located in the skull beneath the brain, like the pituitary gland. Very little is known about this gland. It is thought to be related to sexual growth, because it tends to get smaller at maturity. It produces three important hormones.

Adrenal Glands

Each human body contains two **adrenal glands**. One gland is located on top of each kidney. Each gland has two portions that secrete separate hormones. The hormones stimulate the body to produce energy quickly during an emergency, manage electrolytes in the blood, elevate the blood sugar, and influence the sex hormones.

Gonads

The **gonads** are the male and female sex glands. The female gonads are the **ovaries**, which produce the hormones responsible for female sexual characteristics, menstruation, and pregnancy.

The testes are the male gonads. They produce **testosterone**. This hormone is responsible for secondary male sex characteristics.

Thyroid Gland

The **thyroid gland** has two lobes and is found in the neck, anterior to the larynx. Hormones secreted by this gland regulate metabolism.

Parathyroid Glands

The tiny **parathyroid glands** are embedded in the posterior thyroid gland. The hormone they manufacture helps control the body's use of calcium and phosphorus. Insufficient amounts of calcium result in severe muscle spasms or **tetany**. Untreated tetany can lead to death.

Islets of Langerhans

The **islets of Langerhans** are small groups of cells found within the pancreas. These cells produce two hormones: insulin and glucagon. **Insulin** lowers blood sugar. **Glucagon** elevates blood sugar.

INTEGUMENTARY SYSTEM STRUCTURE AND FUNCTION

The integumentary system (Figure 5-16) includes the skin, hair, nails, sweat glands, oil glands, and nerves in the skin.

The outermost layers of the skin make up the *epidermis*. The dermis lies under the epidermis. The **subcutaneous tissue** that attaches the skin to the muscles lies under the dermis.

The nails are horny cell structures found on the dorsal, distal surfaces of the fingers and toes. They protect the

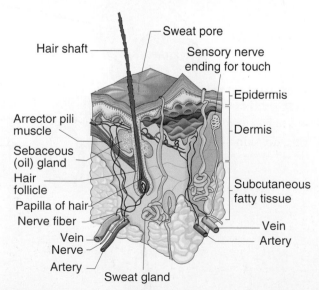

FIGURE 5-16 Cross-section of the skin. (© *Delmar/Cengage Learning*)

sensitive fingers and toes. The teeth are formed from the tissues of the **integument** (body shell).

Epidermis

The **epidermis** consists of dead outer cells that are constantly shed as new cells move upward from the dermis. There are no blood vessels in the epidermis, so injury to this layer does not cause bleeding. Nerve endings in this layer keep us in contact with changes in the environment. The nerves are sense organs. Nerve endings called *receptors* receive information about heat, cold, pain, and pressure.

Dermis

The **dermis** contains blood vessels, nerve fibers, sweat, and oil glands.

Sweat Glands

The sweat glands produce perspiration that reaches the skin surface through tubes that end in openings called *pores*. Heat from deep in the body is brought to the skin by blood vessels. This heat is transferred to the perspiration.

Oil Glands and Hair

Oil glands lubricate and keep the hairs in the skin flexible. Hair covers almost all body surfaces except for the palms of the hands and the soles of the feet.

Skin Functions

The skin performs many functions that are critical to the well-being of the body:

- Protection—forms a continuous membranous covering for the body
- Temperature—helps regulate and maintain body temperature
- Storage—stores fat and vitamins
- Elimination—loses water, salts, and heat through perspiration
- Sensory perception—contains nerve endings that keep us aware of environmental changes

The skin tells us much about the general health of the body:

- Hot, dry skin—may indicate a fever

Critical Information ALERT

Sweat from the apocrine glands (those located mainly in the underarm and genital areas) is odorless. Body odor is caused by the action of the skin's normal bacteria on the sweat. ∎

Critical Information ALERT

The average scalp has about 100,000 hairs. The hair on the head grows at a rate of approximately 1 cm per month (1 centimeter = 0.3937 inch). The average person sheds approximately 50–100 hairs from the head each day. ∎

- Unusual redness—**rubra**, or flushing of the skin
- **Pallor**—less color than normal

The oxygen content of the blood can be noted quickly by the color of the skin. When the oxygen content is very low, the skin appears bluish or cyanotic.

NERVOUS SYSTEM STRUCTURE AND FUNCTION

The nervous system reaches throughout the body, controlling both involuntary and voluntary functions.

Neurons

Cells of the nervous system are called **neurons** (Figure 5-17A). These special cells conduct electrical impulses. The neuron has extensions called **axons** and **dendrites**. Impulses enter the neuron only through the dendrites and leave only through the axon.

Although neurons do not touch each other, the axon of one neuron and the dendrites of another are close to each other. Because of this, impulses follow many pathways by

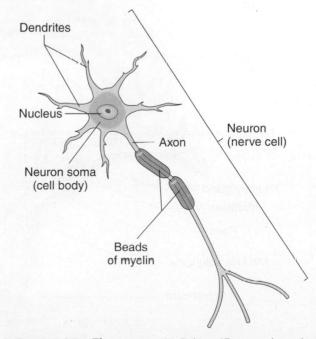

FIGURE 5-17A The neuron. (© *Delmar/Cengage Learning*)

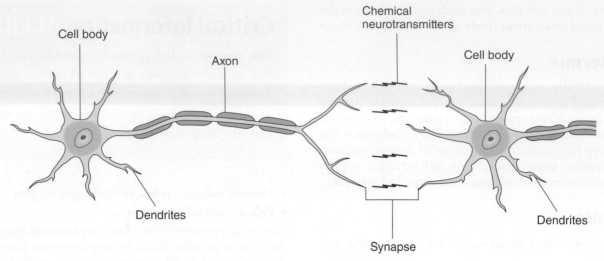

FIGURE 5-17B Chemicals called neurotransmitters help pass a message across the synapse from one neuron to another. (© *Delmar/Cengage Learning*)

jumping from one neuron to another. The space between the axon of one cell and the dendrites of others is called a **synapse**. A sheath called *myelin* acts as insulation for the axons and dendrites.

Neurotransmitters

Neurotransmitters are chemicals that enable messages (nerve impulses) to pass from one cell to another (Figure 5-17B). If the chemicals are not produced in the right amounts, the message pathway becomes confused or blocked.

Nerves

Axons and dendrites of many neurons are found in bundles that are held together by connective tissue. The bundles resemble telephone cables and are called **nerves**. The axons and dendrites are far from the ends of the nerves in clusters called *ganglia*.

Sensory nerves carry messages *in* to the brain and spinal cord from the body. If the impulses are interrupted, feeling is lost. Motor nerves carry messages *out* from the brain and spinal cord to the rest of the body. Paralysis or loss of

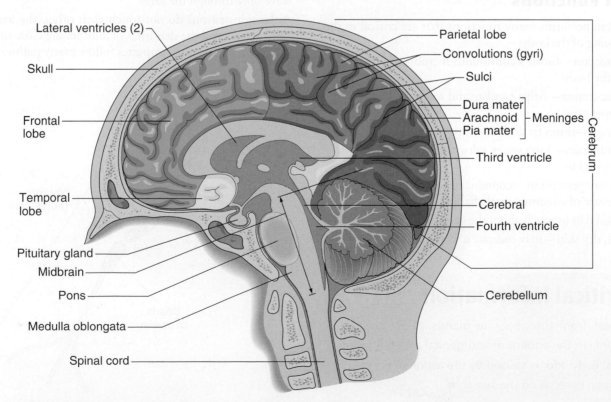

FIGURE 5-18 The central nervous system is composed of the brain and the spinal cord. (© *Delmar/Cengage Learning*)

function occurs when these nerves are damaged. The nervous system is an interwoven system, consisting of millions of neurons. It consists of two parts:

- Central nervous system (CNS)—brain and spinal cord (Figure 5-18)
- Peripheral nervous system (PNS)
  - 12 pairs of cranial nerves
  - 31 pairs of spinal nerves that reach throughout the body (Figure 5-19)

The Central Nervous System

The brain and spinal cord are:

- Surrounded by bone
- Protected by membranes called meninges
- Cushioned by cerebrospinal fluid

The brain and spinal cord are a continuous structure within the skull and spinal canal. Nerves extend from the brain and the spinal cord. The spinal cord is about 17 inches long. It ends just above the small of the back.

The brain The brain is a large, soft mass of nerve tissue inside the skull (cranium). It is composed of gray matter and white matter. Gray matter consists of nerve-cell bodies. White matter consists of nerve cells that form connections between various parts of the brain.

The brain can be further subdivided into the:

- **Cerebrum**—The largest portion of the brain. It is separated into lobes (Figure 5-20). All mental activities

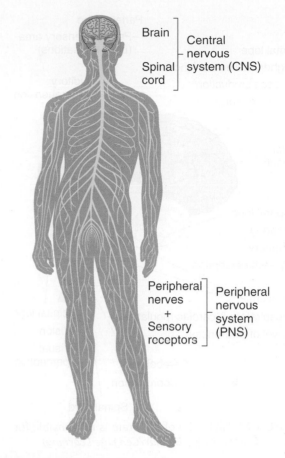

FIGURE 5-19 The peripheral nervous system connects the central nervous system to the various parts of the body. *(© Delmar/Cengage Learning)*

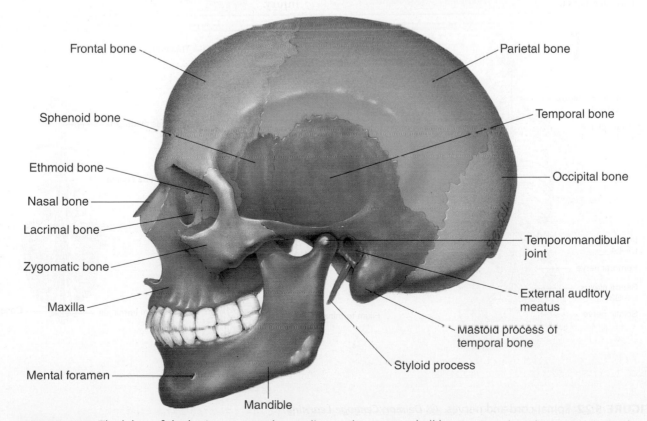

FIGURE 5-20 The lobes of the brain are named according to the nearest skull bones. *(© Delmar/Cengage Learning)*

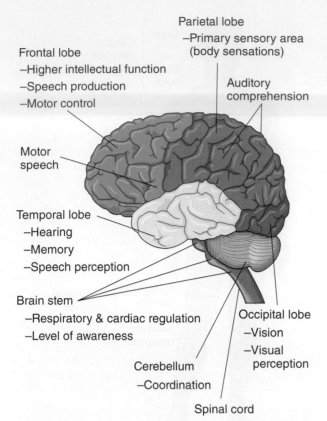

Parietal lobe
–Primary sensory area (body sensations)

Frontal lobe
–Higher intellectual function
–Speech production
–Motor control

Auditory comprehension

Motor speech

Temporal lobe
–Hearing
–Memory
–Speech perception

Brain stem
–Respiratory & cardiac regulation
–Level of awareness

Occipital lobe
–Vision
–Visual perception

Cerebellum
–Coordination

Spinal cord

FIGURE 5-21 Each lobe of the brain is responsible for a different function. (© *Delmar/Cengage Learning*)

are carried out by cerebral cells (Figure 5-21). The right side of the cerebrum controls the left side of the body and vice versa.

- **Cerebellum**—Found beneath the cerebrum. This portion of the brain coordinates muscular activities and balance.
- **Brain stem**—The midbrain, pons, and medulla are in the brain stem. Brain stem injuries are always very serious or fatal because this area controls involuntary movements of the heart, lungs, and other vital parts of the body.

The spinal cord The spinal cord (Figure 5-22) extends from the medulla to the second lumbar vertebra. Nerves entering and leaving the spinal cord carry impulses to and from the control centers. Reflex activities are controlled within the spinal cord. Pulling your hand away from something hot is an example of this type of reflex activity (Figure 5-23).

The meninges Three membranes, called **meninges**, surround both the brain and the spinal cord. They are the:

- Dura mater, or tough outer covering
- Arachnoid mater in the center that is filled with cerebrospinal fluid
- Pia mater in the center. This is a very vascular, delicate layer.

Cerebrospinal fluid *Ventricles* are cavities within the cerebrum that are lined with highly vascular tissue. These tissues produce **cerebrospinal fluid (CSF)**, which flows around the brain and spinal cord. The fluid bathes and cushions the central nervous system against injury.

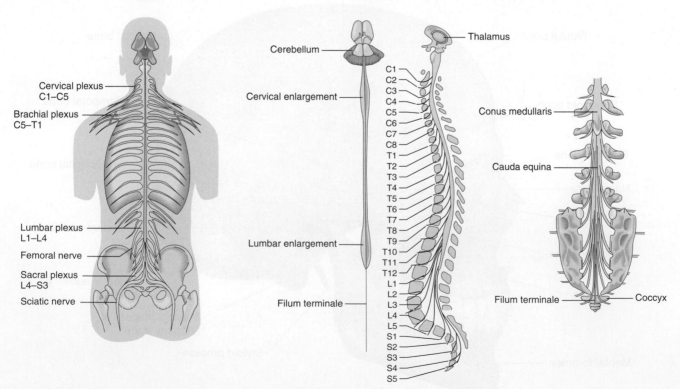

FIGURE 5-22 Spinal cord and nerves. (© *Delmar/Cengage Learning*)

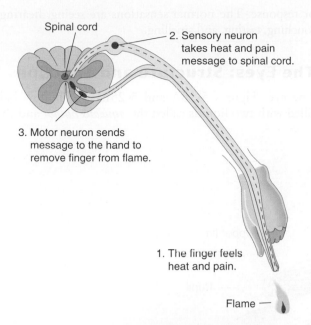

Spinal cord

2. Sensory neuron takes heat and pain message to spinal cord.

3. Motor neuron sends message to the hand to remove finger from flame.

1. The finger feels heat and pain.

Flame —

FIGURE 5-23 Reflex arc. (© Delmar/Cengage Learning)

Special Relationships: The Autonomic Nervous System

The term *autonomic nervous system* (*ANS*) refers to special pathways in cranial and spinal nerves (Figure 5-24). The control center is in the brain stem. The autonomic nervous system consists of two parts:

- Sympathetic fibers, which trigger the "fight or flight" reaction in emergencies.
- Parasympathetic fibers, which control the heartbeat, respiration, and other body functions

Sensory Receptors

The ends of the dendrites carry sensations to the central nervous system from the body. These sensations provide information about position, pain, heat, pressure, cold, smells, and tastes. Sensory dendrites also receive stimulation from the eye and the ear by carrying information about the outside world to the brain. The brain interprets, processes, and responds to the information.

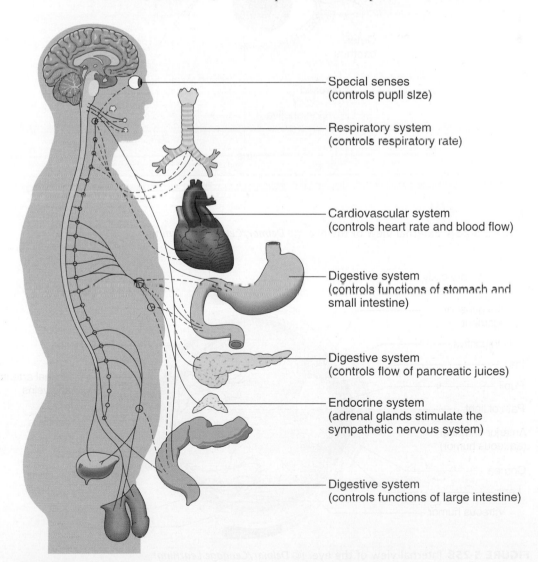

Special senses
(controls pupil size)

Respiratory system
(controls respiratory rate)

Cardiovascular system
(controls heart rate and blood flow)

Digestive system
(controls functions of stomach and small intestine)

Digestive system
(controls flow of pancreatic juices)

Endocrine system
(adrenal glands stimulate the sympathetic nervous system)

Digestive system
(controls functions of large intestine)

FIGURE 5-24 Autonomic nervous system. (© Delmar/Cengage Learning)

THE SENSORY ORGANS

The sensory organs are part of the nervous system, although they may be considered a separate system. The sensory organs are responsible for identification of outside stimuli. Once identified, the nervous system carries a message to the brain for interpretation and further action or response. The normal sensations are seeing, hearing, touching, tasting, and smelling.

The Eyes: Structure and Function

The eye (Figures 5-25A and 5-25B) is a hollow ball filled with two liquids called the *aqueous humor* and the

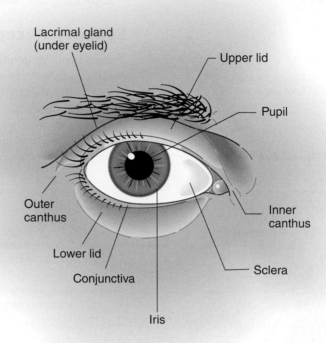

FIGURE 5-25A External view of the eye. (© Delmar/Cengage Learning)

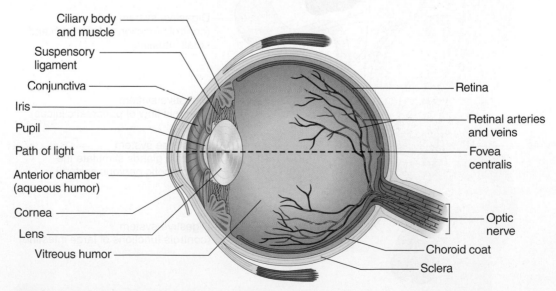

FIGURE 5-25B Internal view of the eye. (© Delmar/Cengage Learning)

vitreous humor. The wall of the eye is made up of three layers:

- The sclera—a tough, white outer coat that is protective. The **cornea** is the transparent portion in the front. Light rays pass through the cornea into the eye.
- The choroid: The nutritive layer found beneath the sclera. The choroid nourishes the eye tissues through its large number of blood vessels.
- The retina: The innermost layer is made up of neurons that are sensitive to light. Nerves carry impulses to the occipital lobe of the cerebrum to let us know what we are seeing.

The eye is responsible for vision. We see as light enters the eye through the cornea. The amount of light that enters is controlled by the **iris**, the colored portion of the eye behind the cornea. Fluid between the cornea and iris helps to bend the light rays and bring them to focus on the retina. The opening in the iris is called the **pupil**. The pupil appears black because there is no light behind it. Directly behind the iris is the lens. The lens changes shape, enabling us to adjust our vision from far to near or from near to far. The eye is:

- Held within the bony socket by muscles that can change its position.
- Covered by the **conjunctiva**, a mucous membrane that lines the eyelids and covers the eye.
- Protected by the eyelids and eyelashes. Tears are manufactured by the **lacrimal glands**, which are beneath the upper lid. Tears protect and wash the eye, keeping it moist. They drain into the nasal cavity.

The Ears: Structure and Function

The ear is sensitive to sound (Figure 5-26) and allows us to hear. It also affects equilibrium (balance). The ear has three parts:

- Outer ear, consisting of the external ear (*pinna*) and a canal, which directs sound waves toward the middle ear.
- Middle ear, which consists of three tiny bones called **ossicles**, which form a chain from the tympanic membrane to an opening in the inner ear. The middle ear also houses the **tympanic membrane** (eardrum), which is at the end of the ear canal. Sound waves cause the eardrum to vibrate. Small tubes, called the **eustachian tubes**, lead from the nasopharynx into the middle ear to equalize pressure on the eardrum. The ossicles vibrate in response to sound, causing fluid movement in the inner ear.
- Inner ear, which is a very complex structure consisting of two main parts. The **cochlea** responds to sound and stimulates the dendrites. An auditory nerve in each ear carries sensations to interpret what we are hearing. Three **semicircular canals** send impulses to the brain about the position of the head, which helps us keep our balance.

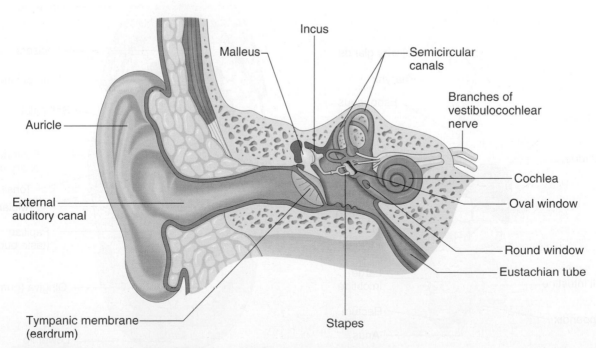

FIGURE 5-26 Internal view of the ear. *(© Delmar/Cengage Learning)*

GASTROINTESTINAL SYSTEM STRUCTURE AND FUNCTION

The gastrointestinal system is also called the GI or digestive tract. It extends from the mouth to the anus and is lined with mucous membrane (Figure 5-27). The organs of the GI system convert food into simple forms that can be used by the body. The nutrients pass through the walls of the small intestine into the circulatory system, where they are carried to body cells. Food changes as it moves through the digestive tract, as a result of mechanical action and chemicals called *enzymes*. The nondigestible portions of what we eat are moved along the intestines and are excreted from the body as feces. Several organs contribute to the digestive process and many disease conditions affect them.

Mouth

In the mouth (Figure 5-28), food is chewed so it can be swallowed easily. The digestive process begins with the:

- Tongue—a muscle that is covered by tastebuds. The tongue pushes the food so it is broken up, and assists in mastication (chewing). The tongue affects swallowing by moving the food back toward the pharynx. It is also important for speech formation.

- Salivary glands—secrete saliva to initiate carbohydrate digestion and help swallowing by moistening food. The average person produces about 1½ quarts of saliva each day.

- Teeth—break up food into smaller particles so it can be swallowed.

- Pharynx—allows the passage of both food and air. It leads to the esophagus.
- Esophagus—a tube that carries food to the stomach. Strong muscular contractions called *peristaltic* waves move the food along the tract.

The tongue has many *papillae*—tiny bumps that are commonly called tastebuds. Humans can detect five known tastes, but this is an area in which further study is needed. The areas that have been identified are:

- Sweet
- Salt
- Bitter
- Sour
- *Umami* (first recognized as a taste in 2000. *Umami* is a Japanese word for a savory, meaty, or protein taste. Examples of umami tastes are steak and sauteed mushrooms.)

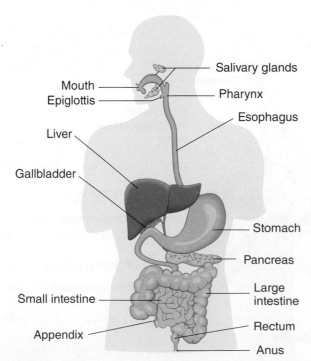

FIGURE 5-27 Digestive system. (© *Delmar/Cengage Learning*)

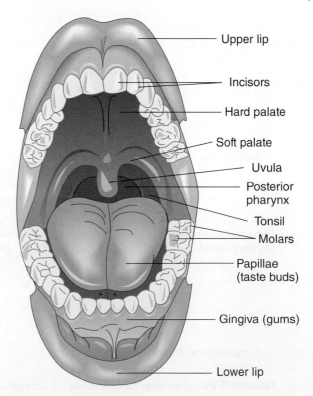

FIGURE 5-28 Mouth. (© *Delmar/Cengage Learning*)

Salt intensifies the response of the tastebuds, probably by acting as an electrical conductor.

Stomach

The stomach is a hollow, muscular organ that has muscles at either end to hold food while it mixes with digestive enzymes.

The Intestines

Food leaves the stomach in a semiliquid state and enters the small intestine, where any undigested nutrients are broken down. The small intestine is about 23 feet long, making it the largest internal organ in the body.

Food continues moving through the intestines by waves of peristalsis. Digestion is completed in the small intestine, where most of the nutrients and food the body needs are absorbed into the bloodstream. The large intestine (colon) is 4 ½ feet long; this is where some vitamins are absorbed, and bacteria act on complex carbohydrates. Any remaining water is absorbed, converting waste to a more solid form. Peristalsis continues to move waste through the large intestine until it reaches the rectum. The rectum absorbs water from the stool. When a certain amount of solid matter has been collected in the rectum, it is eliminated as feces through the anus. This process is called **defecation**.

Appendix

The appendix is located in the lower right quadrant. Its function is not known. *Appendicitis* occurs when it becomes inflamed.

Liver and Gallbladder

The liver is a large gland beneath the diaphragm. It controls protein and sugar in the blood; detoxifies food, medication, and other substances; and produces proteins, which are needed for blood clotting. The liver produces bile, which is used in the digestion of fats.

The gallbladder is attached to the underside of the liver. It holds about two ounces of bile that it receives from the liver. It releases bile into the small intestine to help digest a fatty meal. Bile gives solid wastes their usual brown color.

Pancreas

The pancreas is a glandular organ that produces the digestive enzymes insulin and glucagon, which are needed for blood sugar regulation. It also manufactures pancreatic juice, which aids digestion.

MUSCULOSKELETAL SYSTEM STRUCTURE AND FUNCTION

The *muscular system* and the *skeletal system* are two separate and distinct body systems. However, they work closely together and are often viewed as a single unit called the *musculoskeletal system*.

Bones

Babies are born with 300 bones, but by adulthood we have only 206 in our bodies. Bones come in all shapes and sizes, each with a specific function. Study the skeleton in Figure 5-29 and review the skull in Figure 5-20.

Joints

Joints are points where bones come together. Movable joints are essential for walking, lifting, and sitting. Joints are capable of different movements (Figure 5-30). We use special terms to describe these different movements:

- **Flexion**—decreasing the angle between two bones (Figure 5-31A), such as bending the elbow.
- **Extension**—increasing the angle between two bones (Figure 5-31B), such as straightening the elbow.
- **Rotation**—circular motion in a ball-and-socket joint (Figure 5-31C), such as moving the shoulder in all directions.
- **Abduction**—moving away from the midline (Figure 5-31D).
- **Adduction**—moving toward the midline (Figure 5-31E).

Ligaments are strong bands of fibrous tissues that hold the bones together and support the joints. **Bursae** are small sacs of synovial fluid that are located around joints and help reduce friction.

Muscles

There are about 650 muscles in the body (Figures 5-32A and 5-32B). The muscles work in groups. There are three kinds of muscles:

1. **Cardiac muscle** forms the wall of the heart.
2. **Voluntary muscles** are skeletal muscles that are attached to bones. We use voluntary muscles when we want to pick something up.
3. **Involuntary** or **visceral muscles** form the walls of organs. These muscles operate without our conscious control.

To locate the major muscle groups responsible for an activity, remember that:

- Muscles have two points of attachment to the bone. As they stretch from one point (**origin**) to the other (**insertion**), they cross over one or more joints.

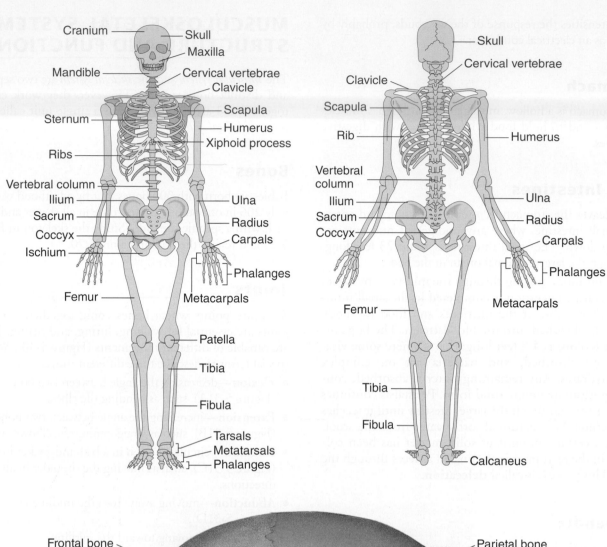

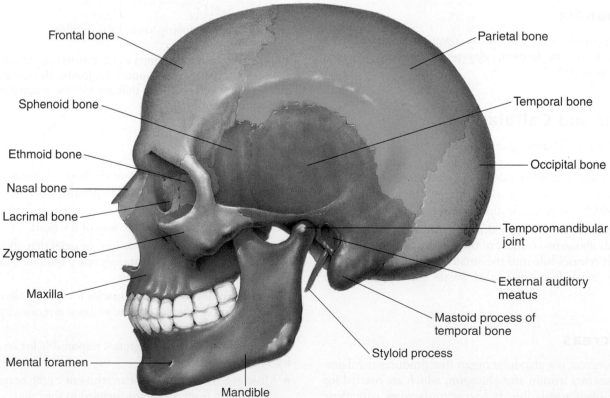

FIGURE 5-29 The human skeleton. (© *Delmar/Cengage Learning*)

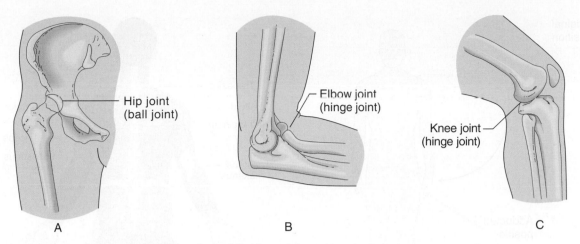

FIGURE 5-30 Types of joints: A. Ball joint. B. and C. Hinge joints. *(© Delmar/Cengage Learning)*

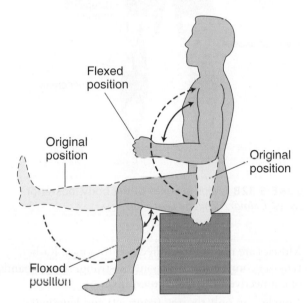

FIGURE 5-31A Flexion—bending a joint.
(© Delmar/Cengage Learning)

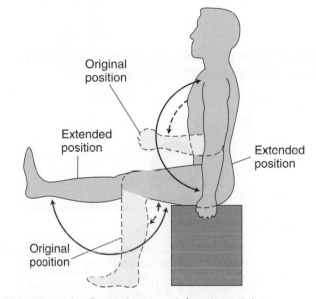

FIGURE 5-31B Extension—straightening a joint.
(© Delmar/Cengage Learning)

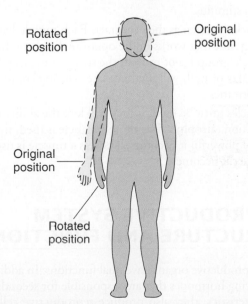

FIGURE 5-31C Rotation—moving a joint in a circular motion.
(© Delmar/Cengage Learning)

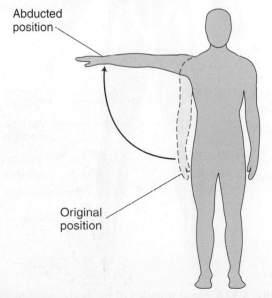

FIGURE 5-31D Abduction—moving an extremity away from the body. *(© Delmar/Cengage Learning)*

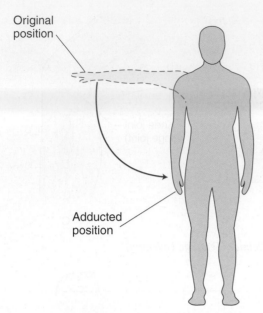

FIGURE 5-31E Adduction—moving an extremity back toward the body. (© Delmar/Cengage Learning)

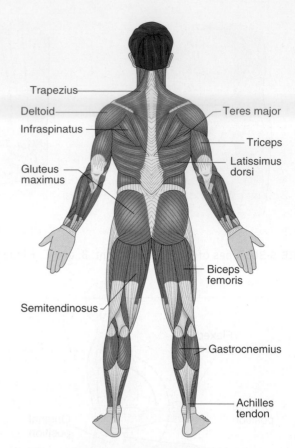

FIGURE 5-32B Major muscles of the body, posterior view. (© Delmar/Cengage Learning)

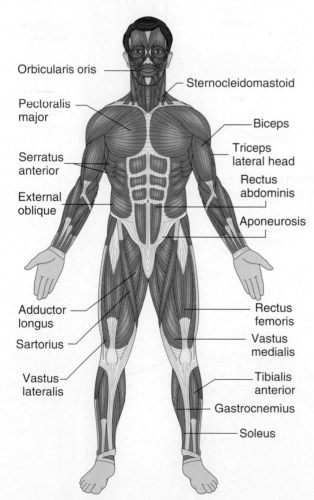

FIGURE 5-32A Major muscles of the body, anterior view. (© Delmar/Cengage Learning)

- Muscles are not inserted directly into bones. Rather, they are connected to the bone by strong, fibrous bands of connective tissue called **tendons**.
- Muscles can only shorten (contract) and lengthen (relax). Contraction occurs when nerves bring a message (**stimulus**) to the muscle cells. Muscles relax when there is no stimulus.
- Muscles shorten as they contract. Each muscle has an antagonist that works in the opposite direction. If a muscle group is not moved, the stronger muscles (those that flex or pull) will predominate, causing contracture deformities.
- Muscles must be used or they will lose the ability to function (atrophy). The more a muscle is used, the more powerful it becomes. The less a muscle is used, the weaker it becomes.

REPRODUCTIVE SYSTEM STRUCTURE AND FUNCTION

The reproductive organs have dual functions. In addition to producing hormones that are responsible for secondary sex characteristics, they also produce reproductive cells. The male produces **sperm**. The female produces the **ovum**.

The Male Reproductive Organs: Structure and Function

The male organs (Figure 5-33) include the:

- **Testes**—two glandular organs that produce sperm and testosterone.
- **Epididymis**—a tube that stores sperm and allows them to mature.
- **Vas deferens**—a tube that carries sperm during ejaculation.
- **Seminal vesicles**—store sperm and contribute nutrients to the seminal fluid.
- **Ejaculatory duct**—carries the fluids that are added as the sperm are propelled forward. The sperm and fluid form the seminal fluid or ejaculate.
- **Prostate gland**—encircles the urethra; secretes fluid that increases motility of the sperm. Prostate enlargement may prevent urine from passing through the urethra. This is common in older men.
- **Cowper's glands**—two glands that produce mucus for lubrication.
- **Penis**—male sex organ that enters the vagina to deposit seminal fluid. Loose-fitting skin (the prepuce or foreskin) covers the penis.

The urethra passes through the penis and carries fluid during intercourse and urine during voiding. These activities cannot occur at the same time because they are under the control of different parts of the nervous system.

The Female Reproductive Organs: Structure and Function

The external female structures (**genitalia**) (Figure 5-34) include the:

- **Vulva**—includes two liplike structures, the **labia majora** and **labia minora**. When the labia are separated, other external structures may be seen.
- **Clitoris**—a sensitive structure that functions during sexual stimulation and is associated with the ability to have orgasm (climax).
- **Urinary meatus**—the opening of the urethra to the outside.
- **Vaginal meatus**—the opening to the vagina or birth canal.

The internal female reproductive organs (Figures 5-35A and 5-35B) include the:

- **Ovaries**—glands that produce hormones and the egg (ovum). About once each month, an ovum is released during a process is called **ovulation**.
- **Fallopian tubes (oviducts)**—tubes that serve as a pathway between the ovary and uterus. Fertilization takes place here.
- **Uterus**—a hollow organ that sheds its lining each month during menstruation. Protects the fetus during pregnancy until the fetus is expelled through the cervix at birth.
- **Vagina**—canal between the urinary bladder and the rectum. Used for sexual activity and birth of an infant.

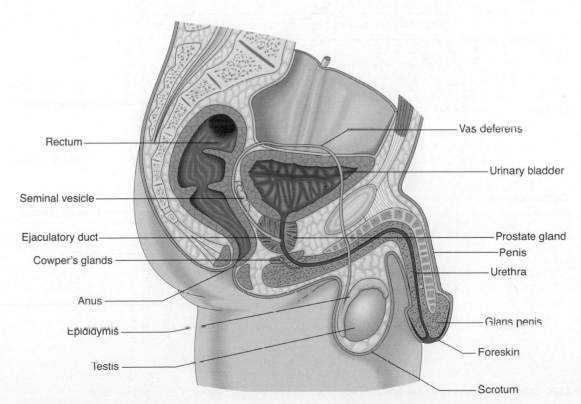

FIGURE 5-33 Cross-section of the male reproductive system. (© *Delmar/Cengage Learning*)

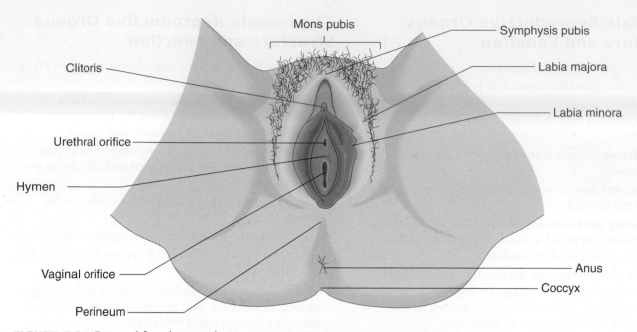

FIGURE 5-34 External female reproductive organs. (© *Delmar/Cengage Learning*)

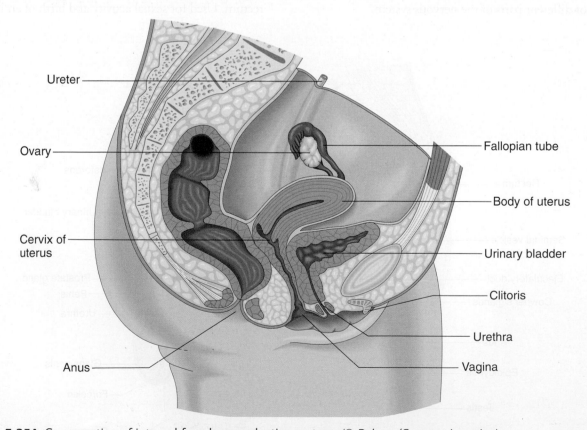

FIGURE 5-35A Cross-section of internal female reproductive system. (© *Delmar/Cengage Learning*)

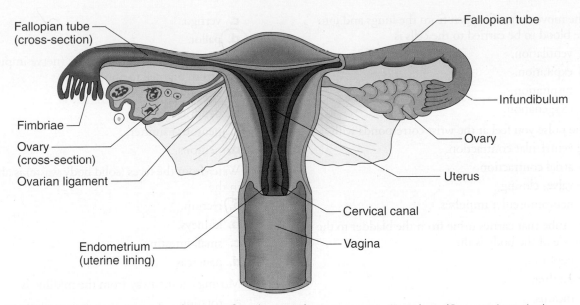

FIGURE 5-35B Anterior view of interior female reproductive organs. (© Delmar/Cengage Learning)

REVIEW

A. Multiple Choice

Select the one best answer for each of the following.

1. When describing the relationship of the hand to the elbow, you should refer to the hand as being
   a. proximal.
   b. posterior.
   c. distal.
   d. anterior.

2. The appendix is located in which quadrant of the abdomen?
   a. URQ
   b. RLQ
   c. ULQ
   d. LLQ

3. The pancreas is part of the
   a. circulatory system.
   b. reproductive system.
   c. endocrine system.
   d. immune system.

4. Which organ pumps blood throughout the body?
   a. lungs
   b. heart
   c. liver
   d. adrenal glands

5. Which of the following is part of the skeletal system?
   a. ureters
   b. sternum

   c. gallbladder
   d. testes

6. The breasts are part of which system?
   a. muscular
   b. urinary
   c. cardiovascular
   d. reproductive

7. A prefix is found
   a. at the beginning of a word.
   b. in the middle of a word.
   c. at the end of a word.
   d. after an abbreviation.

8. The eye and ear are part of which system?
   a. endocrine
   b. nervous
   c. cardiovascular
   d. digestive

9. The endocrine system
   a. reproduces the species.
   b. brings in oxygen.
   c. transports blood.
   d. produces hormones.

10. The human body has
    a. five major body systems.
    b. nine major body systems.
    c. 10 major body systems.
    d. 12 major body systems.

11. The movement of oxygen from the lungs and into the blood to be carried to the cells is
    a. ventilation.
    b. expiration.
    c. inspiration.
    d. oxygenation.

12. The pulse you feel at the wrist corresponds with
    a. ventricular contraction.
    b. atrial contraction.
    c. valves closing.
    d. neuromuscular impulses.

13. The tube that carries urine from the bladder to the outside of the body is the
    a. nephron.
    b. urethra.
    c. meatus.
    d. ureter.

14. The human body produces more than
    a. 20 hormones.
    b. 30 hormones.
    c. 50 hormones.
    d. 80 hormones.

15. Jason, a new nursing assistant, tells you that Mrs. Spitzer looks "white as a ghost." You check the resident and find that her skin is very white and pale. You will inform the nurse that Mrs. Spitzer has
    a. rubra.
    b. cyanosis.

    c. vertigo.
    d. pallor.

16. Chemicals that enable messages (nerve impulses) to pass from one cell to another are
    a. axons.
    b. dendrites.
    c. neurotransmitters.
    d. neurons.

17. Water from the feces (solid body waste) is absorbed in the
    a. rectum.
    b. kidneys.
    c. small intestine.
    d. pancreas.

18. Moving a joint away from the midline is
    a. rotation.
    b. abduction.
    c. extension.
    d. adduction.

19. The gland that encircles the urethra in the male is the
    a. vas deferens.
    b. epididymis.
    c. Cowper's gland.
    d. prostate gland.

B. Nursing Assistant Challenge

Examine the sample care plan and use your understanding of medical science and terminology to define each medical term and abbreviation used on the plan.

1.	**Patient Name** Bruce Tratt	**Age** 47	**Rel** Prot		#876-3291-7	
2.	**Physician** R. Morgan M.D.	**Dx** Splenomegaly—Diabetes Mellitus				
3.		**Orders**				
4.	**Preop orders** 3/18	on call for OR at 8 am 3/19				
5.	Stat CBC, ABG, FBS					
6.	UA					
7.	NG Tube at 6 am 3/19					
8.	Foley cath this pm.					
9.	Surg Prep.					
10.	NPO p̄ midnight					
11.	SSE at 9 pm HS.					
12.	Amb ad lib. this pm.					
13.						
14.	Anesthesiologist will call preop meds.					
15.						

UNIT 6

Classification of Disease

OBJECTIVES

After completing this unit, you will be able to:
- Spell and define terms.
- Define disease and list some possible causes.
- Distinguish between signs and symptoms.
- List ways in which a diagnosis is made.
- Recognize alternative medicine and therapies.
- Understand the body's natural defenses against disease.

VOCABULARY

Learn the meaning and the correct spelling of the following words and phrases:

acute disease	complication	noninvasive	✓ signs
acute exacerbation	etiology	predisposing factor	✓ symptoms
alternatives	invasive	prognosis	therapy
chronic disease	medical diagnosis	protocol	vaccine

INTRODUCTION

The nurse values and uses your observations when making evaluations and planning nursing care for patients, as part of the nursing process. The better you understand the basic principles of disease, the more accurately you can provide information.

DISEASE

The body is a complex chemical factory that needs all of its parts to perform efficiently. It is subject to external and internal forces and stress that can threaten its ability to function properly (Figure 6-1).

Disease is any change from a healthy state. The disease (illness) may be a change in structure or function, or it may be failure of a part of the body to develop properly. Each illness has:
- An **etiology**—cause of the illness or abnormality.
- A usual set of indications. These are called signs and symptoms.
- A usual course or disease progression.
- A **prognosis** or probable outcome of the process.

Predisposing factors to disease are conditions, such as malnutrition, that may contribute to the development of illness. Some diseases have related risk factors. *Risk factors* are behaviors or conditions that tend to promote certain diseases (Figure 6-2). For example, smoking is a risk factor for lung disease or cancer.

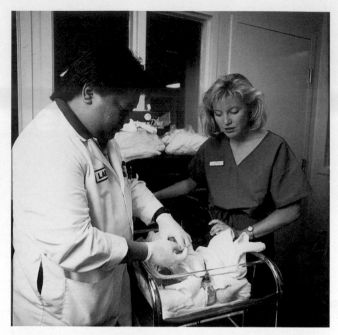

FIGURE 6-1 The laboratory technician draws blood from the heel of this newborn. *(© Delmar/Cengage Learning)*

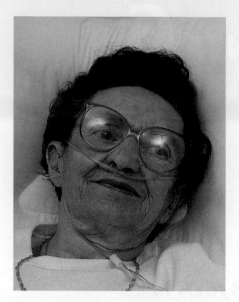

FIGURE 6-2 Advanced age is a risk factor that predisposes people to some diseases. *(© Delmar/Cengage Learning)*

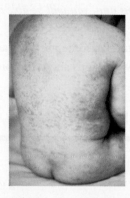

FIGURE 6-3 A maculopapular rash is characteristic of skin changes in measles (rubeola). *(Courtesy of Centers for Disease Control and Prevention)*

Age Appropriate Care ALERT

As a nursing assistant, you will be caring for patients of all ages. You must learn how to provide age-appropriate care to each age group. This means that you will meet the patient's age-related needs for communication, safety and security, and personal care and comfort. These measures vary somewhat for each age group. Avoid treating adults as children, or children as adults. Meet each patient on his or her own level. ■

Signs and Symptoms

Signs of a disease can be seen by others. The color or condition of the skin is an example of a sign of disease (Figure 6-3). **Symptoms** are felt by the patient, who tells us about them. Pain is a symptom common to many illnesses (Figure 6-4).

The Course (Pattern) of Disease

The development and course of different illnesses vary greatly. **Acute disease** develops suddenly, progresses rapidly, and lasts for a predictable period, and then the person recovers (or dies). For example, the signs and symptoms of an infected finger may develop rapidly and last a relatively short period. Then, as the body controls the process, recovery is seen.

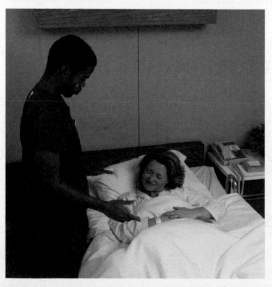

FIGURE 6-4 Sometimes patients communicate pain through their body language. *(© Delmar/Cengage Learning)*

With a **chronic disease**, there are often periods when the patient experiences the signs and symptoms and periods when the disease is less pronounced. Rheumatoid arthritis is such a disease. At times the joints are red, swollen, and painful. At other times, the signs and symptoms seem to go away. An **acute exacerbation** of a chronic disease is when the severity of signs and symptoms increases.

Complications

A **complication** makes the original condition more serious. For example, if a child has measles and develops pneumonia (a serious lung condition), the pneumonia is a complication that makes it more difficult for the child to recover.

DIAGNOSIS

The **medical diagnosis** (the process of identifying and naming the disease) is made by the physician. To do this, the physician examines the person, reviews the patient's past history and the results of various tests. The physician matches the findings to possible diseases, and then names the process to establish the medical diagnosis.

Diagnostic Studies

Laboratory tests (Figure 6-5) and diagnostic studies give the physician valuable information for naming the disease and planning the treatment. The nursing staff prepares the patient for tests and cares for the patient after the tests are completed. You will help give this care and may be assigned to collect certain specimens.

Protocols are procedures for the preparation and care of the patient for each test or study. Protocols must be followed carefully to achieve satisfactory results. Following the instructions correctly to prepare the patient is very important.

Noninvasive tests Some tests and studies are **noninvasive**. This means that they are done without breaking the skin or damaging body tissue. For example, X-rays do not break the skin, but do give information about internal body structures.

Invasive tests Invasive tests penetrate body surfaces. Examples of invasive tests include taking tissue samples and probing into body cavities. Most invasive techniques are carried out in special areas, such as the operating room. The specimens obtained are usually examined in laboratories.

THERAPY

Once the medical diagnosis is known, it is possible to predict its course and a probable prognosis (likely outcome of the disease). The physician then determines the most appropriate **therapy** (treatment). There are four basic approaches to therapy that may be used alone or in combination:

1. Surgery—this form of therapy may remove unhealthy tissue (Figure 6-6); replace unhealthy parts; or repair injured, malformed, or defective areas.
2. Chemotherapy—this form of therapy uses drugs to improve body functions and control pain (Figure 6-7). Medicines (chemicals) are used to treat many conditions.
3. Radiation—this form of therapy uses controlled radiation to destroy tumor cells (cancerous cells).
4. Supportive (palliative) care—this form of therapy supports the patient's body in its attempt to return to health. It also includes comfort, care, and pain control for persons who are not expected to recover.

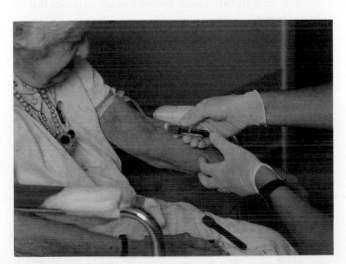

FIGURE 6-5 Blood tests provide information about body chemistry and contribute to a correct medical diagnosis. (© Delmar/Cengage Learning)

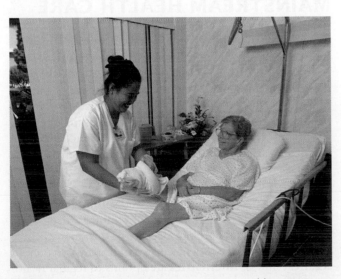

FIGURE 6-6 This patient's leg was amputated because of peripheral vascular disease. (© Delmar/Cengage Learning)

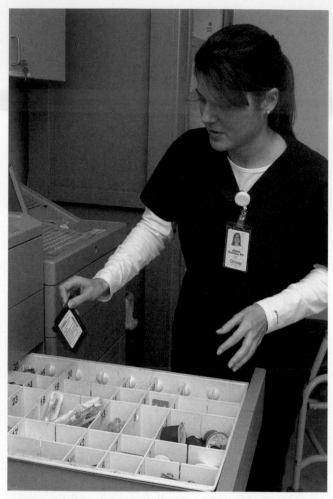

FIGURE 6-7 The nursing assistant reports the patient's complaint to the nurse, who will further assess the patient and provide pain medication. (© Delmar/Cengage Learning)

ALTERNATIVES TO MAINSTREAM HEALTH CARE

When most people in Western society think of medical care, they think of medical, surgical, pharmaceutical, and technological treatment of patients. In the United States, these are the accepted, traditional approaches to patient care and healing of illness. Throughout history, though, people have turned to other means of healing the sick. Egyptian society (Figure 6-8) used very advanced medical practices; Native American tribes had medicine men. These practices were considered mainstream before twentieth-century advances in medicine.

Today, some people prefer natural and spiritual treatments for illness. Others are afraid of the technology, drugs, and surgical procedures of today. Because of this, many people use alternative health care practices and products to prevent and treat illness. **Alternatives** are options to regular health care. Alternative therapies are used to treat every imaginable symptom and condition. Some people use alternatives to

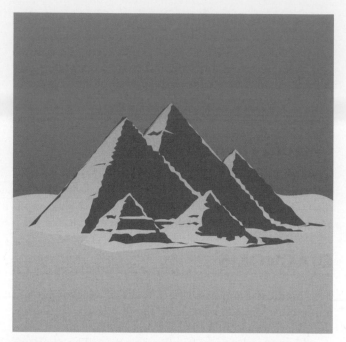

FIGURE 6-8 The ancient Egyptians used many natural substances and medical practices that were advanced for their time. (© Delmar/Cengage Learning)

prevent illness. Others use alternative practices in addition to medical treatment. For safety, an alternative program should be supervised by a physician.

BODY DEFENSES

The body has a natural line of defense against disease. These defenses include:

- Unbroken skin and mucous membranes, which act as mechanical barriers
- Mucus, which traps foreign particles, and cilia (small hairlike structures), which propel foreign particles out of the body
- The acidity of certain body fluids, such as perspiration, saliva, and stomach juices, which slows the growth of microorganisms
- White blood cells, which destroy anything foreign that enters the body
- Inflammation
- The immune response (immunity)

Inflammation

The process of inflammation, which is associated with boils and abscesses, is an important part of the body's natural defenses. When anything foreign enters the body, small blood vessels (capillaries) in the area get bigger (dilate), bringing more blood to the infected part. The blood contains white blood cells and other protective substances. Fluid (serum) and white blood cells pass through the capillary walls and gradually build a wall around the foreign object. As the white blood cells try to destroy the invader, pressure builds up, forcing the material to the body surface. The inflammatory process takes place whenever injury occurs. The signs and symptoms of acute inflammation are:

- Redness
- Swelling
- Heat
- Loss of function
- Pain

Immunity

Immunity protects the body against specific infections by producing chemicals called *antibodies*. For example, a person exposed to the measles becomes ill with the disease. After recovery, the antibodies protect the person from catching measles again.

Vaccines (altered germs or their products) may be given before exposure to a disease. The body can then produce antibodies before actual exposure occurs. You will learn more about vaccines in Unit 12.

REVIEW

A. Multiple Choice

Select the one best answer for each of the following.

1. A sudden flare-up or worsening of a chronic disease is a/an
   a. complication.
   b. exacerbation.
   c. inflammation.
   d. allergic reaction.

2. The medical term for the cause of a disease is a/an
   a. prognosis.
   b. predisposing factor.
   c. risk factor.
   d. etiology.

3. Symptoms are
   a. observations you can see.
   b. things you can measure.
   c. things the patient tells you.
   d. identified only by lab tests.

4. An acute illness
   a. develops suddenly.
   b. is a life-long condition.
   c. always results in death.
   d. is usually painful.

5. The probable outcome of a disease process is the
   a. etiology.
   b. prognosis.
   c. predisposing factor.
   d. risk factor.

6. A noninvasive test
   a. breaks the skin.
   b. must be done in a special area.
   c. does not damage tissue.
   d. provides information about the skin.

7. Chemotherapy
   a. is a form of radiation.
   b. is highly toxic.
   c. involves treatment with chemicals.
   d. must be given by injection only.

8. Signs are
   a. observations you can see.
   b. identified only by using instruments.
   c. things the patient tells you.
   d. identified only by lab tests.

9. A complication of a disease
   a. makes the original condition worse.
   b. suggests that the patient is improving.
   c. is a condition present at birth.
   d. does not affect the outcome.

10. Immunity is a
    a. sign of infection.
    b. type of allergy.
    c. malignancy.
    d. protective reaction.

B. Nursing Assistant Challenge

Read each clinical situation and answer the questions.

11. Your patient is 82 years old, poorly nourished, and has a diagnosis of pneumonia.
    a. Name two risk factors that might predispose your patient to pneumonia.

    _____

    b. Will these factors make recovery more or less difficult?

    _____

    c. How would you classify the illness pneumonia?

    _____

Basic Human Needs and Communication

UNIT 7

Communication Skills

OBJECTIVES

After completing this unit, you will be able to:
- Spell and define terms.
- List the four components of an effective message.
- Explain the types of verbal and nonverbal communication.
- Identify four tools of communication for staff members.
- State the guidelines for communicating effectively with patients.

VOCABULARY

Learn the meaning and the correct spelling of the following words and phrases:

body language	feedback	nonverbal communication	sender
care plan	interpreter	organizational chart	staff development
communication	medical chart	paraphrasing	symbols
ethnic	message	receiver	verbal communication

INTRODUCTION

Communication is a two-way process in which information is shared. Information can be sent orally, in writing, and through body language. Nursing assistants communicate with their patients, with visitors, with their coworkers, and with their supervisors when they are working. As a nursing assistant, you will need to receive and send information:
- About your observations and care of patients
- During interactions with patients and visitors
- About your patients' feelings

This information is received and sent through the process of communication.

ELEMENTS OF COMMUNICATION

Understanding the elements of communication will help you communicate effectively. Each message has four parts (Figure 7-1):
- **Sender**—the person who originates the communication
- **Message**—the information the sender wants to communicate
- **Receiver**—the person for whom the communication is intended
- **Feedback**—confirmation that the message was received as intended

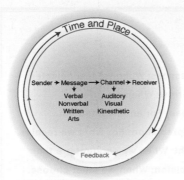

FIGURE 7-1 Nursing assistants communicate with patients in many different ways. However, all messages have a sender, message, and receiver. Feedback is a method of ensuring that the message was received as intended. (© Delmar/Cengage Learning)

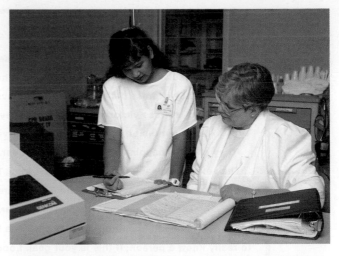

FIGURE 7-2 Verbal communication is the most common way of reporting observations to the nurse. In some cases, you may also provide written information, such as a piece of paper listing a patient's vital signs. (© Delmar/Cengage Learning)

The *channel* is the medium through which the message is sent. Feedback may be verbal or nonverbal. An example of verbal feedback is saying something in response. An example of nonverbal feedback is a nod of the head indicating understanding.

COMMUNICATION IN HEALTH CARE

Communication between staff members must be effective if patients are to receive the safest and best care. Communication with patients and their visitors is also important. You and your patients must understand each other.

Verbal Communication

Verbal communication uses words. They may be spoken or written. You will use words to report your observations (Figure 7-2), as well as written communication in your charting. Written communication also depends on the use of **symbols**. You will use words to answer questions. Choose words carefully so that your message is clear.

Paraphrasing is an effective method of showing that you understand what has been said. When using paraphrasing, restate your understanding of what was said.

Nonverbal Communication

Nonverbal communication is a message that is sent through the use of one's body, rather than through speech or writing. This kind of communication, called **body language**, can tell you a great deal. Nonverbal messages often send even stronger signals than verbal messages.

When speaking with others, always remember the impact of nonverbal communication (Figure 7-3). Your words

> Your message is:
> 7% words + 38% tone of voice
> + 55% body language
> = Total Communication

FIGURE 7-3 Make sure your body language and the tone, pitch, and quality of your voice match the message you intend to send. (© Delmar/Cengage Learning)

constitute only 7% of your message. Your tone of voice represents 38% of the meaning. If the tone and pitch of your voice contradict the spoken words, the tone and pitch will overshadow the intended message. The remainder of the message—55% of your total communication—is conveyed through facial expressions, gestures, and overall body language.

Eye contact makes the biggest impression and will be remembered best (Figure 7-4). You create a positive atmosphere by looking at the other person. In North America, eye contact is very important to communication. This is not true in all cultures. Be sensitive to cultural differences of patients and coworkers.

A patient who is in pain may protect the affected area. Tears or an unwillingness to make eye contact with you may be a sign of depression. Some of the other ways your patients may "talk" to you through their body language include:

• Posture
• Hand and body movements
• Activity level
• Facial expressions
• Overall appearance
• Body position

Messengers

They express anger; That is easily detected. They express hopelessness; When we feel dejected.

They express delight; When we achieve. They express sorrow; When we grieve.

They express victory; When we win. They express forgiveness; For an imagined sin.

They express confusion; When we don't perceive. They express appreciation; For what we receive.

They express happiness; For all we hold dear. They express fright; When we encounter a fear.

They express disappointment; When we lose. They express indecision; When we must choose.

They express patience; For a child. They express excitement; When our imagination runs wild.

They express love; It's perfectly clear. They speak a language; For all to hear.

In one fluid motion; As they part. The hands become Messengers of the heart.

To really know a person; If this is your goal. Look deep into their eyes; The Messengers of the soul.

An original poem by Marilyn Sossaman, LPN. Used with permission.

FIGURE 7-4 An original poem by Marilyn Sossaman, LPN. Used with permission.

COMMUNICATING WITH STAFF MEMBERS

Each health care facility has a line of authority and communication. The **organizational chart** is a guide for communication and spells out the line of authority. Each facility has an organizational chart that illustrates how a department relates to other departments. Some of the larger departments, such as nursing, have their own charts that indicate the line of authority within the department (Figure 7-5). As a nursing assistant, you will need to communicate with other staff members in nursing and other departments.

Answering the Telephone

Many telephone calls come into a health care facility. Nursing assistants are not allowed to take physicians' orders, to take results of diagnostic tests, or to give information to families. You must call the nurse to do this. If you answer the telephone:

- Identify the nursing unit: "third floor, north," for example.
- Identify yourself and your position: "Mary Smith, nursing assistant."
- Ask the caller's name and ask the caller to wait while you locate the person called.
- If the person is unavailable, take a message and write down the following information:
  - date and time of call
  - caller's name and telephone number
  - message left by caller
  - whether the person is to return the call or whether the caller will telephone again later
  - your signature

Most facilities do not allow employees to make or receive personal telephone calls while they are on duty, except in an emergency.

Manuals

All facilities have several manuals that provide information about policies and procedures (Figure 7-6). These may include:

- Employee Personnel Handbook—Describes all personnel policies and benefits
- Safety and Disaster Manual—Gives directions for actions to take in case of fire or other disasters
- Procedure Manual—Gives directions on how all procedures for patients should be performed
- Nursing Policy Manual—Describes rules and regulations pertaining to the care of patients
- Material Safety Data Sheet (MSDS) Manual—Contains information on safe use and handling of substances used in the facility

There may be other manuals for infection control and quality assurance. You are not expected to memorize all the information in these manuals, but you should know where they are kept on the nursing unit and be able to look up information when you need to.

Staff Development

Staff development is a process used to educate staff from all departments in the facility (Figure 7-7). Classes may be given to inform staff of new rules and regulations, new procedures, and how to use new equipment.

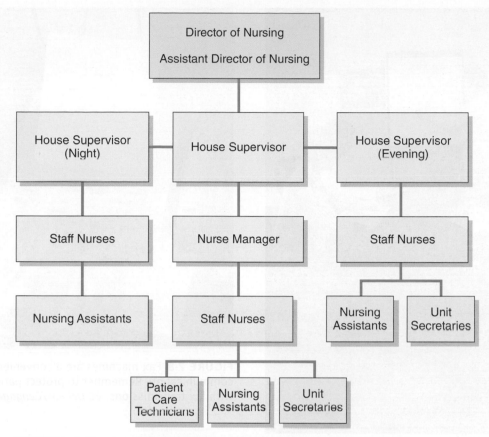

FIGURE 7-5 Nursing department organizational chart. *(© Delmar/Cengage Learning)*

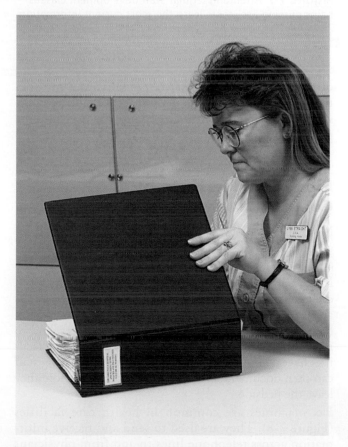

Legal ALERT

Becoming familiar with the location and contents of facility policy and procedure manuals will help you do your job and practice within your scope of responsibility, in keeping with state and federal laws. You must perform procedures according to the guidelines in these manuals. They may be slightly different from those of other facilities. Following your facility policies and procedures will ensure that you give good patient care, and will reduce your risk of legal exposure. ∎

The Patient Care Plan

The interdisciplinary health care team develops an individualized **care plan** for each patient. The care plan describes exactly what care each patient is to receive, and is a good reference if you need information. Unit 8 presents more information on the patient care plan.

The Patient's Medical Chart

Each patient has a **medical chart** or record. The medical chart contains information about the patient, the

FIGURE 7-6 Manuals are an excellent source of information. *(© Delmar/Cengage Learning)*

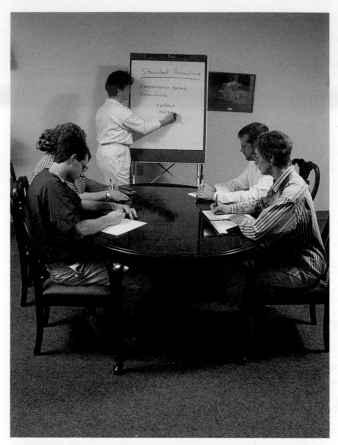

FIGURE 7-7 Attending regular staff development classes helps nursing assistants learn the most current information. (© Delmar/Cengage Learning)

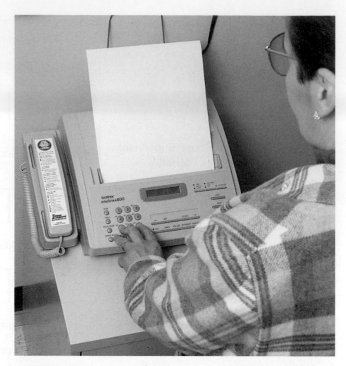

FIGURE 7-8 Fax machines are a convenient means of communication. Remember to protect patient privacy with fax transmissions. (© Delmar/Cengage Learning)

care given, and the patient's response. Unit 8 provides more information on the medical record, and gives instructions for documenting (making notations) on the patient's chart.

Electronic Methods of Communication

Modern technology has increased opportunities for communication. You will see computers at the nurses' station and throughout the building.

Most facilities will have at least one desktop computer in each department. In the nursing department, computers are used to document patient care, to maintain databases, to communicate with physicians' offices, and to maintain records of supplies and equipment. Some facilities have computers in every patient room. Nursing staff can then document appropriate information before they leave the bedside.

Fax machines are common in health care facilities (Figure 7-8). They are used to send and receive information across telephone lines to and from physicians and laboratories.

COMMUNICATING WITH PATIENTS

Your skill in communicating with patients will develop with experience. Often the words we choose are not as important as the way in which we say them. Tone of voice, facial expression, and even the way you touch a patient all communicate a sense of honest caring to the patient. Looking directly at patients as you speak and addressing them respectfully by name are also indications of caring.

Listening actively is a special skill that requires more than just being physically present. When you listen actively, all your attention is focused on the speaker. You maintain eye contact and do not interrupt while the other person is speaking. You ask questions that encourage the speaker to continue and respond to specific questions that he or she asks.

Culture ALERT

Some cultures value periods of silence during conversation or other talks. Allow adequate time. Learn to overcome any personal discomfort with periods of silence. ■

GUIDELINES *for*

Communicating with Patients

- Be sure you have the patient's attention.
- Avoid chewing gum, eating, or covering your mouth with your hand when you speak.
- Use nonthreatening words and gestures that the person is likely to understand.
- Speak clearly and courteously.
- Use a pleasant tone of voice.
- Use appropriate body language.
- Be alert to the patient's needs to communicate with you—allow time for the patient to talk and respond. Show interest and concern (Figure 7-9).
- Do not speak about the patient in front of the patient or other patients.
- Do not interrupt the patient.
- Reflect the patient's feelings and thoughts by rewording his or her statements as questions.
- Ask for clarification if you are unsure of what the patient is saying.
- Give the patient only factual information—not your personal feelings, opinions, or beliefs.
- Information concerning the patient's condition, medications, and treatments should be given only by the physician or nurse, never by the nursing assistant.
- Do not argue with patients.
- Avoid using slang or cultural terms that are not familiar to the patient, and may be misinterpreted.

- Avoid sound-alike words, such as "accept" and "except," and words with a double meaning, such as "haul" and "hall," when possible.
- Do not provide false reassurance, such as "Everything will be all right." The patient will not trust you when she learns you were not sincere.
- Wait long enough for a reply. Patients who are elderly, hard of hearing, or under the effects of certain medications may take longer to process a message and respond.
- Always inform the patient before you leave the room, and be sure the patient has the call signal and other needed items.

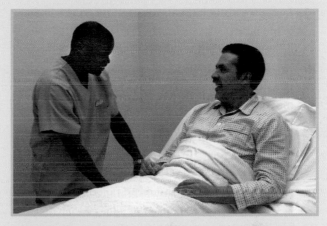

FIGURE 7-9 Recognize the patient's need to communicate with you. *(© Delmar/Cengage Learning)*

Communicating with Patients Who Have Special Needs

There are many reasons why communication with patients may be impaired. The patient may:
- Be hearing impaired
- Be vision impaired
- Have aphasia
- Be disoriented
- Be from a culture different from the nursing assistant's

These patients have special communication needs that should be addressed on the care plan. Always check the care plan before attempting to communicate with a patient who has special communication needs. Specific approaches may be established for all staff members to use with the patient. Lack of consistency in use of these approaches is confusing and frustrating to the patient.

Guidelines for communicating with patients who have special needs can be found in the Online Companion to this book.

Communication HIGHLIGHT

Remember that one of the most important and powerful messages you send to patients is that you care about them. You do this in many ways, including your demeanor when you enter the room, your body language, your tone of voice, and your touch. Verbal communication with some patients will be very limited. Use nonverbal communication to send the message that you care to all patients. ∎

GUIDELINES *for*
Communicating with Patients from Other Cultures

1. Address the person using his or her preferred name.

2. Introduce yourself and identify your position.

3. Plan extra time for the communication if the person is not fluent in your native language. Communicating with persons whose first language is not English will take twice as long as a similar communication with an English-speaking patient.

4. Take responsibility for the communication. Recognize that you are speaking with a person whose culture is different from your own, and that he or she is the cultural expert. Show respect for the person and his or her culture. Be sincere, flexible, tolerant, and empathetic.

5. Avoid stereotyping patients, and recognize your own cultural biases. Consider the individual. Avoid judgments based on your beliefs and stereotypes.

6. Reduce distractions in the environment.

7. Use plain language. This does not mean that you must "dumb down" the message or use overly simple explanations, as you would with a small child. Plain language is clear and effective. Be honest and polite. Apologize if you misunderstand or make a mistake.

8. Pace yourself. Speak slowly and distinctly in short sentences. Adjust the pace of your speech, if necessary. Allow enough time for the person to translate what you have said and formulate a response.

9. Avoid idioms that may be misunderstood. *Idioms* are expressions and phrases that are usually understood only by speakers of your own native language. For example, an expression such as "bite the bullet" is a common English phrase that could be taken literally or misunderstood by persons from other cultures.

10. Be careful when using jokes and humor. A person whose first language is not the same as your own may interpret the message differently.

11. Respect personal space.

12. Monitor your body language.

13. Periodically check the patient's understanding of your message by asking him to paraphrase what you have said.

14. Avoid assumptions. Ask questions if you need clarification. Asking is not offensive and shows that you are making an effort to understand.

15. Avoid discussing or debating whether the person's values and cultural beliefs are right or wrong. Be nonjudgmental.

16. Listen carefully. Give the other person your full attention.

17. Use pictures, gestures, and written words, if appropriate.

18. Stay focused. Discuss only one topic at a time.

Additional information about communications and culturally competent care can be found in Unit 11.

COMMUNICATING WITH PATIENTS FROM A DIFFERENT CULTURE

The persons you care for may come from many different cultures or have different **ethnic** backgrounds. *Ethnic* refers to people who come from other countries and who have different customs, languages, and traditions. For example, in some countries it is considered a sign of disrespect to maintain eye contact when speaking with another person. If you are assigned to care for someone from a different ethnic background, you should be given specific communication guidelines.

Guidelines for caring for and communicating with patients with mental health problems and dementia are found in Units 30 and 31, and in the Online Companion to this book.

Culture ALERT

Patients who are able to speak and read about their care in their native language usually feel more at ease and understand their care better. Some people can read and write in English, but have trouble with verbal communications in English. ∎

WORKING WITH INTERPRETERS

Occasionally, you will care for a patient who does not speak your language at all, and communication may be limited. Gestures and body language can be helpful, but they are not universal. For example, in the United States, we shake the head up and down to mean yes. We move the head from side to side to signify no. In India, these gestures mean just the opposite: Moving the head from side to side means yes, and shaking it up and down means no. Because of differences in culture and language, there may be times when you need the assistance of a communication professional.

An **interpreter** is a communication professional who mediates between speakers of different languages. Interpretation is an activity that consists of establishing, either simultaneously or consecutively, oral or gestural communications between two or more persons who do not speak the same language. Some interpreters speak. Others use sign language. Facilities will use medical interpreters when they are available in the community. Some have a telephone interpreter service. Some can arrange both audio and video interpreter services.

You will find additional information about communication in Units 9, 11, 30, 31, 36, 37, and 38, as well as in the Online Companion to this book.

REVIEW

A. Multiple Choice

Select the one best answer for each of the following.

1. Successful communication is essential for
   a. body language to be meaningful.
   b. patients only.
   c. staff only.
   d. safe care. ✓

2. Verbal communication includes
   a. talking and listening. ✓
   b. facial expressions.
   c. reading reports.
   d. using a fax machine.

3. For successful communication to occur, all of the following elements must be present except
   a. receiver.
   b. hearing. ✓
   c. feedback.
   d. sender.

4. Examples of nonverbal communication include
   a. reading and using the patient's care plan. ✓
   b. answering the telephone.
   c. listening to the shift report.
   d. conversing with patients.

5. Demonstrating your understanding of a message by stating the message in your own words is
   a. channeling.
   b. rephrasing and restating. ✓
   c. paraphrasing. ✓
   d. reorganizing.

6. The portion of communication that has the greatest influence on the receiver's interpretation of the message is the
   a. body language.
   b. tone of voice.
   c. pitch of voice.
   d. eye contact.

7. The document that shows the line of authority for communication is the
   a. staff development chart.
   b. employee personnel handbook.
   c. policy and procedure manual.
   d. organizational chart.

8. Examples of manuals that are found on nursing units include
   a. computer manual, administrative policy manual, quality assurance manual.
   b. procedure manual, infection control manual, disaster manual.
   c. employee assistance program manual, personnel manual, benefits manual.
   d. isolation manual, X-ray manual, nuclear medicine manual.

9. The patient's care plan provides information for
   a. nursing assistant assignments.
   b. employee benefits.
   c. fire drill procedures.
   d. licensed personnel only.

10. The patient's medical record or chart is
    a. used only by the physician.

b. used by all members of the health care team.

c. a temporary record.

d. a report of the nursing assistant's competencies.

11. The patient grimaces and holds his right arm close to his body when he moves. You suspect he may

a. be right-handed.

b. not want to get out of bed.

c. be tired.

d. be having pain.

12. Touching the patient can be a successful method of communication if you

a. ask the family's permission.

b. are not offended by touch.

c. are gentle and caring.

d. always grasp the patient firmly.

B. Nursing Assistant Challenge

Miss Johnson is one of your patients. She is visually impaired and in the hospital because she has a heart problem. Miss Johnson can feed herself and can give herself a bath, brush her teeth, and comb her own hair if she has adequate assistance. Think about suggestions presented in this unit for communicating with persons with visual impairment; then answer the following questions.

13. What can you do to set up meal trays so that Miss Johnson can feed herself?

14. How can you prepare bath items so that she can give herself her bath?

15. What can you do to enable her to comb her own hair and brush her teeth?

16. What other actions can you take to help this patient maintain as much independence as possible?

UNIT 8

Observation, Reporting, and Documentation

OBJECTIVES

After completing this unit, you will be able to:

- Spell and define terms.
- List the components of the nursing process.
- Describe the purpose of the care plan.
- Explain the nursing assistant's responsibilities for each component of the nursing process.
- Describe two observations to make for each body system.

- List three times when oral reports are given.
- Describe the information given when reporting.
- State the purpose of the patient's medical record.
- Explain the rules for documentation.
- State the purpose of the HIPAA laws.

VOCABULARY

Learn the meaning and the correct spelling of the following words and phrases:

approaches	flow sheet	interventions	oral report
care plan conference	goals	Kardex	planning
charting	Health Insurance	nurses' notes	subjective observation
critical (clinical)	Portability and	nursing diagnosis	
pathways	Accountability Act	nursing process	
document	(HIPAA)	objective observation	
evaluation	implementation	observation	

INTRODUCTION

The nursing assistant is responsible for collecting and communicating information about patients. You will gather information by observing the patients and communicate with other team members by reporting and documenting. The mechanism used to carry out these actions is called the **nursing process**.

NURSING PROCESS

To understand the focus of this chapter, you need to know the basic difference between nursing care and medical care. Both medicine and nursing are necessary for positive patient outcomes (Figure 8-1). The physician collects information to diagnose and treat human illnesses. Nurses collect information, then use it to diagnose and treat the

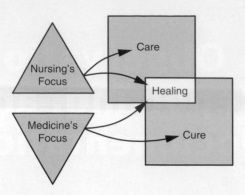

FIGURE 8-1 Medicine and nursing each have a separate focus, but both are essential for patients' well-being if positive outcomes are to be achieved. (© Delmar/Cengage Learning)

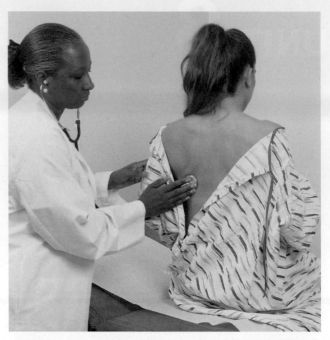

FIGURE 8-2 Part of the nursing assessment involves physical examination. The nurse is auscultating (listening to) the patient's lungs. The admission data are used as a basis for comparison of different assessments. (© Delmar/Cengage Learning)

human response to illness. Nursing diagnoses are very different from medical diagnoses.

The registered nurse is responsible for achieving patient-focused care by using the nursing process. He or she coordinates care and delegates responsibilities to others to achieve this goal. The nursing process consists of five steps:

1. Assessment
2. Problem identification (attaching a nursing diagnosis)
3. Planning
4. Implementation
5. Evaluation

Assessment involves the collection of data (information) about the patient. The registered nurse coordinates all assessments. The data are entered on a special form. Information is obtained from:

- Interviewing the patient
- The medical record
- The patient's family, if the patient is unable to communicate
- Physical examination (Figure 8-2)
- Collection of measurable data and information such as weight and vital signs (these data can be obtained by workers other than the nurse)
- Observations and information provided by other members of the nursing team

Proper use of the nursing process is essential for the delivery of effective health care. Nursing units run more efficiently if all staff understand and adhere to this model of care. If the nursing process breaks down, the risk of negative outcomes is increased. Understanding and fulfilling your role in the nursing process is an important responsibility.

The nursing assistant is responsible for collection of data by making and reporting observations. The nurse analyzes the data, identifies the patient's problems, and formulates nursing diagnoses. A **nursing diagnosis** is the statement of a patient problem and the cause of the problem. For example, the nursing diagnosis may be *impaired physical mobility* (the problem) related to paralysis *due to stroke* (the cause of the problem). Nursing diagnoses may reflect:

- Actual clinical problems
- The risk that certain problems will develop
- Health promotion needs, such as things that will help improve the person's health
- Wellness and teaching objectives

The nursing diagnoses provide the foundation for nursing care. Table 8-1 gives a few examples of nursing diagnoses and what they mean.

Planning for patient care (developing a care plan) is done after the nursing diagnoses are made. The purpose of planning is to:

- Identify possible solutions to the problems (nursing diagnoses).
- Develop **approaches** (what team members are going to do) that will help the patient solve the problems. Approaches may also be called **interventions**.
- Establish measurable **goals** for the patient (a goal is an outcome) so that caregivers will know whether the approaches are successful and whether the problems are being resolved.

Planning may be done at a **care plan conference** (Figure 8-3). This is a meeting of the members of the

TABLE 8-1 EXAMPLES OF NURSING DIAGNOSES AND OBSERVATIONS TO MAKE

Nursing Diagnosis	Observations to Make
Imbalanced nutrition; less than body requirements	<ul><li>Food/fluid intake</li><li>Weight loss</li><li>Inability to eat, dislike or refusal of food or fluids</li><li>Pain in abdomen or mouth</li><li>Sores in mouth</li></ul>
Constipation	<ul><li>Lack of bowel movement or hard, dry stools</li><li>Complaints of feeling full</li><li>Abdomen distended and firm</li><li>Passing flatus (gas)</li></ul>
Impaired skin integrity	<ul><li>Redness or destruction of skin</li></ul>
Ineffective coping	<ul><li>Change in usual communication patterns</li><li>Inability to cope or meet basic needs</li><li>Change in behavior</li></ul>
Impaired physical mobility	<ul><li>Ability to move in bed, range of motion, balance, coordination, endurance</li></ul>
Activity intolerance	<ul><li>Fatigue, weakness, shortness of breath</li><li>Irregular pulse</li></ul>
Disturbed sleep pattern	<ul><li>Inability to sleep at night, or wakes frequently</li><li>Abnormal daytime sleepiness as a result of not sleeping at night</li><li>Changes in behavior or speech</li></ul>
Impaired Comfort (this diagnosis is used to represent any discomfort in response to an unpleasant stimulus or order, such as being hungry and NPO)	<ul><li>Actively complains of pain</li><li>Reports or demonstrates discomfort</li><li>Guarding upon movement</li><li>Facial expression and/or body language suggesting pain</li><li>Nausea and/or vomiting</li></ul>
Anxiety	<ul><li>Shakiness, quivering voice, increased movements</li><li>Poor eye contact, helplessness</li></ul>

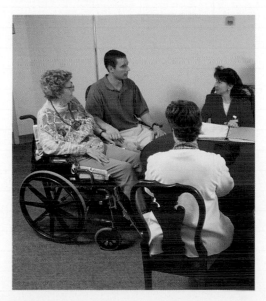

FIGURE 8-3 The care plan is developed during a care conference involving the patient and family member (if desired), and members of the interdisciplinary team. (© Delmar/Cengage Learning)

interdisciplinary team who are involved in the care of the patient. The patient and/or the family (if the patient consents) should be invited to attend the conference. The care plan developed at the conference contains a list of the nursing diagnoses, the approaches, and the patient's goals (Figures 8-4A and 8-4B). The care plan may be kept in the patient's medical record or in a file called a **Kardex** (Figures 8-5A and 8-5B). The nursing assistant is responsible for contributing information (observations) that will help the team develop a workable care plan. Your assignment will involve implementing each patient's care plan approaches. You may be invited to attend the care plan conference.

Implementation is the activation of the care plan. It means following your assignment and carrying out the approaches listed on the care plan in an effort to resolve the problems (nursing diagnoses) and to help the patient reach the goals (Figure 8-6). The approach states:

- Who is to carry out the approach
- When the approach is carried out
- How the approach is carried out

NURSING DIAGNOSIS	NURSING INTERVENTIONS	EVALUATION
Ineffective breathing pattern R/T operative site/incisional pain.	1. Auscultate breath sounds q̄ 4h. & PRN. 2. Assist pt. to turn, cough, and deep breathe q̄ 2h while awake.	1. Lungs clear on auscultation. 2. "It doesn't hurt as much to cough today."
Risk for infection R/T surgical incision & indwelling catheter.	Assess for s/s of infection q̄ 4h	T 100.2°, incision site warm & pink, non-edematous). "It really hurts under the bandage."
Risk for constipation R/T abdominal surgery.	1. Restart oral fluids gradually. Offer clear liquids frequently. 2. Observe for abd. distension & evaluate tolerance when pt. begins taking fluid/foods.	Unable to tolerate oral fluids — vomited p̄ taking ice chips.

FIGURE 8-4A A handwritten care plan, such as the kind used on the Kardex. (© Delmar/Cengage Learning)

PLAN OF CARE

PC: ABDOMINAL SURGERY

PB: TD:____/____Ineffective breathing pattern r/t: op site/incision pain.

EO: Respiratory rate & effort WNL with good chest expansion.

1: Auscultate breath sounds Q4H & PRN. Note diminished/absent sounds, rales, wheezing, crackles, rhonchi. DOCUMENT IN NURSE'S NOTES.

2: Assist pt to turn, cough, and deep breathe Q2H while awake. Support incision. DOCUMENT RESPONSE & EFFORT.

PB: TD:____/____Risk for infection r/t surgical incision/indwelling cath.

EO: Surgical incision healing w/out s/s of infection.

1: Assess for s/s of infection Q4H: (fever, chills, swelling, redness, pain, drainage, increased WBC, etc) DOCUMENT IN NURSE'S NOTES.

PB: TD:____/____Acute pain r/t_____ surgical incision/operative site.

EO: Pt reports pain relieved/ controlled.

1: Implement Patient Controlled Analgesia (PCA) Protocol and PCA Teaching Protocol

PB: TD:____/____Risk for constipation r/t_____surgery.

EO: Pt's bowel elimination is normal within limits of surgical procedure.

1: Restart oral fluids gradually. Offer clear liquids frequently.

2: Observe for abdominal distention & evaluate tolerance when pt begins taking fluid/foods post-op. DOCUMENT IN NURSE'S NOTES.

INT   SIGNATURE

FIGURE 8-4B A computer-generated care plan. Some programs list approaches based on the nursing diagnoses, but the nurse entering the data can reject them or modify them if they are not appropriate. The nurse can also add any relevant personal data to the plan. (*Courtesy of St. Tammany Parish Hospital, Covington, LA*)

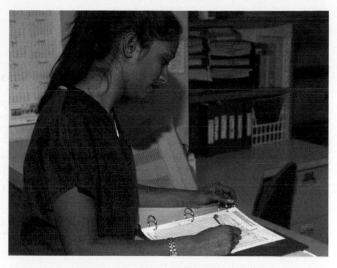

FIGURE 8-5A Care plans are often kept in the Kardex at the nurses' station. (© *Delmar/Cengage Learning*)

See Figure 8-4 for examples of approaches. Nursing assistants are responsible for knowing when and how approaches are to be carried out and for implementing each approach correctly.

Evaluation is the final step of the nursing process, but it is an ongoing activity. The evaluation determines:

• Whether the patient is reaching the goals on the care plan, and if not why

• What should be done to assist the patient to reach the goals

• When goals are reached, whether they should be extended (for example, if the patient reaches the goal of walking 200 feet, it may be increased to 250 feet)

The nursing assistant is responsible for reporting to the nurse when the:

• Approach cannot be carried out for any reason

• Patient is having problems with the approach

• Patient has met a goal

• Patient refuses care listed in the approaches

• Nursing assistant identifies a more effective approach (method of meeting a goal)

Critical (Clinical) Pathways

Many hospitals are using **critical (clinical) pathways** to direct care. The pathways are written documents that detail the expected course of treatment and expected patient outcomes. New goals are set each day. The pathway lists nursing actions to help the patient achieve the goals. The nursing assistant is responsible for many of these interventions. Review the Kardex containing the patient's care plan or critical pathway at the beginning of each shift to help plan your day.

Case Presentation

Mrs. White is admitted with medical diagnoses of hyperglycemia, ketoacidosis, and a history of diabetes mellitus (DM), all diagnostic indicators of diabetic ketoacidosis (DKA). Mrs. White is having labored breathing, vomiting, and weakness. Mr. White states that his wife takes insulin for her diabetes, she doesn't follow her diet, and she has been complaining of thirst and frequent urination. On examination, the patient complains of weakness and abdominal pain, and she has an acetone breath.

White, Mary	F 56
MR#: 000135039	ACCT#: 9710144268
Dr: J. Smith	2/W 402–XX
DX: Diabetic Ketoacidosis (DKA)	DATE: 12/14/XX

SUMMARY: 12/14   0701 to 1501

CILIENT INFORMATION

10/14   ADVANCE DIRECTIVES: No. Advance directive does not exist
10/14   ORGAN DONOR: Unknown
10/14   ADMIT DX: Diabetic Ketoacidosis (DKA)
10/14   ALLERGIES: None Known
10/14   ISOLATION: Not at this time

MISC. CLIENT DATA

10/14   History of Diabetes Mellitus (DM): Insulin-Dependent Diabetic

MEDICAL DIAGNOSES

10/14   PROBLEM # 1: Hyperglycemia
10/14   PROBLEM # 2: Ketoacidosis
10/14   PROBLEM # 3: Hyperventilation
10/14   PROBLEM # 4: Hypovolemia, Hypernatremia
10/14   PROBLEM # 5: Hypotension
10/14   PROBLEM # 6: Hypokalemia

NURSING DIAGNOSES

10/14   PROBLEM 1: Deficient fluid volume r/t osmotic diuresis associated
with hyperglycemia
10/14   PROBLEM 2: Ineffective breathing pattern: Kussmaul respirations/air
hunger r/t metabolic acidosis associated with DKA
10/14   PROBLEM 3: Decreased cardiac output r/t hypokalemia associated
with metabolic acidosis
10/14   PROBLEM 4: Risk for injury: circulatory collapse, renal shutdown,
and coma r/t persistent, untreated hyperglycemia
10/14   PROBLEM 5: Risk for injury: seizure susceptibility if hyperglycemia
is corrected too abruptly
10/14   PROBLEM 6: Ineffective airway clearance: aspiration r/t presence of
vomiting and altered level of conciousness
10/14   PROBLEM 7: Risk for infection r/t invasive procedures
10/14   PROBLEM 8: Altered nutrition: less than body requirements r/t anorexia,
nausea, or vomiting associated with ketoacidosis and hypokalemia
10/14   PROBLEM 9: Deficient knowledge: prevention of DKA r/t proper
management of DM
10/14   PROBLEM 10: Ineffective therapeutic regimen management r/t
inadequate motivation for incorporating strategies for prevention of
DKA into daily living

FIGURE 8-5B Sample computerized care plan, based in part on information from the case presentation. (From Springhouse (2001). *Mastering documentation.* Springhouse, PA: Springhouse; Reiner, A. (Ed.). (2001). *Manual of patient care standards.* Gaithersburg, MD: Aspen; Williams, S. M. (2001). *Decision making in critical care nursing.* Philadelphia, PA: Decker)

ALL CURRENT MEDICAL ORDERS

NURSING ORDERS:

10/14   Activity: Bedrest
          VS: Q15" first 2 Hours, then Q30" until within normal limits, then Q1H
10/14   Telemetry
10/14   Daily Weight: 0600
10/14   Intake & Output: Q 15 min. first 2 hours, then Q 30 min. until output stable at
          30 mL/H, then Q1H
10/14   Urine: Specific Gravity Q1H
10/14   Measure blood glucose levels: Q1H, notify physician when serum
          glucose is less than 300 mg percent
10/14   Oral Hygiene: Q1H
10/14   Monitor for s/s of infection: IV site, triple-lumen, central
          line, right subclavian and indwelling Foley catheter
10/14   Institute fall precautions

SUMMARY: 10/14   0701 to 1501

DIET:

10/14   NPO; Diabetic: 1600 cal., start with breakfast tomorrow

IVS:

10/14   Central line #1...0.9 percent normal saline, 1000 mL @ rate of 1 L/H
          for first 2 H, infusion pump; then decrease infusion of 0.9 percent
          normal saline, 500 mL @ rate of 500 mL/H for the next 2 H; then
          decrease infusion of 0.9 percent normal saline, 250 mL @ rate of 250 mL/H
10/14   Central line #2...50 U of regular insulin to 500 mL normal saline to produce
          a concentration of 0.1 U/mL, infuse @ 7 U/kg per hour, infusion pump
10/14   Administer KCL IV: If serum K^+ is <3.6 give 40 mEq/H; 3.5-5.5 give
          20 mEq/H; >5.5 give no K^+

SCHEDULED MEDICATIONS:

10/14   None

STAT/NOW MEDICATIONS:

10/14   IV bolus of regular insulin of 0.2 U/kg

PRN MEDICATIONS:

10/14   None

LABORATORY:

10/14   Stat Chem Profile 23
          Blood Glucose Q1H
          Stat Arterial Blood Gases
          Urinalysis Now

ANCILLARY:

10/14   Stat EKG
10/14   FSBS PRN s/s hypo/hyperglycemia

Last Page

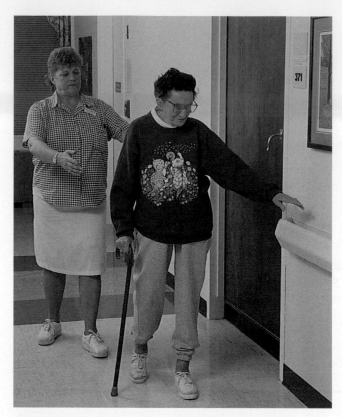

FIGURE 8-6 Nursing assistants are responsible for implementing many of the care plan approaches. (© Delmar/Cengage Learning)

MAKING OBSERVATIONS

An **observation** is information that is obtained by using one's senses: seeing, hearing, smelling, or feeling.

There are two types of observations: subjective and objective. An **objective observation** is factual or measurable in some way. For example, blood in the urine is factual. Blood pressure, temperature, pulse, and respirations are measurable. You make objective observations by using your senses of sight, smell, hearing, and touch. A **subjective observation** is a statement or complaint made by the patient. For example, "I have a headache," or "I feel sick to my stomach" are subjective observations.

Making Initial Observations

To make accurate observations, you must first know what is normal for an individual. For this reason, baseline information is collected at the time of admission. Make observations each time you are in the room. Noting possible signs of injury or skin breakdown is important. Initial status provides a basis for making comparisons. For example, one patient may have a blood pressure of 110/68 on admission. If the patient's blood pressure is 140/88 later in the shift, notify the nurse, because this is not the usual value for this person.

Try to establish a routine way of making observations. Keep in mind the age and known illnesses of the patients. It may be helpful to think of each body system and note the following:

Integumentary system (skin, nails)
- Color: flushed, pale, jaundiced (yellow color), or cyanotic (bluish, ashen, gray color); nails pale, pink, or cyanotic
- Temperature: warm, hot, cool
- Moisture: dry, perspiring
- Abnormalities: rashes, bruises, scars, pressure ulcers, injuries

Musculoskeletal system (muscles, bones, joints)
- Posture: stooped, curled up in bed, straight
- Mobility: ability to move in bed, to get out of bed, to stand, to walk, and to maintain balance
- Range of motion: ability to move all joints (Figure 8-7)

Circulatory system (heart, blood vessels, blood)
- Pulse: strength, regularity, rate
- Skin: (see integumentary system)
- Nails: (see integumentary system)
- Blood pressure
- Swelling of face, hands, lower legs, and/or feet

Respiratory system (nose, throat, trachea, bronchi, lungs)
- Respirations (breathing): rate, regularity, depth, difficulty in breathing, shortness of breath upon exertion or while still, wheezing or crackling heard
- Cough: frequency; dry, loose, productive (coughing up secretions from the lungs); color and consistency of sputum (if any)

Nervous system (brain, spinal cord, nerves)
- Mental status: orientation to time, place, person; ability to make verbal or nonverbal responses
- Coordination: tremors, reaction time
- Paralysis, inability to move a body part

Senses (eyes, ears, nose, sense of touch)
- Eyes: reddened, drainage, pupils equal in size
- Ears: drainage
- Nose: drainage, bleeding
- Sense of touch: ability to feel pressure and pain

Urinary system (kidneys, ureters, bladder, urethra)
- Urination: frequency, amount, color, clarity, odor, presence of blood or sediment (Figure 8-8); ability to hold urine, incontinence
- Pain on urination (dysuria)

Digestive system (mouth, teeth, throat, esophagus, stomach, large and small intestines, gallbladder, liver, pancreas)
- Full or partial dentures
- Dental caries (cavities)

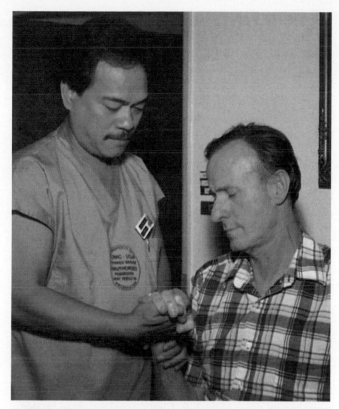

FIGURE 8-7 Report to the nurse if there is a change in the patient's ability to move the joints. *(© Delmar/Cengage Learning)*

- Appetite: amount of fluids and food consumed (Figure 8-9), tolerance of foods, belching (burping)
- Eating: difficulty chewing or swallowing
- Nausea and/or vomiting
- Bowel elimination: frequency, amount, consistency, color of stools; diarrhea, constipation, incontinence, flatus; difficulty in passing stool

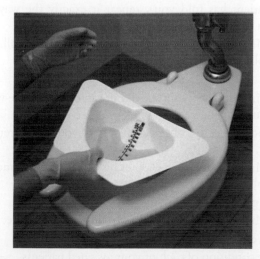

FIGURE 8-8 Check the urine before discarding it. If you observe abnormalities, save it for the nurse to view. *(© Delmar/Cengage Learning)*

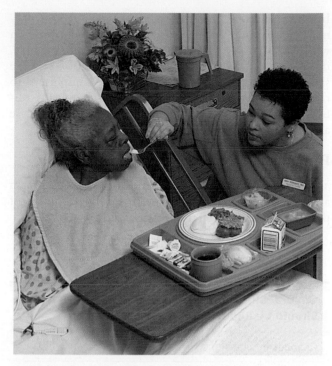

FIGURE 8-9 Monitor and record the amount of food and fluid consumed. *(© Delmar/Cengage Learning)*

Endocrine system (glands)

- Signs and symptoms of diabetes (hypoglycemia, hyperglycemia)

Reproductive system (male and female internal and external sex organs)

- Female
  - Breasts: condition of nipples, presence of lumps, discolorations
  - Menstrual periods: frequency, amount, and character of bleeding; cramping
  - Vaginal drainage: amount, odor, and character
  - Unusual sores or lesions on external genitals (painful or painless)
- Male
  - Testes: lumps
  - Penis: amount and character of drainage
  - Unusual sores or lesions (painful or painless)

In addition to body system observations, you also need to note facts related to pain, behavior, and function.

- Pain: location, type of pain (sharp, dull, aching), constant or intermittent or related to specific activities, time pain started
- Behavior: actions, conduct
- Function: ability to move about and complete tasks such as bathing

When reporting behavior, avoid using "labels" based on your judgment of the patient. Report only what you see and hear.

In some situations, you may be expected to report "normal" observations. This tells the nurse and physician whether the patient's condition is improving. For example, if a patient has had a respiratory tract infection and the signs and symptoms have diminished, it is important to report "no coughing or respiratory distress is noted." Abnormal observations that should be reported to the nurse are listed in Table 8-2.

Pain

You must be very factual in reporting observations of pain and behavior. Avoid judging patients who complain of pain. Pain is discussed in greater detail in Unit 10.

TABLE 8-2 OBSERVATION AND REPORTING GUIDELINES

General Signs and Symptoms of Illness that Should be Reported to the Nurse
Changes in vital signs
Chest pain
Shortness of breath
Difficulty breathing
Weakness or dizziness
Cyanosis or change in color
Profuse sweating
Cough
Nausea or vomiting
Diarrhea
Abnormal appearance of urine or feces
Unusual drainage from a wound or body cavity
Pain
Excessive thirst
Unable to hear blood pressure or palpate pulse
Lethargy
Headache
Change in mental status
Abnormal behavior, including crying
Requests for medication for an acute problem

REPORTING

Your work day will begin and end with a report. Good communication is an essential nursing assistant skill. Workers who are considered "top notch" usually have good organization and communication skills. Reporting is one of the cornerstones that form the foundation of solid nursing practice. The Joint Commission has identified communication failures as a major source of avoidable patient harm. The shift report is probably the most important communication of your work day. The length of the report, its quality, and the depth of information transmitted depend on the communication skills of the entire nursing team on the unit. During the change-of-shift report, you will learn:

- Changes in patients' conditions
- Information about new admissions
- Names of patients who were discharged or died
- Incidents that occurred involving patients
- New physicians' orders affecting nursing care
- Special events for patients that will occur during your shift

Giving an **oral report** is one method of reporting information to other staff members. You will give and receive oral reports several times each shift. Oral reports are given by the:

- Nurse going off duty to the staff coming on duty (Figure 8-10) (in some facilities, the off-going nurse may give a report only to the oncoming nurse)—this is called a *shift report*. Some facilities leave a tape-recorded report for the next shift.
- Nursing assistant to the nurse when leaving the unit for any reason (such as lunch break).
- Nursing assistant to the nurse at the end of the shift.
- Nursing assistant to the nurse if any unusual or new observations are made.

Be specific when reporting your observations. When informing the nurse of a subjective observation (something the patient has told you), repeat it exactly the way the patient told it to you. For example:

Mrs. Goldberg was wandering around in the hall. (objective)

versus

Mrs. Goldberg said she did not know where she was. (subjective)

To report objective observations, state your measurement or fact, such as:

Mr. Hernandez ate 30% of his meal at lunch time. (objective)

Avoid giving your opinion:

Mr. Hernandez probably was not hungry. (subjective)

At the end of your shift, report to the nurse:

- The condition of each of your assigned patients
- The care given to each patient
- Observations you made while giving care

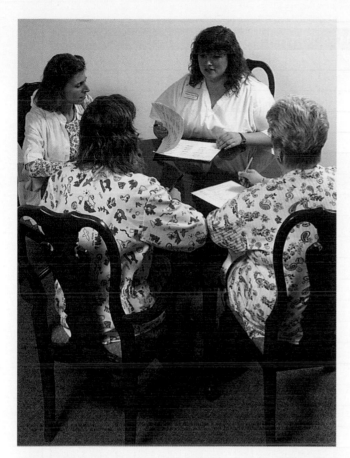

FIGURE 8-10 Report is given to the oncoming shift by the nurse who worked the previous shift. *(© Delmar/Cengage Learning)*

Reporting is an essential part of the job. Preparing to give and receive report are critical activities. Although you may think you are simply transferring information, in most situations you are doing much more than this. You are transferring the responsibility for the patient to another individual, department, or shift. Practice your

observation and reporting skills until you master them. This foundation will serve you well throughout your nursing career.

You will find additional information and guidelines for reporting in the Online Companion to this book.

Seeking Higher Authority

Sometimes a report you make to your immediate supervisor is not taken seriously. Nurses are busy and verbal reports given to them in passing may be forgotten. If the nurse does not respond within a reasonable period of time, try again. If you fail to get a response, but know that the information is very important, move up to the next person in the chain of command. This situation should not occur often, but it can happen.

DOCUMENTATION

You may be expected to record your observations on the patient's medical record (chart) (Figure 8-11). The medical record is a **document**, or legal record of a patient's care. Each patient's permanent medical record contains physician's medical orders and progress notes, diagnostic tests, treatments, medications, medical history and physical examinations, assessments, nursing notes, the care plan, special reports (such as surgical reports), notes from all departments providing patient care, and the patient's response to care.

Recording the patient's care, response to treatment, and progress in the chart is called **charting** or *documentation*. Nursing assistants may document on **flow sheets** (Figure 8-12) in the chart or on the **nurses' notes** (Figure 8-13) (sometimes called nurses' progress notes).

Communication HIGHLIGHT

You will learn when to report your observations about patients as you gain experience. In general, high-priority reporting items are abnormal vital signs, chest pain, difficulty breathing, change in color, change in mental status, bleeding, and pain. If you are in doubt about the urgency of reporting to the nurse, report your observation immediately. If the patient's condition changes after you have reported your observations, inform the nurse again. ▪

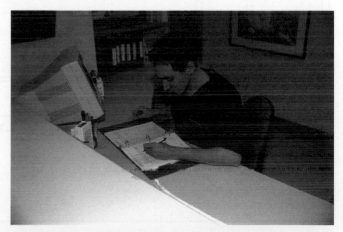

FIGURE 8-11 Observations are recorded in the patient's medical record. *(© Delmar/Cengage Learning)*

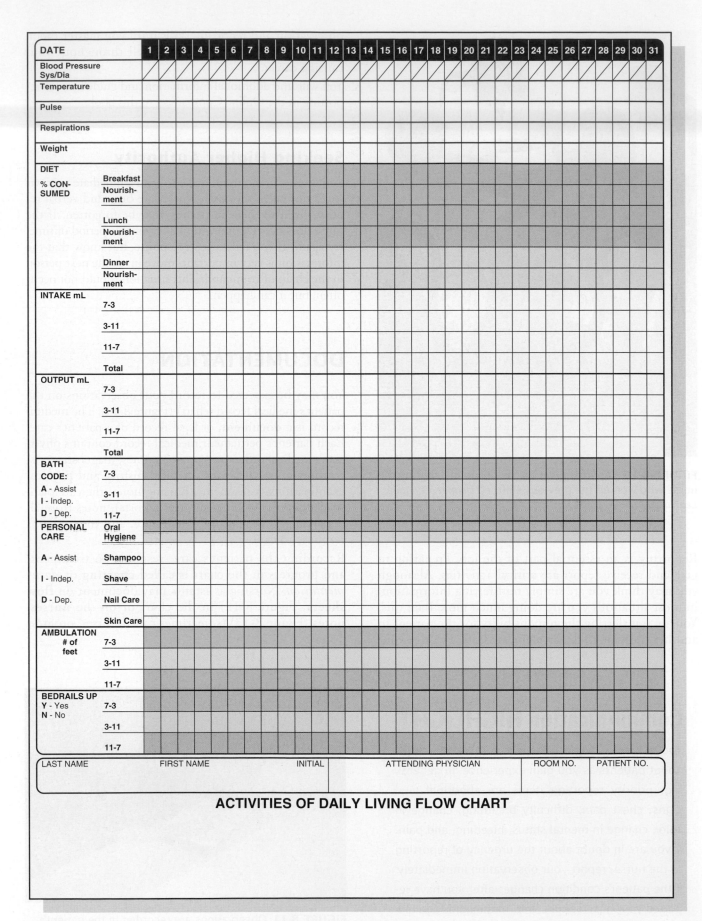

DATE		1	2	3	4	5	6	7	8	9	10	11	12	13	14	15	16	17	18	19	20	21	22	23	24	25	26	27	28	29	30	31
Blood Pressure Sys/Dia																																
Temperature																																	
Pulse																																	
Respirations																																	
Weight																																	
DIET % CONSUMED	Breakfast																																
	Nourishment																																
	Lunch																																
	Nourishment																																
	Dinner																																
	Nourishment																																
INTAKE mL	7-3																																
	3-11																																
	11-7																																
	Total																																
OUTPUT mL	7-3																																
	3-11																																
	11-7																																
	Total																																
BATH CODE: A - Assist I - Indep. D - Dep.	7-3																																
	3-11																																
	11-7																																
PERSONAL CARE A - Assist I - Indep. D - Dep.	Oral Hygiene																																
	Shampoo																																
	Shave																																
	Nail Care																																
	Skin Care																																
AMBULATION # of feet	7-3																																
	3-11																																
	11-7																																
BEDRAILS UP Y - Yes N - No	7-3																																
	3-11																																
	11-7																																

LAST NAME	FIRST NAME	INITIAL	ATTENDING PHYSICIAN	ROOM NO.	PATIENT NO.

ACTIVITIES OF DAILY LIVING FLOW CHART

FIGURE 8-12 You may be expected to document your care and observations on a flow sheet. (*Courtesy of Briggs Corporation*)

DATE		1	2	3	4	5	6	7	8	9	10	11	12	13	14	15	16	17	18	19	20	21	22	23	24	25	26	27	28	29	30	31
UP IN CHAIR A - Assist I - Indep. D - Dep.	7-3																															
	3-11																															
	11-7																															
ROM Exercises A - Active P - Passive	7-3																															
	3-11																															
POSITION changed A - Assist I - Indep. D - Dep.	7-3																															
	3-11																															
	11-7																															
BLADDER ACTION C - Continent I - Incontinent F - Foley # x's	7-3																															
	3-11																															
	11-7																															
BOWEL ACTION C - Continent I - Incontinent # x's	7-3																															
	3-11																															
	11-7																															
CONSISTENCY L - Liquid S - Soft formed H - Hard formed	7-3																															
	3-11																															
	11-7																															
PERI CARE A - Assist I - Indep. D - Dep.	7-3																															
	3-11																															
	11-7																															
RESTRAINT P - Pelvic W - Waist B - Belt G - Geri Chair Check q 1/2 Hr. Release q 2 hrs.	7-3																															
	3-11																															
	11-7																															
Nursing Assistant's Initials	A.M.																															
	P.M.																															
	NOC.																															
Licensed Nurse Initials	A.M.																															
	P.M.																															
	NOC.																															

Nursing Assistant's Initials and Signature

_____ _____   _____ _____   _____ _____   _____ _____

_____ _____   _____ _____   _____ _____   _____ _____

Licensed Nurse Initials and Signature

_____ _____   _____ _____   _____ _____   _____ _____

_____ _____   _____ _____   _____ _____   _____ _____

LAST NAME	FIRST NAME	INITIAL	ATTENDING PHYSICIAN	ROOM NO.	PATIENT NO.

NURSE'S PROGRESS NOTES

DATE AND TIME	NURSING CARE NOTES	SIGNATURE
3-16-XX	2200 Found lying on floor beside bed. Responds verbally. States was "trying to get to the bathroom." Nurse notified immediately.	C. Simmons CNA
	2205 ROM satisfactory. Denies having pain. No injuries noted. ROM wnl. No obvious deformities. Assisted back to bed. Call light within reach. Instructed to use call light when having to go to B.R. Pulse 86, strong and regular. B/P 136/84. Oriented to time, place, person. Incontinent after fall. Pajamas chgd. Dr. Stone & responsible party notified.	
	2300 Sleeping s̄ distress	B. Selici RN
3-17-XX	2400-0200 Sleeping soundly. Respirations regular. Pulse 78 strong and regular.	
	0230 Awake. c/o "arthritis pain" in both hips. Acetaminophen 500 mg tabs ii given with water. Assisted to bathroom. Voided large amt. clear urine.	
	0230-0630 Slept soundly. Pulse 72 strong and regular. B/P 128/80. T 98⁶(0). Denies pain anywhere. No	
3-17-XX	other c/o distress.	P. Hernandez RN
	~~0710 Up to B.R. c̄ assistance~~ ——Error ES	E. Seldes LPN

FIGURE 8-13 The nurse's notes are a narrative record of patient care and observations. (© Delmar/Cengage Learning)

Charting Guidelines

A patient's medical record (chart) may be used in court as evidence. Everything should be correct and legible. Documentation must be clear, simple, and accurate. Entries must be printed or neatly written so that they are not misunderstood. Each patient has an individual chart. Because the chart is about only one person, there is no need to use the term *patient* or to use the patient's name. You should:

- Use phrases and fragments instead of full sentences.
- Avoid erasures and empty spaces on the record.

- Write in permanent black ink; avoid using erasable ink, ink that bleeds, and correction fluid.
- Use the correct medical terms and be sure they are spelled correctly.
- Use abbreviations that have been approved for use by your facility.
- Chart only for yourself. Never agree to document for someone else.
- Note the time when the entry is made.
  - Most health care facilities use international time (Table 8-3) to avoid confusion between AM and PM.

TABLE 8-3 INTERNATIONAL TIME

Standard Clock	International Time	Standard Clock	International Time
AM 12 midnight	2400	PM 12 noon	1200
1	0100	1	1300
2	0200	2	1400
3	0300	3	1500
4	0400	4	1600
5	0500	5	1700
6	0600	6	1800
7	0700	7	1900
8	0800	8	2000
9	0900	9	2100
10	1000	10	2200
11	1100	11	2300

Many facilities use flow sheets for documenting routine patient care. Flow sheets save time and simplify documentation. To avoid problems, you should:

- Understand what you are supposed to be documenting. Read the flow sheet carefully.
- Never initial a procedure or observation that you did not do.
- Initial the right procedure, on the right day, on the right shift.
- Put your complete signature on each flow sheet (usually at the bottom of the page).
- Remember that flow sheets are legal records just like the other forms in the medical record.
- Chart only after an event occurs or care is given. Never chart in advance.
- Notify the RN if something is missing from a computerized flow sheet. He or she will add missing information that is listed on the patient's care plan or critical pathway. For example, your facility routinely charts that patients are turned and repositioned every two hours. You routinely turn and reposition Ms. Avilla, according to her critical pathway. However, there is no place to document this important care on the flow sheet.
- If you forget to chart something or make an error, follow your facility policy for making a late entry note or correcting the error.

CONFIDENTIALITY AND PRIVACY

Each patient has a right to expect that his or her medical information will be private. The medical record is a private and confidential document. All staff must protect patient information and data from access by unauthorized persons. Likewise, avoid reading patient charts out of curiosity. Medical records may be accessed only by those with a need to know the information.

In 1996, Congress passed the **Health Insurance Portability and Accountability Act (HIPAA)**. This law has many provisions. One portion applies to privacy, confidentiality, and medical records.

The HIPAA rules protect all individually identifiable health information in any form. The rules apply to paper, verbal, and electronic documentation; billing records; and clinical (medical) records. Because of this, staff is given information on a "need to know" basis. This means that the person needs the information to carry out his or her duties. For example, the dietary department would need to know if a patient was on a diabetic diet. They would not need to know that the patient has an infectious disease. The nursing assistant would need to know about both the diabetes and the infection. Facilities must monitor how and where patient information is used.

HIPAA affects all health care communication, especially information technology (IT). Because of this, hospital systems have layers of access to patient medical records. If you will be using the computer, you will be able to access the records only for your assigned patients. Information will be limited to that which is essential to patient care. The IT department can track who is accessing any patient's record and can readily identify misuse of the system. If the facility has Internet access, the IT department will construct a firewall to ensure that sensitive patient data are not being broadcast into cyberspace.

Legal ALERT

In health care, there is a saying, "If it's not charted, it wasn't done." The purpose of documentation is to communicate the care given and the patient's response. Documentation is a true record of patient care. Never chart care that you did not provide. For example, some assistants will chart that a patient was "turned every two hours" because they know that this care is *supposed* to be given. Document only the facts. If you are unable to turn the patient every two hours, inform the nurse in advance, so he or she can arrange for help or adjust your assignment, if necessary. Do not be tempted to document this care because it is supposed to be given. Document only what you have actually done. Never document on the medical record in advance. If you forget to document, follow your facility procedure for making a late entry. Clearly mark your documentation as a late entry. ■

Infection Control ALERT

The computer, mouse, and keyboard are potential sources of cross-contamination. Microbes that cause infections can live on these surfaces, including the mouse and keyboard, for a long time. Wash your hands well before and after using the computer. When you have finished, wipe the keyboard and mouse with a disinfectant approved by the facility. Take care to avoid getting liquids inside the mouse and keyboard. If the keyboard is covered with a plastic cover, wipe the surface with a disinfectant when you have finished. ■

Documentation on the Computerized Medical Record

- Do not be afraid of the computer. Make sure you enter the correct identification code for each patient.

- Select a password that is not easily deciphered, and do not give it to anyone. Do not write it down or leave it where it is easily found, such as under the mouse pad, keyboard, or in an electronic file. Change your password promptly if you suspect that it has been compromised.

- Turn or position the monitor so it is not visible to others.

- Document only in areas you are authorized to use.

- Most hospitals have policies about using paper documentation if the computer is down. A notation is made on the electronic record if manual (paper) records are also being used. If this is the case, the records must cross-reference each other.

- Follow any reminders or error codes on the screen.

- Do not print information unnecessarily. If your facility policy requires you to retain hard copies of your documentation, print it at the end of your shift, or according to facility policy (Figure 8-14). Printing after each entry may result in a large number of partial, unusable documents that must subsequently be destroyed.

- Destroy information you have printed that is not needed. Avoid placing printouts in the wastebasket. Records are commonly destroyed by shredding them in a paper shredder.

- Electronic documentation must be signed by the person giving care. Your facility will have a procedure for electronic signatures.

- Always log off when you have finished using the computer.

- Wash your hands after using the computer, even if you type through a plastic cover. Many people use it, so the keyboard is a huge potential source of cross-contamination.

```
                              Longmeadow Subacute Care
Age/Sex: 70 F      Attending:                                                    Page 2
 Unit #: H000133357  Account #: M00850678608
Location: M.C4S      Admitted: 08/01/XX at 2005      **LIVE**        Printed 08/07/XX at 0152
Room/Bed: M. 486-B   Status: ADM IN          NURSING DAILY SUMMARY   24 hours ending 08/06/XX at 2359
```

PATIENT CARE				
	08/06 0332 KSB	08/06 0800 CIB	08/06 1200 CIB	08/06 2231 JRS
DIET				
Meal	Snack	Breakfast	Lunch	Supper
Diet	Soft	Soft	Soft	Soft
% Eaten	100	90	75	65
How Taken	Assisted by Famil	Assisted by Famil	Assisted by Famil	Total Feed by Sta
Diet Intake <50 % x	Y	Y	Y	
HYGIENE				
Bath		Sponge	Sponge	
Assistance		x1 Staff	x1 Staff	
Oral Care	Staff	Staff	Staff	Staff
Skin Care	Staff	Staff	Staff	Staff
Peri Care	Staff	Staff	Staff	Staff
Catheter Care	Not Applicable	Not Applicable	Not Applicable	Not Applicable
ACTIVITY				
Activity	Bedrest	Bedrest	Bedrest	Bedside Commode
Assistance		x1 Staff	x1 Staff	x1 Staff
Time: Hours		5	5	
Minutes				
Distance (ft)				
Tolerated		Good	Good	Fair
Repositioned	Staff	Staff	Staff	Staff
TCDB	Y	Y	Y	
SAFETY				
Siderails	Up X 4	Up X 4	Up X 4	Up X 4
Bed Low Position	Y	Y	Y	Y
Protective/Supporta	N	N	N	N
Call Light in Reach	Y	Y	Y	Y

```
 Recorded       Occurred                               Notes: All Categories
 Date   Time   Date   Time  By                                        Category

08/06/XX 0440 08/06/XX 0436 LRR                                    Nursing Notes
    INCONTINENT OF SOFT STOOL. HAD PRUNE JUICE AT HS. COOPERATIVE WITH CARE.
08/06/XX 1524 08/06/XX 0800 MW                                     Nursing Notes
    DISORIENTED X3. RESPONDS TO VEBRA STIMULI BUT SPEECH SOFT AND UNCLEAR AT TIMES.
08/06/XX 1526 08/06/XX 0800 MW                                     Nursing Notes
    GENERALIZED WEAKNESS AND REQUIRES ASSIST WITH ALL TRANSFERS.
08/06/XX 1529 08/06/XX 0800 MW                                     Nursing Notes
    UP IN CHAIR AT BEDSIDE TOL. FAIR.
08/06/XX 1529 08/06/XX 1030 MW                                     Nursing Notes
    BACK TO BED POSITIONED FOR COMFORT.
08/06/XX 1554 08/06/XX 1552 KM                                Social Service Notes
    ORDERS REC FOR HH TO FOLLOW PT AFTER DISMISSAL. SPOKE W/PT AND REVIEWED CHART. SHE WOULD LIKE SERVICES
    ARRANGED W/HOME CARE. ORDERS AND INFO WILL BE GIVEN TO AGENCY OF PT PREFERENCE CLOSER TO TIME OF DC.
08/06/XX 1732 08/06/XX 1729 BGB                               Social Service Notes
    TEAM CONFERENCE HELD ON 8-5-XX TO DISCUSS PATIENT'S CARE PLAN AND DISCHARGE NEEDS. PATIENT IS HERE FOR THERAPY
    SERVICES FOR HER ACUTE EPISODE OF WEAKNESS RELATED TO PARKINSON'S DISEASE. SHE IS CURRENTLY IN A PROGRESSIVE
    DISEASE PROCESS.. AND IS AT TIMES NOT ORIENTED TO TIME AND PLACE. ORDERS WERE WRITTEN TODAY FOR PATIENT TO
    RETURN HOME WITH HER HUSBAND, SON, AND OTHER FAMILY AND CHURCH MEMBERS TO ASSIST WITH HER CARE. THE FAMILY HAD
    CONSIDERED ASSISTED LIVING PLACEMENT. BUT DECIDED AGAINST THIS. PATIENT WILL BE TRANSPORTED HOME ON FRIDAY BY
    AMBULANCE.
```

FIGURE 8-14 Print a hard copy of your documentation at the end of the shift, or according to facility policy. Sign the document as required. Shred or destroy incomplete print copies of the record that are not needed. *(© Delmar/Cengage Learning)*

GUIDELINES *for*
Charting

- Check for right patient, right chart, right form, right room, right time.
- Fill out new headings completely.
- Use the correct color of ink.
- Date and time each entry using the time the entry is made.
- Chart entries in correct sequence.
- Make entries brief, objective, and accurate.
- Print or write clearly.
- Spell each word correctly.
- Leave no blank spaces or lines between entries.
- Do not use the term *patient*.

- Do not use ditto marks.
- Sign each entry with your first initial, last name, and job title.
- Make corrections by drawing one line through the entry; then print the word "error" on the line and your initials above.
- Make late entries when you have honestly forgotten to document something. Write them in a manner that does not appear to be self-serving. For example: *3/24/xx 1330. Late entry for 3/23/xx 1422. Vomited 150 mL clear yellow liquid. Nurse informed of emesis and documented amount on I&O record. T. Adajian, CNA.*

REVIEW

A. Multiple Choice

Select the one best answer for each of the following.

1. The purpose of the nursing process is to
   a. make a medical diagnosis.
   b. achieve patient focused care.
   c. make assignments.
   d. cure illness.

2. The nursing assistant contributes to the nurse's assessment of the patient by
   a. listening to the heart and lungs.
   b. keeping the environment neat and tidy.
   c. establishing goals for the patient.
   d. reporting observations and vital signs.

3. The statement of a patient's problem and its cause is called
   a. a medical diagnosis.
   b. an approach.
   c. an assessment.
   d. a nursing diagnosis.

4. The purpose of nursing evaluation is to determine whether the
   a. patient is reaching the goals on the care plan.
   b. laboratory and diagnostic tests are accurate.
   c. patient agrees with the critical pathway.
   d. family understands the patient's condition.

5. The purpose of making observations is to
   a. make sure the nurse gets along with the patient.
   b. inform the doctor of how the patient's family is doing.
   c. note changes in condition or new problems developing.
   d. see if the medical diagnosis is accurate.

6. An example of an objective observation is that the patient
   a. complains of abdominal pain.
   b. says she is feeling sad.
   c. has a pulse of 72. ✓
   d. says she is not hungry.

7. When you offer to give Mrs. Jones a bath, she says, "Get out of here and don't come back." You report this to the nurse and say
   a. "Mrs. Jones told me to leave her room and not come back."
   b. "Mrs. Jones is angry today."
   c. "Mrs. Jones is not cooperating with me."
   d. "Mrs. Jones does not want a bath today."

8. The form on which nurses enter daily information about the patient is called the
   a. progress notes.
   b. nurses' notes.
   c. nurses' daily log.
   d. document.

9. Charting should always be
   a. done in pencil.
   b. done after care is given.
   c. signed at least once each day.
   d. done before care is given.

10. In international time, midnight would be called
    a. 12:00 AM.
    b. 2400.
    c. 1200.
    d. 12:00 PM.

11. The HIPAA rules
    a. make it easier to share patient information with other workers.
    b. prohibit the sharing of patient information with unlicensed workers.
    c. empower the physician to specify information to disclose.
    d. restrict the use and disclosure of personal patient information.

12. Medical records and other patient data
    a. may be reviewed by nursing employees who are curious about the patient.
    b. should be accessed only by those with a need to know the information.
    c. must be used only by the physician and the RN.
    d. may be reviewed by the patient's family members, if desired.

B. Nursing Assistant Challenge

Mr. Fensten is a 47-year-old patient on the medical floor. He has had a stroke. These events occur while you are taking care of him:

- He has trouble walking because of hemiparesis (weakness from the stroke) on the right side of his body and almost falls while you are walking him to the bathroom.
- He refuses to eat his breakfast.
- He throws the washcloth across the room when you help him with his bath.
- His B/P is 146/88.
- He smiles and hugs his wife when she comes to visit.
- You do range-of-motion exercises on all joints without any problem.
- You notice a persistent reddened area on his coccyx (tailbone).

13. For each of these observations, write out the documentation exactly as you would on the patient's medical record.

14. Think about these observations and note how many examples of verbal and nonverbal communication are given.

15. Do any of these situations involve Mr. Fensten's rights as a patient? If so, describe them and the rights that apply.

UNIT 9

Meeting Basic Human Needs

OBJECTIVES

After completing this unit, you will be able to:
- Spell and define terms.
- Describe the stages of human growth and development.
- List five physical needs of patients.
- Define self-esteem.

- List nursing assistant actions to ensure that patients have the opportunity for intimacy.
- Explain why cultural and spiritual beliefs influence patients' psychological responses.
- List some guidelines to assist patients in meeting their spiritual needs.

VOCABULARY

Learn the meaning and the correct spelling of the following words and phrases:

adolescence	growth	neonate	sexuality
bisexuality	heterosexuality	personality	tasks
coitus	homosexuality	preadolescence	toddler
continuum	intimacy	reflexes	transgender
development	masturbation	self-esteem	

INTRODUCTION

Each of us has things that we need to live successfully. These are called *needs* simply because we cannot get along without them. When patients are admitted to the hospital, they bring their needs too. The difference now is in the way those needs are expressed and fulfilled. Expression and fulfillment have to be different because of the hospital environment and the illness. Remember that the basic needs remain the same, regardless of how they are expressed or how they have to be met because of an individual's level of development or state of health.

Age Appropriate Care ALERT

Avoid stereotyping patients based on their age or other characteristics, such as skin color, religion, or sexual preference. Provide patient-focused care by treating each patient as an individual. A key part of your job is the ability to recognize each patient's unique needs and abilities. ■

HUMAN GROWTH AND DEVELOPMENT

Human beings change as they age, through the processes of growth and development. **Growth** involves the changes that take place in the body. It is usually measured by height and weight and degree of system maturation. **Development** involves the changes that take place on the social, emotional, and psychological levels. Behavior and interpersonal skills indicate a person's developmental level.

People move from one level of development to the next (Table 9-1). At each level, they change in both the way they look and the way they think and act (Figure 9-1). Each level presents tasks that must be mastered before the person can move on to the next level. The **tasks** to be mastered are those things that lead to healthy and satisfactory participation in society. The tasks are defined by the needs of the individual and the pressures of society.

Growth and development follow a set of basic principles of progression:

- There is continuous movement from simple to more complex. For example, baby sounds progress to speech patterns.
- Development and growth move from head to feet and from torso to limbs. The infant first raises the head, then sits, stands, and finally walks.
- At each stage of development, the person has a set of tasks to master before moving on to the next level.

TABLE 9-1 STAGES OF GROWTH AND DEVELOPMENT

Neonate	Birth to 1 month
Infancy	1 month to 2 years
Toddler	2 years to 3 years
Preschool	3 years to 5 years
School Age	5 years to 12 years
Preadolescence	12 years to 14 years
Adolescence	14 years to 20 years
Adulthood	20 years to 49 years
Middle Age	50 years to 64 years
Later Maturity	65 years to 75 years
Old Age	75 years and beyond
Old Old	Category used by some experts to describe those aged 85 and older

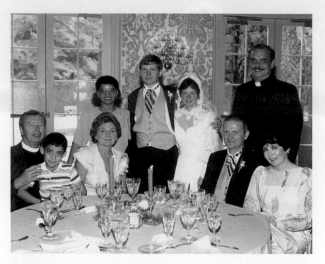

FIGURE 9-1 The characteristics of different age groups are reflected in this family picture. *(Courtesy of Mary Ellen Estes)*

- The rate of progression varies for each person.
- Growth patterns progress at the person's own individual rate.

Review the tables for age-appropriate care in the Online Companion to this book.

Neonatal and Infant Period (Birth to Two Years)

The neonatal and infant period extends through the first two years of life. It is a time of rapid physical growth and development. The infant gradually learns to:

- Sit
- Crawl
- Stand
- Take first steps

Other changes also occur during this period:

- Moves from self-awareness and parental attachment toward ties with others
- Systems that are relatively immature at birth stabilize
- Alertness and activity increase
- Teeth appear (erupt)
- Food intake progresses from milk to solid food
- Verbal skills begin to develop.

Age Appropriate Care ALERT

Communicate with an infant (newborn to 12 months) by smiling, being gentle, hugging, rocking, and touching. Speak softly and slowly or sing quietly during care. ■

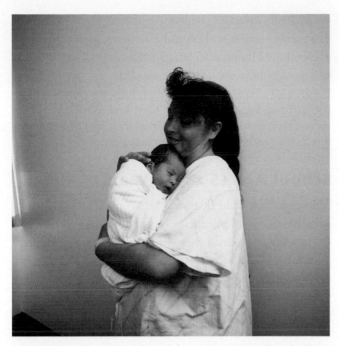

FIGURE 9-2 Newborn infant (neonate). *(© Delmar/Cengage Learning)*

The mother is usually the primary caregiver, or central figure of the infant's emotional attachment. Growth and development progress so rapidly that changes can be seen each month.

The **neonate** (newborn) (Figure 9-2):

- Weighs 7–8 pounds.
- Is approximately 20–21 inches long.
- Has a head that seems disproportionately large compared to the body.
- Has skin that is wrinkled, thin, and red.
- Has an abdomen that seems to stick out (protrude).
- Has dark blue eyes.

In the newborn, the:

- Conversion of cartilage to bone is not complete. This can be seen in the soft spots (fontanels) and suture lines (joints) of the skull.
- The nervous system is not fully developed, so muscular activities are uncoordinated.
- Vision is not clear, but hearing and taste are developed. Certain **reflexes** (automatic responses) are also developed. They are the:
  - Moro reflex—when a loud noise startles the infant, the arms are spread across the chest, the legs are extended, and the head is thrust back. This response is also called the *startle reflex*.
  - Grasp reflex—touching the infant's palm causes the fingers to flex in a grasping motion.
  - Rooting (sucking) reflex—stroking the cheek or side of the lips stimulates the infant to turn its head in the direction of the stroking. This is important in finding the nipple to suck the milk.

- Diet is milk or milk substitute.
- Routine is largely sleeping, eating, and eliminating.

The infant is unable to support her head, so she must be handled carefully and be well supported when held.

A three-month-old infant:

- Can hold her head up and raise her shoulders.
- Has lost the Moro, rooting, and grasp reflexes.
- Produces real tears.
- Can follow objects with the eyes.
- Can smile and coo at the caregiver.

The six-month-old infant:

- Has learned to roll over.
- Can sit for short periods of time.
- Holds things with both hands and directs them toward the mouth.
- Responds with verbal sounds when a caregiver speaks.
- Begins to cut front teeth.
- Eats finger foods and strained fruits and vegetables.
- Recognizes family members.
- Develops fear of strangers.

The nine-month-old infant:

- Crawls and may begin to stand when supported.
- Has more teeth erupt.
- Can respond to her name.
- Says one- and two-syllable words such as "mama."
- Shows a preference for right- or left-hand control.
- Eats junior baby foods.

The one-year-old infant:

- Understands simple commands such as "No."
- Begins to take steps—supported at first, then independently.
- Eats table foods and can hold her own cup.
- Weighs three times the original birth weight.

Toddler Period (Two to Three Years)

The **toddler** period is a busy, active phase. Motor abilities develop (Figure 9-3) and vocabulary and comprehension increase. The toddler:

- Learns to control elimination.
- Starts learning the difference between right and wrong.
- May respond negatively to attempts at socialization and discipline.
- Tolerates brief periods of separation from the mother.
- May play in the company of other children but with no interaction. This age group is very possessive. "No" and "mine" are major parts of their vocabularies.

Reaching the end of this period, the toddler is able to:

- Walk and run.
- Use motor (manual) skills for activities such as feeding and riding toys.

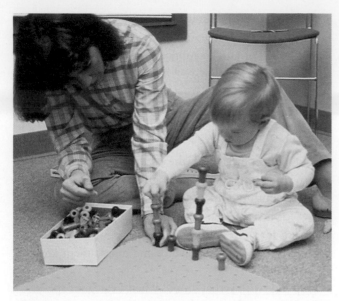

FIGURE 9-3 The toddler begins to develop gross motor skills. *(Photo courtesy of Henrietta Egleston Hospital for Children, Atlanta, GA. Photograph by Ginger Lovering.)*

- Put words together and speak more clearly. The average vocabulary of a two-year-old is about 300 words.

Preschool Years (Three to Five Years)

The three- to five-year-old (Figure 9-4) builds on the motor and verbal skills developed as a toddler. The preschooler:

- Grows less reliant on the mother; begins to recognize his position as a family member and his uniqueness from other members.
- Develops rivalries with siblings and develops greater attachments to the father or alternate caregiver.

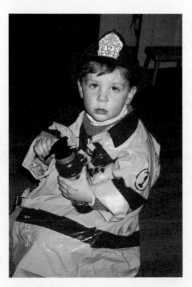

FIGURE 9-4 This child is expanding his awareness of the world. *(© Delmar/Cengage Learning)*

- Gradually increases cooperative play.
- Improves language skills and asks many questions.
- Develops a more active imagination.
- Becomes more sexually curious.

By the end of this period, children have become far more socialized and cooperative than they were as toddlers. They seem eager to follow the rules within limits. They enjoy interacting with family members and peers.

School Age (5 to 12 Years)

The school-age child (Figure 9-5):

- Is able to communicate.
- Has developed small (fine) motor skills that are needed to master tasks such as writing.
- Develops an increased sense of self.
- Establishes peer relationships.
- Reinforces proper social behavior through games, simple tasks, and play.
- Chooses sex-differentiated friends.
- Joins groups like Scouts. This helps the child identify with others of a particular gender, and provides security and a sense of belonging.
- Begins to show concern for other living things (Figure 9-6).

Preadolescence (12 to 14 Years)

Preadolescence is a period of great change and uncertainty. During this period:

- Hormones stimulate the development of secondary sex characteristics.
- The child feels on the threshold of tremendous change, though not yet in a period of sexual functioning.
- Mood swings and feelings of insecurity are common.
- There is a growing awareness of and interest in the opposite sex.
- Arms and legs seem out of proportion to the rest of the body.

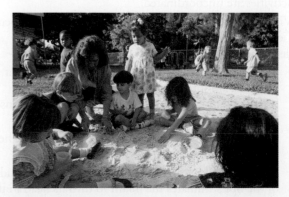

FIGURE 9-5 School-age children like to play in peer groups. *(© Delmar/Cengage Learning)*

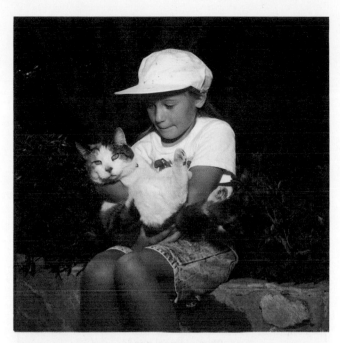

FIGURE 9-6 Young children learn to reach out and have concern for others. (© Delmar/Cengage Learning)

Adolescence (14 to 20 Years)

Adolescence is marked by:

- The gradual development of sexual maturity.
- A greater appreciation of one's own identity as a male or a female person.
- Conflicting desires for the freedom of independence and the security of dependence. This may be a source of conflict.
- The establishment of personal coping systems and the ability to make independent judgments and decisions.
- Gradual success in mastering developmental tasks. The person may compare the values learned at home and school with reality.

Adulthood (20 to 49 Years)

Early adulthood is marked by:

- Independence and personal decision making.
- The choice of a mate.
- Establishment of a career and family life.
- Optimal health.
- The choice of friends to form a support group.

Middle Age (50 to 64 Years)

Middle age is associated with:

- Final career advancement, ending in retirement.
- Children leaving home to enter their own adult period.
- Health that is usually good, although chronic diseases may develop during this period.

- More time for leisure activities.
- More time and money to pursue personal interests.
- Revitalizing one's relationship with a mate.
- Enjoying grandchildren.
- For some middle-aged persons, being a member of the "sandwich" generation—caring for both their own parents and their children or grandchildren.

Later Maturity (65 to 75 Years)

Later maturity is marked by:

- A gradual loss of vitality and stamina.
- Physical changes of aging (for example, sight and hearing diminish).
- Chronic conditions that develop and persist.
- A period of gradual losses: loss of mate, friends, self-esteem, some independence.
- Examination of a lifetime.
- More time to pursue personal interests.
- Fewer responsibilities related to raising a family and holding a job.
- Increased wisdom.

Old Age (75 Years and Beyond)

Old age is frequently characterized by:

- Failing health and growing dependency (Figure 9-7).
- Coping with illness, loneliness, loss of friends and loved ones, and the realization of mortality.

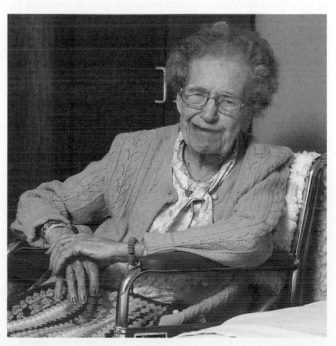

FIGURE 9-7 Physical status often declines in old age. (© Delmar/Cengage Learning)

Successful development in old age depends on the coping mechanisms that the person has developed over a lifetime. Emotional and physical support are also important.

Aging is a gradual process that begins at birth. Old age can be a period of development and enjoyment.

BASIC HUMAN NEEDS

Developmental skills and physical growth may vary during the life span. The basic human needs, however, are much the same for every individual.

Basic human needs are the things and activities that all persons require to successfully and satisfactorily live their lives. These needs are the same for everyone. Culture influences the way in which individuals express these basic needs. *Culture* refers to customs and practices that are common to groups of people. Culture affects language, dialect and accent, dietary habits, health practices, expressions of spirituality, and ways of celebrating. Cultural patterns help to make each person unique and must be considered when providing patient care.

Abraham Maslow and Erik Erikson are two leaders in the field of human behavior. They have helped us understand basic needs and how people go about satisfying them.

Personality

The method each person uses to satisfy personal psychological needs reflects his or her personality. **Personality** is the sum of the ways we react to events in our lives. It develops gradually through experience and is molded by cultural heritage, and through mastery of developmental tasks.

Maslow placed the needs on a **continuum** showing that physical needs must be satisfied before psychological or sociological needs become important (Figure 9-8). This progression is called a *hierarchy of needs.*

 ## PHYSICAL NEEDS

The most basic human needs are physical needs. They include:

- Oxygen
- Nutrition
- Rest
- Shelter
- Elimination
- Activity
- Sexuality

Illness at any age creates stresses that make meeting the needs a challenge for both patient and caregivers.

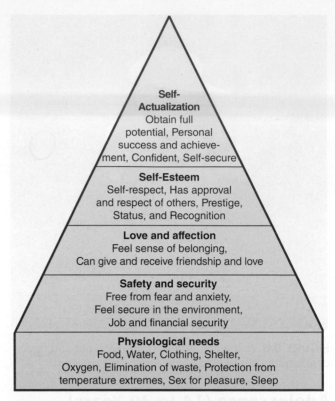

FIGURE 9-8 Maslow's hierarchy of needs. Lower-level needs must be satisfied before higher-level needs become important. (© *Delmar/Cengage Learning*)

Meeting the Patient's Physical Needs

There are times when you must provide for the physical needs of your patients. These include the need to breathe, to eat, to eliminate waste products, to sleep, to be sheltered, and to engage in physical activity.

Oxygen Most of us take breathing for granted. We seldom think of it until it becomes difficult. Many things can cause difficult breathing. When a person has difficulty, the need is always the same. The body cannot live without oxygen, which is found in the air. It may be necessary to give the patient extra oxygen to nourish the body. Oxygen is given through cannula, mask, or another device for this purpose (Figure 9-9). Sometimes the need can be met by supporting the patient with pillows while he or she leans across the overbed table, making breathing easier.

Food Patients may lose their appetites when they are in the hospital. Some patients must be spoon-fed. Others must be given special foods. Some are given liquid nourishment through a feeding tube. Fluid replacement may also be given through a sterile tube into the veins. Because patients receive nourishment in such a variety of ways, you must meet the special needs of each individual. To help ensure that the need for food is met, prepare the patient for meals and assist with toileting. Assist with washing the

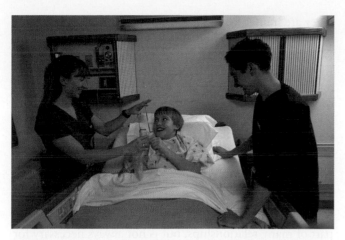

FIGURE 9-9 Allowing a child to play with the equipment before she has to use it is a good approach for decreasing fear. *(Stock image)*

hands and face and providing oral care. Eliminate unpleasant sights and odors, and position the person in a comfortable position with the head elevated as much as possible. Serve food at the proper temperature. Be sure it is accessible by assisting with removing packages, cutting food, and providing condiments as the patient desires. Be sure the person can reach the food. Be available to assist with feeding, if needed.

Elimination To stay healthy, the body must be able to rid itself of waste products, such as perspiration, urine, and feces. You will assist the patient with meeting elimination needs, toileting, and bathing to eliminate waste products from the skin.

Shelter In the health care facility, you meet the patient's need to be sheltered when you help maintain the proper environment. This means keeping the room at the proper temperature, and ensuring that it is safe and comfortable.

Physical activity People, by nature, are active beings. Illness almost always limits activity. Some patients must stay in bed for a long time. Staff must find ways of providing appropriate activity for each person. The patient's ability and treatment goals must be considered when initiating activities.

You may be assigned to assist patients with activities, such as walking (Figure 9-10), getting into and out of bed, and using the bedpan or commode. Review the care plan and become familiar with each patient's abilities, limitations, and the degree and type of activity allowed. Encourage patients to be as independent as possible, but monitor to be sure they do not become stressed or tired.

SECURITY AND SAFETY NEEDS

If physical needs are not met, the person will not be concerned with safety. Once physical needs are met, safety and security become priorities. You will meet security and

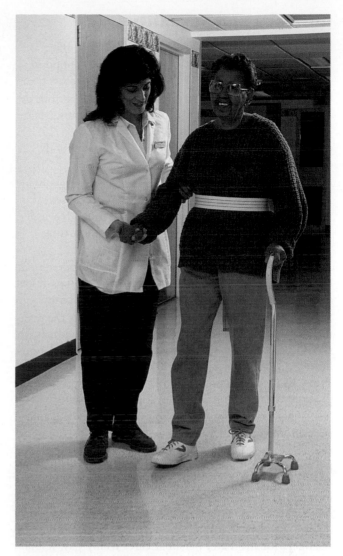

FIGURE 9-10 This patient needs minimal assistance with ambulation. *(© Delmar/Cengage Learning)*

safety needs by maintaining a safe environment, knowing how to respond to emergencies, and implementing the patient's care plan as indicated.

EMOTIONAL NEEDS

The third and fourth levels of Maslow's hierarchy relate to emotional needs, including the need for love and belonging and the need for esteem. Each person has a need to give and receive love and be treated with respect.

All individuals have a mental picture of the image they project or wish to project to others. How we feel about ourselves and the image we believe we project to others is **self-esteem**. A person's self-esteem must be protected at all costs. You will help meet patients' emotional needs by providing privacy when the person wants to be alone or has visitors, and by treating all patients with consideration, respect, and dignity.

Intimacy and Sexuality

Some terms related to human sexual expression are:

- **Heterosexuality**—sexual attraction between opposite sexes.
- **Homosexuality**—sexual attraction between persons of the same sex. Female partners are called lesbians. Male partners are often referred to as gay.
- **Bisexuality**—sexual attraction to members of both sexes.
- **Transgender**—A person whose personal feelings about gender identity do not match the anatomical sex the person was born with. These individuals feel as if they were born with a physical body of the wrong gender.

Intimacy is a feeling of closeness with another human (Figure 9-11). It is a relationship marked by feelings of love and affection. It is an integral part of human response.

Sexuality is a lifelong characteristic that defines the maleness or femaleness of each person. All individuals are sexual, whether or not they have physical sexual relations. Sexuality has to do with the ability to develop relationships, to give of oneself to others, and to appreciate the giving by others. Intimacy is one aspect of sexuality.

Sexual behavior is a personal choice, but intimacy is an important aspect of the human sexual experience. Some patients will have same-sex partners. Others will select a partner of the opposite sex. One's choice of sexual partners and sexual preference is a very complex subject. Avoid judging the patient's choice of a partner. This is especially important with members of the gay, lesbian, and transgender community. Most people worry about depending on strangers for intimate, personal care. Many gay, lesbian, and transgender persons have been insulted, isolated, disrespected, and shunned when seeking health care services, and they fear that they will be treated badly or ignored.

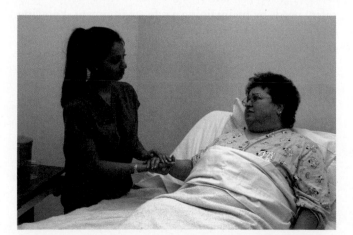

FIGURE 9-11 Everyone needs intimacy and human touch. This is important regardless of the patient's age or appearance. If in doubt about the patient's response, ask her permission to touch or hug her. *(© Delmar/Cengage Learning)*

They are human beings above all else, and as such deserve to be cared for with compassion and respect.

Being old, ill, or disabled does not diminish human sexuality. However, our society tends to associate youth, beauty, and physical agility with sexuality. Remember that the person within a human being does not change. Although the hair is gray, the person inside still has feelings and longing for love, affection, and intimacy.

The range of ways to express love is enormous. Caressing, exchange of loving gestures, talking, hugging, and touching are all ways love is expressed between people. Some people practice **masturbation**, which is self-stimulation for sexual pleasure. **Coitus** (intercourse) may be an enjoyable part of many relationships, but is not always necessary for satisfaction.

It is not always easy to provide opportunities for patients to meet sexual and intimacy needs in a health care setting. Nursing assistants can help patients meet sexual and intimacy needs by:

- Respecting privacy. Always knock and wait before opening a closed door.
- Speaking before opening the bedside curtains.
- Not judging behaviors and practices as wrong.
- Not discussing personal sexual information about a patient with others.

PATIENT PRIVACY

Patients in a health care facility give up a good bit of control over their lives. They put their lives and well-being into the hands of caregivers. In exchange, patients assume that certain of their rights will be assured. These rights include the right to privacy.

Patients must feel certain that their privacy will be protected. Even though you perform the most intimate procedures for them, you must do so in a way that neither exposes them unnecessarily nor embarrasses them.

Assist with meeting privacy needs by knocking and saying the person's name before entering the room. Use curtains and screens around the bed during personal care. Cover the body with a bath blanket and expose only the area you are currently working on. Speak before entering a screened area. Recognize a patient's need for privacy and do your best to provide it.

SPIRITUAL NEEDS

Spiritual beliefs are deeply held by some patients and disregarded by others. Some personal items may have special religious significance and must be treated with respect.

Patients' spiritual needs are often greater when they are fearful and ill (Figure 9-12). Inform the nurse if a patient requests a clergy visit or spiritual support. Do not impose your beliefs on the patient.

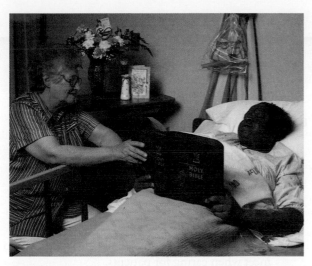

FIGURE 9-12 Spiritual needs may be greater during illness. (© Delmar/Cengage Learning)

Remember that each person has a right to believe in any faith system or to deny the existence of any beliefs. Listen to the patient's thoughts and keep them confidential. Reflect the patient's ideas. Do not try to convince the patient of your own ideas. For example, if the patient asks if you believe in God, reflect the patient's thinking with a statement such as "You have been thinking about God," or "Would you like to talk?" Patients may request clergy visits or ask about chapel services. Know what services are available to your patients. When asked, share this information, but do not recommend any particular service. Provide privacy during clergy visits.

SOCIAL NEEDS

When primary physical, psychological, and spiritual needs have been met, the person is free to pursue the fourth level of social needs and activities that are unique to the individual. These activities make one feel good as a person and increase self-esteem.

One of the most basic needs of all people is the need to understand others and to be understood. We achieve this sense of understanding when we communicate successfully with others. We do this by communicating verbally, with body language, and through touch. Being interested and unhurried in talking with patients makes it easier for patients to say what they need. This approach also makes it easier for the staff to find proper ways to fulfill these needs.

HUMAN TOUCH

The need for human touch is very strong and very important. This pleasurable sensation begins at birth when the mother and child touch one another. The same human feelings are also experienced by adults.

Age Appropriate Care ALERT

You will learn how aging affects each body system, and the person as a whole. Normal changes of aging affect the way the human body functions. Look at each patient *holistically*. This means to look at the entire person and realize that something that affects one part or body system affects the person as a whole. For example, aging changes in vision and hearing may cause an alert person to seem confused and disoriented. Some aging changes cause the person to feel loss of control and loss of self-care ability. Changes in the environment of an elderly person may cause confusion, changes in behavior, feelings of loss of control, stress, and sleep disturbances. (This problem may be referred to as *transfer trauma*.) An acute illness may cause mental confusion, changes in behavior, and loss of self-esteem. The nursing assistant must:

- Report changes in condition to the nurse promptly.
- Understand that aging changes are beyond the patient's control.
- Help the person adapt to aging changes as much as possible, so he or she functions at the highest level possible. ■

As people age, they have fewer opportunities for touch. People may feel deprived and lonely. A friendly hug and smile, a pat on the shoulder, a clasp of a hand, and a backrub are ways that nursing assistants can satisfy the patient's need for human contact. Never force your attentions on a patient, but be open to nonsexual touching. It can mean much to the lives of those in your care.

You will learn that wearing gloves is sometimes necessary for the procedures you must do. Sometimes caregivers apply gloves as soon as they enter the room and wear the gloves for all care. There are times when this is necessary, but wearing gloves is not necessary or desirable in most patient care situations. In fact, wearing the same pair of gloves for many different activities poses a major risk of cross-contamination. Remove used gloves before touching side rails, counters, doorknobs, faucets, and so forth. Wearing gloves may send a message that the patient is undesirable, untouchable, or highly infectious. Avoid offending patients with unnecessary use of gloves. Balance your infection control precautions with patients' emotional needs for love, belonging, and acceptance.

REVIEW

A. Multiple Choice

Select the one best answer for each of the following.

1. Growth and development
   a. move from limbs to torso and feet to head.
   b. involve more complex tasks during growth spurts.
   c. can proceed normally even if tasks are not mastered.
   d. have specific tasks that must be mastered at each stage.

2. The main activity (activities) of the toddler period is (are)
   a. exploration and investigation.
   b. cooperative play.
   c. establishing peer relationships.
   d. showing concern for others.

3. Preschoolers are
   a. less reliant on their mothers.
   b. able to join groups like Scouts.
   c. able to choose sex-differentiated friends.
   d. unable to tolerate brief separation from the mother.

4. The ways in which we react to the events in our lives are called
   a. personality.
   b. self-identity.
   c. tasks of personality development.
   d. hierarchy of needs.

5. The human needs that must be satisfied first, before others become important, are
   a. spiritual.
   b. safety.
   c. mental.
   d. physical.

6. If a patient is masturbating behind the closed bedside curtain, you should
   a. leave the room.
   b. notify the nurse.
   c. tell the patient to stop.
   d. cover the patient with a blanket.

7. Persons in the "later maturity" age group are
   a. 50 to 64 years old.
   b. 65 to 75 years old.

c. 76 to 84 years old.
d. 85 years old and over.

8. Social needs
   a. can be met only after physical, spiritual, and psychological needs have been met.
   b. must be met for the person to have the ability to communicate with others.
   c. are among the most important needs on the second level of the Maslow hierarchy.
   d. are among the most important low-level needs to meet when caring for patients.

9. Elderly patients
   a. usually get mad if they are touched.
   b. have forgotten the meaning of gentle touch.
   c. have few opportunities to be touched.
   d. no longer have the need to be touched.

10. Sexual preference is:
    a. not an issue with elderly persons.
    b. very important to preadolescents.
    c. a low priority in patient care.
    d. unrelated to basic human needs.

B. Nursing Assistant Challenge

Mrs. McClendon is a 35-year-old patient with a diagnosis of breast cancer. She recently had a radical mastectomy (extensive breast and tissue removal). She has lost most of her hair and has no appetite as a result of chemotherapy. Mrs. McClendon has lost weight and has occasional severe pain. She has a husband and three young children. Consider the needs that all people have and think about Mrs. McClendon.

11. Which of this patient's physical needs may be difficult to meet? What can the nursing staff do to help Mrs. McClendon meet these needs?

12. Do you think her need for safety and security will be met? What information do you have indicating that she has reason to feel fear and anxiety?

13. How might Mrs. McClendon's condition affect her relationship with her husband and children?

14. How do you think her sexuality may be affected?

15. Maslow states that human needs are on a hierarchy. Describe how this hierarchy may change throughout the day for Mrs. McClendon.

Comfort, Pain, Rest, and Sleep

OBJECTIVES

After completing this unit, you will be able to:

- Spell and define terms.
- Explain how loud noise affects patients and hospital staff.
- Explain why nursing comfort measures are important to patients' well-being.

- List six observations to make and report for patients having pain.
- State the purpose of the pain rating scale and briefly describe how a pain scale is used.
- Describe nursing assistant measures to increase comfort, relieve pain, and promote rest and sleep.

VOCABULARY

Learn the meaning and the correct spelling of the following words and phrases:

analgesic	guarding	rest
comfort	pain	sleep

 ## PATIENT COMFORT

All humans need comfort, rest, and sleep for physical and emotional well-being, health, and wellness. **Comfort** is a state of physical and emotional well-being. The patient is calm and relaxed, and is not in pain or upset. Assisting patients with their comfort needs is a major nursing assistant responsibility. In fact, assisting patients with physical and emotional comfort needs is at the heart of nursing care.

Many factors affect patient comfort. Environmental factors that interfere with comfort are unfamiliar environment, lack of privacy, noise, odor, temperature, lighting, and ventilation. Personal and uncontrollable factors that may increase or contribute to discomfort include age, activity, injury, illness, surgery, stress, and pain.

As a rule, patients are uncomfortable when their physical and emotional needs are not met. Unmet needs cause tension and anxiety, and interfere with comfort and rest (Figure 10-1). Using basic nursing measures to meet patients' needs promotes comfort, aids in relaxation, and provides a sense of well-being.

NOISE CONTROL

Florence Nightingale is considered the founder of modern nursing. In *Notes on Nursing*, she wrote, "Unnecessary noise is the most cruel abuse of care which can be inflicted on either the sick or the well."[1] Miss Nightingale would be aghast at the high-tech world of the 21st century. We have

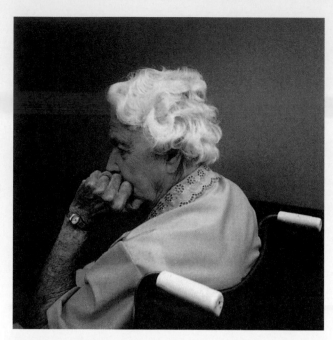

FIGURE 10-1 This patient's body language betrays the anxiety she is feeling. (© *Delmar/Cengage Learning*)

TABLE 10-1 AVERAGE NOISE LEVELS

Noise in Decibels (dB)	Source
194	loudest tone possible
180	rocket launch
165	12-gauge shotgun
140	jet engine at takeoff
120	ambulance siren
110	chainsaw
105	bulldozer, spray painter
96	tractor
90	hair dryer, power lawn mower
80	ringing telephone
60	normal conversation
30	whisper
0	weakest sound heard by the average human ear

Modified from National Institute for Occupational Safety and Health (NIOSH). (2001). General estimates of work-related noises. Retrieved November 15, 2004, from http://www.cdc.gov/niosh/01-104.html.

alarms on most medical equipment and electronic technology that did not exist in the 19th century. Even without considering alarms, some medical equipment is very noisy.

Comfort, rest, and sleep are important for patient well-being. Excessive noise delays healing, impairs immune function, and increases the heart rate and blood pressure. Patients may feel very anxious, and may not realize that noise is the cause of their distress. Patients who do not sleep well at night may be unhappy with care, and may be unable to fully participate in daytime activities and therapy because they are sleepy. Some patients become confused and agitated when deprived of sleep. Confused patients may begin wandering to escape noise.

The Occupational Safety and Health Administration (OSHA) has established noise standards for employee safety. Workers should not be exposed to 90 decibels of sound for more than eight hours. Average noise levels are listed in Table 10-1. The Environmental Protection Agency (EPA) recommends that hospital noise levels not exceed 45 decibels during the day. Examples of various types of noise are pictured in Figure 10-2.

A study done by the staff of one hospital unit has direct application to nursing assistant practice.[2] In this study, nurse researchers were admitted to the hospital as patients. They measured noise levels during the night. The workers on the unit did not know that noise was being measured. During the study, decibel levels as high as 113 were recorded at night. The noisiest time was at shift change. The two "nurse patients" stated that the noise kept them from falling asleep. Other routine noises awakened them at night. Noises that were tolerable during the day were more disruptive at night.

An uncomfortable noise level has been called an invasion of privacy by some patients. This is a concern because the patient is powerless to control the disturbing noise. A 1960 study at Johns Hopkins Hospital revealed that the average noise level was 57 decibels. A repeat study in 2005 found that the noise had increased to 72 decibels.[3] In 1995, the World Health Organization (WHO) recommended keeping noise levels below 35 decibels in hospitals and other health care facilities. However, a study of Houston-area long-term care facilities in 2005 revealed noise levels from 70 to 101 decibels. This is not significantly different from the noise levels in hospitals and other types of facilities. Most of the staff complained of feeling agitated and irritable, and were more likely to make errors when noise was excessive.[4] When the unit is noisy, patients and staff must speak louder to be heard over background noise. Noise contributes to stress and exhaustion.

Active listening requires focusing on the conversation. Health care workers must be active listeners, whether they are listening to patients or coworkers. Active listening is work. Having to speak louder and be even more attentive

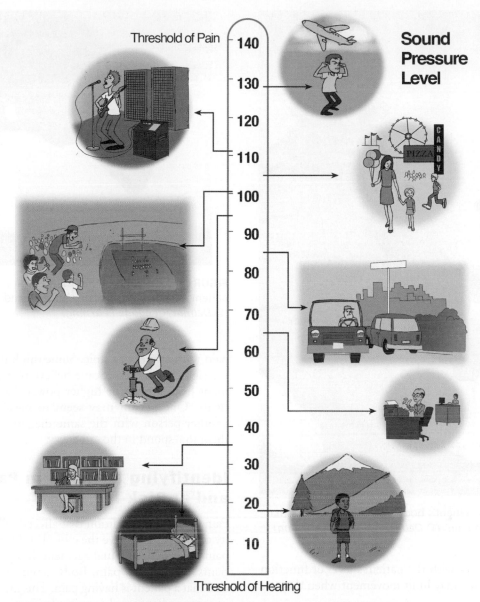

Threshold of Pain

Sound Pressure Level

Threshold of Hearing

FIGURE 10-2 Sound intensity generated by various activities. One study showed that hospital noises during the night were as loud as jackhammers and chainsaws, making it difficult for patients to sleep. Simple steps, such as closing doors to patients' rooms and muffling the clatter of clipboards and metal charts, help reduce noise. (*© Delmar/Cengage Learning*)

when listening are leading causes of staff fatigue. Reducing noise improves working conditions for staff and quality of care for patients. The effects of noise and sleep deprivation are areas in which additional study is needed, but it is safe to say that research proves that noise is disruptive. Do all you can to reduce and manage noise on your unit.

✳ PAIN

Pain (Figure 10-3) is a state of discomfort that is unpleasant for the patient. Pain is always a warning that something

Age Appropriate Care ALERT

The golden rule for pain relief is that whatever is painful to adults is painful to children unless proven otherwise. Never lie to a child when asked if a procedure will hurt. Admit that it will, but reassure the child that you will help make him or her as comfortable as possible. ■

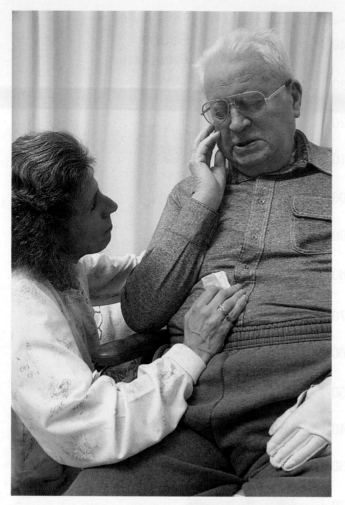

FIGURE 10-3 This patient's body language suggests that he is having severe pain. (© Delmar/Cengage Learning)

is wrong. It interferes with the patient's level of function and self-care. Patients may limit movement when they are having pain.

Pain decreases quality of life, and may cause hopelessness, helplessness, anxiety, and depression. Pain may cause problem behavior in both children and adults. It slows recovery and increases health care costs.

Pain causes stress and interferes with comfort, rest, and sleep (Figure 10-4). Rest and sleep are necessary for the body to repair itself and to restore strength and energy. *Insomnia* (inability to sleep) may be caused by pain.

Patients' Responses to Pain

Patients' responses to pain vary widely. Some do not feel pain as acutely as others. Some try to ignore pain. Other patients may try to deny pain because they are afraid of what it means. Ignoring or denying pain increases the risk of injury because the patient does not act on the warning that pain provides.

Patients' responses to pain may be related to culture. People from some cultures are very emotional when they are in

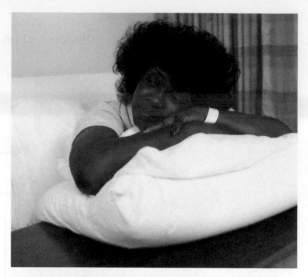

FIGURE 10-4 Although her expression is stoic, the patient cannot sleep because of pain and anxiety. (© Delmar/Cengage Learning)

pain. Others are very stoic. Some think that showing pain is a sign of weakness. Some believe that pain is a punishment from a deity or higher power. Never compare patients. One person may seem to have more pain than another person with the same diagnosis. Do not expect them to respond in the same way.

Identifying Patients in Pain and at Risk for Pain

Pain is a serious condition that affects well-being and quality of life. Patients have the ethical and legal right to timely pain assessment and management. Many factors affect patients' reactions to pain. Body language is often the first clue that a patient is having pain. This may be the only clue in some pediatric and cognitively impaired patients, those from other cultures, and patients who are comatose. Look for pain upon movement, facial expressions, crying, moaning, rigid posture, and guarded positioning. **Guarding** is an unconscious, protective action, position, or movement to shield a painful or injured area. The patient may withdraw when he or she is touched or repositioned. Watch for restlessness, irregular or erratic respirations, intermittent breath holding, dilated pupils, and sweating. The patient may favor one extremity. He or she may become irritable, fatigued, or withdrawn. The patient may refuse to eat for no apparent reason. The patient may act opposite of normal.

Never ignore body language or other signs of pain in patients. Use nursing measures to make the patient comfortable. Always report pain to the nurse. Signs and symptoms of pain to report to the nurse are listed in Table 10-2.

Always suspect pain if the patient's behavior changes. Report your observations to the nurse as comparisons with the normal behavior for the patient. If the behavior

TABLE 10-2 SIGNS AND SYMPTOMS OF PAIN THAT SHOULD BE REPORTED TO THE NURSE IMMEDIATELY

- Chest pain
- Pain that radiates
- Pain upon movement
- Pain during urination
- Pain when having a bowel movement
- Splinting an area upon movement
- Grimacing, or facial expressions suggesting pain
- Body language suggesting pain
- Unrelieved pain after pain medication has been given

changes back to normal after the nurse administers an **analgesic** (pain) medication, this confirms that the change in body language or behavior was caused by pain.

Although many patients with pain display outward signs through their body language and behavior, avoid making assumptions about the presence or absence of pain if the person is laughing, talking, or sleeping. For example, some health care workers assume that patients who are smiling or laughing cannot be in pain. These workers believe that patients who are having pain should be grimacing, frowning, or crying. This is untrue. Some patients may appear comfortable even while they are having severe pain. Vital signs may be normal. Accept that pain is whatever the person says it is.

The patient's self-report is the most accurate and reliable indicator of the existence and intensity of pain, and should be respected and believed. Never question the validity of a patient's complaints. Notify the nurse. Describe the pain using the patient's exact words. When asking about pain, use words the person is likely to understand, and make sure the patient can see and hear you. Allow enough time for the patient to process your questions and respond. Be patient.

Remember that patients may use different words for pain, such as "hurt," "sore," or "tender." Children and patients who are mentally confused may surprise you. Some can describe their pain accurately. Always ask patients who are crying, who display body language suggesting pain, or whose behavior suggests pain.

Pain is *never* normal; *all* complaints of pain should be reported to the nurse promptly.

Pain Assessment Scales

Many different pain scales are used in health care. In most facilities, several different pain scales are available. The scale is a tool for communication. Pain scales use pictures, words, or numbers to help the person describe pain intensity. (The scales shown in Figures 10-5A and 10-5B are only examples.) The patient selects the scale that best helps her describe the pain. Using a pain scale keeps everyone informed as to the level and intensity of the patient's pain.

Many facilities use a 0 to 10 scale, with 0 meaning no pain and 10 meaning intolerable pain. If the patient tells you that she is having pain at "level 5," for example, you must know what this means and report the problem to the nurse. Likewise, if the patient complains of pain at "level 9" an hour after receiving pain medication, this suggests a potentially serious problem and must be reported immediately.

If a patient has been medicated for pain, but continues to complain, inform the nurse. Do not assume that the pain has been relieved after a medication has been given, even if the patient is laughing or talking. Ask the patient. If he or she admits to continued pain, the nurse must assess the patient further.

Avoid judging patients who take narcotic medications to control their pain. Many health care workers try to discourage patients from taking these drugs because of the potential for addiction. Studies have shown that very few patients with severe pain become addicted to these drugs.

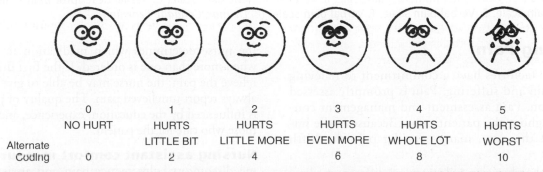

FIGURE 10-5A Each patient will select the pain rating scale that best helps describe the level and intensity of pain. The FACES scale is excellent for children and adults, as well as patients who do not speak English. *(FACES Pain Rating Scale from Hockenberry, M. J., Wilson, D., & Winkelstein, M. L. (2005). Wong's essentials of pediatric nursing, ed. 7. St. Louis: Mosby, p. 1259. Used with permission. Copyright © Mosby.)*

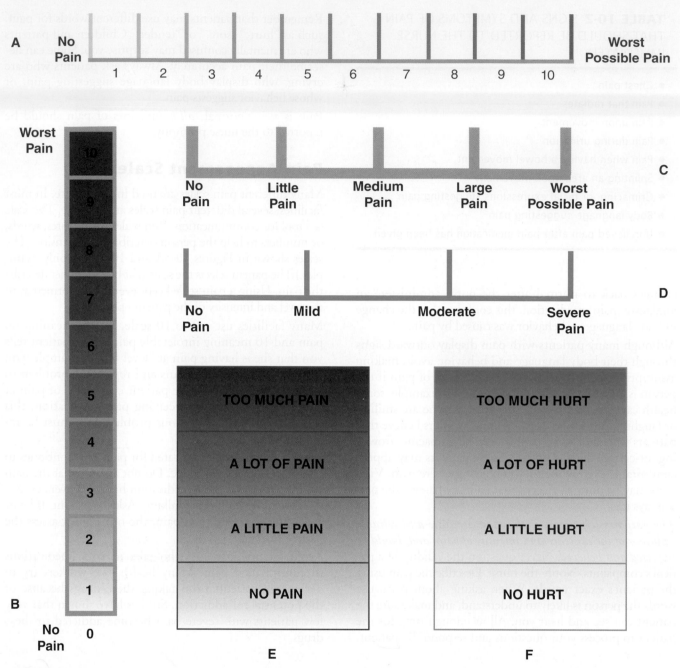

FIGURE 10-5B A. Horizontal numeric pain scale. B. Vertical numeric pain scale. C. Verbal descriptor pain scale. D. Verbal pain scale. E. Verbal pain scale. F. Verbal pain scale. (© *Delmar/Cengage Learning*)

Managing Pain

Health care facilities have a commitment to relieving patients' pain and suffering. Pain is promptly assessed on admission. Pain assessment and management continue throughout the patient's stay. Because of the importance of this care, many consider pain the "fifth vital sign."

Sometimes the physician orders several different medications for a patient's pain. The nurse will select which drug to use based on an assessment of the patient (Figure 10-6). Your observations, the patient's self-report of pain intensity, and nursing assessment findings are all considered when

the nurse determines which medication to administer, when more than one is ordered. If the first drug does not relieve the pain, the nurse may be able to give another, so always report unrelieved pain. The quality of pain control is influenced by the education, experience, and attitude of those who care for the patient.

Nursing assistant comfort measures Relieving discomfort helps reduce pain and anxiety. Nursing assistants can use many basic nursing measures to make a patient more comfortable. These include:

● Assisting the person to assume a comfortable position (Figure 10-7)

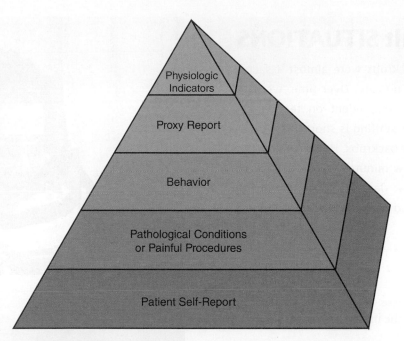

FIGURE 10-6 The hierarchy of pain assessment lists factors that the health professional considers when evaluating pain. Factors at the bottom of the scale are given the most consideration. The importance and weight of each factor decreases progressively to the top. *(© Delmar/Cengage Learning)*

- Repositioning the patient when needed to relieve pain and muscle spasms
- Using pillows and props to support the affected body part(s) (Figure 10-8)
- Changing the angle of the bed to relieve tension on surgical sites and other painful or injured areas
- Avoiding sudden, jerking movements when moving or positioning the patient
- Providing extra pillows and blankets for comfort and support

- Timing patient care to coincide with pain medication and waiting at least 30 minutes after the nurse administers pain medication before moving the patient, performing procedures, or undertaking activities
- Giving a backrub
- Placing a cool, damp washcloth on the patient's forehead
- Playing soft music to distract the patient
- Listening to patients' concerns and emotional support
- Maintaining a comfortable environmental temperature
- Providing a quiet, dark environment

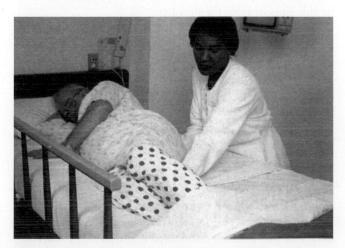

FIGURE 10-7 Assisting the patient into a comfortable position will enable him to relax and rest. *(© Delmar/ Cengage Learning)*

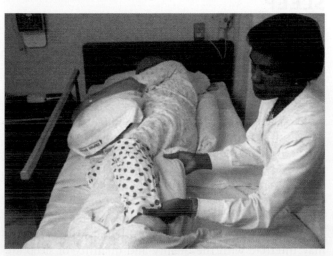

FIGURE 10-8 Support the arm and leg with pillows to relieve discomfort. *(© Delmar/Cengage Learning)*

Difficult SITUATIONS

For many years, backrubs were almost a sacred part of routine nursing care. Over time, we have become much more dependent on technology. When we are busy or staffing is short, it seems as if there is no time for backrubs. However, you may find that taking a few minutes to give a backrub will save you a great deal of time in caring for your patients. A good backrub is comforting and relaxing. ■

Regularly incorporate these steps into your patient care. Follow the directions on the individual patient's care plan.

REST

Rest is a state of mental and physical comfort, calmness, and relaxation. The patient's basic needs of hunger, thirst, elimination, and pain must be met before effective rest is possible. The patient may sit or lie down, or may do things that are pleasant and relaxing (Figure 10-9). Some patients have rituals, such as reading or reciting the rosary.

The environment should be calm and quiet to promote rest. Some patients feel refreshed after 15 minutes of rest. Others need more time. Some patients must rest frequently throughout the day. Plan your schedule and activities to allow for rest periods. Follow the care plan and the nurse's instructions. Evaluate the patient's response to your care.

SLEEP

Sleep is a period of continuous or intermittent unconsciousness in which physical movements are decreased. Sleep is a basic need of all humans, as it allows the mind and body to rest. Adequate sleep is necessary for the body and mind to function properly.

Sleep occurs in a cycle that lasts for several hours at a time. The body repairs itself during sleep. Because movement and activity are limited, the body's metabolic needs are reduced. The patient may become cold and need a blanket because he or she is not moving. It is common for vital signs to decrease during sleep.

Many factors affect sleep. Sleep problems often result from a combination of several factors. Obvious problems that may interfere with the quality and quantity of sleep are pain, hunger, thirst, and need to use the bathroom.

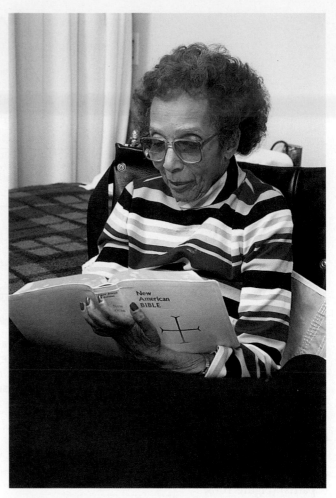

FIGURE 10-9 Reading the Bible is relaxing for this patient. (© Delmar/Cengage Learning)

Worry is another factor that interferes with comfort, rest, and sleep. Patients worry about many things. Although you will not have the answers to their problems and concerns, be a good listener. Sharing concerns with the nurse is not gossiping. The nurse and the other professionals may be able to help solve the problems.

Sleep and the Older Adult

The need for sleep decreases with age. Older persons awaken much more easily with even the slightest noise, whereas younger adults sleep through it. Older patients often have trouble falling asleep, awaken several times during the night, then wake up earlier in the morning than their younger counterparts.

Sleep is important to prevent feelings of fatigue, and for healing of medical and surgical problems. Getting enough sleep and rest allows patients to function at their highest level. Uninterrupted sleep is important. Elderly patients who do not sleep well may become disoriented (Figure 10-10). This correctable problem may be mistaken for confusion! It is corrected by uninterrupted sleep.

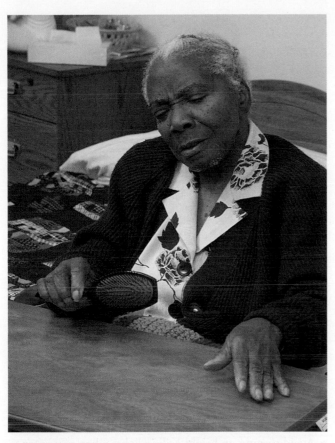

FIGURE 10-10 Lack of sleep can increase confusion and disorientation in elderly adults. (© Delmar/Cengage Learning)

NURSING ASSISTANT MEASURES TO PROMOTE COMFORT, REST, AND SLEEP

Basic nursing comfort measures, such as those used to relieve pain, are also effective in helping patients to rest and sleep. Specific measures for each patient will be listed in the care plan. Measures that promote comfort, rest, and sleep include:

- Help the patient into loose-fitting, comfortable clothing or nightwear.
- Assist with toileting, cleanliness, oral care, and personal hygiene needs.
- Provide a warm bath or shower, if permitted.
- Avoid serving beverages containing caffeine after the evening meal.
- Provide a snack, if desired.
- Straighten the bed.
- Assist the patient into a comfortable position and provide pillows and props as needed for comfort.
- Adjust room temperature and ventilation, if needed.
- Provide an extra blanket, if desired.

Difficult SITUATIONS

Patients always rest better when they are comfortable. Elderly persons are often uncomfortable in a cool environment. The discomfort increases restlessness and decreases patient satisfaction with care. Warmth promotes comfort, rest, and sleep, and reduces pain in elderly persons. Most hospitals have commercial warmers for IV solutions and bath blankets. These are usually in the perioperative department, but may be in other areas as well. If warm blankets are available on your unit, use them! Nurse researchers studied the effects of applying warmed blankets to patients (ages 65 to 98) who were cold, anxious, or uncomfortable. They measured the level of comfort before and one hour after applying a warm blanket. They found that the patients were more comfortable after receiving the warm blanket.[5] Patients who could describe how they felt said they were more comfortable. Nonverbal patients had fewer behavior problems and less body language suggesting discomfort. Offering patients a warmed blanket is a simple nursing measure that the nursing assistant can implement at any time. Helping to relieve pain and suffering is an important part of nursing assistant care. By using simple measures such as a warmed blanket to increase patient comfort, you will be rewarded with improved patient satisfaction, quality of care, and quality of life. ■

- Eliminate unpleasant odors.
- Eliminate and control noise.
- Adjust the lighting to a comfortable level, darkening the room as much as possible for sleep, and provide a nightlight if desired (Figure 10-11).
- If the patient is anxious, listen to what he or she says. Eliminate the cause of the anxiety, if possible (Figure 10-12).
- Avoid startling the patient.
- Handle the patient gently during care.
- Organize routine care to allow the patient uninterrupted sleep or rest.

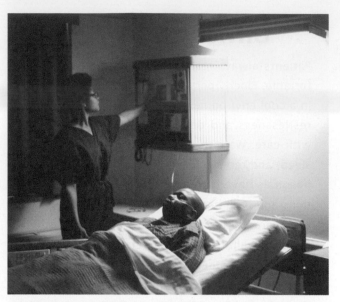

FIGURE 10-11 After the patient is comfortable and settled, turn the light off. *(© Delmar/Cengage Learning)*

- Avoid physical activity or activities that may upset the patient before bedtime.
- Assist with personal bedtime rituals, if any.
- Allow the patient to select his or her own bedtime.
- Allow the patient to read, watch television, or listen to the radio, if desired.

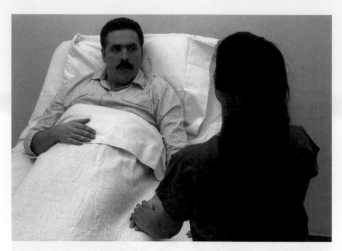

FIGURE 10-12 Listening to the patient's concerns provides emotional support and relieves anxiety. *(© Delmar/Cengage Learning)*

- Assist with relaxation exercises and activities, as directed.
- If the patient receives a sleeping medication, make sure the patient is ready for sleep before the nurse administers the medication.
- Close the door to the patient's room.
- Monitor noise levels in the hallway when patients are asleep.
- Avoid turning on bright ceiling lights when you enter a sleeping patient's room.

REVIEW

A. Multiple Choice

Select the one best answer for each of the following.

1. The WHO recommends a noise level of no more than _____ decibels in hospitals.
   a. 21
   b. 35
   c. 79
   d. 122

2. Loud noise
   a. causes worker stress and fatigue.
   b. is to be expected in large facilities.
   c. can never be controlled.
   d. is therapeutic for most patients.

3. Pain is
   a. the nurses' responsibility.
   b. a sign of something wrong.
   c. an objective sign.
   d. a normal part of illness.

4. Pain
   a. does not interfere with rest and sleep.
   b. is not stressful or worrisome.
   c. negatively affects well-being.
   d. can usually be ignored.

5. If a patient expresses his problems and worries, the nursing assistant should
   a. stay out of the patient's business.
   b. not tell the nurse about the patient's concerns.
   c. be a good listener and allow him to talk about it.
   d. provide answers to the problems.

6. Pain assessment is considered to be the
   a. first vital sign.
   b. frequency at which pain is evaluated.
   c. measurement of the "fifth vital sign."
   d. effectiveness of pain medication.

7. A state of mental calmness, comfort, and relaxation is
   a. comfort.
   b. sleep.

c. leisure.

d. rest.

8. A period of continuous or intermittent unconsciousness in which physical movements are decreased is

a. relaxation.

b. comfort.

c. sleep. ✓

d. diversion.

9. When a patient is sleeping,

a. vital signs may be lower than usual.

b. temperature increases.

c. movement increases.

d. the pulse decreases and respirations increase.

B. Nursing Assistant Challenge

Mr. Huynh is grimacing and supporting his right side with his hands when you enter the room. He smiles and nods at you. Complete the following statements regarding this patient.

10. Can Mr. Huynh smile if he is having pain?

11. If Mr. Huynh's right side hurts, you may be able to position him for comfort and support by using _____.

12. Should Mr. Huynh's body language be reported to the nurse?

13. Should you ask Mr. Huynh if he is having pain?

14. List six nursing assistant measures you can take to make Mr. Huynh more comfortable.

Footnotes

[1] Nightingale, F. (1859). *Notes on nursing*. London: Harrison and Sons.

[2] Cmiel, C. A. et al. (2004). Noise control: A nursing team's approach to sleep promotion. *American Journal of Nursing, 104*(2), 40–48.

[3] Britt, R. R. (2005). Hospitals getting noisier, threatening patient safety. *Live Science*. Retrieved November 22, 2005, from http://www.livescience.com/othernews/051121_noisy_hospitals.html.

[4] McClaugherty, L., Valibhai, F., & Womack, S. (2005). Physiological and psychological effects of noise on healthcare professionals and residents in long-term care facilities and enhancing quality of life. *The Director, 13*(2). Retrieved August 30, 2005, from http://www.nadona.org/noise.htm.

[5] Robinson, S., & Benton, G. (2002). Warmed blankets: An intervention to promote comfort for elderly hospitalized patients. *Geriatric Nursing, 23*, 320–323.

UNIT 11

Developing Cultural Sensitivity

OBJECTIVES

After completing this unit, you will be able to:
- Spell and define terms.
- Name six major cultural groups in the United States.
- Describe ways major cultures may differ in family organization, communication, need for personal space, health practices, religion, and traditions.

- List ways the nursing assistant can help patients in practicing rituals appropriate to their cultures.
- State ways the nursing assistant can demonstrate appreciation of and sensitivity to persons from other cultures.

VOCABULARY

Learn the meaning and the correct spelling of the following words and phrases:

ablutions	mores	ritual	standards
culture	personal space	sensitivity	stereotypes
ethnicity	race	spirituality	

INTRODUCTION

America is a nation of people whose ancestors came primarily from other countries. Each group brought its own cultural heritage with its language, beliefs, and customs. These people are your coworkers and patients. Each is a unique individual whose development is the result of his or her own culture, current lifestyle and community participation, and personal experiences. As a health care provider, you must show sensitivity and respect for the individuality and cultural heritage of each patient. **Sensitivity** is the ability to be aware of and to appreciate the personal characteristics of others.

When members of different groups must live and work together in a community, it is easy for members of each

group to form specific beliefs about the other groups. When these beliefs are rigid and are based on generalizations, they are called **stereotypes**. For example, others may view people of Asian heritage as being present-focused (thinking about immediate rather than long-term goals), not self-expressive, and reluctant to make eye contact. This view is a stereotype when applied to an entire group without consideration of the traditions of the group and individual characteristics. In contrast to these stereotypes, Van, whose heritage is Vietnamese (Figure 11-1), is outgoing, looks directly at a person speaking to her, has a quick smile, and is future-oriented as she studies to become a health care provider.

Health care providers must be careful not to make assumptions about a patient based on stereotypes of the group of

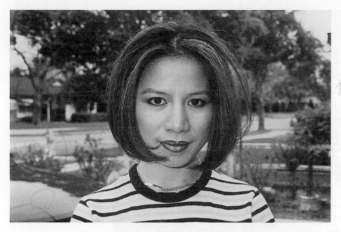

FIGURE 11-1 This young woman, whose parents were Vietnamese immigrants, has absorbed aspects of both her parents' culture and the American culture in which she lives. *(Stock image)*

TABLE 11-1 MAJOR ETHNIC GROUPS IN AMERICA

Group	Some Countries and Areas of Origin
Caucasian	England, Scotland, Ireland, Poland, Scandinavia, Italy, Russia
African American	Africa, Haiti, Jamaica, Dominican Republic
Hispanic	Cuba, Puerto Rico, Mexico, Latin and South America
Asian/Pacific	China, Japan, Philippines, Vietnam, Cambodia, Korea, Hawaii, Samoa
Native American	Hundreds of tribes, such as Cherokee, Apache, Navajo, Blackfoot, Inuit (Alaskan)
Middle Eastern	Egypt, Iran, Yemen, Pakistan, India, Jordan, Saudi Arabia, Kuwait

which the patient is a part. The longer a group is associated with the American culture, the less its members rely on or express the cultural values and traditions of the country of origin. Older people and new immigrants tend to cling more closely to the customs of their homelands.

RACE, ETHNICITY, AND CULTURE

The terms *race, ethnicity,* and *culture* are used to describe groups of people. **Race** is the classification of people according to shared physical characteristics such as skin color, bone structure, facial features, hair texture, and blood type. **Ethnicity** refers to special groups within a race as defined by national origin and/or culture. Members of an ethnic group share a common heritage, social customs, and language. Table 11-1 summarizes the six main ethnic groups in the United States.

Culture

Culture is the way a particular group views the world. Each culture has traditions that are passed from one generation to the next. Culture enforces the **standards** (rules) established by the group based on the values and beliefs.

Cultural **mores** (customs) influence the way people interact. Ethnicity and culture contribute to an individual's sense of self-identity as he or she relates to the group and to other cultures. Culturally sensitive care recognizes the individual within an ethnic and cultural group and provides care that assures cultural and individual acceptance and comfort.

Family organization Families form the basic cultural social groups, but their structure varies from culture to culture. The culture and family organization affect health care decision making.

Health care may be a family responsibility. Figure 11-2 shows an extended family and Figure 11-3 a nuclear family. For example, in Asian families the elderly are given great respect, and caring for them is considered a duty and privilege. In some cultures, caregiving is shared by many family members, including aunts and uncles. In other cultures care of the elderly is given over to others. This may be an economic necessity, because the adults must work to support the household. Leaving a family member in the care of others may cause feelings of worry and guilt.

Personal space needs **Personal space** is the physical closeness that a person is comfortable with when interacting

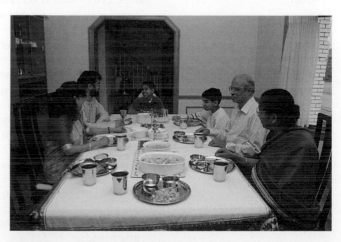

FIGURE 11-2 An extended family. *(Stock image)*

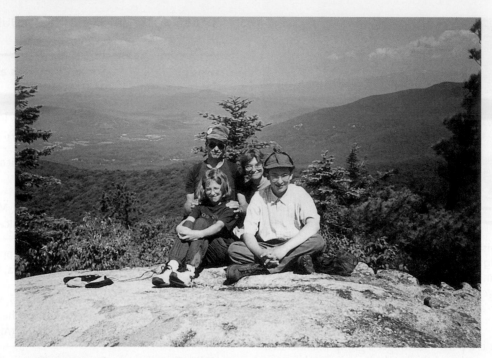

FIGURE 11-3 A nuclear family. *(© Delmar/Cengage Learning)*

with others. Personal space can be invaded by standing too close to another person, or by touch. Eye contact travels through the visual personal space and is interpreted differently by different cultures (see Table 11-2 for examples).

Caucasians and African Americans who were raised in the United States prefer to stand and speak at a distance of about 18 to 36 inches from one another. Space is important to Native Americans but has no specific boundaries. Asians tend to be uncomfortable if standing too close to another person outside of their own culture. In general, this is true of many cultures. Members are accepting of close personal space with members of their own culture. They may be

TABLE 11-2 CULTURAL INTERPRETATION OF NONVERBAL COMMUNICATION AND PERSONAL SPACE

Culture	Nonverbal Communication
American (U.S.) Caucasian and African American	Personal space 18 to 36 inches. Eye contact is acceptable and expected. Lack of eye contact may be interpreted as lack of self-esteem or not telling the truth.
Arab American	Women usually avoid eye contact with males and others whom they do not know well. Close personal space.
Asian	Varies. Eye contact is acceptable in some cultures but avoided in many; close personal space may be acceptable within the cultural group, but avoid touching.
Brazilian	Lack of eye contact is viewed by some as a sign of respect. Close personal space.
Cambodian	Eye contact is acceptable; women may lower eyes slightly; may accept close personal space within the cultural group.
Chinese American	Avoid eye contact with authority figures as a sign of respect; will make eye contact with family and friends. Distant personal space.
Colombian	May avoid eye contact in presence of an authority figure. Close personal space.
Cuban	Eye contact expected during conversation. Close personal space with friends and family.
Ethiopian	Avoid eye contact with those perceived to be in authority. Close personal space with family and friends.

TABLE 11-2 continued

Culture	Nonverbal Communication
European	Eye contact acceptable; distant personal space.
Filipino	May avoid eye contact with authority figures. Close personal space within the culture.
Gypsy (Romany)	Facial expressions reflect mood. Close personal space with family members. Generally avoid contact with non-Gypsies. Also avoid surfaces considered unclean (areas that lower body has touched).
Haitian	Avoid eye contact with those perceived to be in authority.
Hmong	Avoid prolonged eye contact, which is considered rude.
Iranian	Make eye contact only with equals and close family and friends. Close personal space.
Japanese American	Little eye contact. Touching may be considered offensive.
Korean	Little direct eye contact. Touching is considered offensive. Koreans maintain close personal space with family, but consider it disrespectful if an outsider invades their personal space.
Mexican American	Avoid eye contact with those perceived to be in authority. Some may consider touch by strangers to be disrespectful or offensive. Very close personal space.
Native American	Eye contact avoided as a sign of respect. Distant personal space is considered respectful. Comfort with personal space varies with the tribe and individual.
Puerto Rican	Personal space preference varies with age group; generally closer with younger women, more distant with older women.
Russian	Close personal space with family and friends. Direct eye contact acceptable during conversation.
South Asian	May consider direct eye contact with elderly individuals offensive or rude. Close personal space with family members only.
Vietnamese	Avoid eye contact with those perceived to be in authority. Distant personal space.
West Indian	Eye contact is avoided. Distant personal space.

Culture ALERT

Culture affects the type of care the patient expects to receive in the hospital. Patients from some cultures are comfortable doing self-care, if able. However, patients from other cultures may expect total care, even if they do not need it. They believe that they should not expend energy in caring for themselves. In some cultures, family members are expected to care for the patient. In others, only caregivers of the same gender may care for the patient. The care plan should guide you in culturally sensitive care. Consult the nurse if necessary. ■

uncomfortable with close personal space with members of other cultures.

Touch and personal care Touching a person is considered an invasion of personal space in some cultures. Touching the head is unacceptable in many cultures. Some believe the spirit resides in the head. Others believe the head is sacred and unwanted spirits or demons may be imparted through the hands. A handshake is traditional in the United States for both men and women. However, this practice is not acceptable in all cultures.

Touching the body of another person may be even more restricted than the touching of hands in greeting. In Middle Eastern countries, men may not touch females who are not members of their immediate family.

Nursing assistants care for patients during very personal and private moments. Workers may not think about or be troubled by patients' bodies being exposed. However,

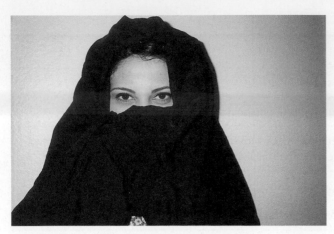

FIGURE 11-4 Traditional Muslim culture requires women to be completely veiled from head to toe. *(Stock image)*

many patients are very modest, and having the body exposed is traumatic. Cultural beliefs about keeping the body covered (Figure 11-4) will affect the care you give. In some cultures, females must be fully covered, even when in bed. Hospital gowns are not adequate. Some hospitals have long-sleeved gowns available that cover the patient from the neck to the ankles. However, these are not available in all facilities. Do whatever you can to keep patients covered and respect their modesty.

Patients who are members of some religions have beliefs about ritualistic washing, water, and personal hygiene. Spiritual **ablutions** and washing are required at certain times of the day. Ablution is the practice of removing sins and diseases and cleansing negative energy from the body, mind, and spirit through the use of ritual washing. Physical cleanliness is associated with spiritual purity. Showering may be preferable to a bath. Patients from some cultures may refuse to eat until they have washed. Water for washing should be available to the patient whenever possible. Members of some cultures use the right hand for eating. The left hand is reserved for personal hygiene and perineal care after toileting.

 Communication   Touching and eye contact are nonverbal forms of communication. A common verbal language is one characteristic of an ethnic group. Silence may be an important part of the language. For example, some Native American groups consider silence to be essential to understanding. Silence does not always mean that the listener has not heard or is inattentive to the speaker.

Communicating in a patient's own language adds greatly to her sense of security. After experiencing a stroke and some other conditions, an elderly person may revert to using a native tongue that he or she spoke many years ago, before coming to this country. The person seems to forget that he or she ever spoke English. When communicating, use a normal tone, speak slowly, and use simple words. Try to obtain feedback to determine the patient's level of understanding.

Monitor your body language and facial expressions to be sure your body is not sending a message that conflicts with your words. Be honest, respectful, and sincere. Review the communication guidelines in Unit 7.

Religious practices   Spirituality and religion are products of an individual's cultural background and experience. Spiritual values and religious beliefs form the rules of what a person considers to be right or wrong.

Many people believe that spirituality and religion are the same thing, but they are not. **Spirituality** is more of an umbrella that defines:

- Our perceptions of our place in the universe
- A higher power (if any)
- Our responsibilities to others
- Our fears and beliefs about living and dying

Religious beliefs provide a person with guidelines for moral behavior. Religious preferences are highly personal and can vary within a given culture. Religion differs from spirituality in that it encompasses beliefs related to both the cause and healing of disease. Religious beliefs vary widely, so making generalizations is difficult. Practitioners of some religions believe that the power of prayer, laying-on of hands, or another ritual is necessary to heal the illness. Religious items and **rituals** (solemn and ceremonial acts that reinforce faith) are meaningful to practitioners. Treat these items and practices with respect.

Special religious rituals and practices related to dying, death, and care of the body after death are discussed in Unit 33. Foods are important in some religions. Food restrictions are discussed in Unit 28.

Nursing Assistant Actions

Health care personnel have a significant role in very personal times of stress and turmoil in patients' lives. Humans are spiritual beings, although we all choose different paths. The need for spiritual caring is important when serious health problems occur. The nursing assistant should:

- Be sensitive to and respectful of each person's paths and choices.
- Avoid judging patients' beliefs, cultures, and health care decisions.
- Pay attention to what the patient is saying. Listen, reflect, and clarify information, if necessary.
- Avoid imposing your beliefs on patients.
- If you do not know an answer, admit it.

Caring for patients during very private moments is a privilege. Do not be so distracted with your workload or the environment that you fail to show sensitivity when patients express cultural and spiritual concerns. Provide privacy and support while they work through challenges to their health and well-being. Nursing assistants have a unique opportunity to learn about other cultures directly from their patients. Always recognize each person as an individual within his or her culture.

REVIEW

A. Multiple Choice

Select the one best answer for each of the following.

1. Awareness and appreciation of the personal characteristics of patients from other cultures is
   a. stereotyping.
   b. ritualism.
   c. sensitivity. ✓
   d. ablution.

2. Classification according to shared physical characteristics such as skin color, bone structure, facial features, and hair texture is
   a. race.
   b. stereotyping.
   c. ethnicity.
   d. mores.

3. The basis for cultural social groups is
   a. race.
   b. the family.
   c. ethnicity. ✓
   d. religious beliefs.

4. Caucasians and African Americans in the United States prefer to stand and speak about
   a. 6 to 10 inches apart.
   b. 18 to 36 inches apart.
   c. 4 to 6 feet apart.
   d. 5 to 8 feet apart.

5. Spirituality
   a. is another word for religion.
   b. determines religious practices. ✓
   c. affects beliefs about dying.
   d. determines one's morality.

6. Your Asian patient looks down and says little when you speak. This is
   a. rude in his culture.
   b. respectful in his culture.

   c. his way of showing anger.
   d. his way of showing fear.

7. Your patient makes direct and prolonged eye contact as you speak. He probably is of what culture?
   a. Asian
   b. Native American
   c. Hispanic
   d. Caucasian

8. Your patient speaks only a few words of English. When you speak to him, you should
   a. raise your voice.
   b. speak slowly.
   c. use slang.
   d. look away.

9. Members of an ethnic group share common
   a. social customs.
   b. religious practices.
   c. stereotypes.
   d. family members.

B. Nursing Assistant Challenge

You have a female patient who is a new immigrant from Iran. She is Islamic and 60 years old. Mark the following true or false.

10. T F She will be comfortable in a short hospital gown.

11. T F She is from the Asian culture.

12. T F Ablutions may be one of her religious practices.

13. T F She prefers distant personal space.

14. T F She probably prefers a female caregiver.

Infection

OBJECTIVES

After completing this unit, you will be able to:
- Spell and define terms.
- Identify the most common microbes and describe some of their characteristics.
- List the links in the chain of infection.
- List the ways in which infectious diseases are spread.
- Define spores and explain how spores differ from other pathogens.
- List natural body defenses against infections.
- Explain why patients are at risk for infections.

VOCABULARY

Learn the meaning and the correct spelling of the following words and phrases:

abscess
acquired immune
   deficiency syndrome
   (AIDS)
airborne transmission
antibodies
antigen
bacteria, bacterium
bedbugs
bioterrorism
carrier
causative agent
chain of infection
contact transmission
contagious
contaminated
droplet transmission

flora
fomites
fungi, fungus
head lice
hepatitis
host
human immunodeficiency
   virus (HIV)
immunity
immunization
infection
infectious
inflammation
jaundice
methicillin-resistant
   Staphylococcus aureus
   (MRSA)

method of transmission
microbe
microorganism
mite
mode of
   transmission
mold
nits
nonpathogen
nosocomial
organism
parasite
pathogen
portal of entry
portal of exit
protozoa, protozoon
reservoir

risk factor
scabies
severe acute respiratory
   syndrome (SARS)
source
spores
susceptible host
transmission
tuberculosis disease
tuberculosis infection
vaccine
vancomycin-resistant
   enterococci (VRE)
vector
virus
yeast

INTRODUCTION

Humans are surrounded by a world of tiny **organisms** (living beings). These beings cannot be seen with the eye. They make their presence known only by their effect, in much the same way we become aware of the wind. We cannot see the wind, but we see its effect on the trees, which bend and sway. These tiny organisms can be seen only with a microscope. They are everywhere—in us, on us, and around us.

Micro means small. Because these organisms (agents) are so tiny, they are called **microorganisms** or **microbes**. They live in relationship to us and to each other.

Microbes that cause disease are called **pathogens** or pathogenic organisms. Pathogens grow best in a warm, moist, dark environment in which they have a food supply and a supply of oxygen. **Infections** occur when the pathogens invade the body and cause disease.

Some microbes are useful. They are called **nonpathogens** because they do not produce disease.

MICROBES

There are many different types of microbes (Figure 12-1) that are pathogenic to human beings. Microbes are classified as bacteria, fungi, viruses, or protozoa.

Bacteria

Bacteria (singular: **bacterium**) are simple one-celled microbes. Some cause infections in the skin, lungs, urinary tract, and bloodstream.

Fungi

Two groups of **fungi** (singular: **fungus**) are most commonly associated with infection in humans. These are

> ### Clinical Information ALERT
>
> The human mouth contains about one hundred million (100,000,000) microbes at any one time. ■

> ### Clinical Information ALERT
>
> Human skin has about 100,000 bacteria per square centimeter (cm). This is a very small area. Ten percent of human dry weight is attributed to bacteria. The normal flora that live on the skin help protect the person from harmful bacteria. *Flora* are the collective bacteria and other microbes that live on a body part. ■

yeasts and **molds**. Both are opportunistic parasites. (A **parasite** (Figure 12-2) lives in or on another organism without benefiting the host organism.) Under normal conditions, these organisms are harmless. However, when the immune system is weakened, they can cause serious infections. For example, a person with AIDS is very susceptible to fungal infections because the immune system is not working properly.

Viruses

A **virus** is the smallest microbe we have been able to identify. Scientists believe that smaller microbes exist, but we cannot see them with the technology available. This is an area of ongoing research.

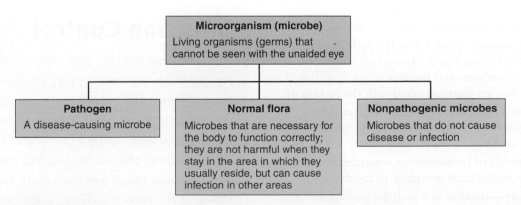

FIGURE 12-1 Various types of microbes. (© *Delmar/Cengage Learning*)

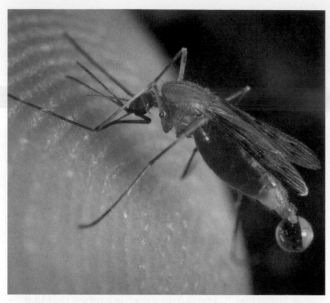

FIGURE 12-2 This female mosquito is a parasite. Females bite as part of the reproduction process. The mosquito is taking a blood meal by pumping the ingested blood through her *labrum*, which is visible here as a thin, red, needle-like structure between the mosquito's head and the skin. The mosquito is so full that clear fluid is spilling from the other end, enabling her to make room for more ingested blood. *(Courtesy of Centers for Disease Control and Prevention)*

Protozoa

Protozoa (singular: **protozoon**) are simple one-celled organisms that live on living matter.

THE CHAIN OF INFECTION

Infections occur when certain conditions exist. These conditions are called the **chain of infection** (Figure 12-3) and include:

- **Causative agent**—pathogen that causes the disease.
- **Reservoir** or **source**—place where the pathogen can live and reproduce, such as in humans or animals, on environmental surfaces, and **fomites** (objects, such as soiled linen, that are **contaminated** with the pathogen).
- **Portal of exit**—place that provides a way for the pathogen to leave the body, such as on the moisture droplets in a sneeze.
- **Method** or **mode of transmission**—manner in which the pathogen moves from one place to another.
- **Portal of entry**—manner in which the pathogen enters another person.
- **Susceptible host** (also called **host**)—a person who cannot resist the pathogen and will become ill from entry of pathogen into the body.

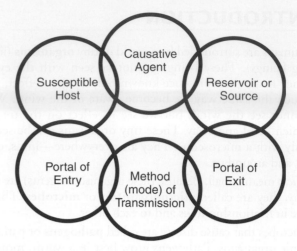

FIGURE 12-3 The chain of infection. *(© Delmar/Cengage Learning)*

Pathogens cause disease by entering the body through a portal of entry. They spread disease to others by leaving the body through a portal of exit and being transmitted to another person, usually on secretions. They enter another person's body through a portal of entry and can cause disease again. The purpose of infection control is to disrupt the chain of infection. Breaking one link (Figure 12-4) is all that is needed to prevent the spread of disease.

A **carrier** is a person who is infectious and can give a disease to others. The person may not know of the infection. The condition is not harmful to the carrier, but may be harmful to others. Another type of carrier is one in whom the organisms are multiplying (incubating) before signs and symptoms develop. This type of carrier can infect many people, because the organisms are passed before the person becomes ill.

Infection Control ALERT

Your bandage scissors and stethoscope can be fomites if they are not kept very clean. As fomites, these personal items may transfer pathogens from one patient to the next. If personal equipment items will be used during a procedure, wash them with an alcohol product or soap and water before and after each use. If you use a cloth stethoscope tubing cover, wash it each day with your uniform. Carry extra covers so you can change the cover if it becomes contaminated. ■

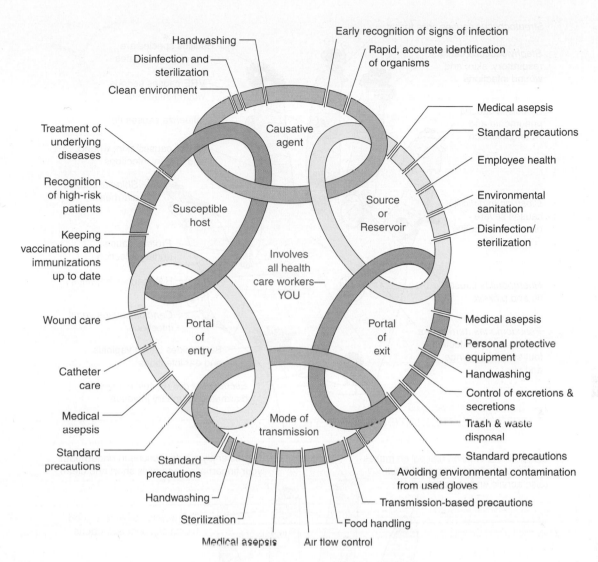

FIGURE 12-4 If one link in the chain is broken, infection cannot spread. This diagram shows the chain of infection, with examples of ways health care workers can break each link. (© *Delmar/Cengage Learning*)

TRANSMISSION OF DISEASE

In infected persons, blood, body fluids, secretions, excretions, and mucus are considered **infectious** or capable of transmitting the disease agent. Not all organisms are transmitted in the same way, and some organisms may be transmitted in more than one way. **Transmission** (spread) of infectious organisms may happen in one of three ways (Table 12-1):

1. **Airborne transmission.** Small particles remain suspended in the air and move with air currents, or become trapped in dust, which is also carried in air currents. The patient breathes in pathogens carried in this manner.

2. **Droplet transmission.** *Droplets* are moist particles produced by people coughing, sneezing, talking, laughing, whistling, spitting, or singing. Pathogens

are transmitted into the air with the droplets. Droplets are believed to stay within three feet of the source of the infection, but this is an area of ongoing study.

3. **Contact transmission.** Transmission occurs when there is direct contact with a person who is the reservoir for the pathogens. The infection is usually passed on the hands (Figure 12-5). Indirect contact occurs when a person touches an item contaminated with pathogens, such as soiled linen.

Nosocomial infections are those acquired during a facility stay. They increase the cost of the stay and can be serious or life-threatening. **Risk factors** are conditions that make a person vulnerable and indicate that a problem may develop, causing the patient's health to worsen. Some risk factors increase the likelihood that the person will develop an infection.

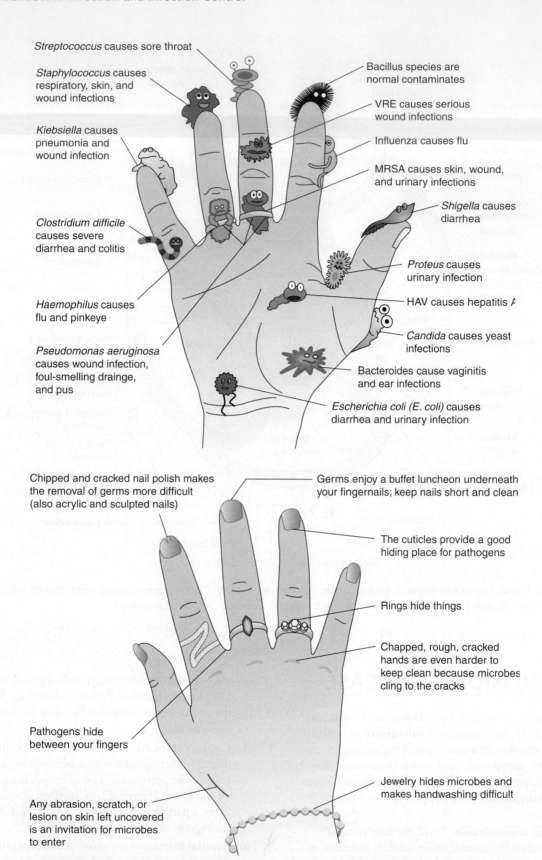

Streptococcus causes sore throat

Staphylococcus causes respiratory, skin, and wound infections

Kiebsiella causes pneumonia and wound infection

Clostridium difficile causes severe diarrhea and colitis

Haemophilus causes flu and pinkeye

Pseudomonas aeruginosa causes wound infection, foul-smelling drainge, and pus

Bacillus species are normal contaminates

VRE causes serious wound infections

Influenza causes flu

MRSA causes skin, wound, and urinary infections

Shigella causes diarrhea

Proteus causes urinary infection

HAV causes hepatitis A

Candida causes yeast infections

Bacteroides cause vaginitis and ear infections

Escherichia coli (E. coli) causes diarrhea and urinary infection

Chipped and cracked nail polish makes the removal of germs more difficult (also acrylic and sculpted nails)

Pathogens hide between your fingers

Any abrasion, scratch, or lesion on skin left uncovered is an invitation for microbes to enter

Germs enjoy a buffet luncheon underneath your fingernails; keep nails short and clean

The cuticles provide a good hiding place for pathogens

Rings hide things

Chapped, rough, cracked hands are even harder to keep clean because microbes cling to the cracks

Jewelry hides microbes and makes handwashing difficult

FIGURE 12-5 A. Many pathogens find their way to workers' hands. These are transferred to patients and environmental surfaces through touch. The worker can introduce them to his own body by touching his eyes, nose, mouth, or other mucous membranes. B. Jewelry worn on hands provides an additional hiding place for pathogens. Practicing good handwashing and not wearing jewelry are the best methods of protecting both workers and patients. *(© Delmar/Cengage Learning)*

CRITICAL THINKING IN ACTION

Marissa Gets the Measles

Marissa has never been immunized. Although she doesn't know it, she is exposed to measles, a disease that is spread by a virus.

Mode of transmission: The measles virus resides in the mucus in the nose and throat of an infected person.

Portal of exit: The disease is usually passed when the infected person coughs or sneezes.

Portal of entry: When an infected person coughs or sneezes, the virus particles are expelled into the air on secretions (droplets from the nose or mouth), and the *susceptible host* (Marissa) inhales them.

Incubation period: Marissa does not get sick immediately. Because she has no signs or symptoms, she does not know that she has been exposed to and infected by a pathogen. However, the measles virus is multiplying inside her body. The period of time from exposure until signs and symptoms develop is called the measles *incubation period.* Marissa is not contagious during the incubation period, so she cannot pass the disease to others until she develops the first signs and symptoms of measles. When this occurs, the cycle begins again.

Signs and symptoms of illness develop: Marissa woke up this morning feeling very ill. She has a high fever, hacking cough, red and watery eyes, and swollen eyelids. These signs and symptoms first occur about 8 to 12 days from the date of exposure.

Mode of transmission and portal of exit: Marissa will also spread the measles through sneezing and coughing. If her close contacts have not been immunized, they will also probably contract measles.

Although Marissa feels very ill, she still may not know that she has the measles. Rash is a late symptom that will show up about four days after the first symptoms develop. Touching a measles rash will not pass the infection, but contacting the rash from some other conditions (such as chickenpox) will spread disease. The mode of transmission for chickenpox is different from the mode of transmission for measles.

Marissa will be highly infectious from the time her first signs and symptoms occur until the rash develops, in about four days after she first feels ill. She will be able to spread the infection for about another four more days after she gets a rash.

Risk factors: Marissa is young, healthy, well-nourished, and has normal fluid intake. She has no known underlying diseases. However, she has never been immunized to prevent the measles. Measles is spread readily, so about 90% of those exposed will develop the disease unless they have been immunized. In this case, the lack of prior immunization is Marissa's only known risk factor for catching measles.

TYPES OF INFECTIONS

Infections can be:

- Local (confined to one area)—such as a boil or skin **abscess**
- Generalized—such as chickenpox (Figure 12-6)
- Systemic—widespread through the bloodstream

Body Flora

Different microbes live in and on our body surfaces. These microbes are called the normal body **flora**. The flora are not the same in all areas of the body. For example, the flora of the intestinal tract are different from those of the respiratory tract. Healthy individuals live in harmony with the normal body flora.

The body functions properly as long as the normal flora remain in the area where they usually reside. However, if flora are transferred to other areas, they may cause an infection. If the organism moves by way of the person's hands,

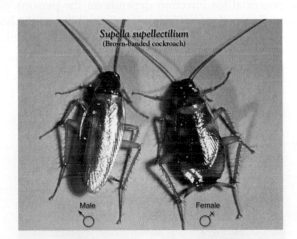

FIGURE 12-6 Insects and animals can transmit pathogens from place to place. Many different types of cockroaches are found living inside human habitations. They live in sewers and bathrooms, kitchens, and areas where food is prepared and stored. They can contaminate food, and have been implicated in the spread of food poisoning, staphylococcus, and other infections. *(Courtesy of Centers for Disease Control and Prevention.)*

TABLE 12-1 WAYS IN WHICH MICROBES ARE SPREAD FROM ONE PERSON TO OTHERS

Airborne Transmission	Droplet Transmission	Contact Transmission
Pathogens carried by moisture or dust particles in air; can be carried long distances	Droplet spread within approximately 3 feet (no personal contact) of infected person (Figure 12-7) by: • Coughing • Sneezing • Spitting • Talking • Laughing • Singing • Whistling	Direct contact with infected person: • Touching • Sexual contact • Blood • Body fluids (drainage, urine, feces, sputum, saliva, vomitus) Indirect contact with infected person: • Clothing • Dressings • Equipment used in care and treatment • Bed linens • Personal belongings • Specimen containers • Instruments used in treatment • Food • Water

Note that pathogens can also be carried by insects and animals (vectors) and passed to humans.

it may be transferred to everything and everyone he or she touches. This is why handwashing is so important after using the bathroom.

HOW PATHOGENS AFFECT THE BODY

The potential for infection depends on the person's risk factors. Two major factors are the susceptibility of the host and the amount of infectious agent that finds a portal of entry into the host. Even then, an infection will not occur unless all elements of the chain of infection are present.

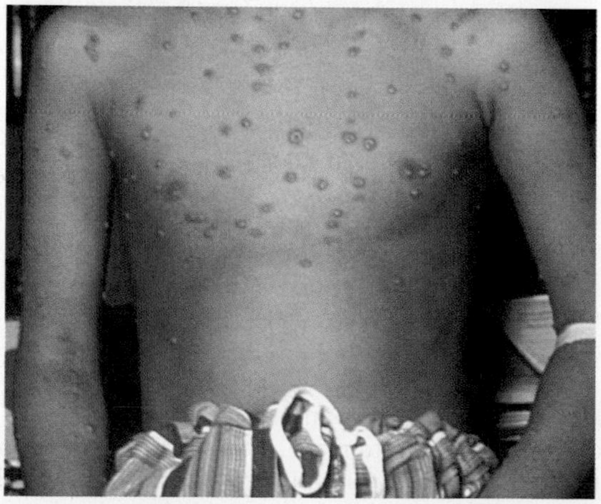

Body Defenses

The body has some natural defenses to protect it from infections. The most important of these is the skin. Intact skin acts as a barrier against the entry of pathogens. When a pathogen penetrates the skin, the affected area becomes swollen, hot, and painful as blood rushes to the area and begins to fight the invading pathogen. This internal defense against infection is called **inflammation** (Figure 12-8).

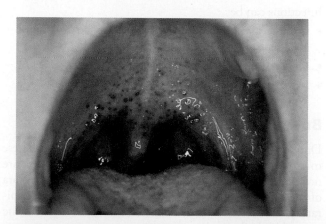

FIGURE 12-7 This child has chickenpox (varicella), which is highly contagious, and spreads via coughing or sneezing. *(Courtesy of Centers for Disease Control and Prevention.)*

FIGURE 12-8 Redness, swelling, heat, and pain are signs of inflammation. A sore throat is an excellent example of painful inflammation. *(Courtesy of Centers for Disease Control and Prevention.)*

Immunity

Immunity is the ability to fight off disease caused by microbes. A pathogenic microbe that enters the body is an **antigen**. In response to this, the blood develops substances called **antibodies**. The antibodies provide immunity (resistance) to the disease caused by that particular antigen. For example, if an individual has measles antigens in the bloodstream, he or she will form antibodies in the blood that prevent the occurrence of measles a second time.

Immunizations

Artificial defenses called **immunizations** protect against specific pathogens. Immunization against viruses is provided by **vaccines** that help the body develop protective antibodies before the need arises. Health workers who have direct contact with patients are advised to take hepatitis B vaccine. You will find a listing of recommended immunizations for health care workers in the Online Companion to this book.

SERIOUS INFECTIONS IN HEALTH CARE FACILITIES

Persons who are very old, very young, ill, frail, or have a weakened immune system are more likely to contract diseases. Signs and symptoms of infection to report to the nurse are listed in Table 12-2.

MRSA and VRE

Two groups of organisms have become resistant to two powerful antibiotics, methicillin and vancomycin. These organisms are:

- **Methicillin-resistant** *Staphylococcus aureus* (MRSA). Staphylococci bacteria are normally found on skin and mucous membranes. (See the Online Companion to this book.)

TABLE 12-2 SIGNS AND SYMPTOMS OF INFECTION THAT SHOULD BE REPORTED TO THE NURSE IMMEDIATELY

- Elevated temperature
- Rapid pulse and/or respirations
- Sweating
- Chills
- Skin hot or cold to touch
- Skin color abnormal—flushed, red, gray, or blue
- Inflammation of skin (redness, swelling, heat, pain)
- Drainage from any skin opening or body cavity
- Any other unusual body discharge, such as mucus or pus
- Other abnormalities specific to body system

- **Vancomycin-resistant enterococci (VRE).** Enterococci are found in the gastrointestinal tract. They are a major cause of infections acquired in health care facilities. Most strains are highly resistant to many antibiotics. Newer strains are resistant to vancomycin.

Additional pathogens are also developing resistance to methicillin and vancomycin. The emergence of these "superbugs" makes eliminating infection very difficult. The drugs used to kill some pathogens are so strong that they have the potential to cause serious complications, such as liver failure, kidney damage, and loss of hearing.

Tuberculosis

Mycobacterium tuberculosis is the bacterium that causes tuberculosis (TB). Before the development of antibiotics, tuberculosis was widespread. In the 1950s, antibiotics (which were new at the time) reduced the numbers of TB cases and deaths. Since 1985, the incidence has increased, in part because new strains of *Mycobacterium tuberculosis* are resistant to the antibiotics used to treat tuberculosis. There has also been an increase in the number of people who are at risk for infection.

Tuberculosis infection Tuberculosis infection occurs when the bacterium enters the body through inhalation. The body usually creates a barrier that confines the infection to the lungs. If the barrier remains intact, the infection is inactive. The person is not **contagious** (capable of passing the infection to others).

Tuberculosis disease Tuberculosis disease develops if the barrier in the lungs breaks down, allowing bacteria to enter the body. This may occur with aging or when the person has another condition that weakens the immune system. The person will show signs and symptoms of illness and can spread the disease to others through respiratory secretions.

The bacteria that cause TB are lightweight and can travel for long distances in air currents and indoor ventilation. Most health care workers must undergo skin testing for tuberculosis before employment, and periodically after that (Figure 12-9).

Infectious Diarrhea

Spores are microscopic reproductive bodies that are responsible for the spread of some diseases. They are similar to seeds that are dispersed from plants, but you cannot see them. Spores are very hearty and difficult to eliminate. Many can survive for long periods of time. They exist in a dormant form until conditions are ideal for reproduction. When this occurs, they multiply and spread infection.

Some spores cause very serious infections, such as botulism. Several forms of infectious diarrhea are spread by spores. Outbreaks of infectious diarrhea have occurred in both hospitals and long-term care facilities. Patients with infectious diseases spread by spores are placed in contact precautions (Unit 13).

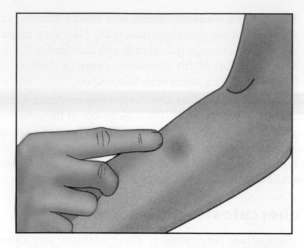

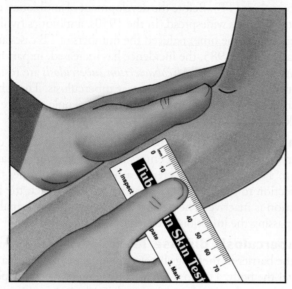

FIGURE 12-9 A positive Mantoux test shows redness and induration (swelling) 48 to 72 hours after the test. *(© Delmar/Cengage Learning)*

Environmental cleanliness When patients have infectious diarrhea or another condition spread by spores, special attention must be paid to hand hygiene and environmental cleanliness. These pathogens have the following features in common:

- Spores are usually plentiful in the environment (room or unit) of patients with infectious diarrhea.
- Spores have been found on the hands and under the fingernails of health care workers who provide care to affected patients or touch items and surfaces in the patient's room.
- Spores are capable of surviving for days to months in the environment.
- Spores are resistant to many chemical disinfectant products, including alcohol.
- Spores are transmitted through the digestive tract (usually entering through the mouth via the hands).
- Studies have shown that environmental surface contamination is a common source of infection.

- Good handwashing—with soap, water, and friction—is required to eliminate pathogens and spores from hands.
- Environmental cleaning is required, with friction and a disinfectant product known to kill the pathogen, such as those containing sodium hypochlorite (bleach).

Viral Infections

Several viral infections are discussed in this section:

- Shingles (herpes zoster)
- Influenza
- Hepatitis
- Acquired immune deficiency syndrome (AIDS)
- Severe acute respiratory syndrome (SARS)

Shingles Shingles (herpes zoster) (Figure 12-10A) occurs in people who were infected by the virus that causes chickenpox. Sometimes these organisms do not leave the body. They remained hidden in the nervous system in a nonactive (dormant) state.

Years later, when the person is in a weakened condition, the organisms become active. Painful blister-like lesions develop in the skin along the paths of sensitive nerves. The blisters contain infectious organisms. Workers who have never had chickenpox, and those who have not been immunized against chickenpox, should not care for a person with shingles. Workers who are pregnant should not enter the room because the fetus is at risk of complications from possible exposure. The patient is no longer infectious and will be removed from isolation when all the lesions have burst and have crusted over (Figure 12-10B).

Influenza Influenza (flu) is caused by a family of viruses. The infection can have serious consequences for elderly or frail people. Each year new types of viruses spread rapidly from person to person by way of respiratory secretions, causing many to become ill. Vaccines offer some protection against influenza viruses and are often given to residents in long-term care.

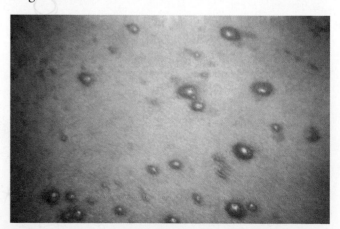

FIGURE 12-10A A rash in a patient with shingles. The blisters are intact, so the patient is infectious. Compare these blisters with the photo of chickenpox. *(Courtesy of Centers for Disease Control and Prevention.)*

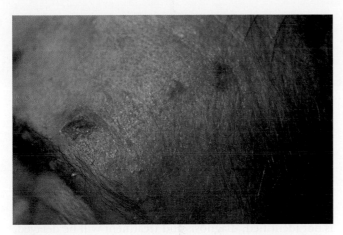

FIGURE 12-10B These shingles blisters have erupted and crusted over into scab-like areas. The patient is no longer infectious when all blisters have ruptured. *(Courtesy of Centers for Disease Control and Prevention.)*

In addition to making the person feel ill, flu viruses may lower the patient's resistance to other pathogens. These other organisms can cause pneumonia and other life-threatening infections. Medicines may be given to limit the effects of the viruses and antibiotics are given to combat bacterial infections that may develop.

You can help protect the patients in your care by:

- Staying healthy
- Not reporting for duty when you are ill
- Carrying out standard precautions faithfully
- Following the facility's policies regarding special precautions when a patient has a respiratory infection

- Encouraging the patient to drink fluids
- Reporting to the charge nurse when a visitor seems to be ill

Hepatitis Hepatitis is an inflammation of the liver caused by several viruses:

- Hepatitis A virus (HAV) is the most common. It is transmitted by feces, saliva, and contaminated food. **Jaundice**, a yellow color of the skin and sclera (Figure 12-11), is a common sign. Some people do not notice any signs of illness.
- Hepatitis B virus (HBV) is very serious. It is transmitted by blood, sexual secretions, feces, and saliva. HBV causes liver cancer and death. Although infectious, some patients have no symptoms. A person with hepatitis B remains infectious for life.
- Hepatitis C virus (HCV) is transmitted through blood and body fluids. The disease may be present for years. It is the leading cause of need for liver transplants in the United States.

Other types of hepatitis are less common. These are hepatitis D, hepatitis E, and hepatitis G. Infection with these organisms is not as serious as the other types. However, any infection of the liver is serious, because the liver is a vital organ. Take hepatitis very seriously, because many persons are infected, and can spread the infection to others. The information in Unit 13 will help you protect yourself and others.

Acquired immune deficiency syndrome (AIDS)

Acquired immune deficiency syndrome (AIDS) is a viral disease. It is transmitted primarily through direct contact with the bodily secretions of an infected person. The virus

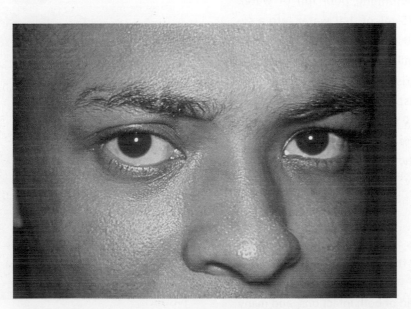

FIGURE 12-11 Jaundice is a yellowing of the skin and whites of the eyes caused by hepatitis and other conditions. *(Courtesy of Centers for Disease Control and Prevention.)*

that causes AIDS is the **human immunodeficiency virus (HIV)**. The hepatitis B virus is passed in the same manner. HIV and HBV are most commonly transmitted by contact with blood, body fluids, nonintact skin, secretions, excretions, and mucous membranes, usually through:

- Needle sharing among drug users
- Prick from a contaminated needle or sharp
- Unprotected vaginal, oral, or anal intercourse when one partner is infected

The AIDS virus (HIV) has many variants, and does not live long outside the body. It is eliminated by common chemicals such as bleach. Once in the body, it depresses the immune system, increasing the risk for infection and causing many complications. The HIV virus destroys white blood cells, which are protective cells used to fight infection. When the level of certain protective white blood cells (*CD4 cells*, also called *T-cells*) decreases to a certain point, the person is said to have progressed from HIV disease to AIDS. Although the person's CD4 count may later improve with treatment, he or she still has AIDS.

Severe acute respiratory syndrome Severe **acute respiratory syndrome (SARS)** was first seen in China in late 2002. It has now spread throughout the world. SARS is a viral respiratory illness caused by a coronavirus that is highly contagious. Distemper shots given to dogs protect the animal from infection with this virus. No such vaccine is available for human use.

Bioterrorism

Bioterrorism is the use of biological agents, such as pathogenic organisms or agricultural pests, for terrorist purposes. Many individuals could be infected by a biological weapon before the problem is identified. Some of the diseases that can be used as biological weapons have not been seen in years. Today's health care professionals may not recognize them. This compounds the problem because if the disease is not identified, diagnosis and treatment will be delayed, and the condition may continue to spread to others. Thus, bioterrorism is a significant threat.

PARASITES

Some insects are parasites because they survive by feeding off another human or animal. Fleas, ticks, lice, mites, and bedbugs are common examples of parasites.

Head Lice

Head lice (Figure 12-12A) are tiny brown parasites about the size of a sesame seed. They spread by direct and indirect

Infection Control ALERT

Hepatitis B is much more contagious than HIV. Imagine that a quarter-teaspoon *(1.25 mL)* of hepatitis B virus is mixed into a 24,000-gallon *(90,849,883 mL)* swimming pool full of water. Someone draws 1.25 mL of that water into a syringe and injects 10 people with it. Despite the amount of dilution, all 10 people will become HBV positive. By comparison, imagine that someone mixes a quarter-teaspoon (1.25 mL) of HIV virus into one quart (1,000 mL) of water. Ten people are injected with a quarter-teaspoon (1.25 mL) of this solution. Statistically, only one person in ten will become HIV positive. As you can see, hepatitis B is a much greater threat to health care workers than HIV.

Because a vaccine is available to protect workers from hepatitis B, the threat can be eliminated completely. Proper use of standard precautions (Unit 13) will prevent the spread of both infections, and many others. ■

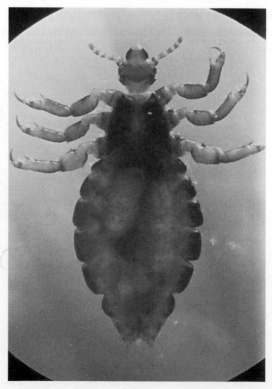

FIGURE 12-12A A magnified view of a head louse. Head lice are tiny, but can be seen with the unaided eye. *(Courtesy of Centers for Disease Control and Prevention.)*

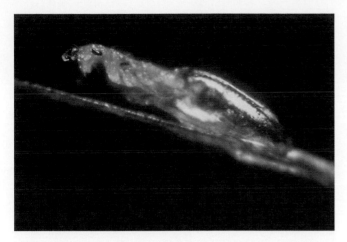

FIGURE 12-12B A head louse hatching from a nit. The empty nit case remains firmly attached to the hair shaft. *(Courtesy of Centers for Disease Control and Prevention.)*

contact with a person or fomite, such as brushes, combs, and bed linen. Head lice do not hop, jump, or fly. They crawl quickly and run away from light. Monitor patients for **nits** (Figure 12-12B). Nits look like dandruff, but firmly adhere to the hair and are very difficult to remove. Dandruff brushes off readily. The nits are eggs that will hatch into live lice. Notify the nurse if you find nits or other abnormalities.

Scabies

Scabies is a highly contagious disease of the skin caused by a parasite called a **mite** (Figure 12-13A). A mite cannot be seen with the eye. Scabies is spread by direct and indirect contact. It causes a rash (Figure 12-13B) and severe itching of the skin. The rash commonly appears in the webs of the fingers, inner wrists, forearms, outer elbows, and underarms. However, the rash may be present anywhere on the

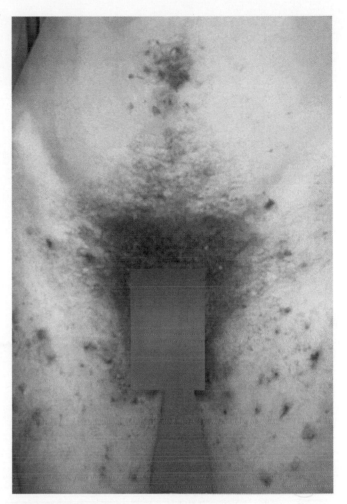

FIGURE 12-13B The scabies rash is often severe in the abdomen, groin, genital area, and knees. *(Courtesy of Centers for Disease Control and Prevention.)*

body. If you notice a rash, notify the nurse immediately. As with head lice, you will be directed to wear a gown and gloves for further patient contact.

Bedbugs

Most people think **bedbugs** (Figure 12-14A) are imaginary pests from a nursery rhyme. In fact, they are real parasites that have been found in hotels, hospitals, and nursing homes. They are usually seen at night, and are stealthy and fast-moving. They can survive in temperature extremes, and can live for up to a year without a blood meal. The bite from a bedbug causes a rash-type area that often causes pain or intense itching.

A bedbug is tiny, flat, and clear or white in appearance before feeding. After eating a blood meal, it develops a redbrown coloration (Figure 12-14B). They leave little excretion droppings on the sheets. Tiny bloodstains on the linen, or dark spots from the droppings, are strong indications that bedbugs are present.

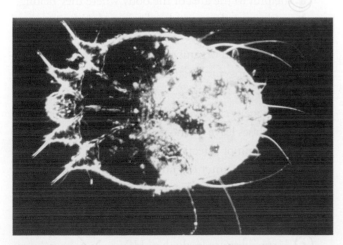

FIGURE 12-13A A microscopic view of the scabies mite, which cannot be seen with the unaided eye. *(Courtesy of Centers for Disease Control and Prevention.)*

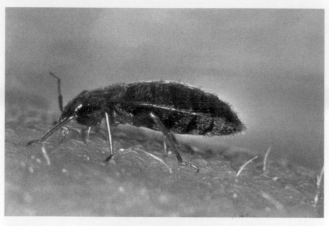

FIGURE 12-14A The bedbug is tiny, but can be seen with the unaided eye. *(Courtesy of Centers for Disease Control and Prevention.)*

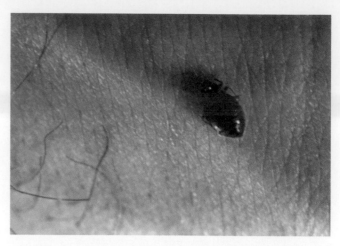

FIGURE 12-14B The bedbug is clear until it ingests a blood meal, which causes it to darken to a red-brown color. *(Courtesy of Centers for Disease Control and Prevention.)*

REVIEW

A. Multiple Choice

Select the one best answer for each of the following.

1. Pathogens grow best if the environment is
   a. cool, dry, and oxygen rich.
   b. warm, dry, and light.
   c. warm, moist, and dark.
   d. cool, moist, and light.

2. Which is an example of a local infection?
   a. hepatitis B
   b. tuberculosis
   c. boil
   d. bedbugs

3. One patient's visitor is coughing and looks flushed. Your best action is to
   a. ask the visitor to leave.
   b. put a mask on the visitor.
   c. put a mask on the patient.
   d. refer the matter to the nurse.

4. You woke up not feeling well this morning. You have an elevated temperature. Your best action is to
   a. call in sick.
   b. go to work.
   c. stay home without notifying the facility.
   d. call a friend to go to work for you.

5. Spores
   a. remain dormant until conditions are ideal for reproduction.
   b. can be eliminated from the environment with alcohol.

   c. are usually responsible for boils and skin abscesses.
   d. can be treated with antibiotics and increased fluids.

6. Bioterrorism is
   a. not a concern in the United States.
   b. the use of chemicals to cause illness.
   c. the use of biological agents for terrorist purposes.
   d. easily detected and treated.

7. Hepatitis B
   a. is spread by oral–fecal transmission.
   b. can be readily cured with antibiotics.
   c. causes visible signs of serious illness.
   d. can be prevented by vaccination.

8. Flora are
   a. helpful to the area of the body where they belong.
   b. pathogens that must be eliminated with antibiotics.
   c. single-celled organisms that cannot reproduce.
   d. nonpathogenic microbes that help the entire body.

9. The reservoir is the place where
   a. pathogens can live and reproduce.
   b. microbes leave the host's body.
   c. the chain of infection is strongest.
   d. pathogens enter the host's body.

10. Hepatitis B
    a. is a weak virus that does not pose a threat.
    b. is readily cured with antibiotics.
    c. is spread more easily than HIV.
    d. is a harmless chronic disease.

B. Nursing Assistant Challenge

Mr. Reynolds is in isolation. The nurse informs you that they are waiting on laboratory tests to confirm the diagnosis, but they suspect he has a type of diarrhea that is spread by spores. She instructs you to use isolation precautions and emphasizes the need for good handwashing several times.

11. Why is good handwashing important?

12. Will you use an alcohol-based hand cleaner? Why or why not?

13. Since the infectious pathogen is spread through the stool, what are the two modes of transmission for this organism?

14. How might Mr. Reynolds have acquired this infection?

Infection Control

OBJECTIVES

After completing this unit, you will be able to:

- Spell and define terms.
- Explain the principles of medical asepsis.
- Explain the components of standard precautions.
- Describe nursing assistant actions related to standard precautions.
- Describe airborne, droplet, and contact precautions.
- List the types of personal protective equipment and discuss the use of each item.
- Demonstrate the following:
  - Procedure 1—Handwashing
  - Procedure 2—Putting on a Mask
  - Procedure 3—Putting on a Gown
  - Procedure 4—Putting on Gloves
  - Procedure 5—Removing Contaminated Gloves
  - Procedure 6—Removing Contaminated Gloves, Eye Protection, Gown, and Mask
  - Procedure 7—Transferring Nondisposable Equipment Outside of the Isolation Unit
  - Procedure 8—Specimen Collection from a Patient in an Isolation Unit
  - Procedure 9—Transporting a Patient to and from the Isolation Unit

VOCABULARY

Learn the meaning and the correct spelling of the following words and phrases:

AII room (A2 room)
airborne precautions
airborne transmission
anteroom
asepsis
autoclave
biohazard
communicable disease
contact precautions
contact transmission
contaminated
dirty
disinfection

disposable
droplet precautions
droplet transmission
exposure incident
face shield
goggles
high-efficiency
  particulate air (HEPA)
  filter mask
isolation
isolation technique
isolation unit
medical asepsis

N95 respirator
National Institute of
  Occupational Safety
  and Health (NIOSH)
negative air pressure
  room
occupational exposure
other potentially
  infectious material
  (OPIM)
personal protective
  equipment (PPE)
PFR95 respirator

sharps
standard precautions
sterile
sterilization
surgical mask
transmission-based
  precautions
ultraviolet germicidal
  irradiation (UVGI)
work practice controls

DISEASE PREVENTION

In Unit 12 you learned what infections are and some of the causes of infection. This unit introduces you to actions and procedures that can help prevent the transmission (spread) of infection, so that you can protect yourself, your coworkers, and those in your care.

MEDICAL ASEPSIS

Asepsis is the absence of disease-producing microorganisms. Medical asepsis and surgical asepsis are the methods used to achieve asepsis in the health care facility.

Medical asepsis refers to practices that prevent the spread of microbes. You will hear the terms *clean* and *dirty* applied to equipment and supplies. Articles that have come into contact with known pathogens or have been exposed to potential pathogens are called **dirty**, soiled, or **contaminated**. Articles that are free of pathogens are considered clean or uncontaminated.

For example, the linen you carry into the patient's room is "clean." Once in the room, though, it is considered "dirty." If it is not used there, it cannot be used for another patient or returned to the clean linen cart; it must be placed in the soiled laundry hamper. Once linen is in a patient's room, it is exposed to the microbes in the environment. Some of these may be pathogens. Keeping each patient's supplies separate from those for other patients is part of medical aseptic technique.

It is not possible to eliminate all microorganisms from our bodies or the environment. However, microbes and the

---

GUIDELINES *for*
Maintaining Medical Asepsis

To maintain medical asepsis, the nursing assistant should:

- Wash hands thoroughly and regularly or use an alcohol-based hand cleaner.
- Treat breaks in the skin by washing, cleaning with an antiseptic, and covering. Report breaks in the skin to your supervisor.
- Use gloves when required.
- Bathe, shower, and wear clean clothing daily. Keep your hair clean and away from your face and shoulders. Avoid artificial nails and acrylic overlays. Keep natural nails short and clean. Do not wear jewelry or rings, other than a plain wedding band.
- Assist patients with their personal hygiene.
- *Never* use one patient's personal items for another patient.
- Keep patient personal care items in the proper areas. Always separate clean and soiled (dirty) items.
- Place personal hygiene (clean) items, such as the toothbrush, in the top drawer of the bedside stand. Keep clean utensils, such as the washbasin, in the second drawer or top shelf of a cupboard-type bedside stand. Store dirty items, such as the bedpan and urinal, in the bottom drawer or on the bottom shelf.
- Disinfect equipment that is used by more than one patient before and after each use.
- Avoid contaminating environmental surfaces by touching them with used gloves.

- Use the overbed table for clean items, such as food trays and the water pitcher.
- Keep the water pitcher covered.
- Keep food trays covered in the hallways. Do not return used trays to the food cart until all clean trays have been delivered to patients.
- Monitor food in patient rooms. Be sure food is wrapped and does not require refrigeration.
- Carry clean and soiled supplies by holding them away from your uniform.
- Do not use anything that has touched the floor without cleaning the item.
- Do not shake linens; this scatters contaminated dust and lint. Fold used linens inward with the dirtiest area toward the center. Keep soiled linen hampers covered. Keep linens (even if soiled) off the floor.
- In the hallway, separate the soiled linen hamper and housekeeping cart from the clean linen cart and food cart by at least one room's width.
- Soiled linen and laundry hampers or barrels must be marked with a biohazard emblem, and stored in the designated area when not in use.
- Clean from least-soiled areas toward the most soiled.
- Keep work areas such as utility rooms clean. Return clean equipment to the proper (clean) storage areas after washing.

risk of infection (Unit 12) can be reduced by always using medical aseptic technique.

Handwashing

Handwashing is the most important method of preventing the spread of infection. Liquid soap is used in health care facilities. Pathogens can grow on wet bar soap and in the soap dish, contaminating the soap.

When washing your hands, keep your fingertips pointed down. Never lean against the sink or touch the inside of the sink with your hands. The most important part of the handwashing procedure is creating friction by rubbing the hands together. Friction loosens and removes microbes from the hands.

Cleansing the hands:

- Is the most important measure for the prevention of nosocomial infection
- Is the most important way of breaking the chain of infection

The technique used depends on the purpose of the handwashing. Hands can usually be washed effectively in 15 to 20 seconds. More time will be needed, however, if hands are visibly soiled (refer to Procedure 1).

Wash your hands:

- At the beginning of your shift
- After picking up any item from the floor
- After personal use of the bathroom
- After handling a sanitary napkin or tampon
- After using a tissue
- After you cough or sneeze
- Before handling a patient's food and drink
- After handling a patient's belongings
- After touching any item or surface that is soiled or in the vicinity of patients
- Before handling clean supplies
- Immediately before touching mucous membranes or nonintact skin; if you are already wearing gloves, change them
- Immediately after accidental contact with blood, moist body fluids, mucous membranes, or nonintact skin
- Before and after contact with your mouth or mucous membranes, such as touching, eating, drinking, smoking, using lip balm, or manipulating contact lenses
- Before and after every patient contact
- Before applying and after removing gloves
- Whenever your hands are visibly soiled
- Any time your gloves become torn
- At the end of your shift before going home

Most facilities do not permit caregivers to wear artificial fingernails or natural nails that extend more than one-quarter inch beyond the fingertips. Long and artificial nails harbor bacteria, and increase the risk of tearing gloves. Facilities may also have restrictions on the types of rings you may wear while on duty. Rings with many stones and elaborate settings can also hold harmful microbes, and are difficult to clean. Rings may also tear gloves. Rings other than flat bands are better left at home.

Hand Lotion and Cream

Select and use hand care products carefully. Lotions and creams from jars or squeeze bottles, where hands touch the dispenser, may become a source of contamination to everyone who uses them. An individual, personal-size bottle is best.

Waterless Hand Cleaners

Many facilities provide dispensers containing waterless hand cleaner throughout the facility. The containers dispense an alcohol-based product in small portions. Most also contain moisturizers that prevent drying of the skin. In most facilities, the alcohol cleaner may be used instead of handwashing during routine patient care. However, you must wash at the sink when your hands are visibly soiled. To use the alcohol product, dispense the proper amount into the palm of your hand. Rub the product into your hands until it dries, making sure to rub all areas and surfaces, including the nail beds and between the fingers. This should take about 15 to 20 seconds.

Protecting Yourself

As you perform your duties, you may contact **other potentially infectious material (OPIM)**, such as blood or other body fluids, that may contain pathogens. This is called **occupational exposure**.

In an **exposure incident**, your eyes, nose, mouth, mucous membranes, or nonintact skin had contact with blood or other potentially infectious material. Flush your eyes, nose, or mouth immediately with clear water. Wash exposed skin and open or cracked areas well with soap and water. Notify your supervisor promptly.

Infection Control ALERT

Always wash your hands with soap and water if a patient has infectious diarrhea or another condition spread by spores. As a general rule, *alcohol-based cleaners will not eliminate spores*. The mechanical action of soap, water, and friction used during handwashing will loosen spores from your hands and flush them down the drain. ■

PROCEDURE

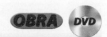

1

HANDWASHING

1. Check that there is an adequate supply of soap and paper towels. A waste container lined with a plastic bag should be in the area near you.

2. Remove rings, if possible, or be sure to lather soap underneath.

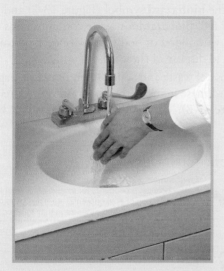

FIGURE 13-1 Keep your fingertips pointed down when washing hands. *(© Delmar/Cengage Learning)*

3. Remove your watch, or push it up over your wrist.

4. Turn on the faucets.

5. Adjust water to a warm temperature. Stand back from the sink to avoid contaminating your uniform. Wet your hands, keeping your fingertips pointed downward (Figure 13-1).

6. Apply soap and lather over your hands and wrists, between fingers, and under rings. Remember to wash your thumbs. Use friction and interlace your fingers (Figure 13-2). Work lather over every part of your hands and wrists. Clean your fingernails by rubbing them against the palm of the other hand to force soap under the nails. Continue rubbing the hands together for 15 to 20 seconds (Figure 13-3).

7. Rinse hands with fingertips pointed down. Do not shake water from hands.

8. Dry hands thoroughly with a clean paper towel.

9. Turn off the faucets with a paper towel (Figure 13-4); drop the used towels in the waste container.

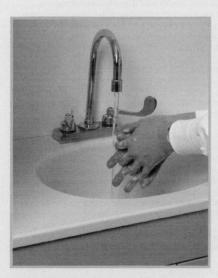

FIGURE 13-2 Interlace the fingers to clean between them. *(© Delmar/Cengage Learning)*

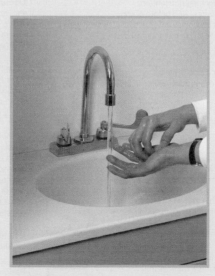

FIGURE 13-3 Rub nails against the palms of the hands to clean under the nails. *(© Delmar/Cengage Learning)*

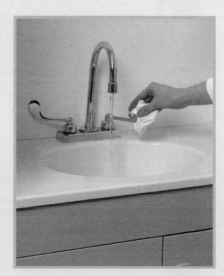

FIGURE 13-4 Use a clean, dry paper towel to turn faucets off. *(© Delmar/Cengage Learning)*

STANDARD PRECAUTIONS

Standard precautions (Figure 13-5) are the infection control actions used with all people receiving care, regardless of the patient's condition or diagnosis. Standard precautions apply to situations in which workers may contact:

- Blood, body fluids (except sweat), secretions, or excretions
- Mucous membranes
- Nonintact skin

Standard precautions stress handwashing and the use of **personal protective equipment (PPE)**: gloves, gown, mask, and goggles or face shield.

All health care workers must follow specific procedures, called **work practice controls**, to prevent the spread of infections.

Other Waste

- Dispose of **sharps**—needles, razors, and other sharp items—in a puncture-resistant, leakproof container near the point of use (Figure 13-6). Do not recap or handle needles before disposal. The container should be labeled with the **biohazard** symbol (Figure 13-7) and color-coded red. Biohazardous waste contains items contaminated with blood or body fluids. Special precautions are taken to dispose of these waste containers.

- Dispose of waste and soiled linen in plastic bags. Discard these items in the biohazardous waste (Figure 13-8). The handling of biohazardous waste is

---

STANDARD PRECAUTIONS FOR INFECTION CONTROL

Wash Hands (Plain soap)
Wash after touching blood, body fluids, secretions, excretions, and contaminated items. Wash immediately after gloves are removed and between patient contacts. Avoid transfer of microorganisms to other patients or environments.

Wear Gloves
Wear when touching blood, body fluids, secretions, excretions, and contaminated items. Put on clean gloves just before touching mucous membranes and nonintact skin. Change gloves between tasks and procedures on the same patient after contact with material that may contain high concentrations of microorganisms. Remove gloves promptly after use, before touching noncontaminated items and environmental surfaces, and before going to another patient, and wash hands immediately to avoid transfer of microorganisms to other patients or environments.

Wear Mask and Eye Protection or Face Shield
Protect mucous membranes of the eyes, nose and mouth during procedures and patient-care activities that are likely to generate splashes or sprays of blood, body fluids, secretions, or excretions.

Wear Gown
Protect skin and prevent soiling of clothing during procedures that are likely to generate splashes or sprays of blood, body fluids, secretions, or excretions. Remove a soiled gown as promptly as possible and wash hands to avoid transfer of microorganisms to other patients or environments.

Patient-Care Equipment
Handle used patient-care equipment soiled with blood, body fluids, secretions, or excretions in a manner that prevents skin and mucous membrane exposures, contamination of clothing, and transfer of microorganisms to other patients and environments. Ensure that reusable equipment is not used for the care of another patient until it has been appropriately cleaned and reprocessed. Ensure that single-use items are properly discarded.

Environmental Control
Follow hospital procedures for routine care, cleaning, and disinfection of environmental surfaces, beds, bed rails, bedside equipment, and other frequently touched surfaces.

Linen
Handle, transport, and process used linen soiled with blood, body fluids, secretions, or excretions in a manner that prevents exposure and contamination of clothing, and avoids transfer of microorganisms to other patients and environments.

Occupational Health and Bloodborne Pathogens
Prevent injuries when using needles, scalpels, and other sharp instruments or devices; when handling sharp instruments after procedures; when cleaning used instruments; and when disposing of used needles.

Never recap used needles using both hands or any other technique that involves directing the point of a needle towards any part of the body; rather, use either a one-handed "scoop" technique or a mechanical device designed for holding the needle sheath.

Do not remove used needles from disposable syringes by hand, and do not bend, break, or otherwise manipulate used needles by hand. Place used disposable syringes and needles, scalpels, blades, and other sharp items in puncture-resistant sharps containers located as close as practical to the area in which the items were used, and place reusable syringes and needles in a puncture-resistant container for transport to the reprocessing area.

Use resuscitation devices as an alternative to mouth-to-mouth resuscitation.

Patient Placement
Use a private room for a patient who contaminates the environment or who does not (or cannot be expected to) assist in maintaining appropriate hygiene or environmental control. Consult Infection Control if a private room is not available.

FIGURE 13-5 Standard precautions. *(Courtesy of BREVIS Corporation, Salt Lake City, UT)*

GUIDELINES *for*
Standard Precautions

1. Wash hands or use an alcohol-based cleanser in the situations listed under "Handwashing."

2. Wear gloves for any contact with blood, body fluids, mucous membranes, or nonintact skin, such as when:
   - Hands are cut, scratched, chapped, or have a rash
   - Cleaning up body fluid spills
   - Cleaning potentially contaminated equipment

3. Gloves are provided in patient rooms, or in wall-mounted dispensers. Carry some in your pocket so they will be available when you need them.

4. If you have a sensitivity to latex gloves, follow your physician's advice.

5. Change gloves and wash hands:
   - After contacting each patient
   - Before touching noncontaminated articles or environmental surfaces
   - Between tasks with the same patient if there has been contact with infectious materials

6. Discard gloves according to facility policy.

7. Wear a waterproof gown for procedures that are likely to produce splashes of blood or other body fluids.

8. Wear a mask and protective eyewear or face shield for procedures that are likely to produce splashes of blood or other body fluids.

9. Wear utility gloves for cleaning soiled utensils and equipment.

10. When using PPE, you should:
    - Know where to obtain these items in your work area.
    - Always remove the items before leaving the work area, whether it is the patient's room, an isolation unit, or the utility room.
    - Place used PPE items in the proper container for laundering, decontamination, or disposal, according to facility policy.
    - Replace supplies that you have used. Never leave gloves or other containers for PPE empty. The next person may need them in a hurry, so they must be readily available.

OSHA ALERT

Most facilities do not permit personnel to wear gloves in the hallway. The OSHA Bloodborne Pathogen Standard states that you must remove PPE before leaving the work area. The patient's room is the work area. Some facilities allow staff to use the one-glove technique to carry wet or soiled linen and other items into the hallway in close proximity to a patient's room. Know and follow your facility policies. ■

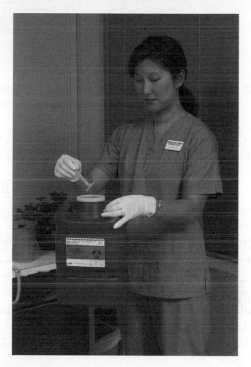

FIGURE 13-6 Carefully discard sharps in a safety container designated for this use. (© Delmar/Cengage Learning)

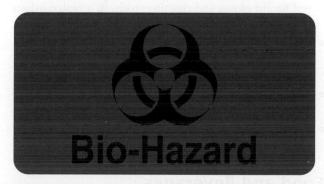

FIGURE 13-7 Containers for contaminated items are identified with the biohazard label. The symbol is black with a red or orange background. (© Delmar/Cengage Learning)

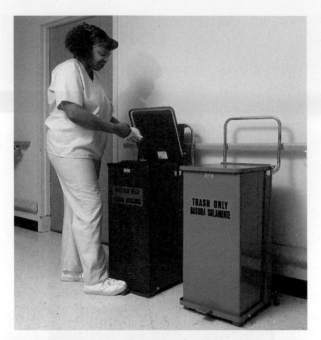

FIGURE 13-8 Discard all potentially infectious materials in the proper container. (© Delmar/Cengage Learning)

very expensive, and storage space is often limited, so do not place packaging and non-biohazardous items in biohazard disposal containers.

- Wipe up blood spills immediately. Disinfect the floor according to facility policy.
  - Use disposable gloves.
  - For small spills, use 1:10 or 1:100 dilution of bleach or facility-approved disinfectant.
  - For larger spills, use a commercial blood cleanup kit. Sprinkle absorbent powder on the spill. The blood will become solid when mixed with the chemical. Clean it up with the scoop provided in the kit. Discard the material and scoop in a biohazard bag (Figure 13-9).
  - Wipe with disinfectant and disposable cleaning cloths.
  - Discard gloves and cleaning cloths in a biohazardous waste container.
- Use a brush and dust pan, tongs, or forceps to clean up broken glass. Wear gloves; clean and disinfect properly. Discard broken glass according to facility policy.
- Liquids may be discarded in a sanitary sewer. Solid items should be discarded in the biohazardous waste.
- Consider laboratory specimens and specimen containers to be potentially infectious materials.

Food and Beverages

Avoid eating, drinking, chewing gum, smoking, applying cosmetics or lip balm, or handling contact lenses in areas where you may be exposed to infectious material. Keep food and drink away from areas where they may be

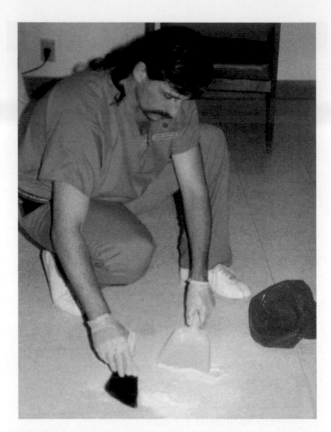

FIGURE 13-9 Clean blood spills immediately and disinfect, using a 1:10 or 1:100 bleach solution or facility-approved disinfectant. For larger spills, you can use a blood spill kit. The powder in the kit solidifies the blood so it can be easily scooped into a plastic biohazard bag. (© Delmar/Cengage Learning)

exposed to laboratory specimens, blood, or other potentially contaminated items.

TRANSMISSION-BASED PRECAUTIONS

Standard precautions do not eliminate the need for other precautions in special situations. A second set of precautions is used with certain highly transmissible diseases. These are called **transmission-based precautions**. They are used to interrupt the mode of transmission. *Standard precautions are always used in addition to transmission-based precautions.*

Diseases may be transferred from one person to another either directly or indirectly. Such diseases are called **communicable diseases**. Specific precautions must be taken to control their spread. Communicable diseases may be spread:

- Through respiratory secretions by **airborne transmission** and **droplet transmission**
- By **contact transmission** (direct contact or indirect contact) with feces or other body fluids, secretions, or excretions
- Through draining wounds or infective material, such as blood, on needles

TABLE 13-1 TRANSMISSION-BASED PRECAUTIONS FOR COMMON DISEASES

Transmission-Based Precautions Category	Disease or Condition
Airborne	Tuberculosis, measles
Airborne and Contact	Chickenpox, widespread shingles
Droplet	German measles, mumps; influenza
Contact	Head or body lice, scabies, impetigo, infected pressure ulcer with heavy drainage

Each mode of transmission requires special precautions to interrupt the movement of microbes from the infected person to others. If a disease can be passed in more than one way, the nurse will consider all methods of transmission when selecting precautions to use. In addition to standard precautions, two types of transmission-based precautions may also be necessary. Table 13-1 lists transmission-based precautions and common diseases in each category.

Isolation

"Isolation" precautions is another term loosely used to refer to transmission-based precautions. **Isolation** means being separated or set apart. The purpose of isolation is to keep the infectious organism separate and contained, to prevent its spread to others.

Psychological Aspects of Isolation

Isolation technique is the name given to the method of caring for patients with easily transmitted diseases. *Transmission-based precautions* refers to the type of isolation precautions being used. Remember that you are isolating the pathogens, not the person. The **isolation unit** is usually a private room.

The patient in isolation fears both the disease and the practices that must be followed for these precautions to be effective. The patient may worry about passing the infection to family and friends. If the patient is confused, he or she may be afraid of the PPE. Patients in isolation require more emotional support and care. Plan your schedule to spend the necessary time with a patient in isolation. If you follow the transmission-based precautions listed for the condition, you need not fear contracting the disease.

Transmission-Based Isolation Precautions

Standard precautions are used with all patients. When patients are known to have or are suspected of having an infectious disease, isolation precautions are always used *in addition to* standard precautions. Guidelines from the Centers for Disease Control and Prevention (CDC) describe the precautions and protective equipment to be used. Review the information about the mode of transmission in Unit 12 for airborne, droplet, and contact spread of pathogens.

Airborne Precautions **Airborne precautions** are used for diseases that are transmitted by air currents. Figure 13-10 shows the required precautions.

Special air handling is necessary when airborne precautions are used. A **negative air pressure room** is commonly used. Your facility may call this an **AII (A2) room** because of the type of air handling used. This means that air leaves the room through a special exhaust system. Air from the isolation room does not circulate into the facility.

Some isolation rooms have special **ultraviolet germicidal irradiation (UVGI)** lights in the air ducts. These are not used for lighting the room. UVGI uses ultraviolet-C light to eliminate pathogens in the upper portion of the room. The lights are not on all the time, and their use is monitored to ensure that the radiation is not a threat to the patient or workers.

Most facilities have an anteroom adjoining an AII room (Figure 13-11). An **anteroom** is a small room just inside the entrance to the patient room. The anteroom serves as a buffer for the changes in air pressure between the patient room and the hallway. When caring for a patient in airborne precautions:

- Keep the door to the room closed.
- Wear a **high-efficiency particulate air (HEPA) filter mask** or other specially filtered mask (Figure 13-12) when entering the room. These filters protect workers from the tiny pathogens present in the environment. A surgical mask does not provide this level of protection. Each worker must be professionally fitted with a HEPA or other filter mask before being permitted to use it. Remove the respirator after leaving the room and closing the door.

Masks that are worn in an airborne precautions room must be approved by the **National Institute of Occupational Safety and Health (NIOSH)**. This agency is part of the CDC, and makes recommendations for preventing work-related disease and injury. The **PFR95 respirator** (Figure 13-13) and the **N95 respirator** (Figure 13-14) are approved alternatives to HEPA masks. Some workers prefer these because they are lighter and more comfortable. The employee must self-test the respirator each time it is applied to be sure there are no air leaks. Figure 13-15 shows the procedure for checking the N95 respirator.

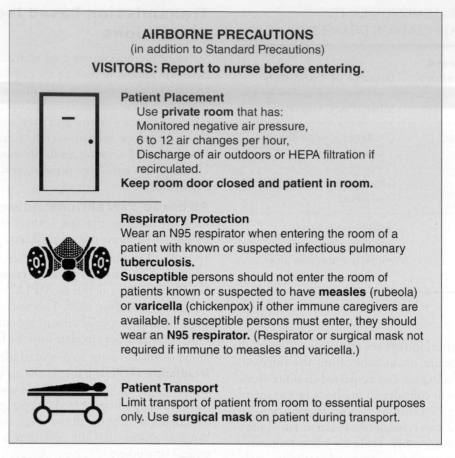

AIRBORNE PRECAUTIONS
(in addition to Standard Precautions)

VISITORS: Report to nurse before entering.

Patient Placement
Use **private room** that has:
Monitored negative air pressure,
6 to 12 air changes per hour,
Discharge of air outdoors or HEPA filtration if recirculated.
Keep room door closed and patient in room.

Respiratory Protection
Wear an N95 respirator when entering the room of a patient with known or suspected infectious pulmonary **tuberculosis.**
Susceptible persons should not enter the room of patients known or suspected to have **measles** (rubeola) or **varicella** (chickenpox) if other immune caregivers are available. If susceptible persons must enter, they should wear an **N95 respirator.** (Respirator or surgical mask not required if immune to measles and varicella.)

Patient Transport
Limit transport of patient from room to essential purposes only. Use **surgical mask** on patient during transport.

FIGURE 13-10 Airborne precautions. *(Courtesy of BREVIS Corporation, Salt Lake City, UT)*

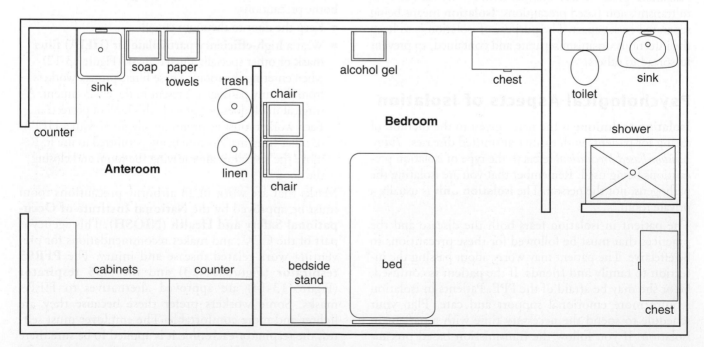

FIGURE 13-11 The floor plan for an isolation room. Note the anteroom, which is an entrance room that is used in negative-pressure rooms. *(© Delmar/Cengage Learning)*

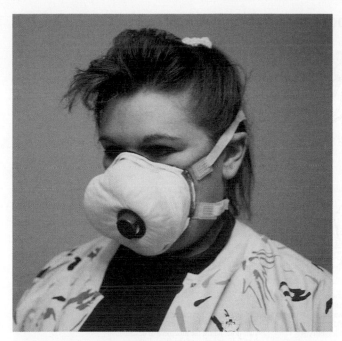

FIGURE 13-12 The HEPA respirator filter is individually fitted to the worker. The respirator is reusable. Store it according to facility policy. (© Delmar/Cengage Learning)

Droplet Precautions Droplet precautions are used for diseases that are spread by droplets in the air. Figure 13-16 shows the requirements for droplet precautions.

- Droplets can be infectious in the air and on contaminated surfaces. Apply a surgical mask when entering the room. In some facilities, gloves and gown are also required. In others, both a mask and eye protection are required. Follow your facility policies.

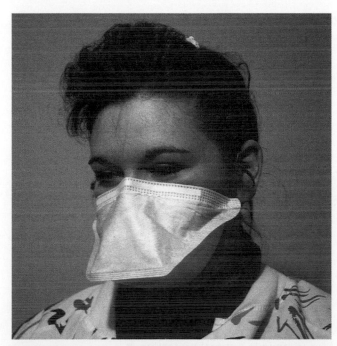

FIGURE 13-13 The PFR95 respirator filter is preferred by many workers because it is lightweight and comfortable. (© Delmar/Cengage Learning)

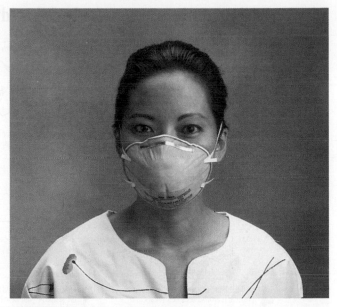

FIGURE 13-14 The N95 respirator is disposable. Some facilities store it for one shift, then discard it. (Courtesy of 3M Health Care, St. Paul, MN)

- The door can be open if the patient desires and the bed is more than three feet from the door.
- The patient must wear a surgical mask (if tolerated) if leaving the room is medically necessary. The person transporting the patient does not wear a mask in the hallway.

Contact Precautions Contact precautions are used when the infection is spread by direct or indirect contact. For example, contact precautions are used for scabies, infected pressure ulcers, and gastroenteritis. Figure 13-17 shows the requirements for contact precautions.

Apply a gown and gloves before entering the room. Change gloves any time you contact contaminated matter in the room. Wash your hands before putting on a new pair of gloves. When finished, remove the PPE and discard it inside the room. Wash your hands. Avoid touching environmental surfaces or other items with your hands or uniform when leaving the room. Use a paper towel to open the door. Discard the towel in the trash container inside the room.

New Precautions and Screening As a result of the 2003 SARS outbreaks, the CDC recommends that measures to prevent the spread of *respiratory infections* begin with the first point of contact with a potentially infected person. The new recommendations are part of standard precautions. Facilities are posting signs at the entrance advising patients and visitors to:

- Notify personnel if symptoms of a respiratory infection are present when they first register for care.
- Practice respiratory hygiene/cough etiquette by covering the nose and mouth when coughing or sneezing, discarding tissues correctly, and cleansing hands after contact with secretions. Facilities are also mounting dispensers of alcohol-based hand cleaner in areas convenient to the public.

Donning instructions (to be followed each time product is worn):

1 Cup the respirator in your hand with the nosepiece at fingertips, allowing the headbands to hang freely below hands.

2 Position the respirator under your chin with the nosepiece up.

3 Pull the top strap over your head so it rests high on the back of head.

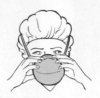
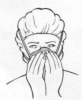

4 Pull the bottom strap over your head and position it around neck below ears.

5 Using two hands, mold the nosepiece to the shape of your nose by pushing inward while moving fingertips down both sides of the nosepiece. Pinching the nosepiece using one hand may result in less effective respirator performance.

6 FACE FIT CHECK
The respirator seal should be checked before each use. To check fit, place both hands completely over the respirator and exhale. If air leaks around your nose, adjust the nosepiece as described in step 5. If air leaks at respirator edges, adjust the straps back along the sides of your head. Recheck.

NOTE: If you cannot achieve proper fit, do not enter the isolation or treatment area. See your supervisor.

Removal instructions:

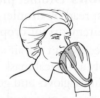

1 Cup the respirator in your hand to maintain position on face. Pull bottom strap over head.

2 Still holding respirator in position, pull top strap over head.

3 Remove respirator from face and discard or store according to your facility's policy.

FIGURE 13-15 Fit-test the respirator each time you wear it. *(Courtesy of 3M Health Care, St. Paul, MN)*

PERSONAL PROTECTIVE EQUIPMENT

Personal protective equipment includes gloves, gown, mask, and goggles or face shield. The following sections describe the correct use of this equipment (see Procedures 2 through 6).

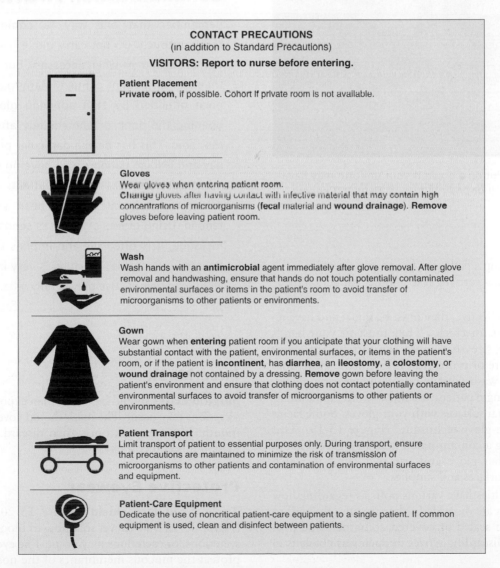

DROPLET PRECAUTIONS
(in addition to Standard Precautions)
VISITORS: Report to nurse before entering.

Patient Placement
Private room, if possible. Cohort or maintain spatial separation of **3 feet** from other patients or visitors if private room is not available.

Mask
Wear mask when working within **3 feet** of patient (or upon entering room).

Patient Transport
Limit transport of patient from room to essential purposes only. Use **surgical mask** on patient during transport.

FIGURE 13-16 Droplet precautions. *(Courtesy of BREVIS Corporation, Salt Lake City, UT)*

Cover Gown

A gown made of a moisture-resistant material is used when soiling or splashing with blood, body fluids, secretions, or excretions is likely (Figure 13-18). Discard gowns after use.

Gloves

The use of gloves prevents the spread of disease. They should be worn for most procedures, and when contact with potentially infectious items is likely. Wear gloves if your hands are chapped, cracked, or have a rash, cuts, or open sores. For routine cleaning procedures, wear utility gloves. *The use of gloves does not reduce the need for hand-washing.* Always wash your hands before and after glove use.

Gloves are used to:

- Protect workers from picking up pathogens from a patient
- Protect patients from picking up a pathogen from workers' hands.

CONTACT PRECAUTIONS
(in addition to Standard Precautions)
VISITORS: Report to nurse before entering.

Patient Placement
Private room, if possible. Cohort if private room is not available.

Gloves
Wear gloves when entering patient room.
Change gloves after having contact with infective material that may contain high concentrations of microorganisms (**fecal** material and **wound drainage**). **Remove** gloves before leaving patient room.

Wash
Wash hands with an **antimicrobial** agent immediately after glove removal. After glove removal and handwashing, ensure that hands do not touch potentially contaminated environmental surfaces or items in the patient's room to avoid transfer of microorganisms to other patients or environments.

Gown
Wear gown when **entering** patient room if you anticipate that your clothing will have substantial contact with the patient, environmental surfaces, or items in the patient's room, or if the patient is **incontinent**, has **diarrhea**, an **ileostomy**, a **colostomy**, or **wound drainage** not contained by a dressing. **Remove** gown before leaving the patient's environment and ensure that clothing does not contact potentially contaminated environmental surfaces to avoid transfer of microorganisms to other patients or environments.

Patient Transport
Limit transport of patient to essential purposes only. During transport, ensure that precautions are maintained to minimize the risk of transmission of microorganisms to other patients and contamination of environmental surfaces and equipment.

Patient-Care Equipment
Dedicate the use of noncritical patient-care equipment to a single patient. If common equipment is used, clean and disinfect between patients.

FIGURE 13-17 Contact precautions. *(Courtesy of BREVIS Corporation, Salt Lake City, UT)*

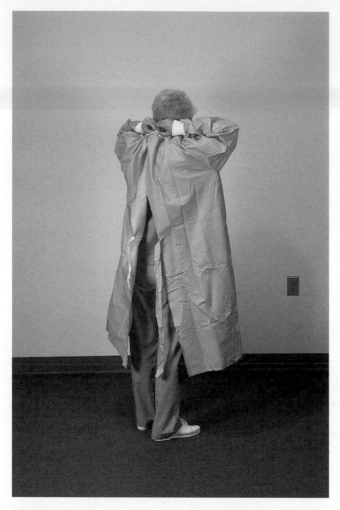

FIGURE 13-18 Put on a gown if your uniform may have contact with blood or body fluids. (© Delmar/Cengage Learning)

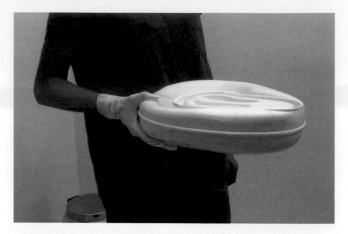

FIGURE 13-19 The one-glove technique is used to carry contaminated items. (© Delmar/Cengage Learning)

- Avoid picking up a pathogen from a patient or his environment and carrying it to another patient on the hands.

For gloves to be effective, they must be intact and have no visible cuts, tears, or cracks. They must fit your hands well. Select the size that most comfortably fits your hands. A measure of protection is lost if the glove does not fit. Do not wash your hands while wearing gloves. Gloves are for single patient use only. Avoid contaminating environmental surfaces with your gloves. Some facilities use the "one-glove technique" (Figure 13-19). This involves carrying a contaminated item in a gloved hand. Remove the other glove and use that hand to touch environmental surfaces and supplies.

Health care facilities have various policies regarding how and where gloves are discarded. Many require the staff to discard gloves in sealed or covered containers and prohibit you from discarding gloves in open wastebaskets in patient rooms.

Communication HIGHLIGHT

Remember that one way to communicate is through touch. Do not carry glove use to the extreme. Use gloves when necessary, but avoid using them for all patient contact. Many patients have been offended by staff applying gloves before opening the door, or immediately after entering the room. This has been a particular problem with gay and lesbian patients who have no evidence of infectious disease. However, patients of all ages, races, and orientation have been similarly offended. Using gloves at all times sends a negative message. It is offensive and implies that the patient is untouchable. Touching is very important to all human beings. Use gloves only when needed. ■

Face Mask

Surgical masks should be worn when exposure to droplet secretions may occur. The mask should cover the nose and mouth. Use the mask once, then discard. Change your mask if it becomes moist.

Protective Eyewear

Apply a full **face shield** (Figure 13-20), or **goggles** (Figure 13-21), whenever splashing of blood, body fluids, secretions, or excretions may occur. The eyewear does not protect the mucous membranes of the nose and mouth,

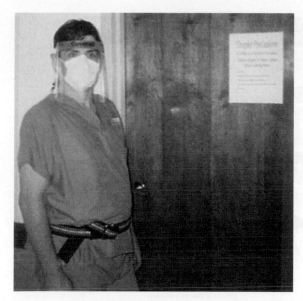

FIGURE 13-20 A surgical mask is always worn under a face shield. (© Delmar/Cengage Learning)

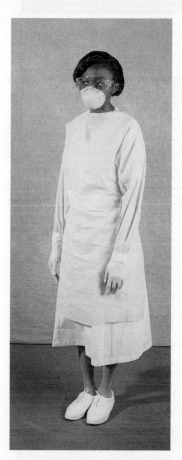

FIGURE 13-21 Always protect your nose and mouth with a mask when wearing goggles. (© Delmar/Cengage Learning)

so a surgical mask is always worn with eyewear. A good rule to follow is that a surgical mask may be worn without protective eyewear, but protective eyewear is never worn without a surgical mask.

Applying and Removing Personal Protective Equipment

Sequence for Applying Personal Protective Equipment
1. Wash hands
2. Gown
3. Mask
4. Goggles or face shield
5. Gloves

Sequence for Removing Personal Protective Equipment
1. Gloves
2. Wash hands
3. Goggles or face shield
4. Gown
5. Mask
6. Wash hands

Figure 13-22 shows the CDC recommendations for application and removal of PPE. Touch only clean areas when removing PPE. Remove PPE at the doorway to the patient room, or in the anteroom. Always wash your hands well or use alcohol-based hand cleaner immediately after removing PPE.

OSHA ALERT

Remember five key points about using PPE:

- Apply PPE before having contact with the patient.
- Use the PPE carefully to prevent spreading contamination.
- When you have finished, remove PPE carefully and discard it properly.
- After removing PPE, wash your hands or use alcohol-based hand cleaner before doing anything else.
- Replace or restock the PPE as necessary. Never leave the supply container or area empty. ■

OSHA ALERT

Always select a gown that fits you correctly. The opening should be in the back and fit securely at the neck and waist. If the gown is too small, wear two gowns. Put the first one on with the opening in the front. Put the second gown on over the first with the opening in the back. ■

SEQUENCE FOR DONNING PERSONAL PROTECTIVE EQUIPMENT (PPE)

The type of PPE used will vary based on the level of precautions required; e.g., Standard and Contact, Droplet or Airborne Infection Isolation.

1. GOWN
- Fully cover torso from neck to knees, arms to end of wrists, and wrap around the back
- Fasten in back of neck and waist

2. MASK OR RESPIRATOR
- Secure ties or elastic bands at middle of head and neck
- Fit flexible band to nose bridge
- Fit snug to face and below chin
- Fit-check respirator

3. GOGGLES OR FACE SHIELD
- Place over face and eyes and adjust to fit

4. GLOVES
- Extend to cover wrist of isolation gown

USE SAFE WORK PRACTICES TO PROTECT YOURSELF AND LIMIT THE SPREAD OF CONTAMINATION

- Keep hands away from face
- Limit surfaces touched
- Change gloves when torn or heavily contaminated
- Perform hand hygiene

SECUENCIA PARA *PONERSE* EL EQUIPO DE PROTECCIÓN PERSONAL (PPE)

El tipo de PPE que se debe utilizar depende del nivel de precaución que sea necesario; por ejemplo, equipo Estándar y de Contacto o de Aislamiento de infecciones transportadas por gotas o por aire.

1. BATA
- Cubra con la bata todo el torso desde el cuello hasta las rodillas, los brazos hasta la muñeca y dóblela alrededor de la espalda
- Átesela por detrás a la altura del cuello y la cintura

2. MÁSCARA O RESPIRADOR
- Asegúrese los cordones o la banda elástica en la mitad de la cabeza y en el cuello
- Ajústese la banda flexible en el puente de la nariz
- Acomódesela en la cara y por debajo del mentón
- Verifique el ajuste del respirador

3. GAFAS PROTECTORAS O CARETAS
- Colóquesela sobre la cara y los ojos y ajústela

4. GUANTES
- Extienda los guantes para que cubran la parte del puño en la bata de aislamiento

UTILICE PRÁCTICAS DE TRABAJO SEGURAS PARA PROTEGERSE USTED MISMO Y LIMITAR LA PROPAGACIÓN DE LA CONTAMINACIÓN

- Mantenga las manos alejadas de la cara
- Limite el contacto con superficies
- Cambie los guantes si se rompen o están demasiado contaminados
- Realice la higiene de las manos

SEQUENCE FOR *REMOVING* PERSONAL PROTECTIVE EQUIPMENT (PPE)

Except for respirator, remove PPE at doorway or in anteroom. Remove respirator after leaving patient room and closing door.

1. GLOVES
- Outside of gloves is contaminated!
- Grasp outside of glove with opposite gloved hand; peel off
- Hold removed glove in gloved hand
- Slide fingers of ungloved hand under remaining glove at wrist
- Peel glove off over first glove
- Discard gloves in waste container

2. GOGGLES OR FACE SHIELD
- Outside of goggles or face shield is contaminated!
- To remove, handle by head band or ear pieces
- Place in designated receptacle for reprocessing or in waste container

3. GOWN
- Gown front and sleeves are contaminated!
- Unfasten ties
- Pull away from neck and shoulders, touching inside of gown only
- Turn gown inside out
- Fold or roll into a bundle and discard

4. MASK OR RESPIRATOR
- Front of mask/respirator is contaminated — DO NOT TOUCH!
- Grasp bottom, then top ties or elastics and remove
- Discard in waste container

PERFORM HAND HYGIENE IMMEDIATELY AFTER REMOVING ALL PPE

SECUENCIA PARA *QUITARSE* EL EQUIPO DE PROTECCIÓN PERSONAL (PPE)

Con la excepción del respirador, quítese el PPE en la entrada de la puerta o en la antesala. Quítese el respirador después de salir de la habitación del paciente y de cerrar la puerta.

1. GUANTES
- ¡El exterior de los guantes está contaminado!
- Agarre la parte exterior del guante con la mano opuesta en la que todavía tiene puesto el guante y quíteselo
- Sostenga el guante que se quitó con la mano enguantada
- Deslice los dedos de la mano sin guante por debajo del otro guante que no se ha quitado todavía a la altura de la muñeca
- Quítese el guante de manera que acabe cubriendo el primer guante
- Arroje los guantes en el recipiente de deshechos

2. GAFAS PROTECTORAS O CARETA
- ¡El exterior de las gafas protectoras o de la careta está contaminado!
- Para quitárselas, tómelas por la parte de la banda de la cabeza o de las piezas de las orejas
- Colóquelas en el recipiente designado para reprocesar materiales o de materiales de deshecho

3. BATA
- ¡La parte delantera de la bata y las mangas están contaminadas!
- Desate los cordones
- Tocando solamente el interior de la bata, pásela por encima del cuello y de los hombros
- Voltee la bata al revés
- Dóblela o enróllela y deséchela

4. MÁSCARA O RESPIRADOR
- La parte delantera de la máscara o respirador está contaminada — ¡NO LA TOQUE!
- Primero agarre la parte de abajo, luego los cordones o banda elástica de arriba y por último quítese la máscara o respirador
- Arrójela en el recipiente de deshechos

EFECTÚE LA HIGIENE DE LAS MANOS INMEDIATAMENTE DESPUÉS DE QUITARSE CUALQUIER EQUIPO DE PROTECCIÓN PERSONAL

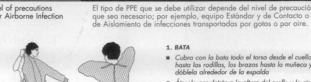
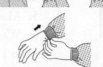
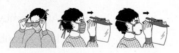
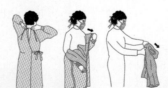
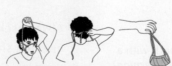

FIGURE 13-22 Sequence for applying and removing personal protective equipment. (*Courtesy of Centers for Disease Control and Prevention*)

PROCEDURE

2

PUTTING ON A MASK

1. Assemble equipment:
   - Mask
2. Tie top strings of mask first, then bottom strings, or slip the elastic ear straps over the ears, depending on the type of mask used.
3. Adjust mask over nose and mouth by fitting the flexible bridge to the nose.

4. Adjust the mask so it fits snugly around the face and chin.
5. Replace your mask if it becomes moist during procedures.
6. Do not reuse a mask and do not let the mask hang around your neck.

PROCEDURE

3

PUTTING ON A GOWN

To be effective, a gown should have long sleeves, be long enough to cover the uniform, and be big enough to overlap in the back. Gowns should be waterproof.

1. Assemble equipment:
   - Clean gown
   - Paper towel
2. Remove wristwatch; place it on a paper towel.
3. Wash hands.
4. Put on the gown outside the patient's room or in the anteroom. Put on gown by slipping your arms into the sleeves (Figure 13-23A).
5. Slip the fingers of both hands under the inside neckband and grasp the ties in back. Secure the neckband (Figure 13-23B).
6. Reach behind and overlap the edges of the gown. Secure the waist ties.
7. Take your watch into the isolation unit, leaving it on the paper towel.

Remember when using gowns:
- A disposable gown is worn only once and then is discarded as infectious waste.
- A reusable cloth gown is worn only once and then is handled as contaminated linen.
- Carry out all procedures in the unit at one time, to save time and unnecessary waste of supplies.

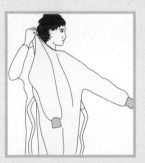 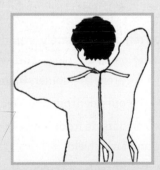

FIGURE 13-23A Select a cover gown that is the right size for you. Unfold the gown, then slip your arms in and pull it up to your shoulders. (*Courtesy of Centers for Disease Control and Prevention*)

FIGURE 13-23B Slip your hands inside, under the neckband, and adust it to fit. Tie the neck ties. Then reach behind, overlapping the edges of the gown so your uniform is completely covered, and tie the waist ties. (*Courtesy of Centers for Disease Control and Prevention*)

PROCEDURE

PUTTING ON GLOVES

1. Assemble equipment:
   - Disposable gloves in correct size

2. Wash your hands.

3. If a gown is required, put gloves on after you have put on the gown.

4. Pick up a glove by the cuff and place it on your hand.

5. Repeat with a glove for the other hand.

6. Interlace fingers to adjust the gloves on your hands.

7. If wearing a gown, pull cuffs of gloves up over the sleeves (Figure 13-24).

8. Remember when using gloves:
   - Wash hands before and after using gloves.
   - Remove gloves if they become torn or soiled. Wash hands and put on a new pair.

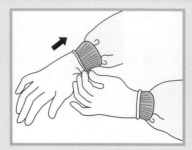

FIGURE 13-24 If you are wearing a gown, pull the cuffs of the gloves up to cover the gown sleeves. (*Courtesy of Centers for Disease Control and Prevention*)

OSHA ALERT

To remove PPE safely, you must be able to identify what parts are clean and what are contaminated. These areas are contaminated:

- The outside front and sleeves of the gown
- The outside front of the goggles, mask, respirator, and face shield
- The outside of the gloves
- Any area with visible blood, body fluids, or soiling

Touch only clean areas when removing PPE. These areas are clean:

- Inside the gloves
- The inside and back of the gown, including the ties
- The ties, elastic, or earpieces of the mask, goggles, and face shield ■

You may remove your PPE after you have finished all tasks in the patient's room. Follow the instructions in Procedures 5 and 6.

EQUIPMENT

Disposable (used once and discarded) patient care equipment is ideal for patients on isolation precautions. Frequently used items remain in the patient's unit. Most articles will not require special handling unless they are contaminated (or likely to be contaminated) with infective material.

Containment of Contaminated Articles

When leaving the patient's room, bag, label, and discard contaminated items in the designated area. A single bag may be used if it is waterproof and contains the article without tearing or contaminating the outside of the bag. (Refer to Procedures 7 and 8.) A label is necessary if the items in the bag have contacted biohazardous materials.

PROCEDURE

5

REMOVING CONTAMINATED GLOVES

1. Grasp the cuff of one glove on the outside with the fingers of the other hand (Figure 13-25A).

2. Pull the cuff of the glove down, drawing it over the glove (Figure 13-25B). Pull that glove off your hand.

3. Hold the glove with the still-gloved hand.

4. Insert the fingers of the ungloved hand under the cuff of the glove on the other hand (Figure 13-25C).

5. Pull the glove off inside out, drawing it over the first glove.

6. Drop both gloves together into the biohazardous waste receptacle (Figure 13-25D).

7. Wash your hands. Dry with a paper towel and discard the towel in the proper container. Use a dry towel to turn off the water faucet. Discard the towel.

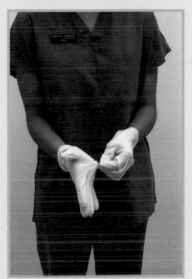

FIGURE 13-25A With the fingers of one glove, grasp the cuff or palm of glove on the other hand. (© Delmar/Cengage Learning)

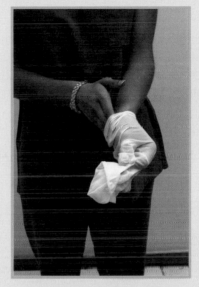

FIGURE 13-25C Hold the glove just removed in the gloved hand. Insert fingers of the ungloved hand inside the cuff of the other glove. (© Delmar/Cengage Learning)

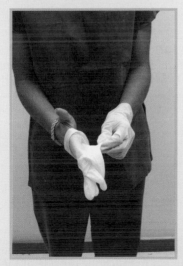

FIGURE 13-25B Pull the cuff of the glove down over the hand and fingers and remove it. (© Delmar/Cengage Learning)

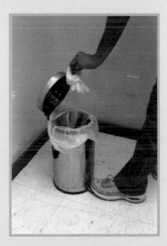

FIGURE 13–25D Pull the glove down over the hand and then pull both gloves off, holding the inside (clean side of glove). Discard the gloves in the proper container. (© Delmar/Cengage Learning)

PROCEDURE

6

REMOVING CONTAMINATED GLOVES, EYE PROTECTION, GOWN, AND MASK

1. Assemble equipment:
   - Biohazardous waste receptacle for disposable items
   - Waste receptacle for gown if it is not disposable
   - Paper towels

2. Undo waist ties of gown, if they are in the front. Follow Procedure 5 for removing contaminated gloves.

3. Grasp the earpieces or head strap of goggles or face shield and lift the eye protection outward, away from the face, and up (Figure 13-26A). Discard or reprocess according to facility policy.

4. Undo waist ties of gown, if they are in the back (Figure 13-26B).

5. Undo the neck ties and loosen gown at shoulders.

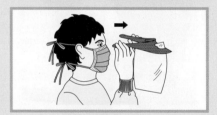

FIGURE 13-26A With ungloved hands, grasp the clean elastic strap or earpiece and lift the eye protection away from the face. (*Courtesy of Centers for Disease Control and Prevention*)

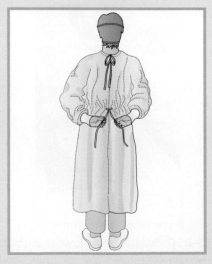

FIGURE 13-26B Untie the gown waist ties. (*Courtesy of Centers for Disease Control and Prevention*)

6. Slip the fingers of your dominant hand inside the cuff of the other hand without touching the outside of the gown (Figure 13-26C).

7. Using the gown-covered hand, pull the gown down over the other hand (Figure 13-26D) and then off both arms.

8. As the gown is removed, fold it away from the body with the contaminated side inward and then roll it up (Figure 13-26E). Dispose of the contaminated gown in the appropriate container.

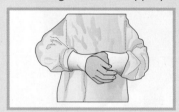

FIGURE 13-26C Slip the fingers of one hand inside the cuff of the other hand. Pull the gown down over the hand. Do not touch the outside of the gown. (*Courtesy of Centers for Disease Control and Prevention*)

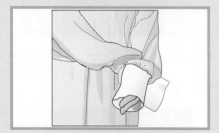

FIGURE 13-26D Using the gown-covered hand, pull the gown down over the other hand. (*Courtesy of Centers for Disease Control and Prevention*)

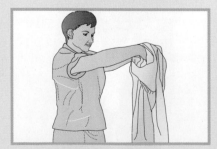

FIGURE 13-26E Pull the gown down off the arms, being careful not to touch the outside of the gown. Hold the gown away from your uniform and roll it with the contaminated side in. (*Courtesy of Centers for Disease Control and Prevention*)

continues

PROCEDURE 6 CONTINUED

9. Turn on faucets with a clean paper towel. Discard the towel.

10. Wash your hands and dry them with a clean paper towel.

11. Use a clean, dry paper towel to turn off the faucet.

12. If you brought a watch into the area (see Procedure 3), remove the watch from the paper towel. Hold the clean side of the paper towel and discard the towel.

13. Use a paper towel to grasp the door handle as you leave the patient's room. Discard the paper towel before leaving the room.

14. Remove mask:
    - Undo the bottom ties first, then the top ties. If the mask has elastic ear straps, remove the strap on one side, then the other.
    - Holding the top ties or one elastic strap, discard the mask in a proper container.

15. Wash your hands.

Soiled linen is a source of pathogens. Transport soiled, wet linen in a leakproof bag. Some facilities place isolation linen in water-soluble bags that melt in the washer. If the bag contains wet linen, place it inside a second plastic bag, because the water-soluble bag will begin to melt if it touches wet linen. The outer bag or container should be labeled with the biohazard emblem.

TRANSPORTING THE PATIENT IN ISOLATION

Sometimes a patient in isolation must go to another area of the facility for treatment or testing. The nursing assistant should:
- Wear PPE when picking up and returning the patient to the isolation room, but not while transporting the patient in the hallway.

PROCEDURE

TRANSFERRING NONDISPOSABLE EQUIPMENT OUTSIDE OF THE ISOLATION UNIT

1. Nondisposable equipment used in a transmission-based precautions area may be dedicated to that patient. The equipment remains in the unit and is used only by that patient. Cleaning is done in the room by the nursing assistant or the housekeeper.

2. If the equipment must be used for other patients, remove it from the isolation unit and disinfect or sterilize it before using it with another patient.

3. Before leaving the isolation unit, wipe the equipment with a disinfectant wipe, if possible.

4. Place the equipment in a biohazard plastic bag. In some facilities, a second person opens a large plastic bag and folds the top over into a cuff to cover his or her hands. The second person stands outside the door and holds the bag open. The person inside the room places the item into the open bag. The second worker fastens the top of the bag.

5. Follow Procedures 5 and 6 for removing contaminated PPE.

6. Pick up the bag containing the equipment and leave the isolation unit.

7. Once outside the unit, disinfect or sterilize the equipment. Apply the PPE necessary for the cleaning procedure.

8. Some equipment may be terminally (finally and completely) cleaned with disinfectant in the patient's unit when isolation is discontinued.

PROCEDURE

8

SPECIMEN COLLECTION FROM A PATIENT IN AN ISOLATION UNIT

1. Outside the isolation unit, assemble equipment:
   * Clean specimen container and cover
   * Paper towel
   * Biohazard bag for specimen container (Figure 13-27)
   * Two completed labels, one for the specimen container and one for the specimen bag

Note: The specimen bag may have a preprinted block that can be completed with the required information. In this case, a second label is not

needed. Prepare the bag before collecting the specimen.

2. Place the equipment on the isolation cart while you put on PPE.

3. The biohazard bag for specimen transport remains outside the isolation unit.

4. Carry the specimen equipment into the isolation unit. Place the container and cover on a paper towel.

5. Identify the patient and explain what you plan to do.

6. Provide privacy.

7. Allow the patient to help as much as possible.

8. Raise the bed to a comfortable working height.

9. Obtain the specimen. Place it into the container without touching the outside of the container.

10. Cover the container and apply a label.

11. Clean the equipment used to obtain the specimen according to facility policy.

12. Carry out all ending procedure actions (see Unit 15).

13. Remove PPE as described in Procedures 5 and 6.

14. Wash your hands.

15. Use a paper towel to pick up the specimen container. Use another paper towel to open the door to leave the isolation unit.

16. Outside the unit, gather the paper towel in your hands so the edges do not hang loosely. Place the specimen container in the biohazard transport bag, being careful not to allow the paper towel to touch the outside of the transport bag.

17. Discard the paper towels in the appropriate receptacle.

18. Follow facility policy for transporting the specimen.

19. Wash your hands.

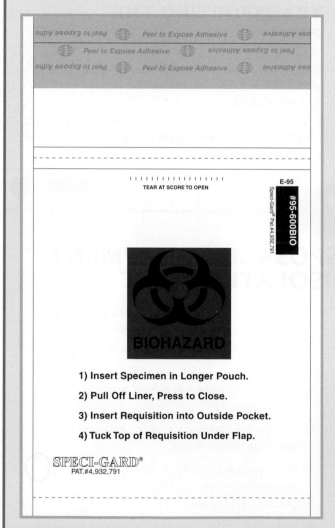

FIGURE 13-27 Transport specimens in the sealed, labeled transport bag. (© *Delmar/Cengage Learning*)

PROCEDURE

9

TRANSPORTING A PATIENT TO AND FROM THE ISOLATION UNIT

1. Wash your hands.

2. Assemble equipment:
   - Transport vehicle (wheelchair or stretcher)
   - Clean sheet
   - Mask for patient, if isolation precautions require it

3. Notify the department where the patient is being transported.

4. If the patient is to be transported by stretcher, ask for assistance in moving the patient to the stretcher.

5. Cover the transport vehicle with a clean sheet. Do not let the sheet touch the floor.

6. Wash your hands.

7. Put on PPE as required by type of precautions being used.

8. Wheel the transport vehicle into the isolation unit.

9. Identify the patient. Explain what you plan to do.

10. Provide privacy.

11. Allow the patient to help as much as possible.

12. If the patient is to be transported by wheelchair, the bed must be in the lowest horizontal position. For transport by stretcher, raise the bed to the same height as the stretcher.

13. Assist the patient into the wheelchair or onto the stretcher.

14. Put a mask on the patient, if required.

15. Wrap the patient in a sheet. Make sure the sheet does not touch the floor.

16. Remove PPE and wash your hands. Open the door and take the patient out of the isolation unit (Figure 13-28).

17. To return a patient to an isolation unit, place the wheelchair or stretcher near the wall of the room as you put on PPE.

18. Enter the isolation unit, unwrap the patient from the sheet, and remove the patient's mask, if used.

19. Assist the patient from the wheelchair or stretcher and return the patient to bed.

20. Carry out ending procedure actions (see Unit 15).

21. Place the sheet in the laundry hamper. Discard the patient's mask in the biohazardous trash.

22. Remove PPE and wash your hands.

23. Remove the transport vehicle from the isolation unit. Clean and store it.

24. Report completion of procedure.

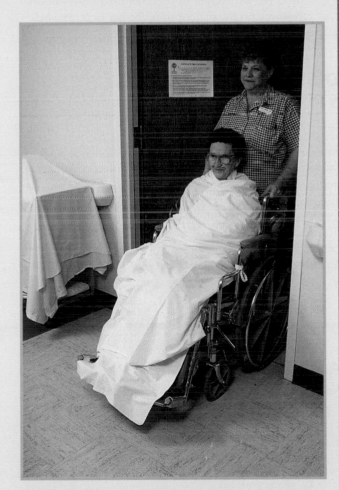

FIGURE 13-28 This patient is leaving her room, where contact precautions are in effect. The receiving area has been notified of her arrival. (© Delmar/Cengage Learning)

- Wash hands or use an alcohol-based hand cleaner after removing PPE.
- Notify the receiving unit of the patient's planned arrival and describe the type of precautions being used.
  - If the patient is on airborne or droplet precautions, the patient should wear a surgical mask while out of the isolation room. (Filter masks are not used on patients.)
  - If the patient is on contact precautions, the infectious area should be covered or contained while the patient is out of the room. In some facilities, the patient is covered with a clean isolation gown or wrapped with a bath blanket before transport. (Refer to Procedure 9.)
- If you will use the elevator during transport, do not allow others to enter when the patient is present, to reduce the risk of spreading infection.
- Don PPE in the new location if you will be assisting with patient care or transfers in that area.
- Disinfect the wheelchair or stretcher used for transport after you return the patient to his or her unit, or when the transport vehicle is no longer needed.

DISINFECTION AND STERILIZATION

Disinfection is the process of eliminating pathogens from equipment and instruments. A chemical called a *disinfectant* is used. You may be required to disinfect personal care items such as wash basins, bedpans, and urinals. You may also use disinfectants to clean wheelchairs and other furniture items. Items are usually washed before they are disinfected. Follow the directions for the product being used. Wear utility gloves and a gown. The chemicals in the disinfectants will damage exam gloves, so they will not

protect you. You may also need a face shield and mask if splashing is likely. Select PPE that is appropriate to the activity or procedure.

SURGICAL ASEPSIS

Surgical asepsis is the means by which an area is kept free of all microbes, both pathogens and nonpathogens. In procedures where surgical asepsis is used, equipment and supplies must be **sterile**.

Sterilization removes all microbes from an item. This process can be completed in an **autoclave**, which uses steam and pressure. Gas sterilization is also used in some facilities. Equipment to be sterilized is specially wrapped. Tape on the outer package changes color when the package is sterilized (Figure 13-29). Do not use the package if the tape has not changed color, or if the package has gotten wet, has been accidentally opened, or is beyond the expiration date.

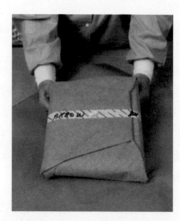

FIGURE 13-29 Before sterilization, the stripes on the tape are not visible. The stripes appear in the autoclave when the tape is exposed to heat and steam. The stripes indicate that the package has been sterilized. *(© Delmar/Cengage Learning)*

REVIEW

A. Multiple Choice

Select the one best answer for each of the following.

1. Housing and caring for a person with an infection is known as
   a. segregation.
   b. isolation.
   c. sequestration.
   d. separation.

2. To remove PPE after caring for a patient in isolation precautions, you should
   a. remove the gown first.
   b. remove the gloves first.

   c. remove the mask first.
   d. remove PPE in any order.

3. The basic foundation of medical asepsis is
   a. handwashing.
   b. wearing goggles.
   c. wearing a mask.
   d. wearing a gown.

4. If there is an exposure incident, you should
   a. ignore the situation.
   b. report it at once to the supervisor.
   c. call the doctor.
   d. tell other nursing assistants.

5. An AII (A2) isolation room
   a. must have the air conditioner on at all times.
   b. has the window cracked open 12 hours a day.
   c. is connected to the facility ventilation system.
   d. uses a negative pressure ventilation system.

6. If a person has signs of respiratory infection upon facility contact, he or she is
   a. instructed to apply a surgical mask.
   b. asked to use respiratory hygiene and cough etiquette.
   c. promptly placed in airborne or droplet precautions.
   d. instructed to leave and return when symptom-free.

7. The most important nursing assistant measure to prevent the spread of infection is
   a. using isolation technique.
   b. good handwashing.
   c. wearing gloves.
   d. using standard precautions.

8. Alcohol-based hand cleaners may be used during routine care except when the hands are visibly soiled or when the
   a. patient is suspected of having an infection spread by spores.
   b. nursing assistant has been caring for a patient in contact precautions.
   c. nursing assistant did not wear gloves during patient contact.
   d. patient is suspected of having an infection caused by drug-resistant pathogens.

9. A room with negative air pressure will be used for Mrs. Wingfield, a new admission who is suspected of having tuberculosis. This room is used for patients in isolation for
   a. universal precautions.
   b. contact precautions.
   c. droplet precautions.
   d. airborne precautions. ✗ *TB*

10. Ultraviolet germicidal irradiation (UVGI) is used to
    a. provide extra lighting to make it easier to see when doing procedures.
    b. lighting the anteroom to kill microbes after patient care.
    c. eliminating pathogens in the upper part of the room and air ducts.
    d. help maintain a negative-pressure environment in the hallway.

11. When a patient is in isolation,
    a. he or she may never leave the isolation room for tests.
    b. standard precautions are used in addition to isolation measures.
    c. the nursing assistant must always apply a mask before entering the room.
    d. he or she must wear a mask while the nursing assistant is giving care.

12. The nursing assistant must apply full PPE in this order:
    a. gown, mask, goggles, gloves.
    b. mask, gown, gloves, goggles.
    c. gloves, goggles, gown, mask.
    d. goggles, mask, gown, gloves.

13. The nursing assistant must remove full PPE in this order:
    a. gown, mask, goggles, gloves.
    b. mask, gown, gloves, goggles.
    c. gloves, goggles, gown, mask.
    d. goggles, mask, gown, gloves.

14. The nursing assistant must select gloves that
    a. fit very tightly.
    b. are the correct size.
    c. are a little too small.
    d. are one size too big.

B. Nursing Assistant Challenge

Mrs. Minion is being transferred to an isolation room. You must set up the room.

15. What equipment should be assembled and where is each item placed?

16. What effect might being placed on isolation have on Mrs. Minion?

17. What might you do to make her adjustment easier?

18. How might her visitors feel?

You are reporting on duty. During your shift, you will be handling food trays, making beds, giving baths, and helping to change a patient who is wet with urine. During your shift you will use a facial tissue and visit the rest room. List six times you will need to wash your hands.

19. _Gloves_
20. _mask_
21. _gown_
22. _____
23. _____
24. _____

Safety and Mobility

Environmental and Nursing Assistant Safety

OBJECTIVES

After completing this unit, you will be able to:
- Spell and define terms.
- Describe the health care facility environment.
- Identify measures to promote environmental safety.
- Describe the elements required for a fire.
- List five measures to prevent fires.
- Describe the procedure to follow if a fire occurs.
- Describe the PASS procedure.
- List at least 10 guidelines for dealing with a violent individual.
- List techniques for using ergonomics on the job.
- Demonstrate appropriate body mechanics.
- Describe the types of information contained in Material Safety Data Sheets.

VOCABULARY

Learn the meaning and the correct spelling of the following words and phrases:

concurrent cleaning	incident report	private room	ward
environmental safety	Material Safety Data	RACE	workplace violence
ergonomics	Sheets (MSDS)	semiprivate room	
incident	PASS	side rails	

INTRODUCTION

The hospital room is the patient's home while he or she is hospitalized (Figure 14-1). The room becomes the patient's world. Cheerful and pleasant surroundings give the patient a better sense of well-being. Attention to safety helps foster feelings of security in this strange environment. *Both* help speed recovery.

The nursing assistant helps keep the patient's unit safe and clean. All health care providers share the task of keeping the entire nursing unit safe and clean.

Environmental safety refers to the condition of an entire facility—patient rooms, hallways, and all departments. Prevention of injuries to patients, visitors, volunteers, and staff members is of primary concern.

Infection Control ALERT

Some hospitals do not permit flowers in areas such as the burn unit, or rooms of patients with weakened immune systems. Flowers increase the risk of spreading infection. Plants and flowers should be cared for by staff who are not involved in patient care, or by the patient or a family member. If you must touch flowers or plants, wear gloves. Perform thorough hand hygiene with soap and water or an alcohol preparation when finished. ■

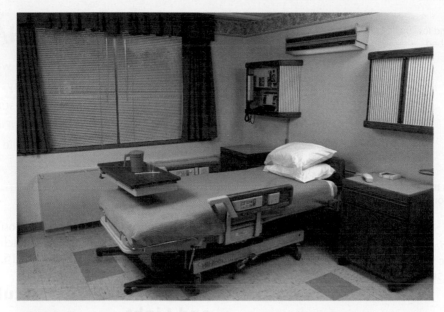

FIGURE 14-1 The patient's unit is home during the hospital stay. (© Delmar/Cengage Learning)

THE PATIENT ENVIRONMENT

In a health care facility, the basic patient unit consists of a/an:

- Hospital bed with rails (Figure 14-2)
- Bedside table
- Chair
- Reading lamp
- Wastebasket
- Overbed table
- Signal cord

A **private room** contains only one bed. **Semiprivate rooms** contain two beds. **Wards** are multiple-bed rooms, usually with three or four beds. Each room and bed are numbered. The beds are marked by letters or numbers. For example, Room 871 in a large medical center may be a four-unit ward. The beds are labeled A, B, C, D (or 1, 2, 3, 4). The patient in the fourth bed is in Unit 871-D or Unit 871-4.

Hospital Beds

Most hospital beds have the same features, but there may be some differences in construction or operation. Hospital beds:

- Differ in how they operate. Most are controlled electrically (Figure 14-3). Some older beds are operated by the turning of cranks or gatch handles (Figure 14-4). These are usually found in home care and some long-term care facilities.

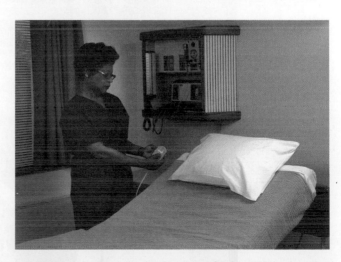

FIGURE 14-2 All hospital beds are equipped with side rails. These are split rails that can be raised and lowered in any combination. (© Delmar/Cengage Learning)

FIGURE 14-3 Some beds also have foot controls that are used to change the angle of the bed. The manual switch controls the head and knee elevation. (© Delmar/Cengage Learning)

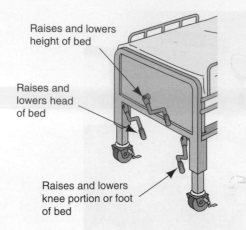

Raises and lowers
height of bed

Raises and
lowers head
of bed

Raises and lowers
knee portion or foot
of bed

FIGURE 14-4 Gatch handles are used to change the position of nonelectric beds. Some stretchers also use handles similar to these. *(© Delmar/Cengage Learning)*

- May be raised to a high horizontal position. This position reduces strain for caregivers. Beds must be returned to the lowest horizontal position when you leave the room.
- Are on wheels, to make it easy to move beds from one place to another. The wheels should always be locked unless the bed is being moved.
- Are jointed in the middle so that the head may be raised.
- Are jointed behind the knees to increase physical comfort for the patient who is confined to bed.

Side rails are attached to the hospital bed. They protect the patient from falling. Side rails are considered to be

OSHA ALERT

Elevating the bed to a proper working height is one of the most important ways to protect your back. For patient safety, make sure you lower the bed when you leave the room. Elevate the rails if you must leave the bedside while the bed is in the high position. ■

restraints in some circumstances. Most health care facilities have policies, procedures, and guidelines describing their use. Side rails are discussed in Unit 15.

Temperature, Air Circulation, and Light

As you adjust and maintain the temperature, light, and ventilation, keep in mind the patient's condition, the patient's personal preference, and the needs of the other patients in the room.

The best temperature is about 72°F (or between 71 to 81°F), according to patient comfort and facility policy. Lower temperatures may cause chilling and higher ones may make patients uncomfortable.

Lighting comes from several sources. Use as much light as needed to safely carry out your job (Figure 14-5). Be careful

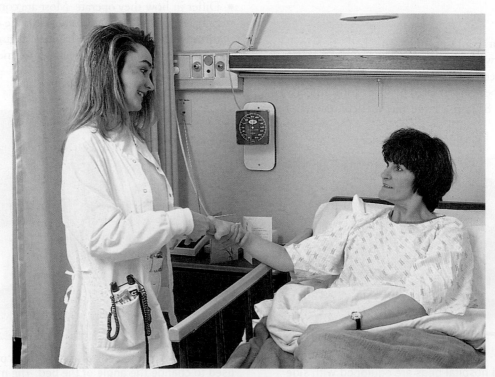

FIGURE 14-5 The overbed light can be adjusted to several different lighting levels. *(© Delmar/Cengage Learning)*

to shield patients' eyes as much as possible. Patients often find it difficult to sleep if lights are too bright. At night, there should be only enough light to enable staff to work safely. If the room does not have a night light, turn the bathroom light on and crack the bathroom door very slightly.

Cleanliness and Noise Reduction

You are responsible for the cleanliness, quiet, and order of the patient units to which you are assigned. Review the information about facility noise in Unit 10.

Nursing assistants are responsible for keeping patients supplied with fresh water, ice, disposable drinking cups, tissues, and straws. Make sure that all necessary hygiene items, such as the wash basin, emesis basin, bedpan, urinal, soap, and towels, are always clean and available (Figure 14-6). These items should be stored in the bedside table.

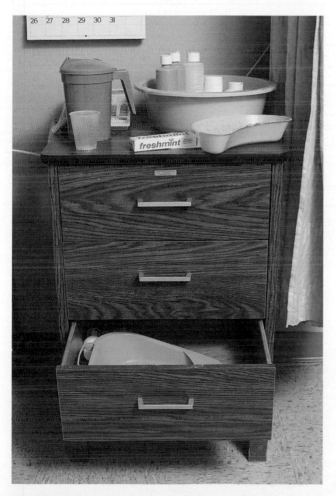

FIGURE 14-6 Personal care supplies are stored in the bedside stand. Items considered clean are stored in shelves or drawers separate from items considered dirty. (© Delmar/Cengage Learning)

Infection Control ALERT

When two or more patients share a room, make sure that all personal care items are labeled with each patient's name. Keep personal care items in the appropriate area. ∎

SAFETY MEASURES

Safety is the responsibility of everyone. A safe environment is essential for both patients and staff. *Safety must be a part of everything you do.* This concern extends to the safety of the unit and the entire environment.

An accident that occurs in the health care facility is referred to as an **incident**. An incident is any unexpected occurrence or event that interrupts normal procedures or causes a crisis. If you see an incident or are involved in one, inform the nurse, who will fill out an **incident report** (Figure 14-7) after obtaining information from the persons involved and witnesses.

Environmental Safety Conditions

Incidents can be prevented by keeping hallways and other walkways free of equipment and clutter. Place equipment

Safety ALERT

Each state has laws governing the water temperature in patient care areas of the facility. In most cases, water temperature at sinks and bathing areas should not exceed 120°F. Some states' laws say that water temperature cannot be higher than 115°F. Unfortunately, regulators sometimes fail, sending excessively hot water into the facility. Water in bath and shower areas must be warm enough to comfortably bathe patients. Comfortable temperature for most people is 95°F to 105°F. Report water in bathing areas that does not warm up enough for comfortable bathing. Also report steaming water or water that feels excessively hot at any faucet in a patient care area. Use bath thermometers to check water temperatures before giving patient care, whenever possible. If no thermometer is available, test water temperature with your elbow. ∎

INCIDENT REPORT

Family Name		First Name		M.I.		Room No.	Hosp. No.

Address		City		State	Zip Code	Age	Sex
							M F

Date of Incident	Time		Place		Attending Physician		
	a.m. p.m.						

Status of person involved: Patient _____   Employee _____   Visitor _____   Other _____

Diagnosis: _____

_____

Describe condition before incident: Disoriented_____   Senile____   Sedated___   Normal___   Other___

_____

Was height of bed adjustable? Yes ___ No ___   Was bed up? Yes___ No___   Was bed down? Yes__ No___
Were bed rails ordered? Yes__ No___   Were they present? Yes__   No___   Were they up? Yes__ No___
Were they down? Yes___ No___ Other_____

Describe incident entirely, include part of body injured and treatment:

_____

_____

_____

_____

_____

_____

_____

_____

_____

_____

Vital Signs: Temp _____   Pulse _____   Resp _____   Blood Pressure_____

Indicate on diagram location of injury

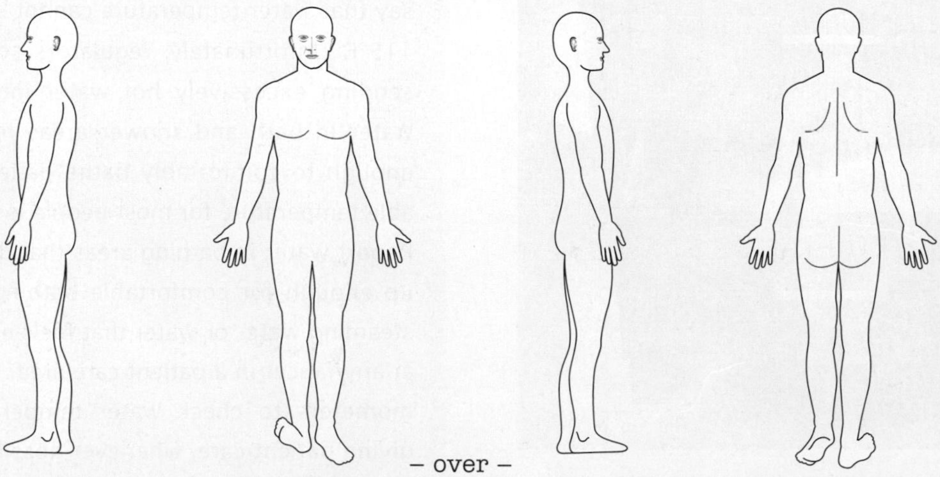

– over –

FIGURE 14-7 A special report is completed any time an incident occurs. (© *Delmar/Cengage Learning*)

continues

Was physician called? Yes _____ No_____ Time_____ a.m. p.m.

Who responded? _____ Time_____ a.m. p.m.

Attending physician_____ On-call physician_____

Statement of physician _____

_____

_____

_____

_____

Was family called? Yes _____ No_____ Time_____ a.m. p.m. Who:_____

Give names, addresses, and phone numbers of any who witnessed incident _____

_____

_____

A copy of this report will be sent to Patient's physician.

Date of Report _____ Signed _____

Signature and title of person preparing report

Nursing Office Review of Incident: Date _____ Signed_____

Comments: _____

_____

_____

_____

FIGURE 14-7 *continued*

and carts on one side of the hallway, leaving the opposite side free so patients can use the hand rail, if needed. This reduces the risk of falls, and means that no one has to navigate through a maze of equipment to walk down the hallway.

EQUIPMENT AND CARE OF EQUIPMENT

The daily or **concurrent cleaning** of equipment is an important part of your job. It contributes to the safety of your patients. The housekeeping department maintains environmental cleanliness. However, spills must be mopped up immediately to avoid falls.

In most health care facilities, equipment is tagged when it needs repair (Figure 14-8). That equipment may not be used again until the tag is removed. Facility policy differs as to who is responsible for applying and removing such tags. Reporting broken or nonfunctioning equipment is the responsibility of everyone.

OSHA ALERT

Handle needles, razors, and other sharp objects with care. Needles are never cut, bent, broken, or recapped by hand. Discard sharp objects in a puncture-resistant "sharps" container. Avoid over-filling the sharps container. Seal the cap when it is three-quarters full. The cap is designed so it cannot be snapped back off after it is closed. The sealed sharps container is stored until it can be picked up with the biohazardous waste. The biohazardous waste disposal area is used for discarding items contaminated with blood or body fluids. Special precautions are taken to contain waste in this area. ■

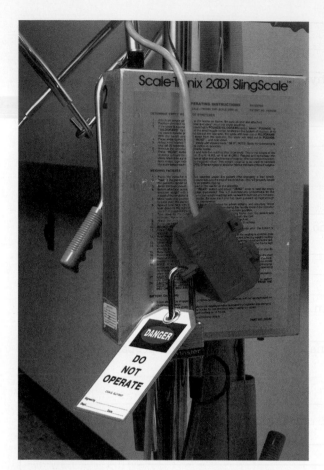

FIGURE 14-8 Unsafe electrical equipment is tagged and locked until it can be repaired. (© Delmar/Cengage Learning)

FIRE SAFETY

It is a scientific fact that if three elements are present in the right proportions (Figure 14-9), there will be a fire. The three elements are heat, fuel, and oxygen.

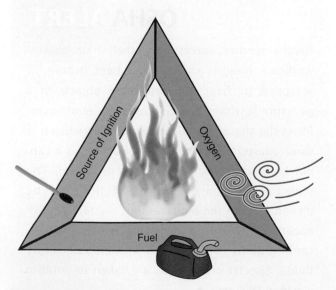

FIGURE 14-9 The fire triangle displays the elements needed to start a fire. (© Delmar/Cengage Learning)

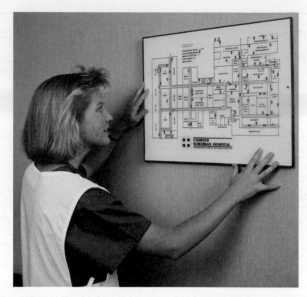

FIGURE 14-10 All personnel must be familiar with the evacuation plan, and must know the location of fire alarms and extinguishers and how to use them. (© Delmar/Cengage Learning)

All staff must know and regularly practice the fire and evacuation plans for the facility.

- Role-play the emergency procedures until you are completely secure.
- Learn the location of escape routes and the location and operation of all fire control equipment (Figure 14-10).
- Know and practice fire drill procedures. These are conducted on a regular basis. Many patients could be injured during a fire because of confusion and their inability to help themselves.
- Keep alert to all possible fire hazards. Promptly report them to the proper person.

Fire Prevention

You and every staff member can do a great deal to prevent the disaster of fire. In general:

- Check for frayed electrical wires.
- Do not overload circuits with too many electrical cords.
- Do not use a lightweight electrical cord with equipment that draws a heavy power load.
- Use three-prong grounded plugs.
- Do not allow clutter to accumulate.
- Empty wastepaper cans into proper receptacles.
- Do not store oily rags or paint rags.
- Report any possible hazards right away.
- Report smoke and/or burning smells.
- Keep all fire exits clear of equipment and debris.
- Know and practice fire safety through fire drills.
- Do not let visitors give cigarettes to patients.

- Notify the nurse if you suspect a patient or visitor is smoking in a patient unit, bathroom, or other restricted area.

Smoking

Smoking in bed should never be permitted. Smoking should be strictly limited to specific areas, if it is permitted at all. Most health care facilities do not permit smoking by anyone in any area.

Oxygen Precautions

The use of oxygen presents a specific hazard. When oxygen is in use:

- Do not use flammable liquids such as oils, alcohol, nail polish, aftershave, lotions, perfume, or hair spray.
- Do not use electrical equipment such as radios, hair dryers, electric razors, heating pads, or toys.
- Post a sign indicating that oxygen is in use. Most facilities use two signs. One is placed on the door to the room, and the other is posted over the bed. Follow your facility policies.
- Use cotton blankets and gowns for the patient.
- In some facilities, the call signal is replaced with a hand bell.
- Wear cotton uniforms and nonwool sweaters when providing care.
- Be certain there are no cigarettes, matches, or lighters in the room.
- Do not adjust the liter flow of oxygen. Know the ordered rate of oxygen and check it each time you are in the room.

RACE System

Become familiar with the fire procedures for your facility. In case of fire, keep calm. Move patients who are in immediate danger to safety, then sound the alarm. Follow the evacuation plan as you have practiced. Patients may be confused and frightened. Therefore, the staff must be calm and in control. In a fire emergency, remember **RACE** as defined here (Figure 14-11):

- R—*Remove patients* from danger by moving them to a safe area.
- A—*Alarm.* Sound the alarm.
- C—*Contain fire.* Close windows and doors to prevent drafts, which cause the fire to spread more rapidly. Before entering a closed door, touch the surface with the back of your hand (Figure 14-12). If the door is hot, do not open it.
- E—*Extinguish* the fire or *evacuate* the area.

Follow the fire emergency plan for your facility:

- Keep calm. Be prepared to follow directions when a person in authority takes charge.
- Shut off air conditioning and other electrical equipment.
- Shut off oxygen.
- Do not use elevators.
- Close all doors into the hallway.
- Remove carts and equipment from the hallway. Get anything that may burn behind a door.

Use of a Fire Extinguisher

When using a fire extinguisher, remember the letters **PASS**.
P—PULL the pin.
A—AIM the nozzle at the base of the fire.
S—SQUEEZE the handle.
S—SWEEP back and forth along the base of the fire.

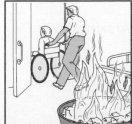 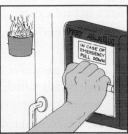 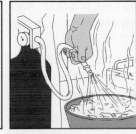 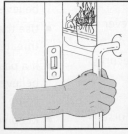 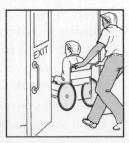

Remove   Activate   Contain or   Extinguish or   Evacuate

FIGURE 14-11 Remember the sequence of critical actions in case of fire. (© *Delmar/Cengage Learning*)

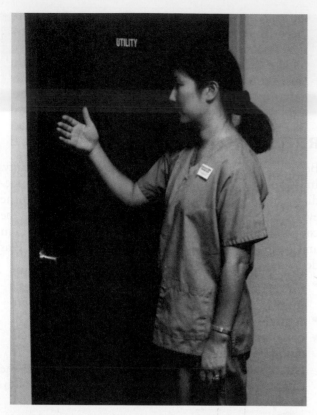

FIGURE 14-12 When you suspect a fire, touch the door with the back of your hand, which is more sensitive to heat than the palm. If the door feels hot, do not open it. (© Delmar/Cengage Learning)

OTHER EMERGENCIES

There may be other disasters for which you and your facility must be prepared. Tornadoes, hurricanes, floods, earthquakes, and bomb threats are examples of such disasters. Each facility has its own policies concerning emergencies. Be sure you are familiar with them.

In all emergency situations, get patients to safety, follow your facility's policy, and keep calm.

VIOLENCE IN THE WORKPLACE

Episodes of violence in the workplace are increasing in our society. Serious violence has occurred in hospitals and long-term care facilities in both rural and urban communities. OSHA has developed guidelines for preventing violence in the health care facility and many employers use these guidelines.

Workplace violence is any physical assault, threatening behavior, or verbal abuse that occurs in the workplace. The workplace includes facility buildings and the surrounding perimeters, parking lots, clients' homes, and traveling to and from work assignments.

GUIDELINES *for*
Violence Prevention

Follow all facility policies and procedures involving safety and security. Other things you can do to prevent potential incidents are:

- Attend continuing education programs to learn how to recognize and manage escalating agitation, assaultive behavior, or criminal intent.
- Attend classes on cultural diversity that offer sensitivity training on racial and ethnic issues and differences.
- If you are responsible for a secured area, control access to the area and keep it locked. Avoid propping locked doors and windows open. Never disable a door alarm.
- Do not leave keys unattended. Never share security alarm codes with unauthorized persons.
- Close shades or curtains at night.
- Report assaults or threats of assaults to the nurse immediately.

- Avoid wearing scarves, necklaces, earrings, and other jewelry that could cause injury if a patient or other individual attacks you.
- Do not carry valuables or large sums of cash to work.
- Avoid remote, dark areas when you are alone.
- Report lights that are burned out and locks that are not working.
- Exercise caution in elevators, stairwells, and unfamiliar areas. Immediately leave the area if you believe that a hazard exists.
- Use the "buddy system" if personal safety may be threatened.
- If a patient or other person is "acting out," or you believe you may be assaulted, do not let the person come between you and the exit.
- Keep your head up, look ahead, and be aware of your surroundings.

continues

GUIDELINES *continued*

- If your facility has security personnel, request that they escort you in dark or potentially dangerous areas. If no security personnel are on duty, ask other staff members to accompany you.
- Park in well-lighted areas. Always lock your car after parking. Look in the car before getting in, then lock the doors after you get in. Do not roll windows down to speak with individuals approaching your car.
- Report suspicious individuals or other potential safety hazards to the proper person. Never approach a suspicious person by yourself.

GUIDELINES *for*

Dealing with a Violent Individual

- Remain calm and avoid raising your voice, which may further agitate the person.
- Speak slowly, softly, and clearly.
- Call for help, if possible, or send someone to get help.
- Move away from heavy or sharp objects that may be used as weapons.
- Monitor your body language and avoid movements that could be perceived as challenging, such as placing your hands on your hips or pointing your finger. Focus your attention on the person so you know what he or she is doing at all times.
- Position yourself at right angles to the person. Avoid standing directly in front of him or her. Estimate the length of the person's arms and stay back as far away from them as you can. Maintain a distance of 3 to 6 feet, if possible.
- Position yourself so that an exit is accessible. Never let the person come between you and the exit.
- Avoid making sudden movements.

- Listen to what the person is saying. Encourage the person to talk, and communicate that you genuinely care and will try to help. Acknowledge that you understand that he or she is upset. Break big problems into smaller, manageable ones.
- Avoid arguing and defensive statements. Accept criticism in a positive way. Ask clarifying questions.
- Ask the person to leave and return when he or she is calmer.
- Ask questions to help regain control of the conversation.
- Avoid challenging, bargaining, or making promises you cannot keep.
- Describe the consequences of abusive behavior.
- Avoid touching an angry person.
- If a weapon is involved, ask the person to place it in a neutral location while you continue talking. Avoid trying to disarm the person, which may put you in danger.

NURSING ASSISTANT SAFETY

The work performed by nursing assistants requires a great deal of lifting and moving of patients, objects, and equipment. It is important that you use your body correctly to avoid injury.

Ergonomics

The field of **ergonomics** concerns adapting the environment and using techniques and equipment to prevent injury. Here are several ergonomic techniques you can use to reduce the risk of injury:

- Use correct body mechanics at all times.
- Raise beds to a comfortable working height (remember to lower the bed when you finish your task).
- Use mechanical lifts and other devices for moving heavy and/or dependent patients.
- Use back supports if this is your preference. The use of back supports is controversial, but many nursing assistants find them helpful (Figure 14-13).

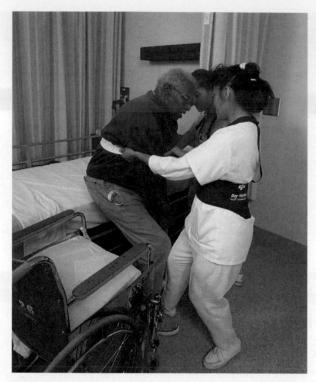

FIGURE 14-13 The back support belt reminds you to use your muscles correctly when lifting and moving patients and heavy objects. Fasten the belt before lifting and moving. Release it when you have finished. (© Delmar/Cengage Learning)

Safety ALERT

Have you ever heard the expression, "When your feet hurt, you hurt all over"? Most experienced health care workers will tell you this old adage is true. Buying a sturdy pair of athletic shoes or duty shoes is one of the best investments you will make in your uniform. ■

- Get another person to help when you need to transfer patients who cannot bear their own weight fully.
- Use a cart to move heavy items.

If you follow these eight commandments for lifting, you will greatly reduce your risk of injury.

1. Plan your lift and test the load (Figure 14-14A).
2. Ask for help (Figure 14-14B).
3. Get a firm footing (Figure 14-14C).
4. Bend your knees (Figure 14-14D).
5. Tighten your abdominal muscles (Figure 14-14E).
6. Lift with your legs (Figure 14-14F).
7. Keep the load close (Figure 14-14G).
8. Keep your back upright (Figure 14-14H).

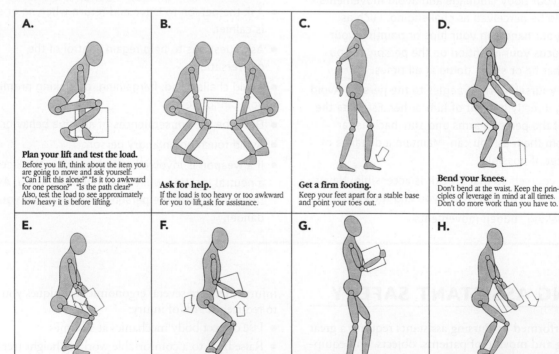

A.

Plan your lift and test the load.
Before you lift, think about the item you are going to move and ask yourself: "Can I lift this alone?" "Is it too awkward for one person?" "Is the path clear?" Also, test the load to see approximately how heavy it is before lifting.

B.

Ask for help.
If the load is too heavy or too awkward for you to lift, ask for assistance.

C.

Get a firm footing.
Keep your feet apart for a stable base and point your toes out.

D.

Bend your knees.
Don't bend at the waist. Keep the principles of leverage in mind at all times. Don't do more work than you have to.

E.

Tighten your stomach muscles.
Use intra-abdominal pressure to support your spine when you lift, offsetting the force of the load. Train your muscles to work together.

F.

Lift with your legs.
Let your leg muscles do the work of lifting. Don't rely on your weaker back muscles.

G.

Keep the load close.
Don't hold the load away from your body. The closer it is to your spine, the less force it exerts on your back.

H.

Keep your back upright.
Whether lifting or putting down the load, don't add the weight of your body to the load. Avoid twisting.

FIGURE 14-14 Eight rules for lifting and moving. (*Reprinted with permission from Ergodyne Corporation, St. Paul, MN*)

Warming up before working is another way to maintain a healthy body. Exercises can be performed before each work shift. Check with your physician before beginning any exercise program.

The Occupational Safety and Health Administration (OSHA) requires that manufacturers of chemical products supply **Material Safety Data Sheets (MSDS)** with any hazardous products they sell. The MSDS provide information that explains:

- Precautions to take in the presence of a hazard
- Instructions for safe use of the potentially dangerous substance
- How to clean up and dispose of the hazardous product
- First aid measures to use if exposure occurs

Safety ALERT

When you are using chemicals in a patient care area, keep them under direct visual control. This means keeping them where you can see them at all times. Do not turn your back on them. ■

Keep hazardous products in their original containers with the original labels intact and legible. Health care facilities must keep all chemicals in locked cupboards.

REVIEW

A. Multiple Choice

Select the one best answer for each of the following.

1. The patient's name is Phe Quan. She is in Room 116–4. From this information, you know that she is occupying a bed in a
   a. private room.
   b. rehabilitation department.
   c. semiprivate room.
   d. ward.

2. Comfortable water temperature for handwashing and bathing is
   a. 55°F to 65°F.
   b. 75°F to 85°F.
   c. 95°F to 105°F.
   d. 115°F to 130°F.

3. The best room temperature is approximately
   a. 45°F.
   b. 65°F.
   c. 72°F.
   d. 88°F.

4. Which of the following represents a fire hazard?
   a. Frayed electrical wire
   b. Using three-prong plugs
   c. Supervised smoking
   d. Using UL-approved items

5. The elements needed to start a fire are
   a. cigarettes, matches, and call signal.
   b. heat, fuel, and oxygen.
   c. electricity, oxygen, and matches.
   d. oxygen, linen, and electricity.

6. Which of the following contributes to unsafe conditions in the facility?
   a. Equipment in the halls
   b. Chemicals in locked cupboards
   c. Allowing patients to smoke with supervision
   d. Teaching patients how to use assistive devices

7. When oxygen is in use, you should not
   a. use cotton blankets on the patient's bed.
   b. remove cigarettes from the room.
   c. adjust the liter flow.
   d. post a sign on the door.

8. Every staff member should know
   a. how to open sealed windows in case of fire.
   b. the RACE procedure.
   c. the distance from the fire department to the facility.
   d. to aim a fire extinguisher at the top of the flames.

9. The word that means adapting the environment to prevent body injury is
   a. body mechanics.
   b. incident.
   c. ergonomics.
   d. RACE.

10. One principle of good body mechanics is to
    a. bend from the waist when lifting.
    b. keep your feet close together when lifting.
    c. use the strong muscles of your legs for lifting.
    d. keep the load as far from your body as possible.

11. MSDS are required to include information on
    a. how to repackage the product.
    b. first aid measures to use if exposure occurs.
    c. how to use the product.
    d. other approved uses of the product.

12. When dealing with a potentially violent individual, the nursing assistant should
    a. speak loudly and clearly.
    b. maintain a distance of two feet.
    c. listen to what the person is saying.
    d. attempt to touch the person gently.

B. Nursing Assistant Challenge

Mary Gonzales is a new nursing assistant at Community Memorial Hospital. She has just completed her CNA course. Consider the information she needs to receive in orientation in order to be a safe and efficient worker.

13. What information does Mary need to learn about the facility to prevent fires and to follow correct procedures in the event of a fire?

14. Mary will need information about the equipment she will be working with. What items of equipment is she likely to be using on her job?

15. Discuss everything Mary can do to prevent work-related injuries.

16. What types of chemicals is she likely to be using?

UNIT 15

Patient Safety and Positioning

OBJECTIVES

After completing this unit, you will be able to:
- Spell and define terms.
- Identify patients who are at risk for having incidents.
- List alternatives to the use of physical restraints.
- Describe the guidelines for the use of restraints.
- Demonstrate the correct application of restraints.
- List the elements that are common to all procedures.
- Describe correct body alignment for the patient.
- List the purposes of repositioning patients.

- Demonstrate these positions using the correct supportive devices: supine, semisupine, prone, semiprone, lateral, Fowler's, and orthopneic.
- Demonstrate the following procedures:
  - Procedure 10 Turning the Patient Toward You
  - Procedure 11 Turning the Patient Away from You
  - Procedure 12 Moving a Patient to the Head of the Bed
  - Procedure 13 Logrolling the Patient

VOCABULARY

Learn the meaning and the correct spelling of the following words and phrases:

ambulate	lateral	physical restraints	splint
aspiration	mobility	postural support	supine
body alignment	modified	pressure ulcer	supportive device
chemical restraints	Trendelenburg	procedure	transfer
contracture	position	prone	trochanter roll
draw sheet	90-90-90 position	semi-Fowler's	turning (moving) sheet
enabler	orthopneic position	semiprone	
Fowler's position	orthotic devices	semisupine	
high Fowler's	(orthoses)	Sims' position	

PATIENT SAFETY

In Unit 14, you learned how to maintain a safe environment and how to avoid personal injuries. The prevention of patient injuries is another very important part of your job as a nursing assistant. Patients in health care facilities are at risk for incidents because of medical problems and other conditions, such as the effects of some medications. Because of these risk factors, the most common incidents in health care facilities are falls.

GUIDELINES *for*

Preventing Patient Falls

- Leave the bed in its lowest horizontal position when you have finished giving care.
- Keep brakes locked on beds at all times except when the bed is being moved.
- Check the care plan to find out whether the side rails are to be raised.
- Check and adjust protruding objects such as bed wheels or gatch handles.
- Do not block or clutter open areas with supplies and equipment.
- Wipe up spills immediately.
- Encourage patients to use the hand rails along corridor walls when walking (Figure 15-1).
- Monitor patients for signs of weakness, fatigue, dizziness, and loss of balance.
- Monitor patients for safe practice if they independently:

    propel their wheelchairs
    transfer (get out of bed)
    ambulate (walk)

- Provide adequate lighting.
- Eliminate noise and other distractions that may increase confusion and create anxiety.
- Avoid leaving patients alone in the tub or shower unless you are given specific permission to do so.
- Check patients' clothing for fit and safety. Loose shoes and laces, long robes, and slacks increase the risk of falling. Footwear should be appropriate for the floor surface. In general, this means using nonskid shoes on tile floor surfaces. However, nonskid shoes may stick to carpeting, causing falls. A leather or synthetic shoe sole may be more appropriate for a carpeted surface.

- Care for the patient's physical needs promptly. Many incidents occur when patients attempt to get out of bed to go to the bathroom.
- Always use the correct techniques for transferring and walking patients.
- Use a gait belt when assisting patients to transfer or ambulate.
- Follow the care plan when assisting patients with transfers and ambulation.
- Elevate the rails if you must leave the bedside while the bed is in the high position.

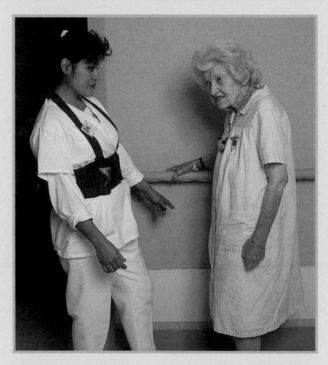

FIGURE 15-1 Encourage patients to hold rails on corridor walls when walking. (© *Delmar/Cengage Learning*)

USE OF PHYSICAL RESTRAINTS

In the past, restraints were routinely used to prevent falls. Research has shown that this approach is ineffective. Many falls occur with side rails up and restraints intact. This can result in serious injury, entrapment, and even death. There are two types of restraints: physical restraints and chemical restraints. **Chemical restraints** are medications that alter the patient's mood and behavior. As a nursing assistant, you will be more concerned with the use of physical restraints. **Physical restraints** are procedures or devices that are attached or next to a person's body that he or she cannot easily remove and that restrict freedom of movement and normal access to the body. There are many complications of restraints. In general, their use is discouraged.

The regulatory and accrediting agencies oversee the use of restraints in health care facilities. If restraints are needed, they are a treatment of last resort and there are many restrictions on use. Generally speaking, the least amount of restraint needed to keep the patient safe should be used for the least amount of time possible. Patients have the right to be free from restraints. Restraints may be used *only* to ensure the immediate physical safety of the patient, a staff member, or others, and must be discontinued at the earliest possible time. A family request or threat regarding the use of restraints is not a justification for actual use.

Examples of physical restraints include:
- Wrist/arm (Figure 15-2) and ankle/leg restraints
- Vests (Figure 15-3)
- Belts
- Jackets (Figure 15-4)
- Hand mitts (Figure 15-5)
- Geriatric and cardiac chairs (Figure 15-6)
- Wheelchair safety belts, bars, and tables (Figure 15-7)
- Bed rails (if they meet the definition of a restraint)

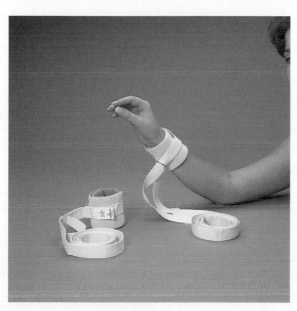

FIGURE 15-2 Wrist restraints may be used to prevent the patient from pulling on IVs and other tubes. (*Courtesy of J.T. Posey Co., Inc., Arcadia, CA*)

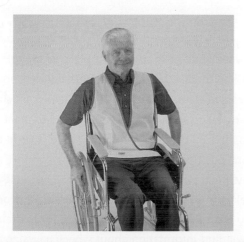

FIGURE 15-3 Vest restraints must be applied as pictured here, with the straps crossed over in front of the patient. Look closely at the strap placement, which is the key to keeping the hips down. The straps are threaded between the seat and the armrests, not through the armrests. (*Courtesy of J.T. Posey Co., Inc., Arcadia, CA*)

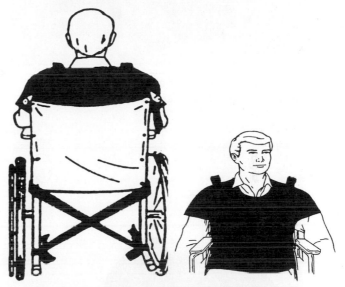

FIGURE 15-4 A jacket restraint has sleeves, whereas a vest does not. However, the straps for both restraints are tied in the same manner. Note the position of the straps. They are threaded through the seat and the armrests, then go around the outside of the side posts. Once the straps are threaded through to the back of the chair, you may loop one strap over the other in the center, if desired. This makes it a little more secure. Then tie each strap in a slip knot on the kickspur on the opposite side. (*Courtesy of J.T. Posey Co., Inc., Arcadia, CA*)

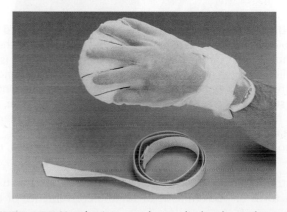

FIGURE 15-5 Hand mitts may be applied to keep the patient from injuring himself (such as by scratching) or pulling on tubes. (*Courtesy of J.T. Posey Co., Inc., Arcadia, CA*)

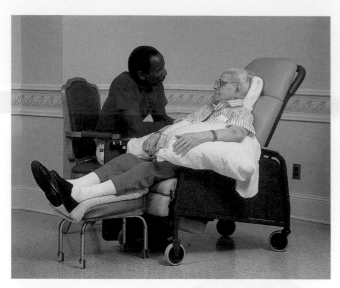

FIGURE 15-6 Geriatric chairs are restraints in some circumstances. (© Delmar/Cengage Learning)

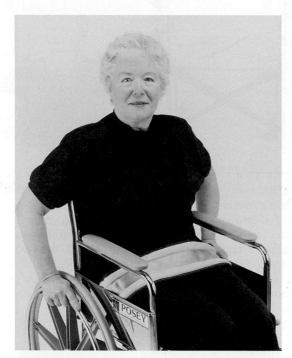

FIGURE 15-7 Most wheelchair safety belts are designed to go over the patient's lap, not around the waist. Check the manufacturer's information if you are unsure. This belt is applied over the lap, then threaded between the seat and armrest. Finish tying it exactly like the vest restraint. Once the straps are threaded through to the back of the chair, you may loop one strap over the other in the center, then tie each strap in a slip knot on the kickspur on the opposite side. (Courtesy of J.T. Posey Co., Inc., Arcadia, CA)

Restraints are medical devices. They should never be used as a form of punishment, or for the convenience of the nursing staff. An example of nursing convenience is when a unit does not have enough staff, or staff do not have enough time to monitor a patient.

Another important concern is restraint size. A restraint that does not fit correctly will not hold the patient securely and increases the risk of injury. Using a restraint that does not fit correctly or is not applied according to manufacturer's directions creates a risk of very serious injuries. Manufacturers provide literature, teaching aids, and guidelines for restraint size, based on patient weight. The color of the trim (piping, binding) on a vest restraint is often a visual key to its size. This color coding does not apply to other types of restraints. Belts are usually one size fits all.

Before restraints are used, the registered nurse must assess the patient's capabilities and the reasons for restraint. If the cause can be identified and corrected, the need for a restraint may be eliminated. For example, an unsteady male patient gets up to use the bathroom at night, but does not call for help. His risk of falls can be modified by making sure a urinal is within reach and emptied regularly.

The care plan will provide information about the type of restraint to use, the time the restraint is to be applied, and other special information and instructions.

Enablers

Enablers are devices that empower patients and assist them to function at their highest possible level. Another term for this type of device is *enhancers*. Devices used as enablers that maintain body position and alignment and support nonfunctioning body parts are called **postural supports**. They give patients a higher degree of independence and enable them to perform tasks they were previously unable to do. For example, a Velcro strap used to hold and support a paralyzed arm to prevent it from sliding off the armrest of a wheelchair is an enabler, not a restraint.

Safety ALERT

The wheelchair is an important piece of equipment in all health care facilities. Patients come in many shapes and sizes. Because of this, wheelchairs come in many sizes, with various accessories to meet the user's medical needs. Attention to wheelchair fit and patient positioning are important for comfort and safety. Restraints are sometimes used because the wheelchair does not fit the patient! Using a proper-fitting chair often eliminates the need for restraints. You will find information about wheelchair size and safety in Unit 17. Always consider the type and size of the wheelchair you are using when determining whether to recommend a restraint! ■

The wheelchair lap tray (Figure 15-8) is a restraint alternative that is also used as an enabler. The tray is attached to the back of the wheelchair with Velcro straps. Patients can lean on it, and its surface can hold personal items or reading and writing supplies. If the tray allows the patient to perform a task, it is an *enabler*. If the person does not have the physical or mental ability to remove the tray, it is a *restraint*. If the person can safely remove the tray, it is a *restraint alternative*.

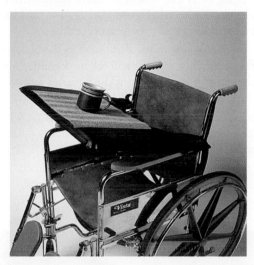

FIGURE 15-8 The lap tray is an *enabler* if it improves function, permitting the patient to eat independently. This tray is lined with gripper, a nonslip surface, to hold the dishes in place. The tray is a *restraint* if it is used to keep the patient in the chair and he cannot remove it by himself. *(Courtesy of Skil-Care Corporation, Yonkers, NY, (800) 431–2972)*

Side Rails as Restraints

Side rails are routinely attached to hospital beds. Rails can be full length, three-quarter length, half length, or quarter length. Half- and quarter-length rails may also be called *split rails*. The rails may be used in any combination. All bed rails can create a hazard in certain circumstances. All are considered restraints in certain situations.

By definition, side rails are restraints. They can also be an enabler. Facilities write their own definitions of restraints. For example, some facilities consider the use of three half-rails an enabler, and four rails a restraint. Some patients pull on rails to position and turn themselves in bed. Others feel more secure if the rails are up. Your facility's policies will define whether rails are restraints or enablers in this situation. Side rails must always be up for patients who are using physical restraints in bed.

Serious injuries can occur if patients attempt to climb over elevated side rails and fall. This is a common cause of hip fractures in confused elderly patients. Leaving the rails down is a much safer alternative. If side rails are raised, monitor the patient frequently.

Monitor the space between the rails, head and footboards, and the mattress. Hospital beds are used for years. Mattresses wear out and are replaced. Patients can become trapped between the mattress, side rails, and other parts of the bed if the replacement mattress is smaller than the original. Make sure that the gap between the mattress and side rails or other parts of the bed is not large enough to cause injury. Figures 15-9A and 15-9B show areas of potential entrapment. If a gap is wide enough to entrap a person or body part, notify the nurse promptly. Another bed can be used or the mattress area modified (Figure 15-10A) to prevent injury.

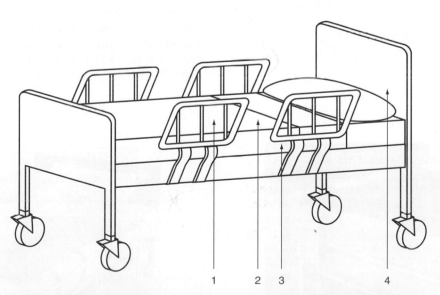

FIGURE 15-9A Entrapment between the mattress and side rails may occur: (1) through the bars of an individual side rail; (2) through the space between split side rails; (3) between the side rail and mattress; or (4) between the headboard or footboard, side rail, and mattress. *(Courtesy of U.S. Food and Drug Administration)*

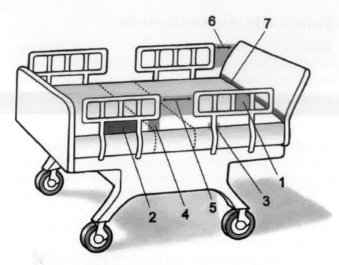

FIGURE 15-9B Seven additional zones of entrapment have been identified. Zone 1: within the rail; Zone 2: between the top of the compressed mattress and the bottom of the rail, between the rail supports; Zone 3: between the rail and the mattress; Zone 4: between the top of the compressed mattress and the bottom of the rail, at the end of the rail; Zone 5: between the split bed rails; Zone 6: between the end of the rail and the side edge of the headboard or footboard; Zone 7: between the headboard or footboard and the mattress end. *(Courtesy of U.S. Food & Drug Administration)*

The nursing orders often specify the use of padded side rails for patients with certain conditions. Using a commercial side rail pad (Figure 15-10B) is the best solution, if they are available in your facility.

Facilities and commercial manufacturers have developed many excellent alternatives to the use of side rails. Possible alternatives to the use of side rails are:

- Beds that can be raised and lowered close to the floor.

- Anticipation of reasons why the patient might get up, including need to use the bathroom, hunger, thirst, restlessness, and pain. Meet these needs and provide calm interventions when you are in the room.
- Use of side rail bolster cushions (Figure 15-11) or body pillows.
- Pressure-sensitive alarms that sound when a patient attempts to get up (Figures 15-12A, 15-12B, and 15-12C).
- Self-release belts that sound an alarm immediately when the closure is released (Figure 15-12D), so staff have time to respond before the person gets up.
- Placement of mats on the floor next to the bed, so that if a fall occurs, the patient will fall on a padded surface. Some mats sound an alarm if the patient's feet or body touch the surface (Figure 15-12E).

Each health care facility has policies addressing when and how side rails may be used. Know and follow your facility policies.

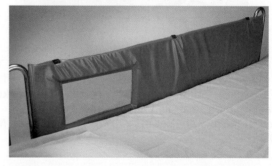

FIGURE 15-10B Padded side rails are a good safety precaution for patients with seizure disorder, as well as patients who might climb through the rail to get out of bed. *(Courtesy of Skil-Care Corporation, Yonkers, NY, (800) 431-2972)*

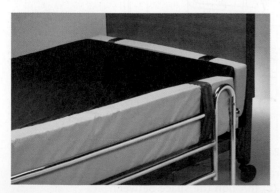

FIGURE 15-10A The mattress can be modified to fit the bed and decrease the risk of injury. *(Courtesy of Skil-Care Corporation, Yonkers, NY, (800) 431-2972)*

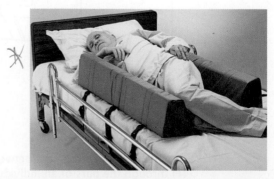

FIGURE 15-11 Bed control bolsters are a good option to use in place of side rails. *(Courtesy of Skil-Care Corporation, Yonkers, NY, (800) 431-2972)*

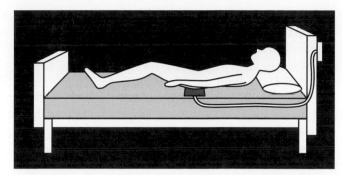

FIGURE 15-12A The pressure-sensitive pad is placed under the sheet. When the patient attempts to stand, an alarm sounds. *(Courtesy of RN+ Systems, Boulder, CO)*

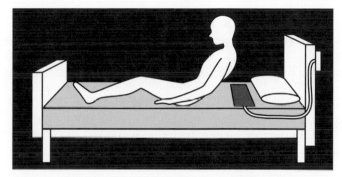

FIGURE 15-12B This pressure-sensitive pad is placed under the sheet beneath the patient's shoulders. When he lifts his upper body off the pad, the alarm will sound. *(Courtesy of RN+ Systems, Boulder, CO)*

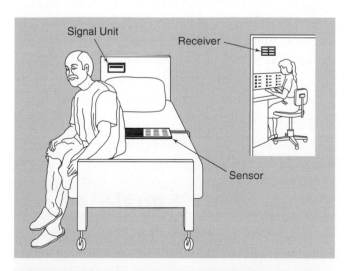

FIGURE 15-12C The pressure-sensitive pad is placed under the sheet. The sensor box is placed in the room. When the patient removes pressure from the pad, a distinctive alarm sounds at the desk. The alarm does not sound in the room. *(Courtesy of RN+ Systems, Boulder, CO)*

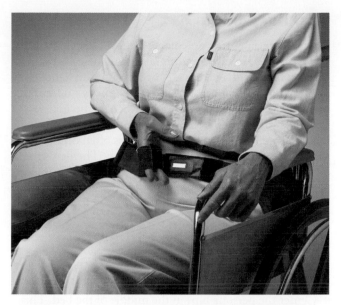

FIGURE 15-12D This self-release belt is a restraint alternative because the patient can remove it. This type of belt is designed to sound an alarm when the patient begins to open the closure, providing time for staff to respond before the patient gets up. *(Courtesy of Skil-Care Corporation, Yonkers, NY, (800) 431-2972)*

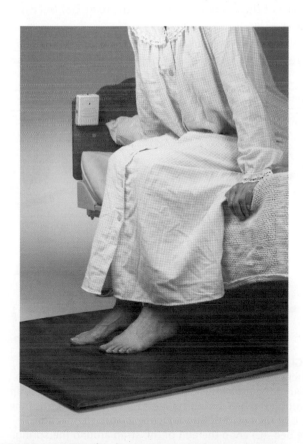

FIGURE 15-12E This battery-operated mat can be placed on one or both sides of the bed. An alarm will sound as soon as the patient's foot touches the mat. *(Courtesy of Skil-Care Corporation, Yonkers, NY, (800) 431-2972)*

Specialty Beds

Health care facilities use many types of specialty beds. Some of these are called *low air loss* beds. These are mattress overlays filled with air that are used for pressure relief. Low air loss mattresses pose a high risk of injury and entrapment if side rails are used. The surface of the mattress is flexible and can easily compress a body part between the mattress and bed frame or side rail. This often occurs when the bed is set for maximum air inflation. The bed should be used at the lowest setting that prevents bottoming-out of the mattress. Closely monitor patients who use low air loss beds.

Applying Restraints in Bed

When applying wrist, vest, poncho, jacket, or belt restraints to a patient in bed:

- Center the person's hips in the middle of the bed. This is where the bed bends when the head is elevated.
- Make sure the straps are not at an angle when extended over the edge of the mattress. If the straps are angled even slightly, they will loosen if the patient moves up or down in bed.
- Wrap the strap around the frame deck (the movable part of the frame that supports the mattress) once or twice (Figure 15-13A).
- Never wrap the strap around the lower frame, or the restraint will tighten and inhibit respiration when the head of the bed is elevated. Never tie the end of the strap to the outside of the frame. This enables the patient to reach down and untie it.
- Thread the strap through the bed springs at least 6 to 8 inches in from the side of the bed and 6 to 8 inches toward the head of the bed (Figure 15-13B). (Manufacturers will supply an adaptor for beds with a solid deck.)
- Loop the end of the strap around the spring (Figure 15-13C).
- Loop the strap around itself again and tighten to form a slip knot (Figure 15-13D).
- Always raise the side rails when a patient is restrained in bed. Never fasten the straps to the side rails or loop or wrap the straps around the side rails.

Alternatives to the Use of Restraints

Alternatives to restraints should be tried before restraints are applied. Restraints are used only as a last resort in situations where the patient may harm himself or others.

If you observe a condition that causes confusion or agitation, or discover an approach that is effective in eliminating or reducing the need for restraints, inform the nurse. Other common restraint alternatives are pictured in Figure 15-14 through Figure 15-20.

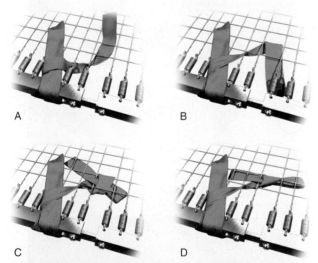

A   B

C   D

FIGURE 15-13 Tie the straps to the inner springs, where the patient cannot reach them. (A) Wrap the strap around the frame deck once or twice. (B) Thread the strap through the bed springs at least 6 to 8 inches in from the side of the bed and 6 to 8 inches toward the head of the bed. (C) Loop the end of the strap around the spring. (D) Loop the strap around itself again and tighten to form a slip knot. For a bed with a solid frame, use the modification for fastening the straps and/or alternate instructions for fastening the straps supplied by the restraint manufacturer. (© *Delmar/Cengage Learning*)

Safety ALERT

When applying restraints to a patient in a chair, make sure the patient's hips are all the way back on the seat. The restraint must keep the hips down. To do this, thread the straps between the seat and the armrest. A common mistake is threading the straps *through the armrests*. Follow the manufacturer's instructions for the type of restraint you are using. ∎

Legal ALERT

Most facilities have restraints from more than one manufacturer, so you must be familiar with the restraints in use. Remember that restraints are not one-size-fits-all devices. You *must* apply the correct size in the proper manner. ∎

GUIDELINES *for*
The Use of Restraints

In addition to the procedures described earlier in this section, follow these guidelines when restraints are necessary:

- Use the right type and size of restraint. Do not use a restraint if it is frayed, torn, has parts missing, or is soiled.
- Apply restraints over clothing, never next to bare skin.
- After application, check the fit. You should be able to slip three fingers between the restraint and the patient's body. The device should never restrict breathing.
- The straps must be smooth and not twisted. Position the straps so the person cannot reach the ties. Tie them with slip knots for quick release in an emergency.
- Be sure the patient has the signal light and other needed items within reach. Visually check the person every 15 to 30 minutes for comfort and safety. Make changes if needed.
- When a person is restrained in a wheelchair, lock the brakes when the chair is parked. Position the large part of the small front wheels facing forward. This changes the center of gravity of the chair, making it more stable and preventing tipping.
- Release the restraint at least every 2 hours for 10 full minutes for toileting, exercise, and/or ambulation. You may release restraints at other times when you are attending to the patient, such as during feeding.
- Maintain good alignment. Position the person in a comfortable, functional position.
- Do not use restraints in moving vehicles or on toilets unless you are sure the device is intended for that use by the manufacturer. (This does not apply to safety restraints that are part of the vehicle. Follow state laws.)

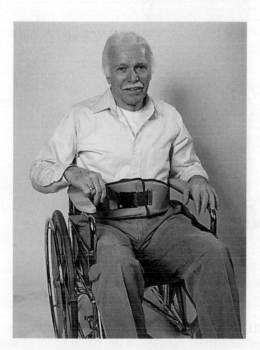

FIGURE 15-14 The self-release belt serves as a reminder to call for help before rising. It Is not a restraint if the patient has the physical and mental ability to release the Velcro fastener. (*Courtesy of Skil-Care Corporation, Yonkers, NY, (800) 431-2972*)

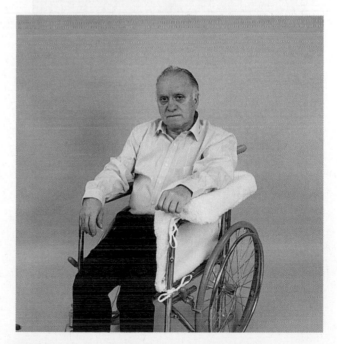

FIGURE 15-15 Some patients lean to the side, necessitating restraint to keep them upright in the chair. The lateral armrest supports the patient and keeps him upright, making restraints unnecessary. (*Courtesy of Skil-Care Corporation, Yonkers, NY, (800) 431-2972*)

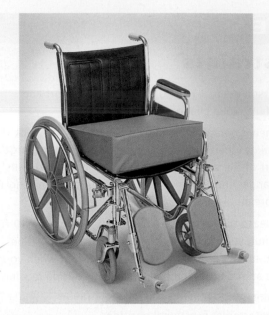

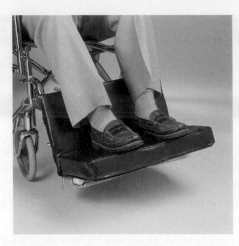

FIGURE 15-18 Proper foot support is essential to good positioning. The feet and legs should never dangle. Unsupported legs are at increased risk of injuries and blood clots. The footrest elevator keeps the patient's legs from dangling and prevents sliding in the chair. (*Courtesy of Skil-Care Corporation, Yonkers, NY, (800) 431-2972*)

FIGURE 15-16 Some patients slide forward to the edge of the chair, and must be restrained to keep their hips back. The wedge cushion prevents sliding. A piece of gripper can be placed under or on top of the wedge for additional security. (*Courtesy of Skil-Care Corporation, Yonkers, NY, (800) 431-2972*)

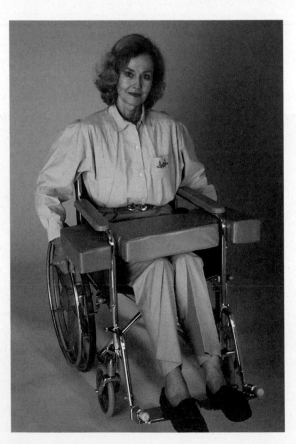

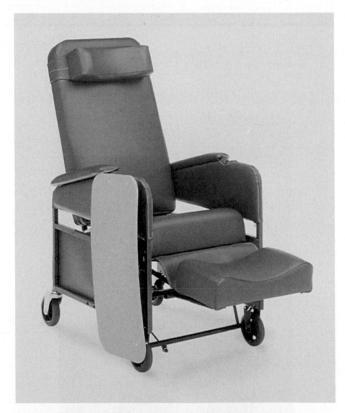

FIGURE 15-17 The lap buddy is foam covered with vinyl. It is lightweight and comfortable and may be used in place of a heavier tray. It is a restraint if the patient cannot remove it. (*Courtesy of Skil-Care Corporation, Yonkers, NY, (800) 431-2972*)

FIGURE 15-19 The geriatric chair can be used as a recliner for patient comfort. If the patient cannot stand, the chair is a restraint when in the reclining position. The tray is locked across the lap to prevent the patient from rising. It cannot be removed independently, so it is considered a restraint. (*Courtesy of Hill-Rom® Long-Term Care Division*)

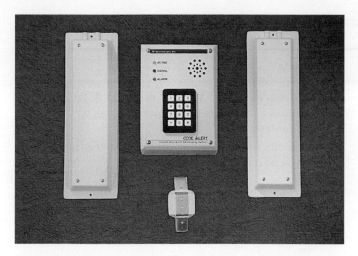

FIGURE 15-20 The magnetic sensor bracelet is placed on the wrist of the patient's dominant hand. It enables cognitively impaired patients to wander freely within the unit. The door alarm will sound if the patient tries to exit. (©1996, RF Technologies. Used with permission)

Infection Control ALERT

Your bandage scissors, stethoscope, and other personal items may transfer pathogens from one patient to the next. If personal equipment items will be used during a procedure, wash them with an alcohol product or soap and water before and after each use. ∎

PREVENTION OF OTHER INCIDENTS

Many situations can result in an incident that may harm the patient. Incidents can be prevented when staff are aware of and follow preventive measures.

Accidental Poisoning

Many common items, such as household chemicals, shaving lotion, plants, and cologne, are poisonous if ingested. Patients who are disoriented may eat or drink any of these items. To prevent accidental poisonings, keep chemicals and cleaning solutions in locked cupboards. Store patients' personal food items in the refrigerator in dated, labeled containers.

Choking ✳

Aspiration is the entry of food, water, gastric contents, or a foreign object into the trachea and lungs. It is usually accidental, such as when the patient "swallows down the wrong tube" or inadvertently inhales food or fluids. Because swallowing becomes less efficient as people age, choking and aspiration occur more often in elderly persons. Those who are disoriented or who have impaired consciousness are also at risk. To prevent choking or aspiration, be aware of which

patients have problems with swallowing. Follow the guidelines for feeding and positioning in Unit 28. Know the procedure to clear an obstructed airway (see Unit 42).

INTRODUCTION TO PROCEDURES

Caring for patients safely means that you must carefully carry out specific routines. The normal manner of carrying out a task is called a **procedure**. *Procedures* are the practices and processes used when following facility policies in patient care. The procedure prioritizes and orders your responsibilities when doing the task.

As you progress in your studies, you will learn the procedures for many nursing assistant tasks. You have already been introduced to the procedures for washing your hands and using PPE. The procedures that follow give you step-by-step directions for carrying out tasks that involve patient care.

Actions that must be done before you begin patient care are called *preprocedure* or *initial procedure actions*. At the end of each procedure, you will carry out a standard series of *ending procedure (procedure completion) actions*. These are important and should not be omitted.

Common Steps in All Procedures

Perform the steps in order, as appropriate to the patient and the procedure. This book calls these steps *initial procedure actions* and *ending procedure actions*.

Initial procedure actions Perform these steps, in order, at the beginning of every procedure.

Initial Procedure Action	Rationale
1. Wash your hands or use an alcohol-based hand cleaner.	Applies the principles of standard precautions. Prevents the spread of microbes and reduces the risk of cross-contamination.
2. Assemble supplies and equipment and bring to the patient's room.	Improves efficiency, organizes your time, and ensures that you do not have to leave the room.
3. Knock on the door and identify yourself (Figure 15-21A).	Respects the patient's right to privacy. Informs the patient who is giving care.
4. Identify the patient according to facility policy (Figure 15-21B).	Ensures that you are caring for the correct patient.

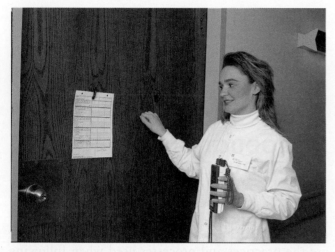

FIGURE 15-21A If the door is closed or the privacy curtains are drawn, knock or speak before entering. Allow enough time for the patient to respond. (© Delmar/Cengage Learning)

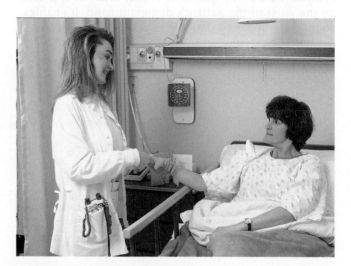

FIGURE 15-21B Identify the patient. (© Delmar/Cengage Learning)

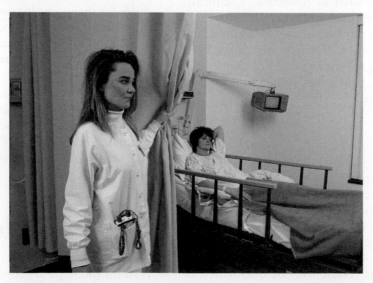

FIGURE 15-21C Draw the curtains for privacy. If the bed is near a window, also close the window curtains. (© Delmar/Cengage Learning)

Initial Procedure Action	Rationale
5. Ask visitors to leave the room and advise where they may wait (as desired by patient).	Respects the patient's right to privacy. Shows respect and courtesy to visitors.
6. Explain what you are going to do and what is expected of the patient. Answer questions. (Maintain a dialogue with the patient during the procedure and repeat explanations and instructions as needed.)	Informs the patient of what is going to be done and what to expect. Provides information about the procedure and shows respect.
7. Provide privacy by closing the door, privacy curtain, and window curtain (Figure 15-21C). (All three should be closed even if the patient is alone in the room.)	Respects the patient's right to privacy. Protects modesty and dignity.
8. Wash your hands or use an alcohol-based hand cleaner.	Applies the principles of standard precautions. Prevents the spread of microbes and reduces the risk of cross-contamination.
9. Set up supplies and equipment at the bedside. (Use an overbed table, if possible, or other clean area. Cover with a clean underpad, according to nursing judgment, to provide a clean work surface.) Open packages. Position items for convenient reach. Position a container for soiled items so that you do not have to cross over clean items to access it.	Prepares for the procedure and helps organize time. Ensures that equipment and supplies are conveniently positioned and readily available. Reduces the risk of cross-contamination.
10. Raise the bed to a comfortable working height.	Prevents back strain and injury caused by bending at the waist.
11. Position the patient for the procedure. Support with pillows and props as needed. Place a clean underpad under the area, as needed. Make sure the patient is comfortable and can maintain the position for the duration of the procedure.	Ensures that the patient is in the correct anatomic position for the procedure. Ensures that the patient is supported, comfortable, and able to maintain the position throughout the procedure.
12. Cover the patient with a bath blanket and drape for modesty. Fold the bath blanket back to expose only the area on which you will be working. (This step is essential even if the door, window, and cubicle curtains are closed.)	Respects the patient's modesty and dignity. Ensures that the patient is warm and comfortable.
13. Apply gloves if contact with blood, moist body fluids (except sweat), secretions, excretions, mucous membranes, or nonintact skin is likely.	Applies the principles of standard precautions. Protects the worker and patient from transfer of pathogens.
14. Apply a gown if your uniform will have substantial contact with linen or other articles contaminated with blood, moist body fluids (except sweat), mucous membranes, secretions, or excretions.	Applies the principles of standard precautions. Protects your uniform and skin from contamination with bloodborne pathogens.
15. Apply a mask and eye protection if splashing of blood or moist body fluids is likely.	Applies the principles of standard precautions. Protects the worker's skin, mucous membranes, and uniform from accidental splashing of bloodborne pathogens.
16. Lower the side rail on the side where you will be working.	Provides an obstacle-free area in which to work.

Ending procedure actions Perform these steps, in order, upon completion of each procedure.

Ending Procedure Action	Rationale
1. Remove gloves.	Prevents contamination of the patient, the environment, and clean supplies from used gloves.
2. Reposition the patient to ensure that he or she is comfortable and in good body alignment.	All body systems function better when the body is correctly aligned. The patient is more comfortable when the body is in good alignment.
3. Replace the bed covers, then remove any drapes used. Place used drapes in plastic bag to discard in trash or soiled linen.	Provides warmth and security. Contains linen and drapes that have been contaminated during the procedure.
4. Elevate the side rails, if used, before leaving the bedside.	Prevents contamination of the side rail from gloves. Ensures patient safety. Prevents falls, accidents, and injuries.
5. Remove other personal protective equipment, if worn, and discard in plastic bag or according to facility policy.	Prevents contamination of the patient, the environment, and clean supplies from used PPE.
6. Wash your hands or use an alcohol-based hand cleaner.	Applies the principles of standard precautions. Prevents the spread of microbes and reduces the risk of cross-contamination.
7. Return the bed to the lowest horizontal position.	Respects patient's right to a safe environment. Ensures patient safety. Prevents falls, accidents, and injuries.
8. Open the privacy and window curtains.	Privacy is no longer necessary unless preferred by the patient.
9. Position the call signal and needed personal items within reach (Figure 15-22A).	Prevents accidents and injuries. Gives the patient a sense of security by ensuring that help is available. Enhances patient convenience. Eliminates the need to call out or reach for needed personal items (which could result in a fall).
10. Wash your hands or use an alcohol-based hand cleaner.	Applies the principles of standard precautions. Prevents the spread of microbes and reduces the risk of cross-contamination. (Although the hands were washed previously, they have contacted the patient and other items in the room. Washing them again before leaving prevents potential transfer of microbes to other patients, equipment, and surfaces outside the patient's unit.)
11. Perform a general safety check of the patient and environment.	Stays consistent with "think safety" motto when entering and leaving the room; decreases exposure to environmental risks and hazards; helps ensure patient safety.

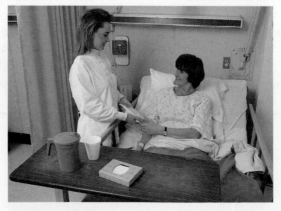

FIGURE 15-22A Lower the bed and place the signal cord within the patient's reach.
(© Delmar/Cengage Learning)

Ending Procedure Action	Rationale
12. Remove procedural trash and contaminated linen when you leave the room. Discard in appropriate container or location, according to facility policy.	Applies the principles of standard precautions. Prevents the spread of microbes and reduces the risk of cross-contamination.
13. Inform visitors that they may return to the room (Figure 15-22B).	Shows respect, courtesy, and hospitality to visitors and patient.
14. Document the procedure, your observations, and the patient's response (Figure 15-22C).	Provides a legal record of ongoing progress and care. Provides a record of what has been done and observations of the patient's condition. Serves as a vehicle for communication for other members of the interdisciplinary team.

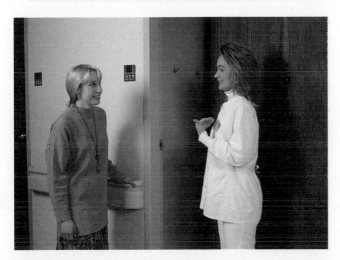

FIGURE 15-22B Let visitors know when they may reenter the room. (© Delmar/Cengage Learning)

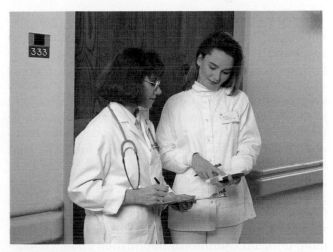

FIGURE 15-22C Report and document your actions and the patient's response. (© Delmar/Cengage Learning)

Because the initial procedure and ending procedure actions are the same for each patient care procedure, they are not restated as individual steps. Rather, a general reference is made to these steps at the beginning and end of each procedure. You must, however, learn and faithfully complete each of these steps for *each* patient care procedure you perform.

BODY MECHANICS FOR THE PATIENT

Body mechanics for the patient are very similar to those for the health care worker. Good posture for the patient means that moving in bed, getting out of bed, standing, and walking are done safely. Patients should be well supported in good body alignment when sitting.

Bed patients tend to slide toward the foot of the bed when the head of the bed is elevated (Figure 15-23). Patients who are dependent are not able to change their position. These patients need extra help to gain and maintain proper alignment.

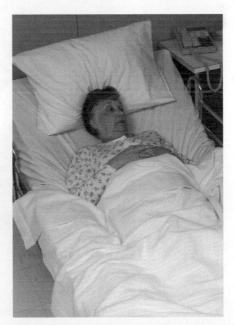

FIGURE 15-23 Patients frequently slide down in bed, causing poor body alignment and increasing the risk for injuries to the skin caused by friction and shearing. (© Delmar/Cengage Learning)

Body Alignment and Positioning

Body alignment means a position in which the body can properly function. Patients who are weak, have impaired consciousness, are disoriented, or are in pain have problems keeping good alignment. Good posture is comfortable for the patient and enables him or her to function at the highest level of ability. Body systems will function more efficiently.

Complications of Incorrect Positioning

The two most common complications of poor positioning are pressure ulcers and contractures. **Pressure ulcers** (bedsores) result when unrelieved pressure on a bony prominence reduces blood flow to the area. Pressure ulcers are dangerous and expensive to treat. (These are discussed in Unit 37.) **Contractures** occur when a joint is allowed to remain in the same position for too long (Figure 15-24). The muscles stiffen and shorten (atrophy), preventing the joint from moving fully. The joint freezes in position and cannot be moved. Usually, the joint becomes fixed in a bent position (position of flexion), but occasionally the joint is frozen in extension. Contractures are painful, permanent, and can interfere with **mobility**. They make caring for the patient much more difficult. (Additional information about contractures can be found in Unit 37.)

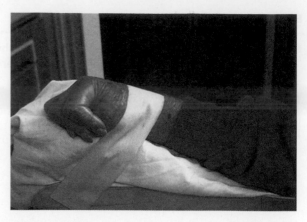

FIGURE 15-24 Contractures occur when joints are allowed to remain in the same position for too long. *(© Delmar/Cengage Learning)*

Supportive Devices

Supportive devices are used to maintain good alignment and body position in bed or in a chair. Supportive devices include:

- Pillows and/or folded sheets, bath blankets, or mattress pads to support the trunk and extremities.
- **Splints** and other specially designed **orthotic devices (orthoses)**. Orthoses restore or improve function and prevent deformity.
- Special boots or shoes that are worn in bed to keep the feet in alignment (Figure 15-25A).

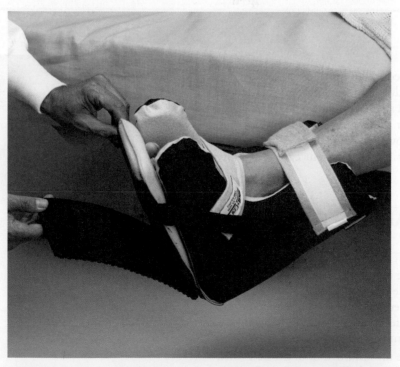

FIGURE 15-25A Special boots will maintain the ankles and feet in good alignment. The boot prevents contractures of the feet and reduces friction and shearing of the skin upon movement *(Courtesy of Skil-Care Corporation, Yonkers, NY, (800) 431-2972)*

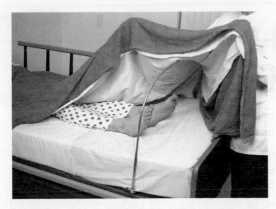

FIGURE 15-25B The weight of the bedding pushes the toes downward, causing discomfort and increasing the risk of contractures. Patients with certain skin conditions also need to keep the bedding off the skin. Bed cradles prevent pressure and elevate the bedding so it does not contact the patient's body. (© Delmar/Cengage Learning)

- Bed cradles, which prevent pressure on the feet from the bed covers (Figure 15-25B).
- Footboards to maintain foot alignment.

BASIC BODY POSITIONS

There are four basic positions, with variations for each one:

- **Prone** (on the abdomen), with a variation of **semiprone**
- **Supine** (on the back), with a variation of **semisupine**
- **Lateral** (on either side), with a variation of **Sims' position**
- **Fowler's position**, with variations of low Fowler's, **semi-Fowler's**, **high Fowler's**, and **orthopneic position**

Changing a patient's position involves these steps:

1. Moving the person into proper body alignment. You may need to move the person up or to one side of the bed. If he will be positioned on the left side, move him to the right side of the bed. Move him to the left side of the bed if you will be turning him to the right. This ensures that he will not be too close to the edge of the bed after he is turned.
2. Turning the patient onto the back, onto the abdomen, or onto the side.
3. Placing the person's trunk and extremities in proper position and maintaining alignment with the use of supportive devices.

Moving Patients

Moving and transporting patients are major responsibilities of the nursing assistant. Using proper body mechanics and following safety rules will protect both you and your

patients from injury. *Always* find out whether you will need help moving a patient before proceeding with your assignment. Check the care plan for special positioning instructions.

A **turning sheet** or **draw sheet** (folded large sheet or half-sheet) may be placed under a heavy or helpless patient to make moving easier. In some facilities, a very large cloth bed protector is used instead of a sheet. All of these methods are effective. To be effective, the sheet must extend from the shoulders to below the hips.

Follow Procedures 10 to 13 for moving patients. Practice the basic rules of good body mechanics you learned in Unit 14.

Positioning the Patient

After you have turned and moved the patient into good alignment, you can place pillows and other supportive devices to help the person maintain the position. Directions are given here for the basic four positions and their variations.

PROCEDURE

OBRA **DVD**

10

TURNING THE PATIENT TOWARD YOU

1. Carry out each initial procedure action.

2. Lower the side rail nearest to you. Cross the patient's far leg over the leg that is nearest to you.

3. Cross the far arm over the patient's chest. Bend the near arm at the elbow, bringing the hand toward the head of the bed.

4. Place your hand nearest the head of the bed on the patient's far shoulder. Place your other hand on the patient's hips on the far side. Brace your thighs against the side of the bed.

5. Roll the patient toward you (Figure 15-26A). Do it slowly, gently, and smoothly. Help the patient bring the upper leg toward you and bend it comfortably.

6. Put up the side rail. Be sure it is secure.

7. Go to the opposite side of the bed.

8. Place your hands under the patient's shoulders and then the hips. Pull toward the center of the bed (Figure 15-26B). This helps the patient maintain the side-lying position. Make sure the patient is not lying directly on the lower arm. The lower shoulder should be tipped slightly, so pressure is not centered directly over the joint.

9. Make sure the patient's body is properly aligned and safely positioned.

10. A pillow may be placed behind the patient's back. Secure it by pushing the near side under the patient to form a roll.

11. If the patient is unable to move independently, position the arms and legs. Support them with pillows between the shoulders, hands and knees, and ankles to prevent friction and contractures (Figure 15-26C). If the patient has an indwelling catheter, make sure the tubing is not between the legs, to prevent traction on the catheter and to prevent pressure ulcers.

12. Carry out each ending procedure action.

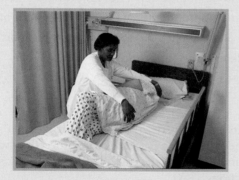

FIGURE 15-26A Place one hand on the patient's far shoulder and hip, then turn the patient toward you. (© Delmar/Cengage Learning)

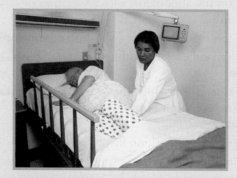

FIGURE 15-26B Move the patient to the center of the bed, keeping your back straight. (© Delmar/Cengage Learning)

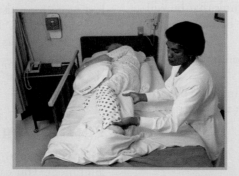

FIGURE 15-26C Place pillows to support the patient's body and maintain good alignment. (© Delmar/Cengage Learning)

PROCEDURE

OBRA

11

TURNING THE PATIENT AWAY FROM YOU

1. Carry out each initial procedure action.

2. Lower the near side rail. Be sure the side rail on the opposite side of the bed is up and secure.

3. Have the patient bend the knees, if able. Cross the arms on the chest.

4. Place your arm nearest the head of the bed under the patient's head and shoulders. Place the other hand and forearm under the small of the back. Bend your body at the hips and knees. Keep your back straight. Pull the patient toward the edge of the bed.

5. Place your forearms under the patient's hips and pull them toward you.

6. Move the ankles and knees toward you by placing one hand under the ankles and one under the knees.

7. Cross the near leg over the other leg at the ankles.

8. Roll the patient slowly and carefully away from you (Figure 15-27) by placing one hand under the shoulder and one hand under the hips.

9. Place your hands under the head and shoulders. Draw them back toward the center of the bed.

10. Move the hips to the center of the bed, as in Step 5.

11. Place a pillow for support behind the back.

12. Make sure that the patient's body is in good alignment. Support the upper leg with a pillow. Place the lower arm in a flexed position. Support the upper arm with a pillow.

13. Replace the side rail on the near side of the bed. Return the bed to the lowest position.

14. Carry out each ending procedure action.

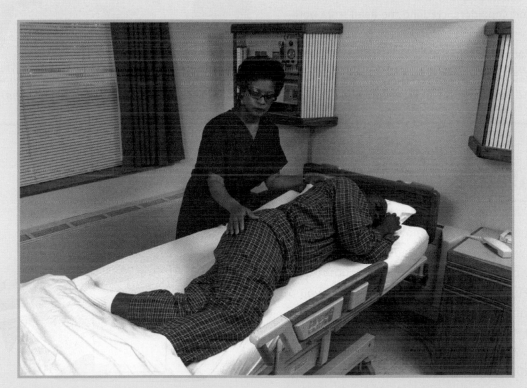

FIGURE 15-27 Roll the patient away from you. (© *Delmar/Cengage Learning*)

PROCEDURE   OBRA DVD

12

MOVING A PATIENT TO THE HEAD OF THE BED

1. Carry out each initial procedure action.

2. Ask a coworker to assist from the opposite side of the bed.

3. Lock the wheels of the bed. Raise the bed to a comfortable horizontal working height. Lower the side rails.

4. Lower the head of the bed if the patient can tolerate this position. Remove the pillow. Place it at the head of the bed, on its edge, for safety.

5. Lift the top bedding and expose the draw sheet. Loosen both sides of the draw sheet.

6. Roll the draw sheet edges close to both sides of the patient's body (Figure 15-28).

7. Face the head of the bed. Grasp the draw sheet with the hand closest to the foot of the bed.

8. Position your feet 12 inches apart, with the foot that is farthest from the bed edge forward.

9. Place your free hand and arm under the patient's neck and shoulders, cradling the head from both sides.

10. Bend your hips slightly.

11. Together, on a count of three, raise the patient's hips and back with the draw sheet, while

supporting the head and shoulders. Move the patient smoothly toward the head of the bed.

12. Replace the pillow under the patient's head.

13. Tighten and tuck in the draw sheet. Adjust the top bedding.

14. Carry out each ending procedure action.

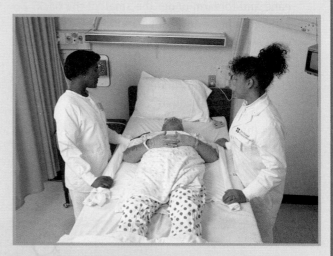

FIGURE 15-28 Using an overhand grasp, roll both edges of the turning (moving) sheet close to the patient's sides. (© Delmar/Cengage Learning)

Clinical Information ALERT

Some beds have an adjustable feature at the foot end of the bed, which makes moving the patient up easier. A switch will tip the bed so the head is slightly downward, in a **modified Trendelenburg position** (Figure 15-29). This position enables you to use gravity to help move and position the bedfast patient. For moving a person up, lowering the head 20° to 30° is sufficient. Use this position only under the direction and supervision of the nurse, because it increases the risk for respiratory complications in some patients. A Gore-Tex or nylon sheet or similar device (see Unit 32) will also make this job easier for you and the patient. ■

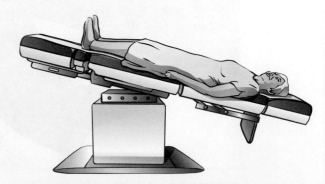

FIGURE 15-29 A variation of the Trendelenburg position is used for some treatments and procedures. Some professionals also use this position to treat patients who are in shock, but this use has fallen out of favor in recent years. (© Delmar/Cengage Learning)

PROCEDURE

13

LOGROLLING THE PATIENT

Note: This procedure is performed when the patient's spinal column must be kept straight, such as following spinal surgery or spinal cord or vertebral column injury. It is a good procedure to use with any dependent patient.

1. Carry out each initial procedure action.

2. Get help from another nursing assistant.

3. Raise the bed to waist-high horizontal position. Lock the wheels.

4. Lower the side rail on the side opposite to which the patient will be turned. Both assistants should be on the same side of the bed.

5. One assistant places hands under the patient's head and shoulders. The second person places

the hands under the hips and legs. Then move the patient as a unit toward you.

6. Place a pillow lengthwise between the legs. Fold the patient's arm over the chest.

7. Raise the side rail. Check for security.

8. Go to the opposite side of the bed and lower the side rail.

9. Turning the patient to the side may be done by:

   a. Using a turning sheet that was previously placed under the patient.

   • Reach over the patient, grasping and rolling the turning sheet toward the patient (Figure 15-30A).

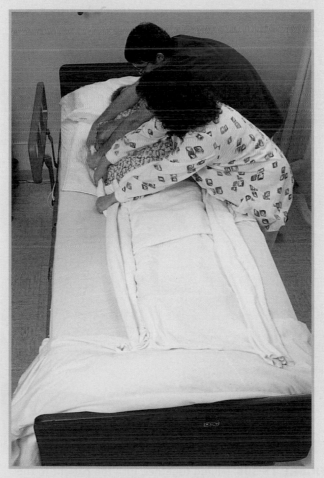

FIGURE 15-30A Roll the turning sheet against the patient. (© Delmar/Cengage Learning)

continues

PROCEDURE 13 CONTINUED

- One nursing assistant should be positioned beside the patient to keep the shoulders and hips straight.
- A second assistant should be positioned to keep the thighs and lower legs straight.

b. If a turning sheet is not in position, the first assistant should position hands on the patient's far shoulder and hips.

- Second assistant positions hands on the patient's far thigh and lower leg.

10. At a specified signal, roll the patient toward both assistants in a single movement, keeping the

spine, head, and legs straight. If a turning sheet is used, grasp the sheet and move the patient as a unit, onto her side (Figure 15-30B).

11. Place additional pillows behind the back to maintain the patient's position. A small pillow or folded bath blanket may be permitted under the patient's head and neck. Leave a pillow between the legs. Position small pillows or folded towels to support the arms.

12. Carry out each ending procedure action.

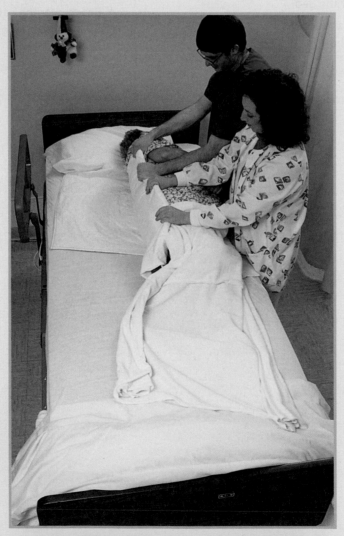

FIGURE 15-30B Pulling together, turn the patient to the side in one smooth motion. (© Delmar/Cengage Learning)

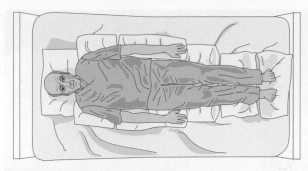

FIGURE 15-31A Supine position. *(© Delmar/Cengage Learning)*

Supine position   For supine position (Figure 15-31A):

1. Start with the bed flat and the patient lying on the back. The patient's head should be about 2 to 3 inches from the head of the bed.

2. Place a pillow under the patient's head. It should extend about 2 inches below the patient's shoulders, with the head in the middle of the pillow.

3. Place a **trochanter roll** along the affected hip or along both hips if the patient has little control over the legs. A trochanter roll is devised by rolling a bath blanket into a shape about 12 inches long. The roll should be just long enough to reach from above the hip to above the knee (Figure 15-31B). The trochanter roll prevents external rotation (Figure 15-31C) of the hip. Make a trochanter roll or support by:

   - Folding a bath blanket lengthwise in thirds.
   - Positioning the patient in the center of the folded bath blanket. The blanket should extend from mid to lower thigh to the waist.

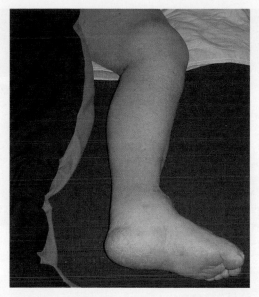

FIGURE 15-31C External rotation of the hip. *(© Delmar/Cengage Learning)*

   - Rolling each side of the blanket under and toward the patient until the blanket roll is firmly against the patient. Then tuck the roll inward toward the bed and patient to maintain the patient's position.

4. Place pillows under the legs to reach from above the back of the knee to the ankle so that the ankles and heels do not rub on the sheets.

5. Lying flat on the back is very uncomfortable for some people. This is especially true for persons with low back pain. Elevating the knees with a foam

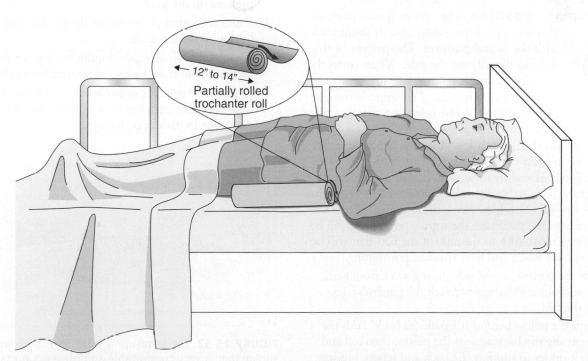

12" to 14"
Partially rolled
trochanter roll

FIGURE 15-31B The trochanter roll should extend from the hip to just above the knee. *(© Delmar/Cengage Learning)*

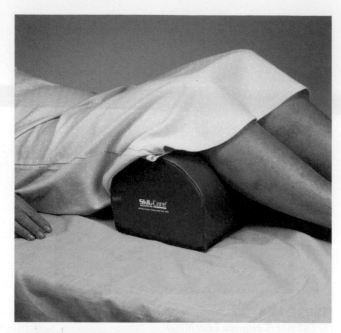

FIGURE 15-31D Supporting the knees relieves pressure and discomfort in the lower back. (*Courtesy of Skil-Care Corporation, Yonkers, NY, (800) 431-2972*)

bolster (Figure 15-31D) or one or more pillows will relieve pressure on the back and reduce discomfort.

6. If the care plan so indicates, position a footboard or place a folded pillow to support the patient's feet. The ankles should be at 90° angles.

7. Extend the patient's arms and place small pillows to reach from the elbow to below the wrist. The hand should be in alignment with the wrist and the palm should be down (Figure 15-31E).

Semisupine position The semisupine position (Figure 15-32) is also called the *tilt position*. It should not be confused with the lateral position. The patient in this position is not lying directly on the side. When correctly used, the semisupine position relieves pressure from the hip, sacrum, coccyx, and buttocks. The spine is straight and the patient is positioned so he is leaning against a pillow for support. Both legs are straight. The top leg is slightly behind the bottom leg. A pillow is placed under the top leg to keep it even with the hip joint. The lower shoulder is pulled slightly forward so that pressure is distributed over the back rather than the shoulder joint. The arms can be at the sides or folded across the abdomen. Begin the procedure with the patient in the supine position. It will be easiest if you move him to the side of the bed that will be behind his back when you have finished positioning.

1. Turn the patient on the side, facing away from you. Leave about a 45° angle between the patient's back and the bed.

2. Position a pillow behind the patient's back. Push the patient slightly back against the pillow, then roll and tuck it under to support the back and relieve pressure on the arm or shoulder.

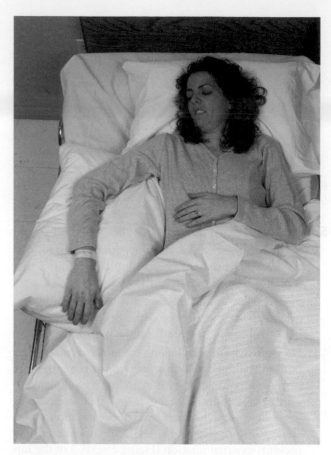

FIGURE 15-31E Pillows support the wrist and arm in good alignment and are more comfortable for the patient. (*© Delmar/Cengage Learning*)

3. Pull the bottom shoulder slightly forward to prevent pressure on the joint.

4. Position another pillow under the patient's top leg, level with the hip joint.

5. Straighten both legs, positioning the top leg slightly behind the bottom leg and supported by a pillow.

6. Position the patient's upper arm in a position of comfort. The wrist may rest on a pillow or the abdomen, according to patient preference.

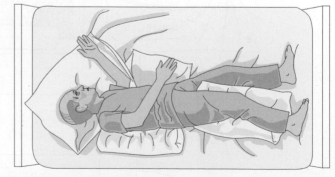

FIGURE 15-32 The semisupine position is a variation of supine that is very comfortable and prevents pressure on the major pressure points. (*© Delmar/Cengage Learning*)

Prone position For prone position (Figure 15-33A), start with the bed flat and the patient lying on the abdomen with the head turned to either side, spine straight and legs extended.

1. Place a small pillow under the head so that it extends to the patient's shoulders and 5 to 6 inches beyond the face.

2. Place a small pillow under the abdomen. This relieves pressure on the lower back and reduces pressure against a female patient's breasts. An alternate method is to roll a towel and place it under the shoulders.

3. Place a pillow under the arms to reach from the elbow to below the wrists. The shoulders and elbows may be flexed or extended, whichever is more comfortable for the patient (Figure 15-33B).

4. Place a pillow under the lower legs to prevent pressure on the toes. The patient may be moved down in bed before starting the procedure, so that the feet extend over the end of the mattress. This allows the foot to assume a normal standing position (Figure 15-33C).

Semiprone position The semiprone position (Figure 15-34) is the opposite of the semisupine position. It is also a very comfortable position. Like the semisupine position,

it eliminates pressure on the major areas at risk for pressure ulcer formation. Breathing is easier in this position than it is in the full prone position.

Begin the procedure by placing the patient prone. Lift the patient's chest and shoulder closest to you and place a pillow under them. Position the opposite arm behind the patient. Fold a second pillow in half and place it under the top leg. Keep the legs and spine straight. Turn the head to

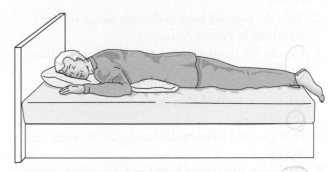

FIGURE 15-33C The patient may be moved down in bed so that the feet hang over the end of the mattress. *(© Delmar/Cengage Learning)*

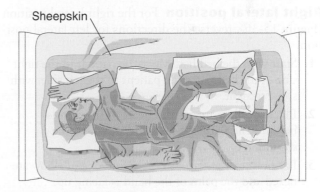

Sheepskin

FIGURE 15-34 The semiprone position is a very comfortable variation of the prone position. *(© Delmar/Cengage Learning)*

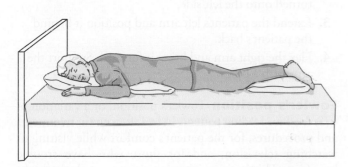

FIGURE 15-33A Prone position. *(© Delmar/Cengage Learning)*

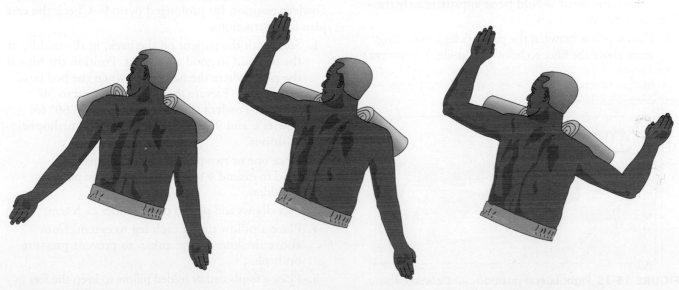

FIGURE 15-33B Position the arms in the way most comfortable for the patient. *(© Delmar/Cengage Learning)*

either side and a position a small pillow for comfort. Follow your facility policy for use of the semiprone position. Like the prone position, some facilities require a doctor's order, because lying on the abdomen may make breathing more difficult for some patients. When this position is used, check the patient every 15 minutes to be sure he or she can tolerate the position.

1. Turn the patient into the prone position as described earlier.

2. Turn the patient's head to the side facing you, or according to patient preference.

3. Gently lift the patient's near shoulder. Position a pillow under the chest and shoulder, with the arm resting on the pillow. Position the other arm behind (but not underneath) the patient.

4. Fold a second pillow in half and place it under the top leg.

5. Straighten and extend both legs for comfort.

6. Monitor the patient frequently for signs of respiratory distress.

Right lateral position For the right lateral position (Figure 15-35), reverse the directions for left lateral position.

1. Start with the bed flat. Move the patient to the right side of the bed. Turn the patient to the left side, with spine straight.

2. Place a pillow under the head so it extends beyond the patient's face and down to the shoulders.

3. Position the right arm so the shoulder and elbow are flexed and the palm of the hand is facing up.

4. Place the left arm so it is extended or only slightly flexed and rest it on the hip, or bring it forward and place it on a pillow. The patient's shoulder, elbow, and wrist should be at approximately the same height.

5. Place a pillow between the patient's legs, extending from above the knee to below the ankle. The patient's

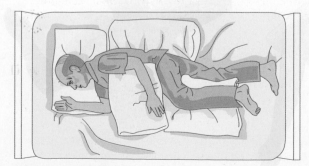

FIGURE 15-35 Right lateral position. (© Delmar/ Cengage Learning)

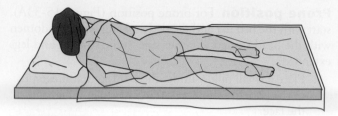

FIGURE 15-36 Sims' position. (© Delmar/Cengage Learning)

hip, knee, and ankle should be at approximately the same height.

6. A pillow may be placed behind the patient to help maintain the position.

Sims' position Sims' position (Figure 15-36) is a variation of the lateral position, with the patient on the left side, left leg extended and right leg flexed. This position is often used for rectal examinations and treatments and enemas.

1. Place a pillow under the patient's head as for lateral position.

2. Start with the bed flat and the patient moved and turned onto the left side.

3. Extend the patient's left arm and position it behind the patient's back.

4. Flex the right arm and bring it forward. Support the arm with a pillow.

Fowler's position Fowler's position, or a variation of it, is used for feeding patients in bed, for certain treatments and procedures, for the patient's comfort while visiting or watching television, and for those who have trouble breathing. This position increases pressure on the buttocks and increases the risk of skin breakdown and pressure ulcers. Because of this, patients should not be left in Fowler's position for prolonged periods. Check the care plan for instructions.

1. Start with the patient on the back, in the middle of the bed and in good alignment. Position the hips at the place where the bed bends when the bed head is rolled up. Elevate the head of the bed to 30° for semi-Fowler's (Figure 15-37), 45° to 60° for Fowler's, and 90° for high Fowler's and orthopneic positions.

2. Place one or two pillows behind the patient's head to extend 4 to 5 inches below the patient's shoulders.

3. Flex elbows and place a pillow under each arm.

4. Place a pillow under each leg to extend from above the knee to the ankle, to prevent pressure on heels.

5. Place a footboard or folded pillow to keep the feet in position, if necessary.

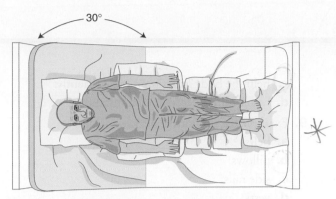

FIGURE 15-37 Semi-Fowler's position. (© Delmar/ Cengage Learning)

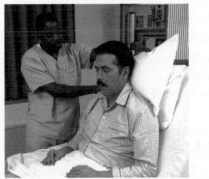

FIGURE 15-38 Orthopneic position. (© Delmar/Cengage Learning)

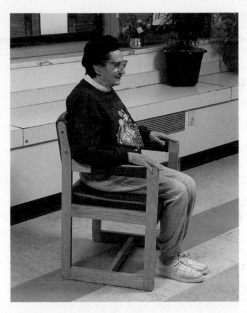

FIGURE 15-39A Maintaining good body alignment is important when patients are sitting in chairs. (© Delmar/Cengage Learning)

Orthopneic position Orthopneic position (Figure 15-38) is a variation of high Fowler's position and is used for patients who have difficulty breathing. Like Fowler's position, the orthopneic position increases the risk of pressure ulcers. Special skin care may be necessary. Check the care plan or ask the nurse for further instructions.

1. The position of the bed remains the same as for high Fowler's. (The head of the bed is raised as high as it will go.)
2. Assist the patient to sit as upright as possible.
3. Have the patient lean slightly forward, supporting himself with the forearms. Placing the overbed table in front of the patient and extending the arms over it provides a good means of support and helps ease respirations. This makes the thorax larger, enabling the patient to inhale more air.
4. Place another pillow behind the patient's low back for support.

Sitting position Patients should be positioned in a comfortable, well-constructed chair, so that the head and spine are erect (Figure 15-39A). The back and buttocks should be against the chair back. Stabilizing the feet on the floor or footrests is the first step in good positioning. Solid foot support also prevents forward sliding. For good posture and even weight distribution, position the feet at a 90° angle

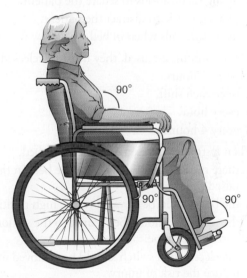

FIGURE 15-39B Remember the 90-90-90 position when positioning patients in chairs. The feet must be well supported at a 90° angle to the lower legs. The lower legs should be at a 90° angle to the thighs. The thighs should be at a 90° angle to the torso. (© Delmar/Cengage Learning)

to the lower legs. Position the lower legs at a 90° angle to the thighs. The thighs should be at a 90° angle to the torso. This is called the **90-90-90 position** (Figure 15-39B).

1. Pillows or postural supports may be needed to maintain the position.
2. A small pillow may be folded and placed at the small of the back to add comfort and support.
3. Do not permit the back of the patient's knees to rest against the chair.

REVIEW

A. Multiple Choice

Select the one best answer for each of the following.

1. Patients may be at risk for incidents because they
   a. ambulate in the hallway.
   b. use a wheelchair for long distances.
   c. keep one side rail up for turning independently when in bed.
   d. receive medications affecting coordination and mental status.

2. Patient falls can be prevented by
   a. encouraging patients to remain in bed.
   b. using restraints when the patient is up.
   c. keeping the side rails up at all times.
   d. meeting the patient's needs promptly.

3. Alternatives to restraints include
   a. taking patients to the bathroom regularly.
   b. giving medications to sedate the patient.
   c. playing music to distract the patient.
   d. using side rails when in bed.

4. When restraints are used, they must be released
   a. every 2 hours.
   b. once each shift.
   c. every hour.
   d. every 4 hours.

5. When restraints are used on patients in bed,
   a. there must be full side rails on the bed, in the raised position.
   b. the bed should be elevated to the high position.
   c. the restraints should be secured to the stationary part of the frame.
   d. the electric bed switch should be removed to reduce the risk of injury.

6. Injuries caused by sitting in the same position for too long are called
   a. lacerations.
   b. bruises.
   c. pressure ulcers.
   d. aspiration.

7. Initial procedure actions include
   a. handwashing.
   b. raising side rails.
   c. placing the call signal within reach.
   d. opening the door.

8. Correct body alignment will
   a. heal disease.
   b. prevent infection.
   c. help the body function more efficiently.
   d. be harmful in certain circumstances.

9. Examples of supportive devices include
   a. belts.
   b. pillows.
   c. side rails.
   d. vests.

10. Supine position is
    a. lying on the back.
    b. lying on the abdomen.
    c. lying on the side.
    d. sitting in the chair.

11. A position used for patients who have trouble breathing is
    a. orthopneic.
    b. semiprone.
    c. lateral.
    d. supine.

12. Logrolling is a procedure performed for
    a. persons who have had both legs amputated.
    b. ambulatory patients.
    c. all conscious patients.
    d. patients who have had spinal surgery.

13. A trochanter roll is used to
    a. maintain the hip in alignment.
    b. maintain the feet in alignment.
    c. support the patient's back.
    d. prevent contractures of the hand.

B. Nursing Assistant Challenge

Sara Abrams is 76 years old, has Parkinson's disease, and is a resident in a long-term care facility. She is ambulatory, with a shuffling walk, and has tremors of her hands related to the Parkinson's. She is disoriented and frequently walks into other residents' rooms.

14. Discuss safety issues related to Ms. Abrams's condition.

15. Which of the Patients' Rights may be a special issue in this situation?

16. What steps can you take to meet Ms. Abrams's physical needs? Will doing so reduce her risk of falling?

17. How can you incorporate exercise into her daily routine?

18. What types of activities might interest Ms. Abrams?

19. Are there actions that can be taken to avoid restraint use and falls?

UNIT 16

The Patient's Mobility: Transfer Skills

OBJECTIVES

After completing this unit, you will be able to:

- Spell and define terms.
- Apply the principles of good body mechanics and ergonomics to moving and transferring patients.
- Describe the difference between a standing transfer and a sitting transfer.
- List at least seven factors to consider before moving a patient, to determine whether additional equipment or assistance is necessary.
- List the guidelines for safe transfers.
- Demonstrate correct application of a transfer belt.
- Demonstrate the following procedures:
  - Procedure 14 Applying a Transfer Belt
  - Procedure 15 Transferring the Patient from Bed to Chair or Wheelchair and Back—One Assistant
  - Procedure 16 Transferring the Patient from Bed to Chair or Wheelchair and Back—Two Assistants
  - Procedure 17 Sliding-Board Transfer from Bed to Wheelchair
  - Procedure 18 Independent Transfer, Standby Assist
  - Procedure 19 Transferring the Patient from Bed to Stretcher
  - Procedure 20 Transferring the Patient with a Mechanical Lift
  - Procedure 21 Transferring the Patient onto and off the Toilet

VOCABULARY

Learn the meaning and the correct spelling of the following words and phrases:

contraindication	mechanical lift	pivot	standing transfer
full weight-bearing	nonweight-bearing	sitting (lateral) transfer	transfer belt
gait belt	partial weight-bearing	sliding board	weight-bearing
manual patient handling			

INTRODUCTION

As a nursing assistant, you will work with many patients who have impaired mobility. In Unit 15 you learned how to move and position patients in bed. In this unit you will learn how to transfer patients (move them from one place to another).

NURSING ASSISTANT SAFETY

Nursing work is always listed as one of the top 10 occupations for work-related musculoskeletal injuries. Having a previous history of back injury was identified as the biggest risk factor for either a new back injury or back pain. The rate of back injury in workers with a history of injury is about twice as high as the rate among workers with no history of back problems.

In 2005, the state of Texas passed the first state law requiring hospitals to implement safe patient handling and movement programs. By the end of 2008, nine states had passed laws related to safe patient handling. Still, the different state laws vary widely in scope and strength. The American Nurses' Association (ANA) is working hard to get legislation on safe patient handling passed in all states.

Moving patients is the task with the highest risk of injury. Workers often find themselves in awkward positions and confined spaces, and must bend or reach while the back is flexed. High-risk patient handling tasks vary by clinical setting.

To reduce the risk of worker injury, facilities have implemented various programs, such as lift teams. These are specially trained personnel who do all patient moving in the facility. Some facilities have "no-lift" policies. This does not mean that workers should never lift a patient, heavy box, or equipment. Instead, it means that no manual lifting should be done. Facilities with no-lift policies usually depend on mechanical aids for moving patients. Some have mechanical, electrical, and ceiling-mounted lifts for moving patients vertically. Many require workers to use gait belts and other aids for moving patients and heavy items. A no-lift policy is a pledge from management that equipment and/or personnel will be available to help with the task and reduce the risk of injury associated with manual patient handling. **Manual patient handling** is moving a person by hand or bodily force, including pushing, pulling, carrying, holding, or supporting the patient or a patient's body part.

The procedures in this chapter are an overview of the basic methods for lifting, moving, and transferring patients. You must learn these before you can safely use a mechanical or friction-reducing device to assist with patient movement. Many new devices are available for lifting, moving, and repositioning patients, to reduce the risk of worker injury. However, their availability varies widely from one facility to the next. You must adapt the procedures in this book to the policies, procedures, and equipment available in your facility for moving patients and protecting your back.

In addition, practicing and using proper body mechanics is key to injury prevention. Before performing the procedures

in this chapter, review and master the information on ergonomics, body mechanics, and safe patient handling in Unit 14. Also, OSHA and ANA have many additional resources related to ergonomics and patient handling.

TYPES OF TRANSFERS

There are basically two types of transfers. In a **standing transfer**, the patient stands during the transfer with the help of one or two nursing assistants. In a **sitting (lateral) transfer**, the patient sits throughout the transfer, such as when a sliding board is used (see Procedure 17). A **sliding board** is a slippery plastic or wooden board about 2 feet long. A sliding board is used for a sitting, *lateral* transfer. A mechanical lift may also be used for sitting transfers, but this device is for *vertical* movement. One type of electrical lift is available for assisted standing transfers. The **mechanical lift** is typically a manually operated hydraulic lift. Many facilities have electrically (or battery) operated lifts or ceiling-mounted electrical lifts available. The electrical or mechanical lift is used to transfer dependent or heavy patients from one surface to another.

The nurse or the physical therapist determines which method is used to transfer a patient (Figure 16-1). It is important to follow instructions carefully to avoid injury. The method selected depends on:

- The patient's physical condition.
- The patient's strength, endurance, and balance.

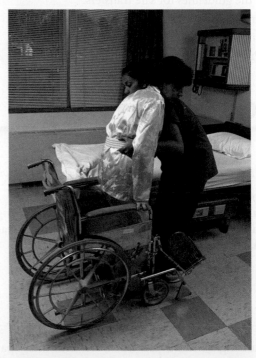

FIGURE 16-1 The nurse or physical therapist determines the method of transfer, but you must also use good judgment, such as deciding that more help will be needed in the current situation. (© *Delmar/Cengage Learning*)

- The patient's ability to stand on one or both legs. This is called **weight-bearing**. For example, a patient may not be able to place full weight on a paralyzed leg. The physician may order the patient to be **nonweight-bearing** or **partial weight-bearing** if the person has had hip surgery. The ability to stand on both legs is called **full weight-bearing**. For a standing transfer, the patient must be able to stand and bear weight on one leg.

- The patient's mental condition and ability to understand, cooperate, and follow instructions.

- The patient's size. For example, transfer of a very tall or large person who cannot bear full weight would require two assistants or a mechanical lift.

You must use good judgment and determine if another person or special equipment are necessary to assist you and ensure a safe transfer. Key elements to consider first are:

- Patient's ability to cooperate and assist with the procedure.
- Patient's ability to bear weight.

GUIDELINES *for*

Safe Patient Transfers

When moving dependent patients, follow these safety measures:

- Use the method of transfer listed on the care plan. Never take shortcuts.
- Tell the patient what you are doing and how he can help.
- Test the patient's understanding and make sure she knows what you expect her to do during the transfer.
- Use correct body mechanics.
- Place the bed in the low position. Make sure all wheels are locked before the move. Elevating the head of the bed may be helpful for bed-to-chair transfers.
- *Never allow patients to place their hands on your body during a transfer.*
- *Never place your hands under a patient's arms or shoulders.* The joints are fragile, and you may injure the patient if you try to lift there.
- Use a transfer belt unless contraindicated.
- Make sure the patient's shoes are appropriate to the floor surface and that clothing does not drag on the floor.
- Avoid pulling on tubes, orthoses, or other items during the transfer. Tubing must move with you so it is not dislodged. One person may be needed to move the tubing.
- Encourage the patient to keep his head up, which will enable him to see the surface to which he is being transferred.
- Transfer the patient toward his or her strongest side, if possible.

- Stand close to the patient during the transfer.
- Brace the knee of a weak or paralyzed leg with your knee or leg. Support a paralyzed arm during the transfer.
- Give only the assistance the patient needs.
- Position the small, front caster wheels with the large part facing forward; lock the brakes during transfers and when the wheelchair is parked (Figure 16-2).

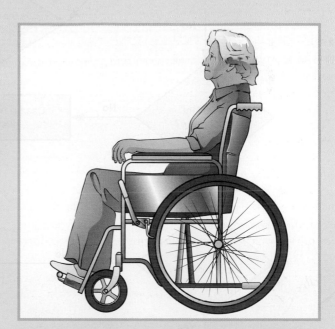

FIGURE 16-2 The large part of the small, front caster wheels must face forward during transfers and when the chair is parked. Changing the position of the front wheels changes the center of gravity of the chair and makes the chair more stable. Tipping is less likely when the large part of the wheels faces forward and the brakes are locked. (© *Delmar/Cengage Learning*)

- Patient's upper-extremity strength, if upper arms are used in the transfer.
- Patient's size (height and weight) compared with your size. In general, if the patient is larger than you are, you will need help, especially if you are unfamiliar with the patient. You may also need help moving dependent and mentally confused patients, even if they are smaller than you are.
- Always get help if there is danger of pulling on or displacing a tube during the transfer.
- Follow special orders for transfers and positioning, such as you would see for a patient who has had hip surgery.

Use the information in Figure 16-3 to help identify the safest method for making the transfer. You will find additional information in the appendix of the Online Companion to this book.

✗ Transfer Belts

A **transfer belt** is an assistive and safety device used to transfer or ambulate patients who need help. (Refer to Procedure 14.) The webbed belt is 1½ to 2 inches wide and about 54 to 60 inches long. Belts are available up to 72 inches long for use on large patients. When it is used to assist a patient with ambulation, it is called a **gait belt**. Using the belt makes it easier to guide and assist the person without pulling on his or her body. It enables you to have more control in directing the transfer. The belt is not used to "lift" a patient. If the person has no ability to bear weight, use another method for transfers. **Contraindications** (situations in which something is not indicated, inappropriate, or potentially dangerous) for use of the transfer belt include:

- Abdominal, back, or rib injuries, fractures, or recent surgery
- Abdominal pacemakers

Transfer to and from: Bed to Chair, Chair to Toilet, Chair to Chair, or Car to Chair

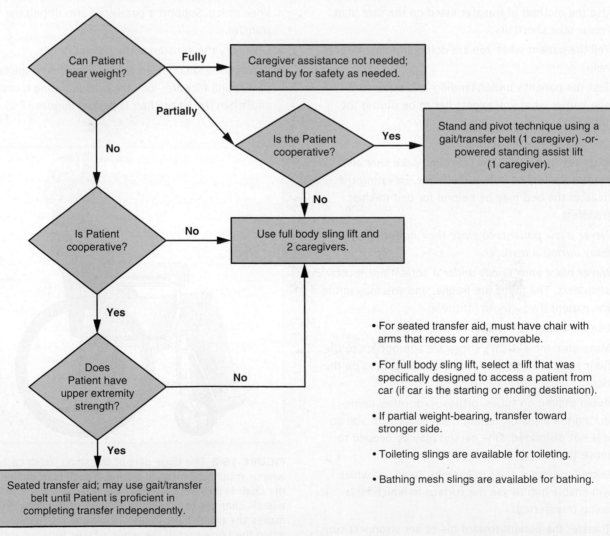

FIGURE 16-3 This algorithm helps you decide when extra help or a lifting device is needed during transfers onto a chair or toilet. *(The Patient Safety Center of Inquiry (Tampa, FL), Veterans Health Administration & Department of Defense (October 2001))*

- Advanced heart or lung disease
- Abdominal aneurysms
- Pregnancy
- Colostomy
- Gastrostomy tube or feeding tube
- Recently implanted abdominal or spinal medication pumps
- Other devices implanted into the spine, such as spinal catheters or spinal stimulators

Medication pumps may be implanted under the skin of the abdomen in some patients. A tiny catheter leads from the pump to the spine, where the medication is delivered. If the surgical site is well healed, it is probably safe to use the transfer belt. However, always follow the care plan or check with the nurse before using a transfer belt to move a patient with any type of implantable device. Many individual variables must be considered when determining the method of transfer.

OSHA ALERT

Each year, more than 12.8 million Americans consult their doctors about back problems. In fact, as many as 8 out of 10 individuals will suffer back pain during their lifetime. A transfer belt is an inexpensive item that helps protect you from injury and makes transfers safer and more secure for patients. Never use a patient's belt or pull on the belt loops of a patient's pants. Make the transfer belt a permanent part of your uniform. Wear it when you are on duty so it is readily available when needed to move a patient. ■

PROCEDURE

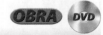

APPLYING A TRANSFER BELT

1. Carry out initial procedure actions.

2. Assemble equipment:
   - Transfer belt

3. Explain the procedure. Tell the patient that the belt is a safety device that will be removed as soon as the transfer is completed.

4. Apply the belt over the patient's clothing (Figure 16-4A). Never apply it to bare skin.

5. If the patient is going to transfer from bed to chair, the belt may be applied after the patient comes to a sitting position on the edge of the bed. If he or she has poor balance, apply the belt while the patient is still lying down in bed. Readjust the belt after the patient sits up, if needed.

6. Keep the belt at the patient's waist level. Make sure the belt is right side out and is not twisted.

7. Buckle the belt in front by threading the belt end through the teeth side of the buckle first and then through both openings (Figure 16-4B). The buckle must be in front.

8. Check female patients to be sure the breasts are not under the belt.

9. The belt should be snug, but not tight (Figure 16-4C). Check the fit by placing three fingers under it. Your fingers should fit comfortably

10. Be sure the patient's feet are flat on the floor before moving. If not, use the belt to assist the patient to the edge of the bed.

11. If you are transferring a patient into or out of a wheelchair, lock the wheelchair brakes and keep the footrests out of the way during the transfer. Be sure the small front wheels face forward. After the patient is seated, the legs should not dangle. Position the feet on the floor or on the wheelchair footrests.

12. Teach the patient to assist by pushing off the bed or arms of the chair with her hands when you count to three.

13. Use an underhand grasp when holding the belt. For transfers, place one hand on each side of the buckle in front.

14. Avoid pulling the patient up with force.

15. When the patient is standing, **pivot** (turn the entire body as one unit) to transfer.

continues

PROCEDURE 14 CONTINUED

16. The chair should be close enough so the patient can feel it with her hands after you pivot.

17. Remove the belt after the patient is safely seated.

18. Carry out ending procedure actions.

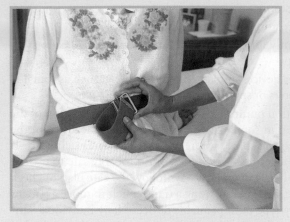

FIGURE 16-4B Thread the belt through the teeth side of the buckle first. (© Delmar/Cengage Learning)

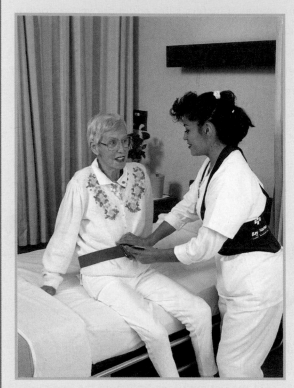

FIGURE 16-4A Always apply the transfer belt over clothing. (© Delmar/Cengage Learning)

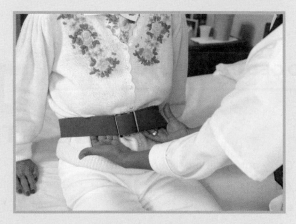

FIGURE 16-4C The belt should be snug but not tight. (© Delmar/Cengage Learning)

PROCEDURE

15

 OBRA DVD

TRANSFERRING THE PATIENT FROM BED TO CHAIR OR WHEELCHAIR AND BACK—ONE ASSISTANT

1. Carry out initial procedure actions.

2. Assemble equipment:
   - Transfer belt
   - Chair for patient
   - Bath blanket
   - Robe or clothing
   - Shoes and socks

3. Position the chair parallel with the bed so that the patient moves toward his or her strongest side. Position the large part of the small front wheels

PROCEDURE **15** CONTINUED

facing forward. Lock the brakes and raise or remove the footrests (Figure 16-5A). Cover the chair with a bath blanket, unless the patient is fully clothed. Apply the transfer belt.

4. Lower the bed to the lowest horizontal position and lock the wheels.

These instructions are for getting out of the right side (patient's right side) of the bed.

5. Stand against the right side (the patient's right, or left side of the bed). Put the side rail down. Ask the patient to slide toward the right side of the bed.

6. Have the patient roll over onto her right side, flexing the knees and bending the right arm so it can be used for propping the upper body. Bend the elbow of the left arm so this hand can be used to push off from the bed.

7. Instruct the patient to use the elbow of her right arm to raise the upper body and to push with the hand of the right arm so she comes to an upright position (Figure 16-5B).

8. Instruct the patient to let her legs slide off the bed at the same time.

9. If assistance is needed, place one arm under the shoulders (not the neck) and one arm over and around the knees (Figure 16-5C). Raise the patient's upper body at the same time you move the legs off the bed.

10. Give the patient time to adjust to sitting up. Adjust the transfer belt, and check the fit with your fingers so it is snug, but not too tight. Assist the patient to put on shoes and socks. (You can put the shoes and socks on while the patient is lying down in bed, as permitted, or if the patient has problems with balance.)

11. Do not let a weak or paralyzed arm hang during the transfer. Put that hand in the patient's pocket, have her cradle the weak arm with her strong arm, or carefully tuck the weaker hand in the transfer belt or waist of the pants until she is seated.

12. When the patient is ready to transfer:
    - Assist the patient to the edge of the mattress. Have her spread the knees, lean forward from the waist, and place the feet slightly back.
    - Place a weak or nonweight-bearing leg in front. Position the strong leg slightly back.
    - Spread your feet apart and bend your knees and hips, keeping your back straight.
    - Hold the belt with an underhand grasp, one hand on each side of the buckle.
    - Press your knee against the weak knee, or block the patient's foot with yours to prevent the weaker leg from sliding out from under her.
    - Tell the patient to press into the mattress, straighten the elbows and knees, and come to a standing position on the count of three (Figure 16-5D).

13. If patient cannot walk, have her pivot around to the front of the chair until the chair is touching the backs of her legs.

14. Instruct the patient to place her hands on the arms of the chair (if able), to bend her knees, and to gently lower herself into the chair as you ease her downward (Figure 16-5E). Replace the footrests.

15. Position the patient comfortably. Place the signal light within easy reach.

16. Straighten the bed and prepare it for the patient's return.

17. Carry out ending procedure actions.

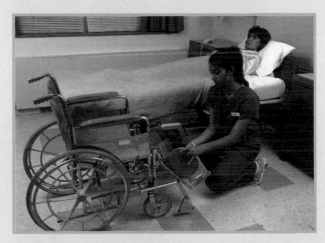

FIGURE 16-5A Lock the wheelchair and lift or remove the footrests before the patient transfers. (© Delmar/ Cengage Learning)

continues

PROCEDURE 15 CONTINUED

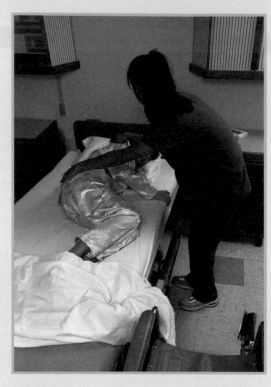

FIGURE 16-5B Instruct the patient to use her hands to push to the sitting position. (© Delmar/Cengage Learning)

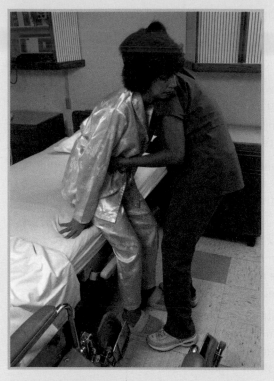

FIGURE 16-5D Tell the patient to straighten her elbows and knees to come to a standing position. (© Delmar/Cengage Learning)

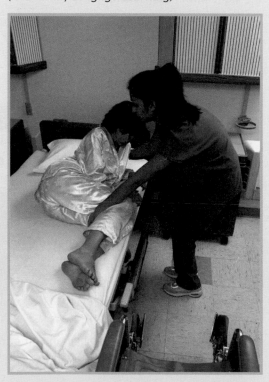

FIGURE 16-5C Place one arm under the patient's shoulders and one arm over and around the knees. (© Delmar/Cengage Learning)

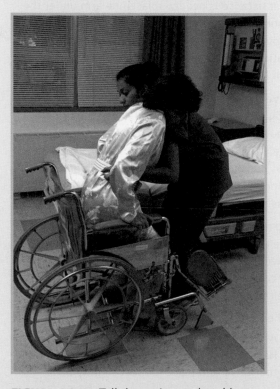

FIGURE 16-5E Tell the patient to bend her knees and lower herself into the chair. (© Delmar/Cengage Learning)

PROCEDURE 15 CONTINUED

Returning the Patient to Bed

18. Carry out initial procedure actions.

19. Assemble equipment:
    - Transfer belt

20. Place chair parallel with bed so the patient moves toward his or her strongest side.

21. Move the bed to the lowest horizontal position and lock the wheels. Fanfold top covers to the foot of the bed if necessary and raise the opposite side rail.

22. Position the large part of the small, front caster wheels facing forward. Lock the wheelchair brakes and raise or remove the footrests.

23. Have the patient place both feet flat on the floor.

24. Place the transfer belt around the patient's waist.

25. Instruct the patient to move forward in the chair, to bend forward, and to spread the knees. Both feet should be back, with the stronger foot slightly behind the weaker foot. Both of the patient's hands should be on the arms of the chair (Figure 16-6).

26. Hold the transfer belt with an underhand grasp. Brace the weaker leg with your knee or leg. Ask the patient to push off on the count of three and to stand up as you provide the necessary assistance.

27. Allow the patient to remain standing for a time to stabilize position. Keep your grasp on the transfer belt and continue to brace the weak leg if necessary.

28. To complete the transfer, instruct the patient to step or pivot around, facing away from the bed. Assist him to sit when he feels the edge of the mattress on the back of the legs. To sit, have the patient bend forward slightly, bend the knees, and lower himself onto the mattress.

29. When the patient is safely in bed, remove the transfer belt.

30. Remove the patient's slippers and robe. Assist the patient to lie down. Assist with positioning as necessary. Cover the patient. Fold the bath blanket (if used) and return it to the bedside stand. Place the signal light within reach.

31. Move the wheelchair out of the way.

32. Carry out ending procedure actions.

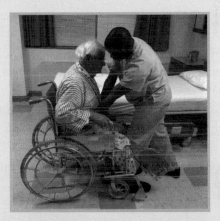

FIGURE 16-6 Instruct the patient to assist by holding the arms of the chair with both hands. (© Delmar/Cengage Learning)

PROCEDURE

16

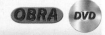

TRANSFERRING THE PATIENT FROM BED TO CHAIR OR WHEELCHAIR AND BACK—TWO ASSISTANTS

Two people may be needed to transfer patients who are weak, disoriented, have limited weight-bearing ability, or are very large. Directions are given for transferring toward the patient's right side.

1. Follow steps 1 through 11 in Procedure 15.

2. The nursing assistants stand one on each side, facing the patient.

continues

PROCEDURE 16 CONTINUED

3. Each assistant places the hand closest to the patient through the front of the belt, with an underhand grasp. The assistants grasp the back of the belt with the other hand. Coordinate your movements (Figure 16-7A).

4. The nursing assistant closest to the chair (on the patient's right side) stands in a position to step or pivot around smoothly to allow the patient access to the chair. This person stands with the left leg further back than the right leg.

5. The other nursing assistant uses the left knee to brace the patient's weaker left leg. This assistant's left leg is further back than the right leg.

6. Have the patient spread the knees spread apart, with both feet back and the stronger foot slightly in back of the weaker foot.

7. Instruct the patient to bend forward and place the palms of the hands on the edge of the mattress to push off on the count of three.

8. The nursing assistants bend their knees and give a broad base of support.

9. On the count of three, the patient stands. Allow him to stand for a moment and bear weight. Tell

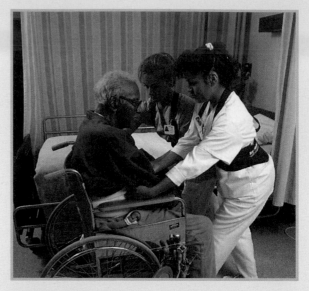

FIGURE 16-7B Instruct the patient to reach for the arms of the chair with both hands. *(© Delmar/ Cengage Learning)*

him to keep his head up. Both nursing assistants help the patient pivot by slowly and smoothly pivoting their feet, legs, and hips to their left.

10. To sit, have the patient bend forward slightly, bend the knees, and lower onto the chair. At the same time, have him reach for the arms of the chair with both hands (Figure 16-7B).

11. Complete the procedure as described for a one-assistant transfer (Procedure 15).

Returning the Patient to Bed

The directions given here are for moving the patient toward the left side.

12. Follow instructions 18 through 25 in Procedure 15.

13. Each nursing assistant places the hand closest to the patient through the front of the belt with an underhand grasp; the other hand goes toward the back.

14. The nursing assistant closest to the bed (on the patient's left side) stands in a position to step or pivot around smoothly to allow the patient access to the bed. This person stands with the right leg further back than the left leg.

15. The other nursing assistant uses the left knee to brace the patient's weaker right leg.

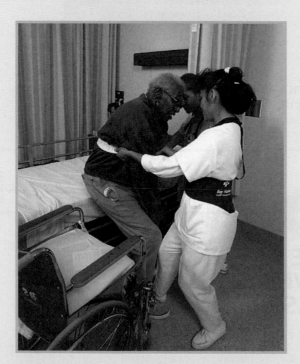

FIGURE 16-7A Coordination of movement is necessary. *(© Delmar/Cengage Learning)*

PROCEDURE 16 CONTINUED

This person's right leg is further back than the left one (Figure 16-8A).

16. Ask the patient to push off from the chair on the count of three and to stand up as you provide the necessary assistance.

17. Allow the patient to remain standing for a time to stabilize position. Keep your hands on the transfer belt and continue to brace the weak leg, if necessary.

18. To complete the transfer, instruct the patient to step or pivot around to stand in front of the bed, facing away from it. Assist him to sit when he feels the edge of the mattress on the back of the legs. To sit, have the patient bend forward slightly, bend the knees, and lower himself onto the mattress (Figure 16-8B).

19. When the patient is safely in bed, remove the transfer belt.

20. Remove the patient's slippers and robe. Assist the patient to lie down. Assist with positioning as necessary. Cover the patient. Fold the bath blanket (if used) and return it to the bedside stand. Place the signal light within reach.

21. Move the wheelchair out of the way.

22. Carry out ending procedure actions.

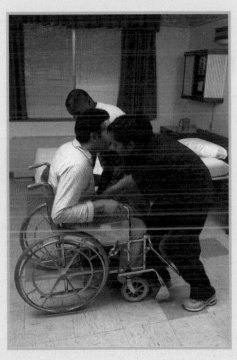

FIGURE 16-8A The nursing assistant uses the knee to support the patient's weaker leg. *(© Delmar/Cengage Learning)*

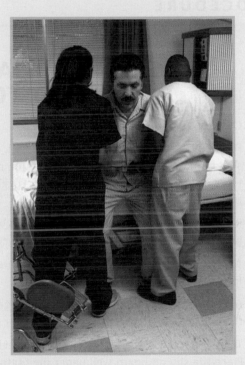

FIGURE 16-8B Tell the patient to bend forward, bend the knees, and lower himself onto the mattress. *(© Delmar/ Cengage Learning)*

Sliding-Board Transfers

A sliding-board (Figure 16-9) transfer is used for patients with good upper body strength and sitting balance. This type of transfer is commonly used for patients with paraplegia, or weakness in both legs, such as those with post polio syndrome and other neuromuscular diseases. The procedure is performed by doing a series of push-ups. The patient locks the elbows and pushes with the hands. To transfer, the patient must be able to lift the buttocks off the bed. After lifting the buttocks, he or she lowers onto the sliding board, then lifts and slides until the transfer is complete. Some patients perform this transfer independently, whereas others need help. If you will be assisting, always use a transfer belt.

To use a sliding board for transfers, a wheelchair with removable armrests must be used. The chair must also have

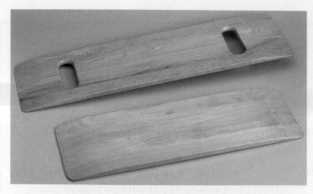

FIGURE 16-9 The sliding board is used when the wheelchair has removable arms and swing-away leg rests. Some fabrics tend to stick to the board. Make sure the patient is wearing pants that will slide across the board easily. (*Photo courtesy of Briggs Corporation*)

removable or swing-away leg rests. The patient must have clothing on the lower half of the body. Bare skin will stick to the board, creating friction and shearing and making the transfer very difficult or impossible. Blue jeans do not slide well on the board. Cotton or synthetic slacks are best. If the patient has difficulty sliding on the board, it may help to drape a pillowcase across the board. (Do not encase the board in the pillowcase as you would a pillow.) A wooden board can be waxed to maintain a slippery surface. Some special boards are available, such as the type with a disk in a track through the center of the board. The patient sits on the disk and slides it down the track to the opposite end of the board. Another type is available that secures to the toilet for bathroom transfers, which are difficult or impossible with a regular sliding board. Curved boards are also available to fit around the large wheelchair wheel.

PROCEDURE   **OBRA**

17

SLIDING-BOARD TRANSFER FROM BED TO WHEELCHAIR

1. Carry out initial procedure actions.

2. Position the wheelchair parallel to the bed, or at a slight (about 35°) angle. Position the large part of the small front wheels facing forward. Lock the brakes.

3. Remove the arm of the wheelchair closest to the bed. Remove the leg rests or fold them back.

4. Apply a transfer belt. Check the fit with three fingers.

5. Assist the patient to move close to the edge of the bed.

6. Tell the patient to lean away from the wheelchair. Place the sliding board well under the buttocks, with the beveled side of the board facing up. Avoid pinching the patient's skin between the board and the bed.

7. Place the opposite end of the board well onto the seat of the wheelchair.

8. Instruct the patient to push up with the hands, lock the elbows, and move across the board. Repeat until the patient is seated in the chair with one buttock on the board. You will assist by grasping the transfer belt with an underhand grasp and sliding laterally when the patient pushes down on the bed.

   - The patient may pull on the opposite armrest of the wheelchair with one hand when she has moved close enough to reach it. This will help her slide across the board. Pushing against the opposite armrest will also help her achieve greater height in the push-ups. The patient may also push with one hand on the board. Caution the patient to avoid placing the fingers under the edges of the board.

9. Be prepared to assist with sliding the patient's buttocks by guiding them with the transfer belt. If the patient is having trouble balancing, place your hands on the patient's shoulders for support. Stop and allow the patient to balance before proceeding.

10. Support and move the patient's legs with your hands, if necessary.

11. Instruct the patient to lean away from the bed. Remove the board.

12. Remove the transfer belt.

13. Replace the arm of the wheelchair. Position the patient's legs on the leg rests, or as instructed.

14. Assist the patient with positioning in good body alignment, as needed.

15. Perform ending procedure actions.

16. Reverse the procedure to return the patient to bed.

PROCEDURE

18

OBRA

INDEPENDENT TRANSFER, STANDBY ASSIST

This method is appropriate for the patient who has good balance and strength and can understand instructions. Put a transfer belt on the patient the first time this is attempted, in accordance with facility policies and as instructed by the care plan.

1. Follow the instructions for getting the patient to a sitting position on the side of the bed. (See Procedure 15.) For an independent transfer, the patient should be able to do this without help.

2. Have the patient place the strongest foot slightly in back of the other foot. Advise the patient to spread the knees slightly apart.

3. Instruct the patient to place the palms of the hands at the edge of the bed and to lean slightly forward.

4. Tell the patient to press the hands into the bed to push off, while straightening the legs, to assume a standing position.

5. Once standing, have the patient reach for the far arm of the chair and then step or pivot to stand in front of the chair. Instruct the patient to sit when he or she feels the edge of the seat against the back of the legs.

6. Carry out ending procedure actions.

Reverse these directions when transferring from chair to bed.

Stretcher Transfers

This procedure is used to move a patient from her room to another room for surgery, treatments, or diagnostic tests. Use all safety features on the stretcher, such as safety belts and side rails. These are not restraints when used during stretcher transport. Never leave a patient on a stretcher unattended.

Note: Procedure 19 is for moving an unconscious or semiconscious patient. For alert, fully awake patients, two people may be able to perform this procedure with one person against the stretcher and the other person on the opposite side of the bed. Instruct the patient how to help you.

PROCEDURE

19

OBRA

TRANSFERRING THE PATIENT FROM BED TO STRETCHER AND BACK

1. Carry out initial procedure actions.

2. Assemble equipment:
   - Stretcher
   - Bath blanket

3. You will need three to four people for transferring an unconscious or comatose patient from bed to stretcher.

4. Lock the wheels of the bed. Raise the bed to a horizontal position equal to the height of the stretcher. Lower the side rails.

5. Place a bath blanket over the patient and fanfold top covers to the foot of the bed, out of the way.

6. Roll the turning sheet up against the patient on both sides. The sheet should be long enough to

continues

PROCEDURE 19 CONTINUED

support the patient's head and shoulders during the move.

7. Position the stretcher close to the bed. Lock stretcher wheels.

8. Two or three people stand along the open side of the stretcher. The other person stands on the open side of the bed. This assistant may need to get on the bed, on her knees, to avoid overstretching her back.

Note: Use an overhand grasp on the moving sheet to avoid wrist strain. Using a friction-reducing sheet, roller, lifting pad (Figure 16-10A), or air-transfer device (Unit 32) will make this task much easier and reduce the risk of personal injury.

- The assistant at the end of the bed grasps the moving sheet by placing one hand by the patient's legs and the other hand by the patient's hips.
- The middle assistant grasps the moving sheet by placing one hand by the patient's hips and the other hand by the patient's shoulders.
- The assistant at the head of the bed grasps the turning sheet by the patient's shoulder and head.
- On the count of three, all persons slide the moving sheet from bed to stretcher (Figure 16-10B).

9. Center the patient on the stretcher in good body alignment. Secure the stretcher safety belt. Raise the side rails of the stretcher.

10. Transport the patient as directed.

11. Upon return to the unit, prepare the bed for the patient's return.

12. Carry out ending procedure actions.

Returning the Patient to Bed

13. Carry out initial procedure actions.

14. Assemble equipment:
- Stretcher
- Bath blanket (patient should already be covered with one on the stretcher)

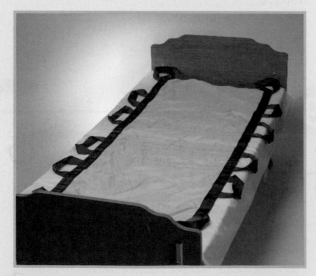

FIGURE 16-10A The surface of the lifting pad slides readily and makes the transfer easier for the staff and more comfortable for the patient. *(Courtesy of Skil-Care Corporation, Yonkers, NY, (800) 431-2972)*

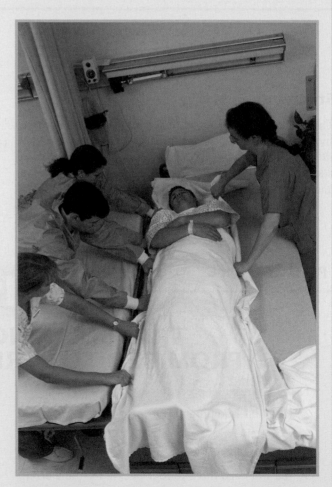

FIGURE 16-10B All persons slide the lifting sheet from bed to stretcher. *(© Delmar/Cengage Learning)*

PROCEDURE 19 CONTINUED

15. You will need three or four people to transfer an unconscious or comatose patient from stretcher to bed.

16. Lock the wheels of the bed. Raise the bed to a horizontal position equal to the height of the stretcher. Lower the side rails. Fanfold top covers to the foot of the bed, out of the way.

17. Place a bath blanket over the patient, if necessary.

18. Roll the turning sheet up against the patient on both sides. The sheet should be long enough to support the patient's head and shoulders during the move.

19. Position the stretcher close to the bed. Lock the wheels and lower the side rails.

20. One person stands along the open side of the stretcher. The other two or three people stand on the open side of the bed. These assistants may need to get on the bed, on their knees, to avoid overstretching their backs. On the count of three, all persons slide the moving sheet from stretcher to bed (Figure 16-11).

21. Center the patient on the bed in good body alignment. Position the patient properly. Raise the side rails of the bed if ordered.

22. Carry out ending procedure actions.

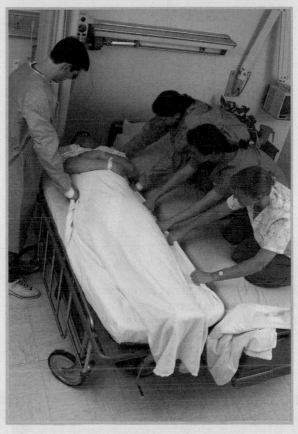

FIGURE 16-11 All persons slide the lifting sheet from stretcher to bed. (© Delmar/Cengage Learning)

Moving the Patient with a Mechanical Lift

The **mechanical lift** is used for moving heavy or dependent patients who have little or no ability to assist. Using a mechanical lift for transfers is safer for both the patient and the nursing assistant. Various types of seats are available so the patient can be moved in the sitting or supine position. Some mechanical lifts may be used to weigh bedfast patients.

Several types of mechanical lifts are available. The most common is the manual hydraulic lift. It is used when a patient is heavy, unable to assist, unbalanced, or has an amputation or other condition that makes transfer with a belt difficult or impossible. Patients are typically transferred from bed to chair. Position the chair next to the bed, facing the head or foot of the bed, according to facility policy. For safety reasons, the manual hydraulic lift should be operated by two or more nursing assistants. Never attempt to operate

Safety ALERT

Some portable lifts are wheeled to the bedside. Some operate by using a ceiling-mounted hoist (Figure 16-12). However, the manual hydraulic lift is still in widespread use. The principles of use are the same for all lifts, and showing instructions for every lift on the market is impossible. The principles of patient safety and movement given here apply to other lifts with a sling seat. Never use an electrical or mechanical lift until you have been instructed in its use and are approved to use the device. ■

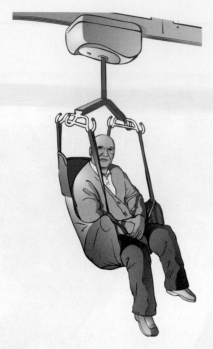

FIGURE 16-12 Some facilities permanently mount a ceiling hoist in certain rooms. These rooms are reserved for patients who are dependent for transfers, such as those with paralysis. (© *Delmar/Cengage Learning*)

it alone. Some electric and battery-operated lifts can safely be used by one person. Know and follow your facility policy for the type of lift you are using.

OSHA ALERT

Many health care facility bathrooms meet the OSHA criteria for confined spaces. Confined spaces cause nursing assistants to work in awkward positions and use forceful movements because the spaces are small, crowded, or have obstructions. Moving a patient in a confined space increases your risk of injury. You may need to use a creative method of doing toilet transfers, such as using a ceiling-mounted lift or by transferring the patient to a shower chair outside the bathroom, then wheeling the chair in and positioning it over the toilet. Two or more workers will probably be necessary for this procedure. ■

PROCEDURE

 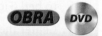

20

TRANSFERRING THE PATIENT WITH A MECHANICAL LIFT

This procedure is used for heavy patients who have little or no weight-bearing ability.

📝 **Note:** Check slings, chains, and straps for frayed areas or clasps that do not close properly. Check the hydraulic lift and the leg spreader to make sure they are both working. Do not use if there is oil on the floor or if equipment is defective. Report the need for repair and obtain safe equipment.

1. Carry out initial procedure actions.

2. Assemble equipment:
   - Mechanical lift
   - Chains, straps, and support bars for the sling
   - Sling
   - Chair

3. Place a wheelchair or other chair with arms parallel to the foot of the bed, facing the head or foot of the bed. Lock the wheelchair.

4. Elevate the bed to a comfortable working height. Lock the bed wheels. Lower the nearest side rail. Roll the patient toward you.

5. Position the sling beneath the patient's body behind shoulder, thighs, and buttocks. Be sure the sling is smooth (Figure 16-13A).

6. Roll the patient back onto the sling and position properly (Figure 16-13B). If the sling has inserts for metal bars, insert them now.

7. Position the lift frame over the bed with base legs in the maximum open position, and lock the lift legs (Figure 16-13C).

8. Attach suspension straps or chains to the sling (Figure 16-13D). Check fasteners for security.

📝 **Note:** Be sure that the correct end of the strap or chain is hooked to the correct place on the sling. Always hook straps or chains from inside to

PROCEDURE **20** CONTINUED

outside so the open part of the hook faces away from the patient.

9. Position the patient's crossed arms inside the straps.

10. Secure straps or chains if necessary.

11. One assistant operates the lift and the other assistant guides the movement of the patient. Lock the hydraulic mechanism, and slowly raise the boom of the lift until the patient is suspended over the bed. Talk to the patient while slowly lifting him free of the bed.

12. Guide the lift away from the bed.

13. Position the patient and lift over the chair or wheelchair (Figure 16-13E). Make sure that the wheels of the wheelchair are locked.

14. Slowly lower the patient into the chair or wheelchair. Pay attention to the position of the

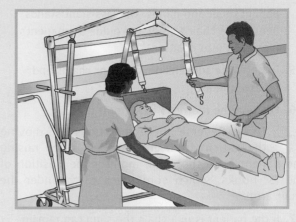

FIGURE 16-13C Position the lift frame over the bed. *(© Delmar/Cengage Learning)*

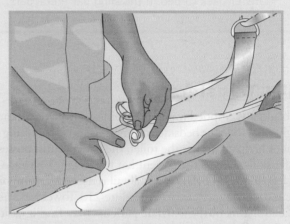

FIGURE 16-13D Attach the straps or chains to the sling. *(© Delmar/Cengage Learning)*

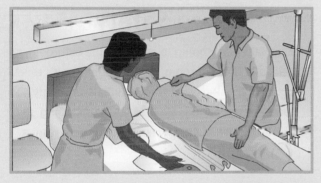

FIGURE 16-13A Position the sling under the patient. *(© Delmar/Cengage Learning)*

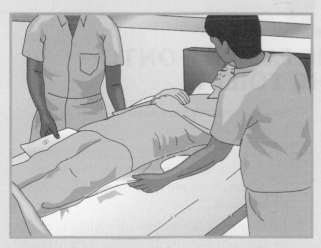

FIGURE 16-13B Roll the patient back onto the sling. *(© Delmar/Cengage Learning)*

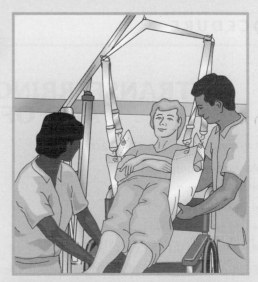

FIGURE 16-13E Position the lift frame over the chair. *(© Delmar/Cengage Learning)*

continues

PROCEDURE 20 CONTINUED

patient's feet and hands. One assistant stands behind the chair to pull and guide the patient's hips back into position.

15. Unhook the suspension straps or chains and remove the lift.

16. Position the footrests to support the feet.

Note: Reverse these directions for moving the patient from chair to bed. When raising the patient from the chair, monitor the position of the "S" hooks, which sometimes catch under the chair arms.

17. If the patient is in a chair, the sling can remain underneath the patient so it is in position for transfer back to bed. If the sling has metal bars,

remove them and make sure the sling is smooth and wrinkle-free. Make sure the signal light is within reach.

18. Remove the sling after the patient has returned to bed. Position the patient and pull the top covers up. Raise both side rails if necessary. Make sure the signal light is within reach.

Note: The method for raising and lowering the lift and for moving the base legs varies for different types of equipment. Read the manufacturer's directions and practice using equipment before using it with patients.

19. Carry out ending procedure actions.

Toilet Transfers

The bladder is emptied much more efficiently if patients are upright on a toilet or bedside commode, rather than using a urinal or bedpan. To use the toilet, the patient must possess transfer skills. Unless the patient has full weight-bearing on both legs and good balance, a wall rail is needed for support while transferring. (Refer to Procedure 21.) Towel racks are not safe for this purpose. Male patients may find it easier and safer to sit rather than stand while urinating.

Safety ALERT

Many falls occur going to and from the bathroom, as well as in the bathroom. Assist patients with toileting regularly. Respond to call signals promptly. Do not leave the patient alone if you think doing so is unsafe. Follow facility policies and the care plan. ■

PROCEDURE

21

TRANSFERRING THE PATIENT ONTO AND OFF THE TOILET

OBRA

1. Carry out initial procedure actions.

2. Assemble equipment:
   - Toilet tissue
   - Transfer belt
   - Disposable gloves
   - Commode if toilet is not available

3. Position the wheelchair at a right angle to the toilet or commode, facing the wall rail. Position the large part of the front caster wheels facing

forward, and lock the wheels. Raise or remove footrests.

4. Place a transfer belt around the patient's waist. Use an underhand grasp with one hand toward the patient's back and the other hand toward the patient's front.

5. Tell the patient to lean forward slightly, to place the strongest foot slightly behind the other foot, to bring herself to a standing position by pushing

PROCEDURE 21 CONTINUED

off from the wheelchair, and to grasp the wall rail with both hands (Figure 16-14A).

6. Have the patient pivot or step around until she feels the toilet against the back of her legs.

7. Slide the pants and underwear down over the patient's knees. You may need to keep one hand on the transfer belt and use the other hand to manipulate the patient's clothing (Figure 16-14B).

8. Assist the patient to a sitting position on the toilet and allow her time to eliminate.

9. When the patient is finished, put on the disposable gloves. Instruct the patient to stand and to reach for the wall rail. Use the toilet tissue to clean the patient if she was unable to do this herself. If the patient is steady, remove and

dispose of your gloves. Then pull the patient's pants or underwear up.

10. If the sink is close enough, the patient can pivot or step to the sink to wash her hands before sitting down in the wheelchair. Otherwise, help her to sit in the wheelchair; then unlock the wheelchair, replace the footrests, and move the wheelchair to the sink so this step can be completed while the patient is seated.

11. Wash your hands.

12. Assist the patient to leave the bathroom. Make sure she is comfortable and has a signal light within reach.

13. Carry out ending procedure actions.

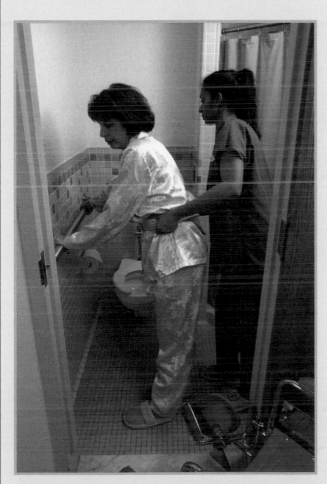

FIGURE 16-14A Tell the patient to grasp the wall rail with both hands. (© *Delmar/Cengage Learning*)

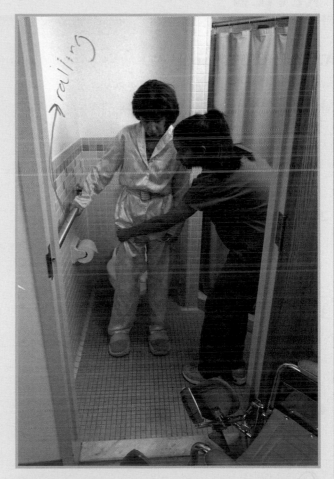

FIGURE 16-14B Keep one hand on the transfer belt and adjust the patient's clothing. (© *Delmar/Cengage Learning*)

Tub Transfers

In the institutional setting, a shower with chair or tub with hydraulic lift is available. If the patient is at home, a tub chair, rail on the wall beside the tub, and slip-proof mats in the tub are needed for safety. Add water to the tub after the patient has safely transferred, with cold water turned on first and off last. A hand-held shower attached to the faucet is safer and easier for self-bathing.

Car Transfers

You may need to assist a patient to transfer into a car when he is discharged from the facility. If you are working in the patient's home, you may need to help the patient into and out of the car. A two-door car makes the transfer easier because the door is wider and more room is available for moving into and out of the car. The patient should always transfer onto the front seat. The front door is usually wider and opens wider.

Safety ALERT

Transfers into and out of vehicles are high-risk tasks, especially if the person is very weak, confused, or acutely ill. Another concern is having to transfer a patient with one-sided weakness or paralysis toward the weaker side. (For most transfers, the stronger side is the leading side.) Make sure you have enough help and supplies, such as a transfer belt, friction-reducing sheet, or other special items, before transferring the patient. ■

REVIEW

A. Multiple Choice

Select the one best answer for each of the following.

1. The method used for transferring a patient depends on
   a. the availability of two nursing assistants.
   b. the patient's personal preference.
   c. the patient's size, strength, and balance.
   d. where the patient is going.

2. A transfer belt should never be used on patients who
   a. have had hip surgery.
   b. have a colostomy.
   c. can stand on their feet.
   d. have an IV or catheter.

3. During a transfer, the patient should never
   a. be allowed to help in the move.
   b. place his hands on your body.
   c. wear shoes.
   d. be allowed to stand.

4. When transferring a patient, you should never place your hands under a patient's arms because the
   a. patient may not want you to stand so close.
   b. patient cannot see where she is going.
   c. patient's joints are fragile.
   d. patient may be ticklish.

5. Using a manual mechanical lift requires that
   a. two or more persons do the procedure.
   b. the patient be able to assist in the move.

   c. the patient be mentally alert.
   d. the patient weigh at least 300 pounds.

6. When transferring a patient from bed to a wheelchair,
   a. the small front caster wheels should be facing sideways.
   b. the large part of the front wheels should face forward.
   c. the drive wheels should face forward.
   d. the drive wheels should be engaged.

7. Before transferring a patient to a wheelchair for the first time,
   a. test the patient's ability to help and follow directions.
   b. ask the patient if she wants you to use a transfer belt.
   c. unlock the wheels of the bed and wheelchair.
   d. clamp or remove all tubing to prevent traction.

8. The patient's left leg is weak, so the nursing assistant will
   a. use his left knee to brace the patient's right leg.
   b. make sure the patient is wearing slippers.
   c. use his right knee to support the patient's left leg.
   d. ask the nurse for further instructions.

9. When using the hydraulic mechanical lift, the open end of the "S" hooks should face
   a. inward.
   b. outward.

c. the patient.

d. the nursing assistant.

10. When a patient is on a stretcher,

    a. the side rails and belts are considered restraints.

    b. apply a vest restraint for extra security.

    c. the safety belt and rails are not restraints.

    d. push the stretcher from the foot end.

B. Nursing Assistant Challenge

You are assigned to Mrs. McNeely, who is scheduled for surgery. She is alert and able to follow your directions. You know that when she returns from surgery she will be semiconscious from the medications and anesthesia. Consider the differences in procedures when she goes to surgery and when she returns to her room.

11. What instructions will you give Mrs. McNeely when she transfers from her bed to the surgical stretcher?

12. What will you need to do to transfer her back to bed after the surgery?

UNIT 17

The Patient's Mobility: Ambulation

OBJECTIVES

After completing this unit, you will be able to:
- Spell and define terms.
- State the purpose of assistive devices used in ambulation.
- List safety measures for using assistive devices.
- Describe safety measures for using a wheelchair.
- Describe nursing assistant actions for:
    - Ambulating a patient using a gait belt.
    - Propelling a patient in a wheelchair.

- Positioning a patient in a wheelchair.
- Transporting a patient on a stretcher.
- Demonstrate the following procedures:
    - Procedure 22 Assisting the Patient to Walk with a Cane and Two-Point Gait
    - Procedure 23 Assisting the Patient to Walk with a Walker and Three-Point Gait
    - Procedure 24 Assisting the Falling Patient

VOCABULARY

Learn the meaning and the correct spelling of the following words and phrases:

ambulate	assistive device	gait	gait training

AMBULATION

The term **ambulate** means to walk. Patients who cannot walk may be able to self-propel their wheelchairs to increase their independence.

The term **gait** refers to the way in which a person walks. Many disorders can affect a person's gait.

Evaluation for Ambulation

Before initiating an ambulation program, the nurse or physical therapist (Figure 17-1) will evaluate the patient's safety awareness, ability to move in bed, transfer, and ambulate. He or she will develop a mobility and/or therapy plan based on this information.

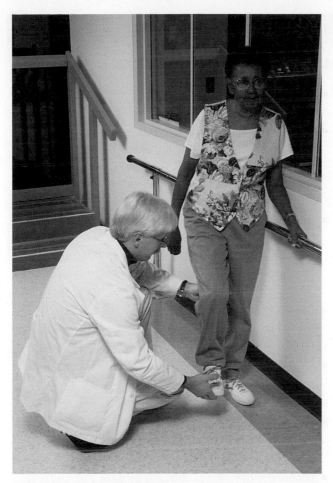

FIGURE 17-1 The physical therapist evaluates the patient's ability to ambulate and need for assistive devices. (© Delmar/Cengage Learning)

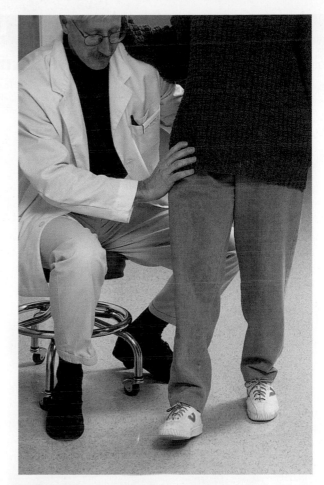

FIGURE 17-2 Walking begins with the ankle in dorsiflexion and the heel striking the floor first. (© Delmar/Cengage Learning)

Normal Gait Pattern

There are two phases to a normal gait (walking). The leg is on the floor during the first phase and the leg is brought forward during the second phase. Walking begins with the ankle in *dorsiflexion* (toes pulled toward shin) and the heel striking the floor first (Figure 17-2), then rolling onto the ball of the foot. The person must be able to stand on this leg while bringing the other leg forward. Each arm swings slightly in the same direction as the opposite leg. To walk safely, the person must have good strength and joint motion in the hips and knees. A physical therapist may work with a patient before the patient starts walking.

Gait Training

The physical therapist may work with a patient on **gait training** (teaching the patient to walk). The therapist

also teaches the staff measures to assist the patient and special safety precautions to follow during nursing care, if needed.

ASSISTIVE DEVICES

An **assistive device** is often prescribed to aid persons who have problems with walking. The device is selected according to the person's needs and the cause of the problem. A walker or crutches are usually ordered if a person has partial weight-bearing on one leg. Canes are ordered for persons who have balance problems. The nurse or physical therapist will adjust the device to fit the patient. The gait is selected by the therapist and depends on the cause of the problem, the patient's abilities, and the type of device being used. Help the patient use the device correctly during ambulation.

GUIDELINES *for*

Safe Ambulation

- Encourage patients to use the hand rail when walking.
- Always stand on the patient's affected (weak) side when walking.
- Use a gait belt if the person needs assistance with ambulation. Grasp the center back of the belt with an underhand grip (Figure 17-3).
- Be sure the shoes are appropriate to the floor surface and clothing is not dragging on the floor.

- Check the floor for clutter or puddles that could cause a fall.
- If you are unsure of the patient's endurance or balance, ask another nursing assistant to follow behind you with a wheelchair. If the patient becomes weak, dizzy, or tired, he or she can sit in the wheelchair.
- Check rubber handgrips and tips on bottoms of canes, crutches, and walkers. Replace if they are cracked, loose, or worn down. If the ridges are filled with debris, use alcohol and cotton swabs to clean them.
- Check screws, nuts, and bolts on assistive devices for tightness. Do not use any device that appears unsafe. Report the problem to the proper person.
- Practice good body mechanics for both yourself and the patient.
- Teach the patient to practice safety.
- Position your body so it moves with the patient's body. Match the patient's stride and avoid interfering with the patient's movement.
- Encourage the patient to stand upright and erect when walking.
- Encourage the patient to take large, even steps while maintaining a wide base of support. The distance between the feet should be equal to the patient's shoulder width.
- Allow adequate time for ambulation. Avoid making the patient feel rushed.
- Allow the patient time to rest, if necessary.
- Provide only the amount of assistance needed.
- Stop ambulation immediately if the patient shows signs of illness, pain, extreme fatigue, shortness of breath, dizziness, sweating, or anxiety. Notify the nurse.
- Never leave a patient standing unattended. Assist the patient to a chair when finished.

Before leaving, quickly check the room for safety, such as items on the floor. Place the call signal and needed personal items within the patient's reach and remind her to call for help, if needed.

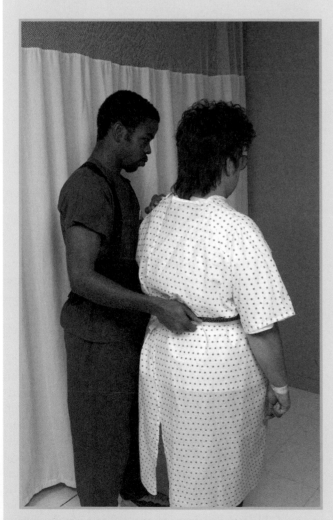

FIGURE 17-3 Hold the gait belt in back, using an underhand grip. (© *Delmar/Cengage Learning*)

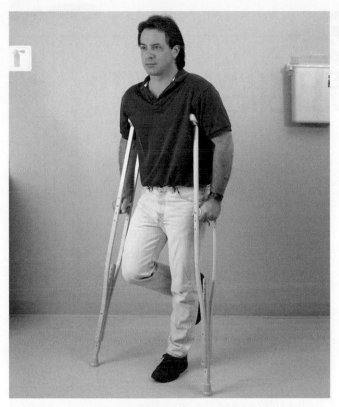

FIGURE 17-4 Standard crutches are usually not appropriate for older patients. *(© Delmar/Cengage Learning)*

Use of Crutches

Standard crutches (Figure 17-4) require good balance and two strong arms. They are seldom recommended for older adults. Metal forearm crutches may be used by persons who have weakness of both legs. The cuff of the crutch encloses the forearm so the patient can release that hand without dropping the crutch (Figure 17-5).

Use of Canes

Several types of canes are available to meet patients' balance needs:

- Quad canes and tripod canes provide a wide base of support.

Safety ALERT

You may observe a patient using an ambulation device incorrectly. For example, the patient may hold the walker when standing, or carry the walker during ambulation. Assistive devices are used for ambulation. Using them for any other purposes may be unsafe. Inform the nurse, who will determine the best way of meeting the patient's mobility needs. ■

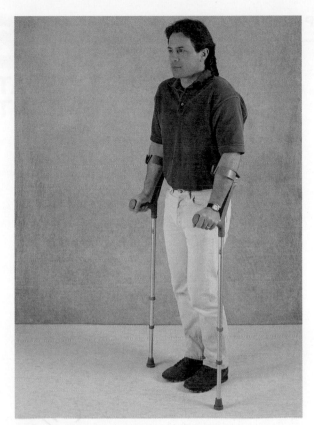

FIGURE 17-5 Forearm crutches can be released to free the hand without dropping the crutch. *(© Delmar/Cengage Learning)*

- Four-pronged pyramid canes have a broad base, and are narrower at the top.
- Single-prong canes with T-handles or J-handles have straight handles and are easier to hold than half-circle handled canes.

For proper fit, the wrist must be even with the hip joint, with the elbow flexed 30°. Remind the patient to hold the

Safety ALERT

The procedures in this chapter assume that the facility has a tile or linoleum floor. You are instructed to apply nonslip footwear to the patient. If your facility is carpeted, shoes with a leather, synthetic, or plastic bottom may be more appropriate. Nonslip soles tend to stick to carpeting, and may cause a weak or uncoordinated patient to stumble. The therapist may slice tennis balls and cap the rear wheels of a wheeled walker to make it easier for the patient to walk on carpeting. As you can see, this is an area where individual, assessment-based care is very important!. ■

PROCEDURE

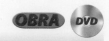

22

ASSISTING THE PATIENT TO WALK WITH A CANE AND TWO-POINT GAIT

1. Carry out initial procedure actions.

2. Assemble equipment:
   - Cane as ordered
   - Gait belt

3. Make sure the patient has on sturdy shoes with nonslip soles. Check clothing to be sure it does not hang down over shoes.

4. Place the bed in the lowest horizontal position, with brakes locked. Assist the patient to sit on the edge of the bed. Place a gait belt on the patient and assist the patient to a standing position. Stand on the patient's affected side. Place your closest hand in the gait belt, using an underhand grip.

5. Instruct the patient to hold the cane on the stronger side, with the tip about 4 inches to the side of the stronger foot. The patient's weight should be distributed evenly between her feet and the cane (Figure 17-6).

6. Tell the patient to move the cane and weaker leg forward at the same time, while her weight is on the stronger leg (Figure 17-7).

7. Instruct the patient to shift her weight to the weak leg and cane, then move the stronger leg forward.

8. Repeat this pattern while the patient is walking.

9. Note the patient's endurance, balance, and strength while walking. Stop immediately if the patient has trouble and help her to the closest chair. Call the nurse.

10. Assist the patient to sit in the chair or to lie down in bed. Remove the gait belt. Store the cane in an appropriate area.

11. Document the distance the patient ambulated and her tolerance of the procedure.

12. Carry out ending procedure actions.

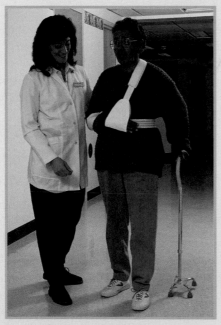

FIGURE 17-6 The patient holds the cane on the strong side of the body. The patient's weight should be distributed evenly between her feet and the cane before she starts to walk. (© Delmar/Cengage Learning)

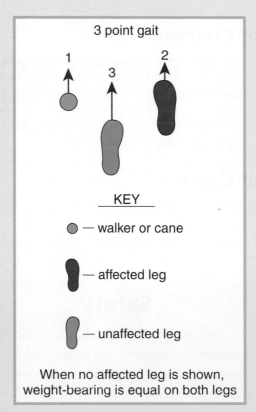

FIGURE 17-7 Three-point gait. (© Delmar/Cengage Learning)

cane on the *strong* side of the body. The therapist will develop a plan for safe ambulation.

Use of Walkers

Walkers are recommended for persons who have weakness of both legs, partial weight-bearing on one leg, or mild balance problems. The patient needs strength in both arms to pick up the walker. Various widths are available. The walker should be wide enough to allow the person to walk into it. With a proper fit, the elbows are flexed 30° when the hands are on the handgrips, and the top of the walker reaches the hip joint. Most walkers are adjustable. The nurse or physical therapist will make any necessary changes. Walkers are available with a variety of features to meet patient needs.

PROCEDURE

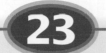

ASSISTING THE PATIENT TO WALK WITH A WALKER AND THREE-POINT GAIT

1. Carry out beginning procedure actions.

2. Assemble equipment:
   - Walker as ordered
   - Gait belt

3. Make sure the patient has on sturdy shoes with nonslip soles. Check clothing to be sure it does not hang down over shoes.

4. Place a gait belt on the patient and assist her to a standing position. Place the walker in front of the patient and have her grasp the walker with both hands. Stand on the patient's affected (weak) side. Place your closest hand in the center back of the gait belt, using an underhand grip (Figure 17-8).

   Note: The walker is not a transfer device and should not be used to help the patient stand up. The patient grasps the walker *after* standing. To sit, the patient releases the grip on the walker while still standing, and then places his or her hands on the arms of the chair before sitting.

5. Instruct the patient to stand with her weight evenly distributed between the walker and both legs, with the walker in front of her.

6. Have the patient shift her weight to the strong leg as she lifts and moves the walker 6 to 8 inches ahead. All four legs of the walker should strike the floor at the same time.

7. Instruct the patient to bring her weak foot forward into the walker.

8. Now have her bring her strong foot forward even with the weak foot.

9. Repeat this process while the patient is walking.

10. Note the patient's endurance, balance, and strength while walking. Stop immediately if the

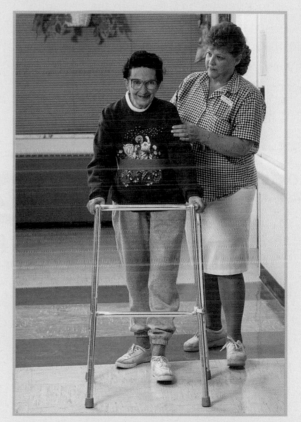

FIGURE 17-8 Stand on the patient's affected side while she grasps the walker with both hands. *(© Delmar/Cengage Learning)*

patient has trouble and help her to the closest chair. Call the nurse.

11. Upon completion of the activity, assist the patient to sit in the chair or to lie down in bed. Remove the gait belt. Store the walker in an appropriate area.

12. Document the distance the patient ambulated and her tolerance of the procedure.

13. Carry out ending procedure actions.

THE FALLING PATIENT

If a patient starts to fall during ambulation, do not try to hold her upright. This will strain your back and may injure the patient. *If a patient does fall, call the nurse to assess the patient for injuries before she is moved.*

Safety ALERT

If you find a patient on the floor, remain in the room and call for help. Leave the patient on the floor. Provide any emergency measures that you are qualified to provide. If the nurse suspects a fracture, she will instruct you on how to return the person to bed. Rolling the patient onto a sheet or blanket will make the transfer less traumatic. After emergency treatment and positioning on a lifting sheet or other device, the patient is lifted back to bed. ∎

WHEELCHAIR MOBILITY

The wheelchair is an essential item in the health care facility. Many patients use wheelchairs for mobility. Some will progress to ambulation. Others will always use the wheelchair to move about. Whenever possible, the facility will restore the patient's ability to ambulate. Because patients spend so much time in wheelchairs, it is important to pay careful attention to fitting the chair to the patient; the chair fit affects comfort, safety, good body mechanics, ease of mobility, pressure ulcer prevention, and restraint elimination. Sometimes wheelchairs are ordered or modified to meet special patient needs. For example, some patients with paralysis on one side of the body can propel the wheelchair by removing one leg rest and using the strong arm on the wheel and pushing the strong leg on the floor. Other adaptations may be needed to enable a patient to be independent when using a wheelchair for ambulation.

The wheelchair is a mobility device, not a transportation device. Propelling the wheelchair is good exercise. Having the ability to move about independently enhances confidence, facilitates communication, and provides opportunities for

PROCEDURE

24

ASSISTING THE FALLING PATIENT

1. Keep your back straight, bend from the hips and knees, and maintain a broad base of support as you assist the falling patient. Maintain your grasp on the transfer belt.

2. Ease the patient to the floor, protecting her head.

3. As you ease the patient to the floor, bend your knees and go down with the patient (Figure 17-9).

4. Call for help, and follow the nurse's instructions.

5. Assist in returning the patient to bed or chair.

6. Carry out ending procedure actions.

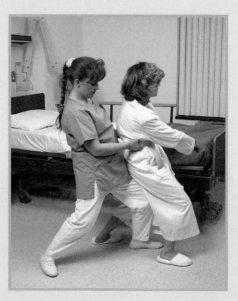

FIGURE 17-9 Ease the falling patient to the floor; bend your knees and go down with the patient. (© Delmar/ Cengage Learning)

the need for restraints, positioning aids, and body supports. The chair will be more comfortable, and reduce the risk of skin breakdown. If the chair fits correctly, there will be:

- About 4 inches between the top of the back and the patient's axillae (armpits).
- Armrests that support the arms without pushing the shoulders up or forcing them to hang.
- Two to three inches clearance between the front edge of the seat and the back of the patient's knee.
- Enough space between the patient's torso and the chair to slide your hand between the patient's hips on each side and the side of the wheelchair.
- Two inches between the bottom of the footrests and the floor.
- 90° angles between the feet and the legs, whether they are on the footrests or on the floor (when the footrests have been removed).

If the wheelchair does not fit the patient, check with the nurse or physical therapist to see how you can use pads or other devices to adapt the chair to the patient.

patients to make choices and decisions. A facility emphasis on efficiency may prevent patients from benefiting from wheelchair independence. Pushing the wheelchairs is faster and more productive for staff. Some patients cannot propel their wheelchairs because the chair does not fit correctly. The therapy and restorative nursing departments will work with patients to fit their chairs correctly, make special adaptations if needed, and teach patients to move the wheelchair independently. Assist and encourage patients with independence whenever possible.

Wheelchair Size and Fit

A wheelchair should fit the person who is using it. Correct fit and body alignment (Figure 17-10) will reduce

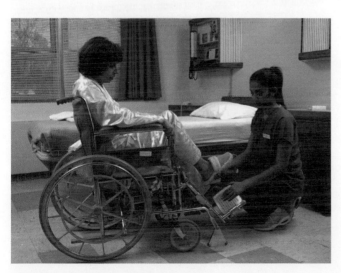

FIGURE 17-10 The wheelchair must fit the patient. *(© Delmar/Cengage Learning)*

GUIDELINES *for*

Wheelchair and Stretcher Safety

- Check the wheelchair or stretcher to see that the brakes are working and wheels are securely attached. If the patient needs footrests, make sure they are in place.

- The small, front caster wheels of the wheelchair provide the ability to move in all directions. The large part of the wheel faces back when the chair is moving. When the chair is parked, the large part of the front wheel should face forward and the brakes should be locked. This changes the center of gravity in the chair, making it more stable and reducing the risk of tipping.

- Position the patient in the 90–90–90 position in a wheelchair, with the feet supported and the knees lower than the hips. Use pillows or props, if needed to enable the patient to sit upright.

- Lock the brakes and lift footrests out of the way when the patient is getting in or out of the wheelchair.

- Instruct the patient not to try to pick up an object off the floor.

- Cover the patient with clothing or a bath blanket for dignity and modesty during transport in the hallways.

- Prevent bath blankets, lap robes, or clothing from getting caught in wheels.

- Guide the wheelchair from behind, grasping both handgrips (Figure 17-11). Guide a stretcher from the head end.

- Approach corners slowly and look before going around them.

- Take care when approaching swinging doors. Prop the door open to enter. If this is not possible, back through swinging doors.

- Back the wheelchair and stretcher over the threshold in doorways and elevators (Figure 17-12).

- When leaving an elevator, push the stop button and ask others to step out. Turn the wheelchair around and back it out the door. Push a stretcher from the head so the feet exit first. If the threshold is uneven, go to the foot end and pull the stretcher out of the elevator.

- Walk backward and slowly pull the wheelchair or stretcher when moving down a ramp or incline. Periodically look over your shoulder, as you would when backing up a car, to make sure that the path is clear.

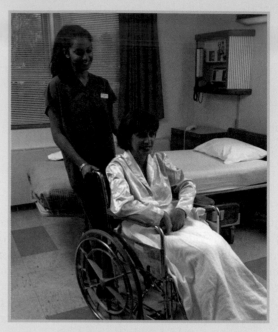

FIGURE 17-11 Guide the wheelchair from behind, grasping both hand grips. (© *Delmar/Cengage Learning*)

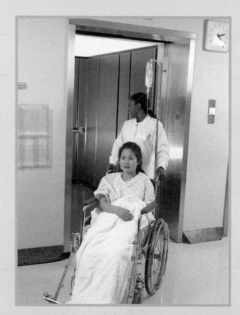

FIGURE 17-12 Always back over the threshold when entering doorways and elevators. (*Stock image*)

- When parking a wheelchair or stretcher, avoid blocking a doorway. Apply the brakes.

- Use all safety belts and side rails when transporting a patient by stretcher. Never leave the patient unattended on a stretcher.

POSITIONING A DEPENDENT PATIENT IN A CHAIR OR WHEELCHAIR

Position patients in the 90–90–90 position in the chair or wheelchair. Follow the care plan and provide props to support the person's body, if needed. The dependent person may slide down in the wheelchair, requiring assistance to regain good alignment. Monitor the patient's body alignment periodically while he is in the wheelchair and assist with repositioning when necessary. Lock the drive wheels and position the caster wheels in the forward position before repositioning the patient.

Several procedures can be used to correct the dependent patient's position:

1. Stand in front of the patient; make sure that the feet are in alignment and the arms are on the armrests. Help the patient lean forward and push with the hands and legs as you push against the patient's knees (Figure 17-13).

2. For an alternate method, place a soft towel or small sheet under the patient's buttocks and use this as a pull sheet to move the patient up in the chair. This requires two people (Figure 17-14).

3. Another method involves using a manual lifting device, such as the TLC pad (Figure 17-15). The number of persons needed to lift is determined by patient

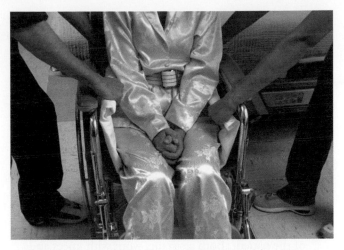

FIGURE 17-14 A draw sheet or lifting pad may be used to correct the patient's body alignment. *(© Delmar/Cengage Learning)*

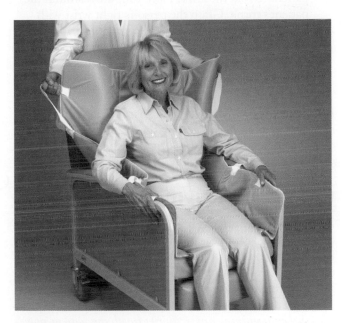

FIGURE 17-15 One worker can move a small or average-size patient up in the geriatric chair by pulling the handles of the TLC pad up and out. If you are unsure about your ability to move the patient, always have help on standby. It is better to ask for help than to injure your back. *(Courtesy of Skil-Care Corporation, Yonkers, NY, (800) 431–2972)*

size, medical (physical) need, and the device you are using. One person may be able to move an average-size patient by using the TLC pad. Do not substitute a sheet for a manual lifting pad. The handles are necessary to coordinate the move and pull the patient safely. If the patient is uncooperative or heavy, two or more caregivers will be necessary. The TLC pad may also be used to turn a patient to the side or pull her up in bed. The pad is left in place when the patient is in a chair. You may use your discretion as to whether it is left in place when the patient is in bed. The pad is soft

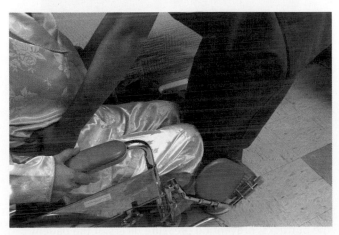

FIGURE 17-13 Push against the patient's knees as she pushes with her hands and legs. *(© Delmar/Cengage Learning)*

and will not injure the skin, and the fabric is quite absorbent and washable in the event of incontinence.

4. This method also requires two people. Place the transfer belt around the patient's waist. One assistant stands in back of the wheelchair and grasps the transfer belt with one hand on each side of the patient. The other assistant stands in front of the patient and places her hands and arms under the patient's knees. On the count of three, this assistant supports the lower extremities while the other one moves the patient back in the chair (Figure 17-16). This is not recommended for a heavy patient.

5. This method also requires two people. Stand in back of the wheelchair and have another assistant in front of the patient. Both assistants work with knees and hips bent and backs straight. Lean forward with your head over the patient's shoulder. Instruct the patient to fold the arms. Place your arms around the patient's trunk. Grasp the person's right wrist with your left hand and grasp the left wrist with your right hand. The other assistant encircles the patient's knees with hands and arms. On the count of three, both assistants lift and move the person back (Figure 17-17).

If the patient can bear weight, assist the patient to stand and then sit back down, getting the hips to the back of the chair. Wedge cushions placed in the wheelchair will prevent the patient from thrusting and sliding forward.

Wheelchair Activity

Pressure on the buttocks is greatly increased when the patient is sitting. Patients can and do develop pressure ulcers from sitting in chairs. Teach the patient (and provide assistance if necessary) to periodically relieve the pressure by shifting weight every 15 minutes. *Be sure the wheelchair brakes are locked, with the caster wheels in the forward position, before beginning any activities involving patient movement in the chair.*

Pressure Relief

Patients can be taught to use "wheelchair pushups" to relieve pressure when sitting in a wheelchair for long periods of time. To do wheelchair pushups:

- Position the caster wheels correctly, with brakes locked. If possible, position the patient's feet on the floor rather than the footrests.
- Teach the patient to place one hand on each armrest, keeping both elbows bent.
- Have the person lean forward slightly, pushing on the armrests and straightening the elbows while lifting the buttocks off the seat. Instruct the person to hold this position to the count of five, if possible (Figure 17-18).

If the person cannot do push-ups, have her place the hands on the armrests or thighs and lean forward slightly. Teach her to lean to each side to relieve pressure on the buttocks.

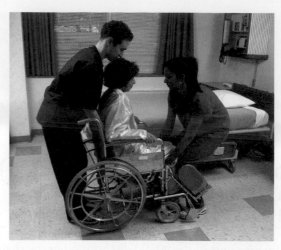

FIGURE 17-16 One assistant supports the lower extremities while the other uses the transfer belt to move the patient back in the chair. (© *Delmar/Cengage Learning*)

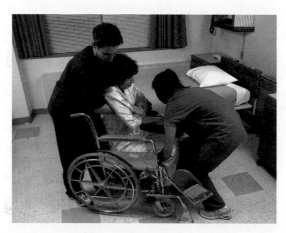

FIGURE 17-17 One assistant encircles the patient's legs with her hands and arms. (© *Delmar/Cengage Learning*)

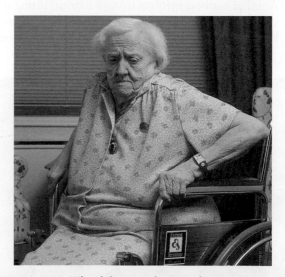

FIGURE 17-18 Wheelchair push-ups relieve pressure on the buttocks, preventing pressure ulcers. If the patient cannot lift up enough to relieve the pressure every 15 minutes, the care plan will list instructions and times for staff to move the patient to alleviate pressure. (© *Delmar/Cengage Learning*)

GUIDELINES *for*
Chair and Wheelchair Positioning

- The patient's head should be upright and erect (or supported), and facing forward.

- If the patient leans to the side, make sure the chair fits correctly. Provide support with pillows, foam, or other props to support the patient upright.

- Position the arms on the armrests if this does not push the shoulders up. If the shoulders are elevated, adding a seat cushion will boost the patient, preventing shoulder strain.

- If the patient's shoulders are hanging, support the arms on pillows, foam, or other props.

- Position the hands on the armrests, or folded over the patient's lap. Place a small pillow for support and comfort, if needed.

- The upper back of the wheelchair should be at the bottom of the shoulder blades.

- Place a folded bath blanket, bed protector, or cloth-covered cushion in the seat of the chair if the patient is wearing a hospital gown.

- Use a pressure-relieving pad in the seat if the person will up for a long time.

  - The sling seat of a wheelchair tends to hammock (sag) in the center when a patient sits on it. The sagging causes rotation of the inner thighs, which increases pressure on the coccyx and buttocks, two common sites of pressure ulcers.

  - Hammocking of the seat promotes sliding; the leveling pad at the bottom of many cushions corrects the sagging, distributing weight more evenly and reducing pressure. Never use a leveling pad alone; it should always be enclosed in a cushion.

  - Although foam is comfortable and reduces pressure, it also traps heat, which increases the potential for skin damage. Using a cushion with a gel layer on top will provide a cooling effect for the skin (Figure 17-19).

  - The gel moves with the patient, reducing friction and shearing.

- Position the hips near the back of the chair at a 90° angle.

- The patient's hips should be near the back of the chair. The front of the seat should end 2 to 3 inches before the back of the knees. A short seat is

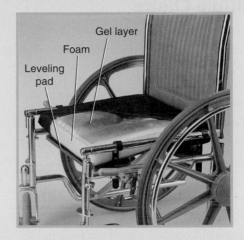

FIGURE 17-19 A pressure-relieving gel and foam pad is very comfortable and is important for preventing breakdown and maintaining skin integrity. *(Courtesy of Skil-Care Corporation, Yonkers, NY, (800) 431–2972)*

uncomfortable for tall patients. If the seat is too long, the weight of the torso shifts toward the sacrum. This is painful and increases the risk of skin breakdown. A long seat will also make it difficult for the patient to propel the chair. He or she will slide forward to the front edge of the chair.

  - Check the depth of the chair if the person's hips slide forward. If the depth is correct, consult the nurse about use of postural supports, a wedge cushion, or restraint alternatives. A gripper or wedge cushion (Unit 15) may be placed on the seat to keep the patient from sliding.

- Avoid pressure on the backs of the knees by ensuring there is at least 2 inches between the backs of the knees and the seat of the chair.

- Support the patient's weight with the legs and buttocks. Distribute weight equally on both sides.

- When positioning the male patient, make sure the scrotum is in front of the body, not underneath the patient.

- Support the feet on the floor or the footrests. If the person's legs dangle:

  - Elevate the feet on a stool when the chair is parked.

  - Use a commercial foot elevator.

  - See if the leg rests can be shortened to fit.

REVIEW

A. Multiple Choice

Select the one best answer for each of the following.

1. When ambulating a patient who has a weak right side, you should stand

   stand on weak side

   a. in back of the patient.
   b. on the patient's right side.
   c. on the patient's left side.
   d. in front of the patient.

2. When ambulating a patient, you should hold the gait belt with

   a. an overhand grasp in back of the patient.
   b. an underhand grasp in back of the patient.
   c. one hand on each side of the patient.
   d. one hand in front of the patient.

3. Before helping a patient to walk with a cane or walker, you should check the

   a. distance between the patient's feet.
   b. screws and bolts for tightness.
   c. height of the walker.
   d. length of each step.

4. The cane is always held

   a. on the patient's weaker side.
   b. on the patient's stronger side.   *stronger side*
   c. in the dominant hand.
   d. in the nondominant hand.

5. When using a two-point gait with a cane, the patient will

   weaker cane stronger

   a. place the strong foot forward, then the cane, then the weaker foot.
   b. place the strong foot and cane forward at the same time and then the weaker foot.
   c. place the weaker foot and cane forward at the same time and then the stronger foot.
   d. place the weaker foot forward, then the stronger foot, and then the cane.

6. If a patient starts to fall, you should

   a. try to hold the patient upright to prevent the fall.
   b. let go of the patient immediately, to avoid back strain.
   c. ease the patient to the floor.
   d. leave the patient and go for help.

7. When using a walker, the walker is set down so that

   a. the front legs strike the floor first and then the back legs.
   b. the back legs strike the floor first and then the front legs.
   c. all four legs strike the floor at the same time.
   d. how the walker is set down depends on the patient's problem.

8. When transporting a patient in a wheelchair, always

   a. stay to the right in corridors.
   b. guide the wheelchair from the front going down ramps.
   c. push the patient into an elevator frontwards.
   d. position the patient's feet at a 45° angle.

9. When a patient is using a wheelchair,

   a. position him in the 90–90–90 position.
   b. keep the small front caster wheels turned sideways.
   c. apply a leveling pad covered with a blanket.
   d. reposition the patient every 4 hours.

10. Assistive devices are usually selected by the

    a. nursing assistant.
    b. physician.
    c. physical therapist.
    d. patient's family.

B. Nursing Assistant Challenge

Mr. Santozi is 76 years old and has had right hip surgery. His physician does not want him to bear full weight on the affected leg. He uses a walker to assist his ambulation. When you help him out of bed, he reaches for the walker to help pull himself up from the bed. As you watch him walk down the hall, you note that he is setting the walker down by the front legs first and then the back legs. When he walks, he moves the walker and his strong leg ahead at the same time.

11. What errors is Mr. Santozi making, and how can you help him?

   * hip surgery
   * reaches walker
   * front leg

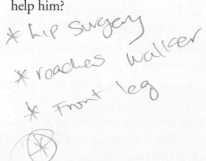

SECTION 6

Measuring and Recording Vital Signs, Height, and Weight

UNIT 18

Body Temperature

OBJECTIVES

After completing this unit, you will be able to:
- Spell and define terms.
- Name and identify the types of clinical thermometers and describe their uses.
- Read a thermometer.
- Identify the range of normal temperature values.

- Demonstrate the following procedures:
  - Procedure 25 Measuring an Oral Temperature
  - Procedure 26 Measuring a Rectal Temperature
  - Procedure 27 Measuring an Axillary Temperature
  - Procedure 28 Measuring a Tympanic Temperature
  - Procedure 29 Measuring a Temporal Artery Temperature

VOCABULARY

Learn the meaning and the correct spelling of the following words and phrases:

Celsius scale	electronic thermometer	probe	tympanic thermometer
clinical thermometer	Fahrenheit scale	temporal artery	vital signs
digital thermometer	flagged	thermometer (TAT)	

INTRODUCTION

Measurement of body temperature is a common nursing assistant task. Body temperature is one of the **vital** (living) **signs**. The patient's other vital signs include pulse, respiration, and blood pressure.

Vital signs must be measured accurately because they tell us a great deal about the patient's condition. If the patient questions you about the results, inform him that you will ask the nurse to discuss the results with him.

Although they are usually determined as a combined procedure, each vital sign is discussed in a separate unit. Many facilities use electronic equipment that automatically registers the four vital signs simultaneously. Measurement of height and weight is discussed in Unit 21.

TEMPERATURE VALUES

Temperature values may be expressed in either of two scales:
- **Fahrenheit scale**, which is indicated by an *F.*
- **Celsius scale** (centigrade scale), which is indicated by a *C.*

A small ° symbol before either capital letter indicates degrees (levels of temperature).

Definition of Body Temperature

Temperature is the measurement of body heat. It is the balance between heat produced and heat lost. Excessive body temperature puts stress on vital body organs.

Temperature Control

Special cells in the brain control and regulate body temperature. The average oral temperature range is 96.8°F (36°C) to 100.4°F (38°C). The average temperature is 98.6°F (37°C). Reportable values for adults are listed in Table 18-1. Normal values for children are listed in Table 18-2.

Measuring Body Temperature

Temperature is usually measured in one of five body areas:

- Mouth (oral)—most common.
- Ear (aural or tympanic)—a rapid method, but with wide variations and a high margin of error related to user technique.

TABLE 18-1 TEMPERATURE VALUES FOR ADULTS

Type	Report Values Normal	Below	Above
Oral	98.6°F	97°F	100°F
Axillary	97.6°F	96°F	99°F
Rectal	99.6°F	98°F	101°F
Temporal Artery	99.6°F	98°F	101°F
Tympanic	Tympanic values are set as oral or rectal equivalents. Use the reporting values for oral or rectal settings.		

TABLE 18-2 AVERAGE TEMPERATURES FOR INFANTS AND CHILDREN

Age	Temperature
3 months	99.4°F
6 months	99.5°F
1 year	99.7°F
3 years	99.0°F
5 years	98.6°F
7 years	98.3°F
9 years	98.1°F
11 years	98.0°F
13 years	97.8°F

- Temporal artery (forehead)—a rapid, accurate method ✓ that has recently become popular.
- Rectal—believed to be the most accurate of commonly used internal sites (mouth, rectal, axillary); rectal temperature registers 1°F higher than oral.
- Axillary or groin—least accurate; measures skin temperature under the arm or at the groin. (This method is used only when the patient's condition or equipment available prevents the use of other methods.) An axillary or groin temperature registers 1°F (or 0.6°C) lower than oral temperature.

Facilities using the temporal artery method commonly use it for all patients except those who require special internal monitoring. If the temporal method is not used in the facility, evaluate the patient's condition to determine which is the best site for measuring temperature. The site used most often is the mouth. It is not, however, always the best or safest site. In some situations, it is wiser to use another site.

Clinical Thermometers

A patient's temperature is determined by using a **clinical thermometer**. There are several types of clinical thermometers.

Glass Clinical Thermometer The glass clinical thermometer is a slender glass tube containing liquid; the liquid expands and moves up or down the tube when exposed to heat. Two types of glass clinical thermometers are commonly used (Figure 18-1): the security thermometer and the rectal thermometer. They differ mainly in the size and shape of the bulb. The *bulb* is the end that is inserted into the patient. When only the security or stubby type is in use, the rectal thermometers are marked with a red dot at the end of the stem. Oral thermometers are marked with a blue dot.

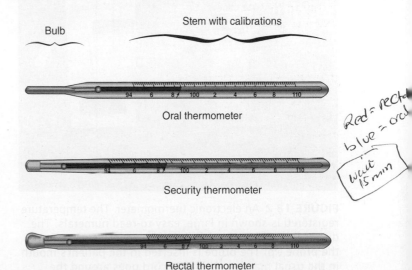

FIGURE 18-1 Clinical thermometers (from top to bottom): oral, security, rectal. (© Delmar/Cengage Learning)

Safety ALERT

Thermometers containing mercury have been used for many years. However, mercury can be very toxic to humans and wildlife, if the product is broken. This is true even if mercury exposure occurs in very small amounts. Alternative products are now being used in glass thermometers because of the potential for toxicity. Some states have banned the use of mercury entirely, and most facilities have stopped using mercury thermometers. However, some mercury thermometers remain in use and other hospital equipment may still contain mercury. Mercury is very toxic if it vaporizes and is inhaled. If you accidentally break a thermometer or other device containing mercury, follow your facility policies and procedures for making notifications and cleaning the spill. ■

Electronic Thermometer The **electronic thermometer** (Figure 18-2) is used in many hospitals. One unit can serve many patients because the nursing assistant simply changes the disposable cover that fits over the probe.

- The electronic thermometer is battery-operated. It registers the temperature on the viewing screen in a few seconds.

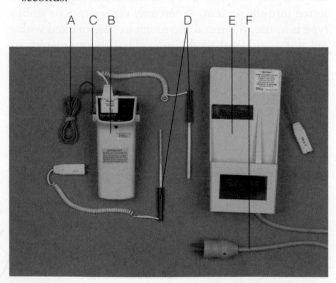

FIGURE 18-2 An electronic thermometer. The temperature registered is shown in large, easy-to-read numerals. The disposable protective sheath (probe cover) is placed over the probe tip. The probe is inserted in the patient's mouth in the usual manner. (A) Plastic cord goes around the nursing assistant's neck when carrying the thermometer. (B) Thermometer. (C) Box of disposable probe covers. (D) Probe (blue = oral, red = rectal). (E) Charging unit. (F) Probe cord. (G) Disposable probe cover. *(Stock image)*

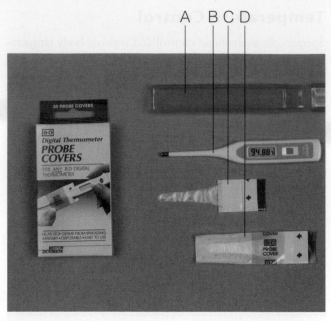

FIGURE 18-3 (A) Carrying case. (B) Digital thermometer. (C) Probe cover without backing. (D) Probe cover with backing. *(Stock image)*

- The portion called the **probe** is inserted into the patient.
- The probes are colored red for rectal use and blue for oral or axillary use.
- The probe is covered by a plastic cover. The cover is discarded after one use.

Digital Thermometer **Digital thermometers** are hand-held and have a probe that is inserted into the patient's mouth, rectum, or underarm area (Figure 18-3). Sheaths are used to cover the probe before use and are discarded after use. The unit is battery-operated. After the sheath-covered probe is inserted, the temperature can be read within 20 to 60 seconds. The temperature is shown as a digital (number) display.

Disposable Oral Thermometers Plastic or paper thermometers (Figure 18-4) are used for taking oral temperatures in some facilities and clinics. They are used once and discarded. The dots on the thermometer change color from brown to blue, according to the patient's temperature.

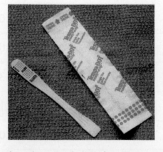

FIGURE 18-4 The chemical dot thermometer is used only for oral temperatures. It is used once, then discarded. *(Stock image)*

Tympanic Thermometer The **tympanic thermometer** measures the temperature from blood vessels in the tympanic membrane (eardrum) in the ear (Figure 18-5). The value is close to the core body temperature. To obtain an accurate reading, gently place the probe into the ear canal, gently sealing the canal. Press the button to activate the instrument. Within a few seconds, it registers the temperature of the blood flowing through the vessels in the eardrum. When this thermometer was first introduced, it became instantly popular. However, many facilities stopped using it because user technique must be precise to obtain accurate values, and the margin of error is great.

Temporal Artery Thermometer The heart, lungs, and brain are vital organs. Blood flow to these organs is normally rich. During illness, blood flow to less essential areas slows to ensure that the vital organs are protected. The ideal location for measuring temperature is in the heart, but doing so is not possible. The temporal artery is a major artery in the head. This is the only major artery in the body that is close enough to the surface of the skin to obtain an accurate temperature. The temporal artery is also close to the heart and has a high blood flow, making it well suited for measuring temperature. The **temporal artery thermometer (TAT)** is battery-operated. It measures the temperature of the skin surface over the temporal artery.

The temporal artery thermometer has a wider range than other types of clinical thermometers, and can measure temperatures from 60°F to 107.5°F. This is especially helpful for monitoring patients with below-normal temperatures or cold exposure. Special error codes will appear on the screen to alert the user to values that are dangerously high or low.

When using the TAT, measure an area of the head that is not covered by a hat or blanket. If the patient's head has been covered, wait at least 10 minutes for it to cool before proceeding. In a stable patient, the temporal artery temperature is approximately 0.8°F higher than an oral temperature, and is about the same as a rectal temperature. If the patient has a fever, the difference may be greater.

This thermometer is more accurate than other types because it is subject to less interference. Many factors interfere with the ability to obtain an accurate oral or rectal value during acute illness.

Other Types of Thermometers A number of different thermometers are available. Many of these were designed with children in mind. For example, there is a pacifier thermometer and a thermometer tape that reads the skin temperature on the forehead. These thermometers are primarily for home use.

Using the Glass Thermometer

The glass thermometer is a long, cylindrical, calibrated tube that contains a column of heat-sensitive liquid (Figure 18-6).

- Starting with 94°F (34°C), each long line indicates a one-degree elevation in temperature.
- Every other degree is marked with a number.
- In between each long line are four shorter lines.
- Each shorter line equals two-tenths (2/10 or 0.2) of 1 degree.

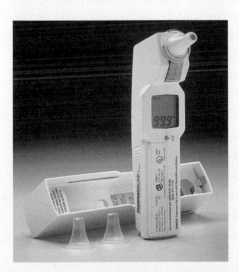

FIGURE 18-5 Cordless, hand-held tympanic thermometer that measures the temperature of the tympanic membrane in the ear. The window on the handset indicates the digital temperature reading. The thermometer can be set to provide an oral, rectal, Fahrenheit, or Celsius equivalent reading. *(Courtesy of Thermoscan® Inc., San Diego, CA)*

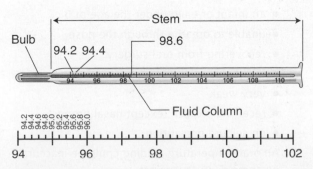

FIGURE 18-6 Reading a thermometer. This thermometer reads 98.6°F. Most Fahrenheit thermometers have an arrow indicating 98.6°F. *(© Delmar/Cengage Learning)*

Clinical Information ALERT

Each facility has policies and procedures about taking an oral temperature when the patient is using oxygen. In general, if the patient is using oxygen by mask, you should avoid taking an oral temperature. The temporal artery and tympanic thermometers are ideal for such patients because the values are not altered by the use of oxygen. Consult the nurse if you are unsure of the method to use for taking the temperature of a patient who is using oxygen. ■

Age Appropriate Care ALERT

When a tympanic thermometer is used for children under the age of 3, pull the pinna down and back. In children over age 3, pull the pinna up and back. This straightens the ear canal, enabling the sensor to detect heat in the eardrum. When the probe is positioned correctly, the probe tip will point at the midpoint between the eyebrow and sideburn on the opposite side of the face. ■

The liquid (the solid color line shown in Figure 18-6) in the bulb of the thermometer rises in the hollow center of the stem as heat is registered. To read the thermometer:

- Hold it at eye level.
- Find the solid column in the center.
- Look along the sharper edge between the numbers and lines.
- Read at the point at which the liquid ends.
- If it falls between two lines, read it to the closest line.

Documentation

In many facilities, temperatures are recorded on a clipboard, then transferred to the individual patient charts. Changes in readings may be **flagged** (specially noted) by placing a circle around the reading or a star beside it. Report any changes from previous temperature readings directly to the nurse. Your accurate observations, reporting, and documentation contribute to the nurses' evaluation and assessment of the patient.

GUIDELINES *for*

Using an Oral or Rectal Thermometer

Oral Thermometer

1. Do not use if the patient is:
   - uncooperative
   - restless
   - unconscious
   - chilled
   - confused or disoriented
   - coughing
   - an infant or child under the age of 6
   - unable to breathe through the nose
   - recovering from oral surgery
   - irrational
   - very weak
   - receiving oxygen (except nasal prongs)
   - on seizure precautions
2. An oral temperature reading could be inaccurate on some denture wearers.

3. If the person has been smoking, eating, or drinking, wait 15 minutes before taking the temperature.

Rectal Thermometer

1. Do not use if the patient has:
   - diarrhea
   - fecal impaction
   - combative behavior
   - rectal bleeding
   - hemorrhoids
   - had rectal surgery or rectal or colonic disease
   - recently had a heart attack
   - recently had prostate surgery
   - a colostomy
2. Always hold a rectal thermometer in place the entire time.

GUIDELINES *for*

Safe Use of a Glass Thermometer

- Make sure the thermometer is clean.
- Wear disposable gloves when measuring oral and rectal temperatures.
- Check glass thermometers for chips.
- Shake the thermometer down before use. Shake away from the patient and hard objects.
- Cover the thermometer with a disposable plastic sheath.
- Do not leave the patient alone with a thermometer in place.
- Allow a glass thermometer to register for at least 3 minutes for oral and rectal temperatures, and 10 minutes for an axillary temperature.

- Hold rectal and axillary thermometers in place.
- When using a rectal thermometer, lubricate the bulb end of the thermometer before inserting it into the rectum. Some sheaths are prelubricated.
- After removing the thermometer and before reading it, wipe the thermometer from end to tip with an alcohol wipe or cotton ball.
- Do not touch a bulb end or disposable sheath that has been in a patient's mouth (oral thermometer) or anus (rectal thermometer).
- Discard the sheath according to facility policy after use.
- Clean and disinfect the thermometer after use.

GUIDELINES *for*

Measuring Temperature Using a Sheath-Covered Glass or Digital Thermometer

Note: These guidelines vary slightly from state to state, and from one facility to the next. Your instructor will inform you if the sequence in your state or facility differs from the guidelines listed here. Know and follow the required sequence for your facility and state.

- Carry out initial procedure actions.
- Assemble equipment:
  - Gloves (standard precautions)
  - Clinical thermometer, glass or digital
  - Protective sheath (unopened package)
  - Pad and pencil
- Have the patient rest in a comfortable position.
- Ask the patient if he or she has had anything to eat or drink or has smoked within the last 15 minutes. If so, wait 15 minutes before taking an oral temperature.
- Apply gloves.
- Shake the glass thermometer down to below 96°F.
- Holding the thermometer in one hand, insert it into the marked end of a protective sheath wrapper (Figure 18-7A).

- Holding onto the sheath tab on the stem end of the thermometer, peel back the paper cover to expose the plastic sheath (Figure 18-7B).
- Hold the paper wrapper in one hand (Figure 18-7C). Twist the paper wrapper to break the seal with the tab and remove the paper wrapper, leaving the plastic sheath on the thermometer (Figure 18-7D).
- Keeping the protective sheath over the thermometer, insert the bulb end of the thermometer under the patient's tongue, toward the side of the mouth.
- Tell the patient to hold the thermometer gently, with lips closed, for 3 minutes.
- After 3 minutes, remove the thermometer and discard the used sheath. Read and shake down. Record on notepad.
- The thermometer can be stored in the patient's bedside stand for reuse with a new sheath.
- Remove gloves and discard according to facility policy.
- Carry out ending procedure actions.
- Report any unusual variations to the nurse at once.

continues

GUIDELINES *continued*

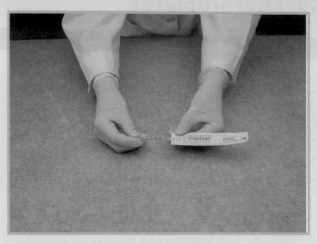

FIGURE 18-7A Inserting a thermometer into a disposable thermometer sheath. *(© Delmar/Cengage Learning)*

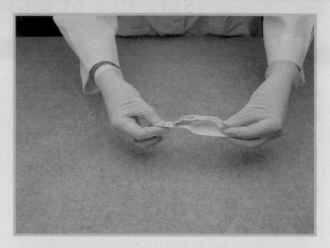

FIGURE 18-7C Grasp the outer paper wrapper. *(© Delmar/Cengage Learning)*

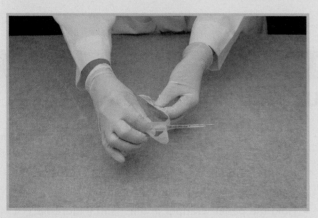

FIGURE 18-7B To remove the sheath, peel back the outer paper wrapper to expose the inner plastic sheath. *(© Delmar/Cengage Learning)*

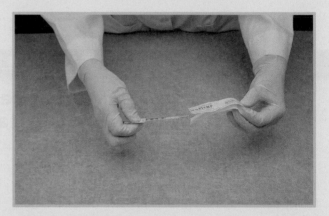

FIGURE 18-7D Holding onto the paper tab with one hand, twist and remove the outer paper wrapper. *(© Delmar/Cengage Learning)*

PROCEDURE

25

MEASURING AN ORAL TEMPERATURE

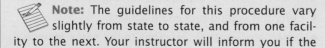

Note: The guidelines for this procedure vary slightly from state to state, and from one facility to the next. Your instructor will inform you if the sequence in your state or facility differs from the procedure listed here. Know and follow the required sequence for your facility and state.

continues

PROCEDURE 25 CONTINUED

1. Carry out initial procedure actions.

2. Assemble equipment on a tray:
   - Gloves
   - Glass or digital thermometer or electronic thermometer with oral (blue) probe
   - Probe cover or plastic sheath

3. Obtain an oral thermometer, disposable sheath or probe cover, and gloves, if this is your facility policy. If using a glass thermometer, rinse the disinfectant off and dry the thermometer. Shake the thermometer down to 96°F.

4. Ask the patient if he or she has had anything to eat or drink or has smoked within the last 15 minutes. If so, wait 15 minutes before taking an oral temperature.

5. Apply a plastic sheath cover to the glass or digital thermometer, or a plastic cover to the blue probe of the electronic thermometer.

6. Insert the covered thermometer or probe under the patient's tongue toward the side of the mouth (Figure 18-8A).

7. Hold the thermometer or probe in position, if needed. Ask the patient to close the mouth and breathe through the nose.

8. When a buzzer signals that the temperature has been determined, remove the probe from the patient's mouth.

9. After the prescribed length of time (3 minutes for glass, or when the electronic thermometer beeps), remove the device from the patient's mouth. Discard the cover in the appropriate container (Figure 18-8B). Hold the glass thermometer at eye level and read the mercury column or read the digital display of the electronic thermometer. Note the reading. Remove gloves, if used, and discard according to facility policy.

10. Shake the glass thermometer down to 96°F. Place the thermometer in the container for used thermometers, or disinfect it according to facility policy, or return the probe to its proper position.

11. Record the temperature on your pad.

12. Return the electronic thermometer unit to the charger.

13. Carry out ending procedure actions.

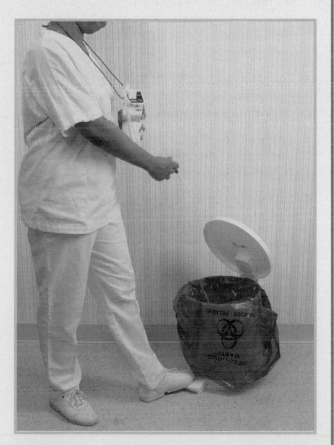

FIGURE 18-8B Discard the used probe cover according to facility policy. (© *Delmar/Cengage Learning*)

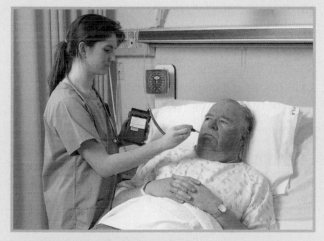

FIGURE 18-8A The thermometer probe is placed to one side of the patient's mouth and positioned under the tongue. (© *Delmar/Cengage Learning*)

PROCEDURE

MEASURING A RECTAL TEMPERATURE

Note: The guidelines for this procedure vary slightly from state to state, and from one facility to the next. Your instructor will inform you if the sequence in your state or facility differs from the procedure listed here. Know and follow the required sequence for your facility and state.

1. Carry out initial procedure actions.

2. Assemble equipment on a tray:
   - Gloves
   - Glass or digital thermometer or electronic thermometer with rectal (red) probe
   - Probe cover or plastic sheath
   - Lubricant

3. If using a glass thermometer, rinse the disinfectant off and dry the thermometer. Shake the glass thermometer down to 96°F. Cover the thermometer or probe with a plastic sheath or probe cover.

4. Lower the backrest of the bed. Ask the patient to turn on his side. Position the patient in the Sims' position. Assist if necessary.

5. Apply gloves. Place a small amount of lubricant on the tip of the sheath or probe cover (Figure 18-9).

6. Fold the top bedclothes back to expose the patient's anal area.

7. Separate the buttocks with one hand. Insert the covered thermometer or probe about 1 inch into the rectum, or as recommended by the thermometer manufacturer. With many electronic and digital thermometers, the rectal probe is inserted approximately 1/4 inch. Hold the thermometer or probe in place. Replace the bedclothes for privacy as soon as the thermometer is inserted. Remove the glass thermometer after 3 minutes, or when the

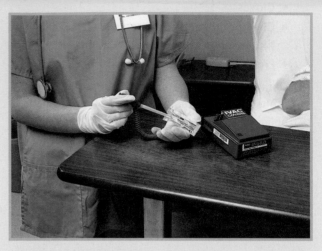

FIGURE 18-9 Apply a small amount of lubricant to the tip of the sheath. (© Delmar/Cengage Learning)

alarm sounds on the electronic or digital thermometer. Discard the cover.

8. Hold the glass thermometer at eye level and read the mercury column, or read the digital display of the electronic thermometer. Note the reading. Return the probe to its proper position.

9. Wipe the lubricant from the patient. Discard the used tissue.

10. Shake the glass thermometer down to 96°F. Place the thermometer in the container for used thermometers, or disinfect it according to facility policy.

11. Remove and dispose of gloves according to facility policy.

12. Record the temperature on your pad.

13. Return the thermometer unit to the charger.

14. Carry out ending procedure actions.

PROCEDURE

27
MEASURING AN AXILLARY TEMPERATURE

Note: The guidelines for this procedure vary slightly from state to state, and from one facility to the next. Your instructor will inform you if the sequence in your state or facility differs from the procedure listed here. Know and follow the required sequence for your facility and state.

1. Carry out initial procedure actions.

2. Assemble equipment on a tray:
   - Gloves, if needed
   - Hand towel
   - Glass or digital thermometer or electronic thermometer with oral (blue) probe
   - Probe cover or plastic sheath

3. If using a glass thermometer, rinse the disinfectant off and dry the thermometer. Shake the glass thermometer down to 96°F.

4. Cover the thermometer with a plastic sheath or probe cover.

5. Apply gloves, if this is your facility policy.

6. Dry the axilla with a hand towel.

7. Insert the thermometer into the center of the axilla, then lower the patient's arm and bend it across the abdomen. Hold the thermometer in place, if this is your facility policy.

8. Leave the thermometer in place for 10 full minutes or until the thermometer alarm sounds. Remove the thermometer from the patient's axilla.

9. Discard the sheath or probe cover according to facility policy.

10. Hold the glass thermometer at eye level and read the mercury column, or read the digital display of the electronic thermometer. Note the reading.

11. Shake the glass thermometer down to 96°F. Place the thermometer in the container for used thermometers or disinfect it according to facility policy, or place the probe for the electronic thermometer in the probe holder.

12. Remove your gloves and discard them according to facility policy.

13. Record the temperature reading.

14. Carry out procedure completion actions.

PROCEDURE

28
MEASURING A TYMPANIC TEMPERATURE

Note: The guidelines for this procedure vary slightly from state to state, and from one facility to the next. Your instructor will inform you if the sequence in your state or facility differs from the procedure listed here. Know and follow the required sequence for your facility and state.

1. Carry out initial procedure actions.

2. Assemble equipment:
   - Disposable gloves if there may be contact with blood or body fluids, open lesions, or wet linens
   - Tympanic thermometer
   - Probe covers

3. Check the lens to make sure it is clean and intact (Figure 18-10A).

4. Select the appropriate mode on the thermometer.

5. Place a clean probe cover on the probe.

6. Put on disposable gloves if you may have contact with blood or body fluids, open lesions, or wet linens.

continues

PROCEDURE 28 CONTINUED

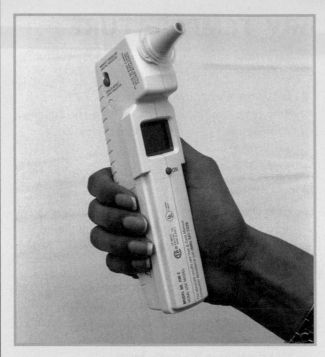

FIGURE 18-10A Check the lens of the tympanic thermometer to make sure it is clean and intact. *(© Delmar/Cengage Learning)*

7. Position the patient so you have access to the ear you will be using.

8. Gently pull the ear pinna back and up (Figure 18-10B). This straightens the ear canal so the thermometer can be placed for an accurate reading.
   - If the patient is a child under age 3, pull the pinna down and back.
   - If the patient is a child over age 3, pull the pinna up and back.

9. Place the probe in the patient's ear, aiming it toward the tympanic membrane. Insert the probe until it seals the ear canal (Figure 18-10C). Do not apply pressure.
   - Check the position of the probe. The tip should be at an imaginary location inside the ear opposite the midpoint between the eyebrow and sideburn on the opposite side of the face.

10. Rotate the probe handle slightly until it is aligned with the jaw, as though the patient were speaking on the telephone.

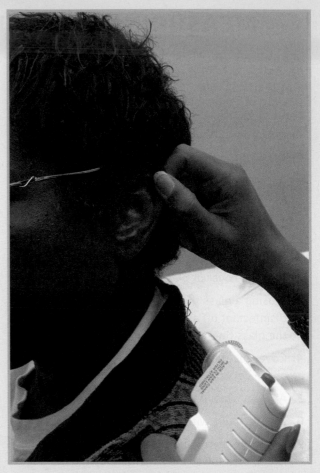

FIGURE 18-10B Gently pull the ear pinna back and up. *(© Delmar/Cengage Learning)*

11. Quickly press the activation button (Figure 18-10D). Leave the thermometer in the ear for the time recommended by the manufacturer.

TABLE 18-3 NORMAL RANGES FOR TYMPANIC TEMPERATURES

Years of Age	Fahrenheit Values
0–2	97.5–100.4°F
3–10	97.0–100.0°F
11–65	96.6–99.7°F
>65	96.4–99.5°F

continues

PROCEDURE 28 CONTINUED

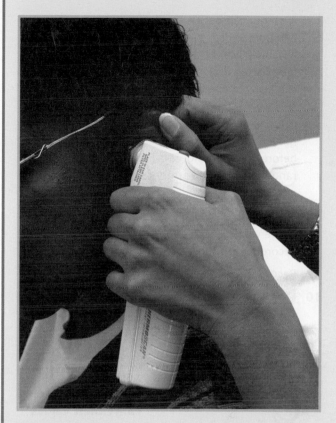

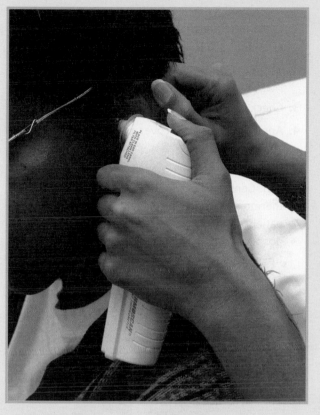

FIGURE 18-10C Place the covered probe in the patient's ear, aiming it toward the tympanic membrane. Insert the probe until it seals in the ear canal, then rotate the handle until it is positioned like a telephone. (© *Delmar/Cengage Learning*)

FIGURE 18-10D Press the activation button and leave the thermometer in the ear for the time recommended by the manufacturer. (© *Delmar/Cengage Learning*)

12. When you have a reading, remove the probe from the patient's ear and dispose of the cover. See Table 18-3 for normal ranges of tympanic temperatures by age group.

13. Record the temperature on your pad.

14. Return the thermometer unit to the charger.

15. Carry out ending procedure actions.

PROCEDURE

29

MEASURING A TEMPORAL ARTERY TEMPERATURE

Note: The guidelines for this procedure vary slightly from state to state, and from one facility to the next. Your instructor will inform you if the sequence in your state or facility differs from the procedure listed here. Know and follow the required sequence for your facility and state.

1. Carry out initial procedure actions.

2. Assemble equipment:
   - Disposable gloves if there may be contact with blood or body fluids, open lesions, or wet linens (Gloves are not necessary unless

continues

PROCEDURE 29 CONTINUED

required by facility policy or potential exposure to body fluids.)

- Temporal artery thermometer
- Probe covers, alcohol sponges, or disinfectant wipes, according to facility policy

3. Check the lens to make sure it is clean and intact.

4. Apply a clean probe cover, or wipe the probe with alcohol or a disinfectant wipe.

5. Hold the thermometer as you would a pencil or pen. Gently press the probe (head) of the thermometer against the center of the patient's forehead. Push the switch to the "ON" position with your thumb (Figure 18-11A). Keep this button depressed.

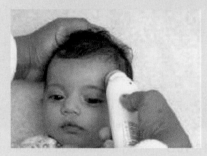

FIGURE 18-11A Hold the button down while moving the probe to the temple area. (© Delmar/Cengage Learning)

6. Slowly move the probe across the forehead to the hair line on one side of the head (Figure 18-11B).

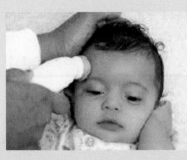

FIGURE 18-11B Push the hair back to maintain good skin contact. (© Delmar/Cengage Learning)

7. Push the hair back slightly with the opposite hand, if needed, then lift the probe slightly. Quickly place the probe down just behind the ear lobe on the neck. (Use the area in which perfume is usually applied.) Release the button and remove the thermometer. Note and remember the value on the digital display. The value should remain on the display for about 30 seconds before disappearing. See Table 18-4 for normal ranges of temporal artery temperatures by age group.

8. Discard the disposable probe cover, or wipe the probe with an alcohol or disinfectant wipe, according to facility policy.

9. Record the temperature on your pad.

10. Carry out ending procedure actions.

TABLE 18-4 NORMAL RANGES FOR TEMPORAL ARTERY TEMPERATURES

Age	Fahrenheit Values
0–2 months	98.3°F–100.7°F
3–47 months	98.3°F–100.3°F
4–9 years	97.8°F–100.1°F
10–18 years	97.4°F–100.1°F
Over 18 years	97.2°F–100.1°F

REVIEW

A. Multiple Choice

Select the one best answer for each of the following.

1. You are about to measure a rectal temperature with a glass thermometer. You find a small chip in the glass. What should you do?
   a. Use the thermometer, because it is just a small chip.
   b. Throw the thermometer in the wastepaper basket.
   c. Break the thermometer in half so no one else will use it.
   d. Discard the <u>chipped thermometer in</u> the sharps container and use another thermometer.

2. You are assigned to measure your patient's rectal temperature using a glass thermometer. How long should you hold the thermometer in place?
   a. 3 minutes
   b. 10 minutes
   c. 15 minutes
   d. 20 minutes

 3 minute

3. Measuring the function of vital organs of the body is called taking
   a. vital statistics.
   b. vital signs.
   c. blood pressure.
   d. pulse.

4. When reading the glass thermometer, each long line represents
   a. one degree.
   b. one-tenth of a degree.
   c. two-tenths of a degree.
   d. five-tenths of a degree.

5. An oral temperature should *not* be used for the patient who
   a. has dentures.
   b. is a mouth <u>breather</u>.
   c. has eaten in the past hour.
   d. used oxygen yesterday.

6. The thermometer must be lubricated before taking a/an
   a. axillary temperature.
   b. temporal artery temperature.

 rectal

   c. rectal temperature.
   d. tympanic temperature.

7. What should you do when the temperature measurement is abnormally high or low?
   a. Record the measurements on the chart at the end of your shift.
   b. Alert the nurse immediately to the abnormal measurements.
   c. Tell the patient and ask what he would like you to do.
   d. Report it to the nurse at the end of your shift.

8. Oral temperatures should not be taken on patients
   a. over the age of 80.
   b. with colostomies.
   c. with seizure disorder. ✓
   d. who are alert.

9. Rectal temperatures should not be taken on patients
   a. with respiratory disease.
   b. with fecal impaction.
   c. using oxygen.
   d. who have been vomiting.

B. Nursing Assistant Challenge

Mrs. LeJune is having difficulty breathing and is very restless. She is hot to the touch. The nurse instructs you to measure her temperature.

10. To obtain the most accurate value, which type of thermometer will you choose if all are available?
    a. Glass oral thermometer
    b. Glass rectal thermometer
    c. Electronic oral thermometer
    d. Tympanic thermometer
    e. Temporal artery thermometer

11. You find that Mrs. LeJune has a temperature of 103.8°F according to the method you selected. The temperature board shows that her temperature was 97.6°F near the end of the previous shift. What action will you take?

Recheck it and check it with the nurse

UNIT 19

Pulse and Respiration

OBJECTIVES

After completing this unit, you will be able to:
- Spell and define terms.
- Define pulse.
- Explain the importance of monitoring a pulse rate.
- Locate the pulse sites.
- Identify the range of normal pulse and respiratory rates.
- Measure the pulse at different locations.
- List the characteristics of the pulse and respiration.
- List eight guidelines for using a stethoscope.
- Demonstrate the following procedures:
  - Procedure 30 Counting the Radial Pulse
  - Procedure 31 Counting the Apical-Radial Pulse
  - Procedure 32 Counting Respirations

VOCABULARY

Learn the meaning and the correct spelling of the following words and phrases:

accelerated	cyanosis	radial pulse	symmetry
apical pulse	dyspnea	rate	tachycardia
apnea	expiration	respiration	tachypnea
bradycardia	inspiration	rhythm	volume
Cheyne-Stokes	pulse	stertorous	
respirations	pulse deficit	stethoscope	

Pressure against arteries

INTRODUCTION

The pulse and respirations are usually counted during the same procedure. Because breathing is partly under voluntary control, a person is able to stop or alter breathing temporarily for a short period. To avoid this, the nursing assistant counts respirations immediately following the pulse count, without telling the patient. You keep the patient's hand in the same position, and your fingers remain on the pulse point so that you seem to be still taking the pulse.

THE PULSE

The **pulse** is:
- The pressure of the blood felt against the wall of an artery as the heart alternately contracts (beats) and relaxes (rests).
- More easily felt in arteries that are close to the skin and can be gently pressed against a bone.
- The same in all arteries throughout the body.
- An indication of how the cardiovascular system is meeting the body's needs.

Clinical Information ALERT

When taking a patient's pulse, check the rate, rhythm, and quality. The *rhythm* is the pattern that you feel, with pulsations and pauses between them. If the pulse is normal, the length of the beat will be approximately equal to the length of the pause. The *quality* of the pulse is the volume you palpate. You can tell from touch whether it is weak, strong, or thready. ■

TABLE 19-1 AVERAGE PULSE RATES

Patient	Beats per Minute
Adult men	60–70
Adult women	65–80
Teenagers	60–90
Children over 7 years of age	75–100
Preschoolers	80–110
Toddlers	90–140
Infants	120–160

Radial Pulse

The **radial pulse** is the most commonly measured pulse. It is measured at the radial artery in the wrist. Figure 19-1 shows areas of the body where other large blood vessels come close enough to the surface to be used as sites for counting the pulse. Check the pulse of unconscious patients at the carotid artery or apically (over the heart).

Pulse measurement includes determining the:

1. Rate or speed
   a. **Bradycardia**—an unusually slow pulse (below 60 beats per minute)
   b. **Tachycardia**—an unusually fast pulse (more than 100 beats per minute)
2. Character
   a. **Rhythm**—regularity
   b. Volume or fullness

Report:
- Pulse rates over 100 beats per minute (bpm) (tachycardia)
- Pulse rates under 60 bpm (bradycardia)
- Irregularities in character (rhythm and volume)

Table 19-1 shows average pulse rates.

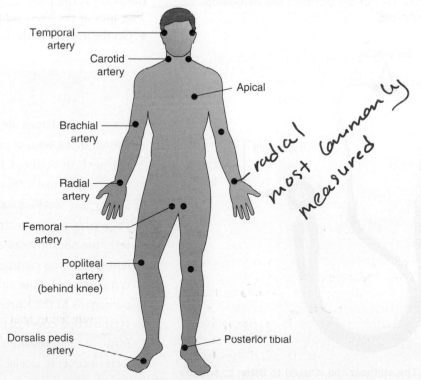

Temporal artery

Carotid artery

Apical

Brachial artery

Radial artery

Femoral artery

Popliteal artery (behind knee)

Dorsalis pedis artery

Posterior tibial

radial most commonly measured

FIGURE 19-1 Common pulse sites of the body. (© *Delmar/Cengage Learning*)

PROCEDURE   OBRA DVD

30
COUNTING THE RADIAL PULSE

1. Carry out initial procedure actions.

2. Position the patient in a comfortable position. The palm of the hand should be down and the arm should rest on a flat surface.

3. Locate the pulse on the thumb side of the wrist with the tips of your first three fingers (Figure 19-2). Do not use your thumb—it contains a pulse that may be confused with the patient's pulse.

4. When the pulse is felt, exert slight pressure. Count for one minute, using the second hand of your watch for timing. Some facilities permit staff to count for one-half minute and multiply by two, and to record that figure as the rate for one minute. A one-minute count is preferred and must be done if the pulse is irregular.

5. Remember the reading. Record the reading on your pad as soon as you have finished counting respirations.

6. Carry out ending procedure actions.

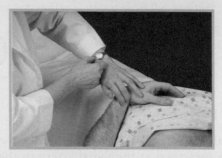

FIGURE 19-2 Locate the pulse on the thumb side of the wrist with the tips of your first three fingers. *(© Delmar/Cengage Learning)*

Using a Stethoscope

A **stethoscope** is an instrument used to listen to sounds inside the body. The parts of the stethoscope are seen in Figure 19-3. Many health care workers use stethoscopes on many patients. This creates a risk of infection in both workers and patients. Always disinfect the stethoscope before and after using it.

The Apical Pulse ✳

An **apical pulse** is measured by counting the heart contractions. The stethoscope is placed over the apex (tip) of the heart. Listen for the heart sounds that occur as the heart pumps blood into the arteries. The rate should be the same as the pulse that is felt elsewhere in the body. The apex of the heart is found:

• On the left side of the front of the chest

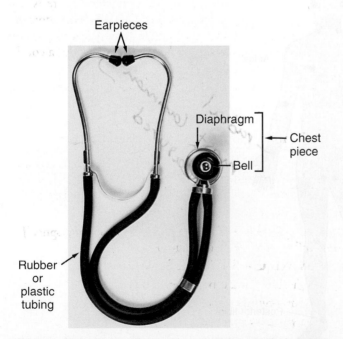

Earpieces

Diaphragm

Chest piece

Bell

Rubber or plastic tubing

FIGURE 19-3 The stethoscope is used to listen to sounds inside the body. *(© Delmar/Cengage Learning)*

OSHA ALERT

Many stethoscopes are made of latex. Nursing personnel often wear a personal stethoscope around the neck throughout the shift, removing it when they need to use it. To reduce the risk of latex exposure, many workers have purchased or made cloth covers for the stethoscope tubing. The cover contacts the neck instead of the latex. This is an excellent idea, but a caution is in order. The cloth cover is a potential fomite and can transmit microbes and pathogens to the worker and the patients. Wash the stethoscope cover daily when you wash your uniform, or keep several covers and alternate them so a clean cover is available each day. ■

GUIDELINES *for*
Using a Stethoscope

- Clean the earpieces and diaphragm of the stethoscope before and after using it.
- Clean the stethoscope tubing if it contacts the patient or bed linen.
- Check the earpieces of the stethoscope for wax, and remove it if present.
- Check the stethoscope tubing. Do not use if it has cracks or holes in it.
- The earpieces of the stethoscope should face forward.
- The diaphragm of the stethoscope should not come in contact with the patient's clothing, blood pressure cuff, or other device.
- Place the diaphragm of the stethoscope flat against the patient's skin and hold it in place. If the diaphragm is at an angle, you will not be able to hear the sounds.
- Apply firm but gentle pressure when holding the diaphragm in place. If you press too hard, you may be unable to hear the sound.

- Between the fifth and sixth ribs
- Just below the left nipple
- In women, under the left breast

Listen carefully for two heart sounds: lub dub. The louder sound (lub) corresponds to the contraction of the ventricles pushing the blood into the arteries, and the closing of the valves. This is the sound to be counted. The softer sound (dub) is heard when the ventricles relax as they fill with blood. When documenting an apical pulse reading, write "AP" after the value.

Apical-Radial Pulse Rate

The apical and radial pulse rate is a comparison of the apical rate and the radial rate. They should be the same.

Sometimes the contraction of the heart is so weak that it fails to send enough blood to the arteries to expand them. When this happens, no pulse is felt. In this case, the number of loud sounds does not correspond with the number of pulses felt in the radial artery.

The difference between the apical pulse (the loud sounds heard over the heart) and the radial pulse (the expansion felt over the radial pulse) is called a **pulse deficit**. Pulse deficits are found in some forms of heart disease. Two people measure the heart rate and the

Clinical Information ALERT

Activity increases the pulse, respirations, and blood pressure. For accurate values, wait at least 30 minutes to take vital signs on patients who have participated in therapy, exercised, or have engaged in another activity, such as ambulating in the hallway, bathing, or showering. ∎

---

radial pulse at the same time. (See Procedure 31.) The nurse measures the apical pulse while the second person counts the radial pulse for one minute. The rates are then compared.

Apical pulse rates are checked:

- Before the registered nurse administers drugs that alter the heart rate or rhythm
- In children whose rapid rates might be difficult to count at the radial artery, and any child aged 12 months or younger
- For one full minute
- Whenever you are uncertain of the accuracy of the radial pulse or it is irregular

RESPIRATION

The main function of **respiration** is to supply the cells in the body with oxygen and to rid the body of excess carbon dioxide. When respirations are inefficient, there is less oxygen in the blood available for body needs. In addition, carbon dioxide is released less efficiently. The skin takes on a bluish or dusky color and the patient develops a condition known as **cyanosis**.

There are two parts to each respiration: one **inspiration** (inhalation) followed by one **expiration** (exhalation). Special terms describe different breathing patterns:

- Normal—regular, 12 to 20 breaths per minute
- **Tachypnea**—rapid, shallow breathing
- **Dyspnea**—difficult or labored breathing
- Shallow—breaths that only partially fill the lungs
- **Apnea**—a period of no respirations
- **Cheyne-Stokes respirations**—a period of dyspnea followed by periods of apnea
- **Stertorous**—Snoring-like respirations

Respirations should be checked for:

- **Rate**—number of respirations per minute
- Rhythm—regularity
- **Symmetry**—equal expansion on both sides of the chest
- **Volume**—depth of respiration

PROCEDURE

31

COUNTING THE APICAL-RADIAL PULSE

1. Carry out initial procedure actions.

2. Clean the stethoscope earpieces and diaphragm with disinfectant.

3. Place the stethoscope earpieces in your ears with tips facing slightly forward for better fit.

4. Place the stethoscope diaphragm over the apex of the patient's heart. If it is cold, warm the diaphragm by rubbing it with your hands before placing it on the patient's chest.

5. Listen carefully for the heartbeat.

6. Count the louder-sounding beats for one minute.

7. Check the radial pulse for one minute. The best way to obtain these numbers is to have the nurse count the apical pulse while you take the radial pulse (Figure 19-4).

8. Note results on a pad for comparison.

9. Clean the earpieces and bell of the stethoscope with disinfectant.

10. Carry out ending procedure actions.
    Example: Apical pulse = 108
    Radial pulse = 82
    Pulse deficit = 26 (108 – 82 = 26)

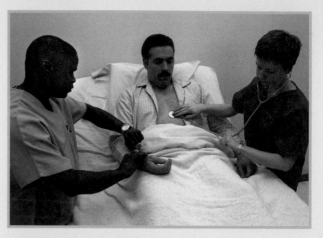

FIGURE 19-4 The nurse takes the apical pulse while the nursing assistant takes the radial pulse.
(© Delmar/Cengage Learning)

Clinical Information ALERT

When counting respirations, note whether the patient's breathing is normal (easy) or labored (dyspneic), shallow or deep, and quiet or noisy. Check the muscles of the neck and abdomen. If the patient is using these muscles to assist in breathing, inform the nurse. ∎

- Character—terms used to describe the character of respirations include:
  - Regular
  - Irregular
  - Shallow
  - Deep
  - Labored (difficult)

The rate of respiration is determined by counting the rise or fall of the chest for one minute, using a watch equipped with a second hand. (See Procedure 32.)

- The average rate for adults is 12 to 20 respirations per minute.

- If the rate is more than 25 per minute, it is said to be **accelerated**. Accelerated respirations should be reported.
- If the rate is less than 12 per minute, it is too slow. This should be reported.

Average respiratory rates are listed in Table 19-2.

Temperature, pulse, and respiration (TPR) rates and character are recorded in a notebook or on a clipboard and then transferred to the patient's chart (Figure 19-6).

TABLE 19-2 AVERAGE RESPIRATORY RATES

Age	Normal Respiratory Rate per Minute
Infant	30–60
Toddler	24–40
Preschool child	22–34
School-age child	18–30
Teenager	12–24
Adult	12–20

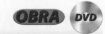

PROCEDURE

32

COUNTING RESPIRATIONS

1. After counting the pulse, leave your fingers in place. Begin counting the number of times the chest rises and falls during one minute (Figure 19-5). Count one inhalation and one exhalation as one respiration.

2. Note the depth and regularity of respirations.

3. Record the time, rate, depth, and regularity of respirations.

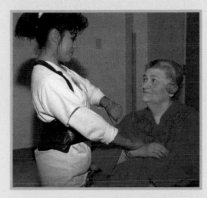

FIGURE 19-5 Leave your fingers on the radial pulse while counting respirations. (© Delmar/Cengage Learning)

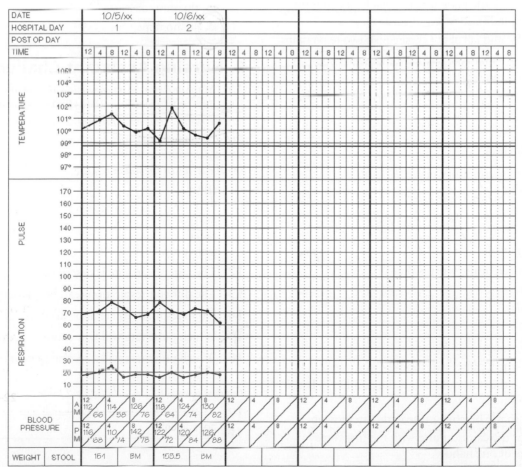

GRAPHIC RECORD

DATE	10/5/xx	10/6/xx
HOSPITAL DAY	1	2

FIGURE 19-6 TPR readings are recorded in the patient's medical record. (© Delmar/Cengage Learning)

REVIEW

A. Multiple Choice

Select the one best answer for each of the following.

1. The rhythmic expansion and contraction of an artery is called the
   a. rate.
   b. pulse.
   c. volume.
   d. blood pressure.

2. Mrs. Wherry's pulse is 120. This is
   a. bradycardia.
   b. normal.
   c. tachycardia.
   d. hypertension.

3. Which of the following is true about counting the patient's respirations?
   a. Respirations are counted by watching the rise and fall of the chest.
   b. Counting of respirations is done simultaneously with counting the pulse.
   c. Always tell the patient when you begin counting the respirations.
   d. One rise and fall of the chest equals two respirations.

4. What body system are you checking when you measure the pulse?
   a. Respiratory
   b. Digestive
   c. Circulatory
   d. Elimination

5. Mr. Rapini's respiratory rate is 20. This is
   a. normal.
   b. tachycardia.
   c. dyspnea.
   d. tachypnea.

6. The pulse felt at the wrist is the
   a. carotid.
   b. brachial.
   c. apical.
   d. radial.

7. When taking a pulse, you should
   a. palpate the pulse and count the number of beats per minute.
   b. listen to the brachial pulse with a stethoscope.
   c. feel for the carotid pulse with the first three fingers of one hand.
   d. count the femoral pulse for 30 seconds and multiply times 4.

8. Difficulty breathing and shortness of breath is
   a. dyspnea.
   b. apnea.
   c. expiration.
   d. aspiration.

9. The act of breathing air out is
   a. aspiration.
   b. inhalation.
   c. expiration.
   d. bradycardia.

10. A pulse rate below 60 beats per minute is
    a. hypertension.
    b. tachycardia.
    c. hypotension.
    d. bradycardia.

11. The instrument used to listen to sounds within the body is the
    a. sphygmomanometer.
    b. monitor.
    c. thermometer.
    d. stethoscope.

B. Nursing Assistant Challenge

Mrs. Morgan has a heart condition that makes her heart rate irregular and faster than normal. Her respirations are difficult or rapid, labored, and moist. She receives a medication that profoundly alters her heart action. Your orders are to assist in determining the pulse deficit. Answer the statements using the terms in the following list.

    apical
    dyspnea
    tachycardia
    radial
    tachypnea

12. The faster heart rate is described as _tach_.

13. The difficult respirations can be charted as _dyspnea_.

14. Rapid respirations are also called _tachy_.

15. Which pulse rate will you count? _radial_.

16. Which pulse rate will a second person count? _apical_.

List two reasons why a radial-apical pulse rate would be ordered.

17. _heart rate problem_

18. _____

Blood Pressure

OBJECTIVES

After completing this unit, you will be able to:

- Spell and define terms.
- Identify the range of normal blood pressure values.
- Identify the causes of inaccurate blood pressure readings.
- Select the proper size blood pressure cuff.
- List precautions associated with use of the sphygmomanometer.

- Describe the use of a pulse oximeter.
- Demonstrate the following procedures:
  - Procedure 33 Taking Blood Pressure
  - Procedure 34 Taking Blood Pressure with an Electronic Blood Pressure Apparatus

VOCABULARY

Learn the meaning and the correct spelling of the following words and phrases:

aneroid gauge	diastole	hypotension	systole
auscultatory gap	diastolic pressure	pulse pressure	systolic pressure
blood pressure	elasticity	sphygmomanometer	
brachial artery	hypertension		

INTRODUCTION

Blood pressure is the fourth vital sign. It is the measure of the force of the blood against the walls of the arteries. Blood pressure depends on the:

- Volume (amount of blood in the circulatory system).
- Force of the heartbeat.

- Condition of the arteries. Arteries that have lost their **elasticity** (stretch) give more resistance. The pressure is greater in these arteries.
- Distance from the heart. Blood pressure in the legs is lower than in the arms.

Pressure varies with contraction (**systole**) and relaxation (**diastole**) of the ventricles of the heart. The systolic blood

TABLE 20-1 AVERAGE BLOOD PRESSURE VALUES

Age	Approximate Blood Pressure Value	
	Systolic	*Diastolic*
2–6 months	91	50 to 53
7–11 months	90	47 + age in months
1–5 years	90 + age in years	56
6–18 years	83 + (2 × age in years)	52 + age in years
Over age 18	120	80

pressure is the working pressure. The diastolic blood pressure is the resting pressure. Average blood pressure values are listed in Table 20-1.

EQUIPMENT

The **sphygmomanometer** (blood pressure measuring apparatus) consists of:

- A cuff that fits around the patient's arm (different sizes are available). There is a rubber bladder inside the cuff. A pressure control button is attached to the cuff. For accurate readings, the cuff must be the correct size. Cuffs that are too wide or too narrow will give

Clinical Information ALERT

Taking accurate blood pressures and reporting and documenting abnormal values saves health care dollars and improves patients' health. For example, the physician will treat high blood pressure values leading to renal failure. High blood pressure causes 80% of all kidney failure. The annual cost of treating renal failure is approximately $20 billion. Controlling high blood pressure can delay the onset of renal failure by 4.5 years. Dialysis costs about $50,000 a year, so this control alone is a potential savings of $225,000. Even more important, being in good health and not using dialysis maintains the patient's quality of life. ■

inaccurate readings (Figure 20-1). To check the size of the cuff, compare the length of the rubber bladder inside the cuff with the patient's arm circumference. The bladder should be at least 80% of the circumference of the arm. The width of the bladder should be about 40% the circumference of the arm. If it is larger or smaller, obtain a different size cuff.

- Two tubes. One tube is connected to the pressure control bulb and to the bladder inside the cuff. The other tube is connected to the pressure gauge.
- A pressure gauge, which may be a column of mercury (Figure 20-2A) or a round **aneroid gauge** (Figure 20-2B)

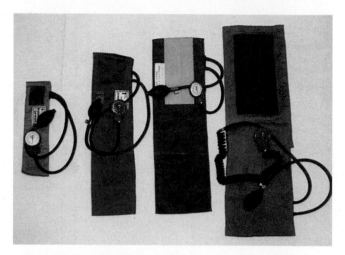

FIGURE 20-1 The cuff must fit properly for accurate readings. A variety of cuff sizes are available. (© Delmar/ Cengage Learning)

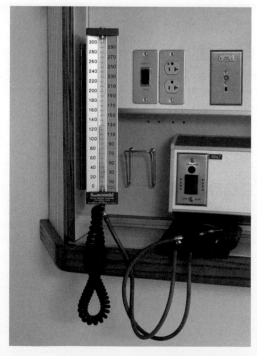

FIGURE 20-2A A mercury gravity sphygmomanometer. (© Delmar/Cengage Learning)

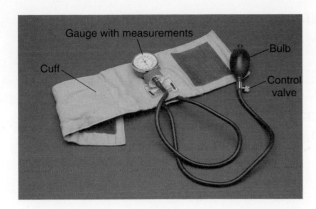

FIGURE 20-2B A dial (aneroid) sphygmomanometer. *(© Delmar/Cengage Learning)*

dial. Both are marked with numbers. Although some states do not permit the sale of new mercury-filled devices, many facilities still use existing mercury pressure gauges.

The stethoscope magnifies sounds. It consists of:

- A bell or diaphragm.
- Tubing that carries sounds to the listener.
- Earpieces that direct the sounds into the listener's ears. The earpieces and diaphragm must be cleaned with antiseptic before and after each use to prevent transmission of disease.

Electronic sphygmomanometers with attached cuffs are used in some facilities. You do not have to use a stethoscope with these units, because they automatically register the readings on a digital display. Follow the manufacturer's directions for the type of unit you are using. Some facilities use an instrument that measures pulse rate, temperature, and blood pressure (Figure 20-3).

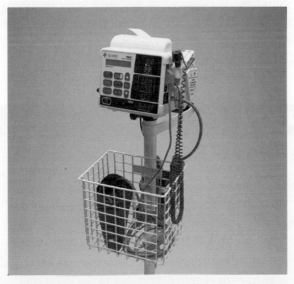

FIGURE 20-3 All vital signs may be checked with a single instrume. *(Vital·Check® patient monitor, photo courtesy of Alaris Medical Systems, Inc., San Diego, CA)*

Clinical Information ALERT

Some facilities prefer to measure the blood pressure in the left arm, if possible, because it is closest to the heart. ■

MEASURING THE BLOOD PRESSURE

Blood pressure is usually measured in the upper arm over the brachial artery. Check with the nurse before taking blood pressure readings anywhere else. The values are recorded in millimeters of mercury (mm Hg). Here are the steps for measuring brachial artery blood pressure:

1. Apply the cuff smoothly, directly over the **brachial artery** (1 inch above the *antecubital* area).

2. Place the stethoscope diaphragm over the brachial artery.

3. Apply pressure by inflating the rubber bladder in the cuff to stop the flow of blood through the artery.

4. Slowly release the pressure at a rate of about 2 to 3 mm per second. You will hear the sounds of heart valves closing. The sounds correspond to pressure changes in the blood.

5. The blood pressure is measured:
   a. At its highest point as the **systolic pressure.** This will be the first regular sound you will hear.
   b. At its lowest point as the **diastolic pressure**. This will be the change or last sound you will hear.
   c. The difference between systolic and diastolic pressure is called **pulse pressure**. The pulse pressure gives important information about the health of the arteries. The average pulse pressure in a healthy adult is about 40 millimeters (mm) of mercury (Hg) (range 30–50 mm Hg). However, factors in both health and disease can alter the pulse pressure. An increase in blood volume or heart rate or a decrease in the ability of the arteries to expand may result in an increased pulse pressure.

6. Record blood pressure values as an improper fraction; for example, systolic/diastolic or 130/92. This means the systolic pressure is 130 and the diastolic pressure is 92. Both numbers in the blood pressure are important, but for people who are 50 or older, systolic pressure gives the most accurate diagnosis of high blood pressure.

7. Blood pressure values:
   a. Average resting adult brachial artery pressure is less than 120 millimeters of mercury (mm Hg)

systolic and less than 80 millimeters of mercury (mm Hg) diastolic.

b. *Prehypertension* is a condition in which the person is likely to develop high blood pressure in the future. In this condition, blood pressure is between 120/80 mm Hg and 139/89 mm Hg. People with prehypertension can take steps to decrease their risk.

c. <u>Hypertension</u> (high blood pressure) exists when values are greater than 140 mm Hg systolic and 90 mm Hg diastolic.

d. <u>Hypotension</u> (low blood pressure) exists when values are less than 100 mm Hg systolic and 60 mm Hg diastolic. Excessive hypotension can lead to shock.

e. For either hypertension or hypotension, unusual or changed readings must be recorded and reported. (See Procedure 33.)

TABLE 20-2 BLOOD PRESSURE CLASSIFICATIONS

Blood Pressure Level (mm Hg)

Category	Systolic		Diastolic
Hypotension	<100	and	<60
Normal	<120	and	<80
Prehypertension	120–139	or	80–89
High blood pressure			
● Stage I hypertension	140–159	or	90–99
● Stage II hypertension	≥160	or	≥100

Note: < means less than; ≥ means greater than or equal to.

f. High blood pressure is a dangerous condition. There are no signs and symptoms. It increases the risk of several serious diseases (Unit 36). It can also cause complications of conditions such as diabetes. People with prehypertension and hypertension require regular blood pressure monitoring.

g. Blood pressure classifications are listed in Table 20-2. When systolic and diastolic blood pressures fall into different categories, the higher category is used to classify blood pressure level. For example, 172/78 mm Hg would be stage 2 hypertension (high blood pressure).

Clinical Information ALERT

Activity increases the pulse, respirations, and blood pressure. For accurate values, wait at least 30 minutes to take vital signs on patients who have participated in therapy, exercised, or have engaged in another activity, such as ambulating in the hallway, bathing, or showering. ■

Infection Control ALERT

Your bandage scissors, stethoscope, and other personal items may transfer pathogens from one patient to the next. If personal equipment items will be used during a procedure, wash them with an alcohol product or soap and water before and after each use. If you use a cloth stethoscope tubing cover, wash it each day with your uniform. Carry extra covers so you can change a cover if it becomes contaminated. ■

GUIDELINES *for*

Preparing to Measure Blood Pressure

Before using the stethoscope:

1. Clean the earpieces with an alcohol wipe (Figure 20-4A) and clean the diaphragm with a different alcohol wipe.

2. Point the earpieces forward when inserting them in your ears.

3. Use the diaphragm portion of the stethoscope.

4. Be sure the diaphragm portion is open so you will hear the beats.

Before using a sphygmomanometer:

● If using a mercury manometer—if the mercury moves up the column very slowly (Figure 20-4B), it may have oxidized. Report this to the nurse and use another sphygmomanometer.

continues

GUIDELINES *continued*

- If using an aneroid manometer—make sure the needle is on zero before you inflate the cuff (Figure 20-4C). If it is not, report this to the nurse and use another sphygmomanometer. Protect the gauge. Banging and bumping it will affect the accuracy of the gauge.

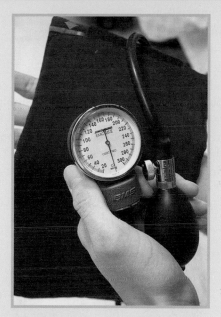

FIGURE 20-4C Make sure the needle is on zero before inflating the cuff on the aneroid sphygmomanometer. *(© Delmar/Cengage Learning)*

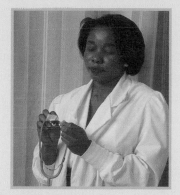

FIGURE 20-4A Clean the earpieces with an alcohol sponge before and after use. *(© Delmar/Cengage Learning)*

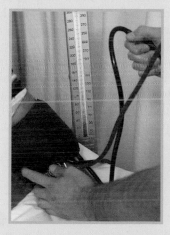

FIGURE 20-4B Do not use the sphygmomanometer if the mercury moves up the column slowly. *(© Delmar/Cengage Learning)*

Generally:

- Turn off radio and television when taking blood pressure. Ask the patient not to talk.

- Do not take blood pressure on an arm that:
  - Is paralyzed
  - Is the site of an intravenous infusion (IV)
  - Has a pulse oximeter on it
  - Has impaired circulation
  - Is the site of a dialysis access device
  - Is fractured
  - Is burned
  - Is on the same side as a recent mastectomy or other surgical procedure site

Inaccurate Blood Pressure Readings

Causes of inaccurate blood pressure readings include:

- Use of a wrong-size cuff
- An improperly wrapped cuff
- Incorrect positioning of arm
- Not using the same arm for all readings
- Not having the gauge at eye level
- Deflating the cuff too slowly
- Mistaking an **auscultatory gap** (sound fadeout for 10 to 15 mm Hg which then begins again) as the diastolic pressure

How to Read the Gauge

The gauges on sphygmomanometers are marked with a series of lines. The large lines are at increments of

10 millimeters of mercury pressure. The shorter lines are at 2-mm intervals. For example, the first small line above 80 mm is 82 mm. The first small line below 80 mm is 78 mm (Figure 20-5).

To properly read the mercury gauge:

- It should be at eye level.
- It should not be tilted.
- The reading should be taken at the top of the column of mercury. It should not be taken at the "hump" in the middle of the mercury when you hear the first sound.

To properly read the aneroid gauge, observe the gauge at eye level. Do not read it at an angle.

Following completion of the blood pressure measurement, you will record and report the following:

- If you were unable to hear the reading

- If blood pressure is higher than in a previous reading
- If blood pressure is lower than in a previous reading
- If the site where you took the reading was other than the brachial artery

Infection Control ALERT

Clean the manual or electronic blood pressure cuff and tubing with a facility-approved disinfectant after each patient. Alternatives are to use a disposable cuff that is issued to each patient and used throughout the hospital stay, or to cover the cuff with a disposable sleeve. ∎

PULSE OXIMETERS

Some electronic vital-signs monitors also measure the pulse oximeter value (Unit 36). The nursing assistant slips a spring clip over the patient's fingertip, and the unit displays the value. If the unit you are using also measures the pulse oximeter value, apply the spring finger clip to the hand on the *opposite side* from the blood pressure cuff. (Applying it to an arm with an inflated blood pressure cuff will cause inaccurate values.) The spring finger clip *may be* applied to an arm with an IV, dialysis access device, or the side affected by a stroke or mastectomy without causing injury. The unit will obtain a reading quickly, usually within a few seconds. If the value is below 95, have the patient take a few deep breaths, and then check the reading again. You may remove the spring clip as soon as the reading is obtained.

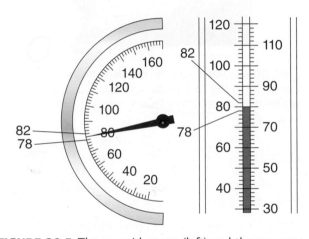

FIGURE 20-5 The aneroid gauge (left) and the mercury gauge (right). Take the reading at the closest line. (© Delmar/Cengage Learning)

PROCEDURE

33

TAKING BLOOD PRESSURE

Note: This is the "two-step" procedure recommended by the American Heart Association (AHA) beginning in 1993. The AHA considers the two-step procedure the most reliable for normal blood pressure measurement. (The most accurate values are obtained by internal monitoring, in which a catheter is placed in an artery. The internal method is not practical for most clinical situations.) In some facilities and states, nursing assistants use a one-step procedure for

measuring blood pressure. For more information, see the appendix in the Online Companion to this book.

1. Carry out initial procedure actions.

2. Assemble equipment:

- Sphygmomanometer with appropriate size cuff
- Stethoscope
- Alcohol wipes

PROCEDURE **33** CONTINUED

3. Remove the patient's arm from sleeve or roll the sleeve 5 inches above the elbow; it should not be tight or binding.

4. Locate the brachial artery with your fingertips (Figure 20-6A).

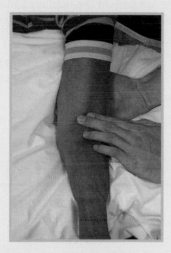

FIGURE 20-6A Locate the brachial artery with your fingertips. (© *Delmar/Cengage Learning*)

5. Place the patient's arm palm upward, supported on the bed or a table, at heart level.

6. Wrap the cuff smoothly and snugly around the arm. Center the bladder over the brachial artery. The bottom of the cuff should be one inch above the antecubital space (inner elbow) (Figure 20-6B). The clothing should not come into contact with the cuff or stethoscope.

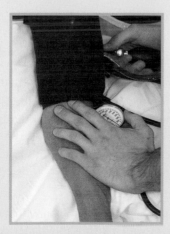

FIGURE 20-6B The bottom of the cuff should be at least 1 inch above the antecubital space (inner elbow). (© *Delmar/Cengage Learning*)

7. Place the bulb in your dominant hand and feel for the radial pulse with the fingers of your other hand (Figure 20-6C). To find out how high to pump the cuff:

- Rapidly inflate the cuff until you no longer feel the radial pulse.

- Add 30 mm to that reading. (For example, if you no longer feel the pulse when the mercury or needle reaches 130, add 30 mm for a reading of 160.) Note that point.

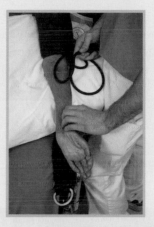

FIGURE 20-6C Hold the bulb in your dominant hand and feel for the brachial pulse with the fingers of the other hand. (© *Delmar/Cengage Learning*)

8. Quickly and steadily deflate the cuff. Wait 15 to 30 seconds.

9. Place the stethoscope over the brachial artery (Figure 20-6D).

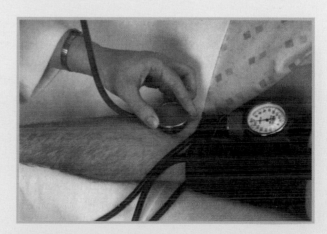

FIGURE 20-6D Hold the stethoscope bell securely over the brachial artery. (© *Delmar/Cengage Learning*)

continues

PROCEDURE 33 CONTINUED

10. Reinflate the cuff quickly and steadily to the level you calculated (in the example in Step 7, to 160).

11. Release the air at an even pace, about 2 to 3 mm per second. Keep your eyes on the needle or the mercury.

12. Listen for the onset of at least two consecutive beats. Note where the needle is on the sphygmomanometer when you first hear the sound. (Do not stop deflating the cuff.) This is your systolic reading.

13. Continue deflating the cuff. The last sound you hear is the diastolic reading. Continue to deflate and to listen for 10 to 20 mm more to make sure you have the correct diastolic reading.

14. Record the reading (blood pressure is always recorded in even numbers, with the systolic on top and the diastolic on the bottom; e.g., 128/82). Indicate the arm used and the patient's position (sitting, lying down, or standing).

15. If you are not sure of the reading and need to retake the blood pressure, wait 1 to 2 minutes before repeating the procedure.

16. Clean the earpieces of the stethoscope with alcohol wipes. If the tubing has contacted the patient or linen, wipe it as well.

17. Return equipment to the appropriate area.

18. Carry out ending procedure actions.

GUIDELINES *for*

Electronic Blood Pressure Monitoring

Patient Selection (refer to Figure 20-7)

• You can do this procedure on patients of all ages and sizes, but you *must* use appropriately sized cuffs.

• At least one blood pressure reading should be taken using the auscultation method before an electronic blood pressure device is used. The auscultation reading is needed as a baseline with which to compare the values from the electronic device.

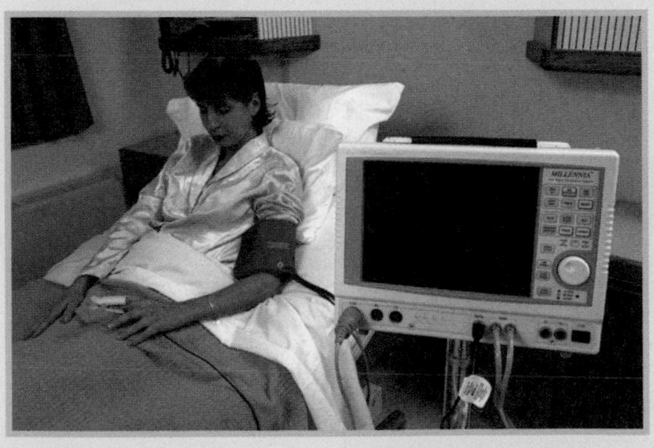

The procedure is contraindicated in patients with:

• Extreme hypertension or hypotension

• Very rapid heart rates

• Excessive body movement or tremors

• Irregular heart rhythms or atrial dysrhythmias

Patients for whom electronic blood pressure monitoring is not acceptable should be known to all caregivers and identified on the care plan or Kardex. If in doubt, check with the nurse for instructions.

Application of the Cuff

• Select the proper cuff size. Clean with a disinfectant wipe or cover with a disposable paper cover.

• The upper arm is the preferred location for the monitoring cuff. Check with the nurse before using other areas.

FIGURE 20-7 The electronic blood pressure monitoring unit takes the blood pressure automatically. (© *Delmar/Cengage Learning*)

PROCEDURE

34

TAKING BLOOD PRESSURE WITH AN ELECTRONIC BLOOD PRESSURE APPARATUS

1. Carry out initial procedure actions.

2. Assemble equipment:
   - Electronic blood pressure device
   - Assortment of cuffs and tubes

3. Wipe the tubing and cuff with a disinfectant wipe. Apply a disposable sleeve over the cuff, if used. Bring the electronic blood pressure unit to the bedside. Place it near the patient and plug it into a source of electricity.

4. Locate the on/off switch and turn the machine on.

5. Select the appropriate cuff for the machine and size for the patient's extremity.

6. Remove restrictive clothing.

7. Squeeze excess air out of the cuff.

8. Connect the cuff to the connector hose.

9. Wrap the cuff snugly around the patient's extremity, verifying that only one finger can fit between the cuff and the patient's skin. Make sure the "artery" arrow marked on the outside of

the cuff is correctly placed over the brachial artery.

10. Verify that the connector hose between the cuff and the machine is not kinked.

11. Set the frequency control for automatic or manual.

12. Press the start button.

13. If the cuff will take periodic, automatic measurements, set the designated frequency of blood pressure measurements.

14. Set upper and lower alarm limits for systolic, diastolic, and mean blood pressure readings.

15. Remove the cuff at least every 2 hours and rotate sites, if possible. Evaluate the skin for redness and irritation. Report abnormalities to the nurse.

16. Wipe the tubing and cuff with a disinfectant wipe. Discard the disposable sleeve, if used.

17. Carry out ending procedure actions.

REVIEW

A. Multiple Choice

Select the one best answer for each of the following.

1. Do not apply a blood pressure cuff
   a. when pulse oximeter values are being checked.
   b. to an arm with a dialysis access device.
   c. above the antecubital space.
   d. that is less than 50% of the arm diameter.

2. Measurement of the amount of force exerted on the walls of the arteries as blood flows through is
   a. pulse.
   b. blood pressure.
   c. pressure factor.
   d. arterial pulse.

3. The patient's blood pressure reading is 130/84. The diastolic reading is
   a. 214.
   b. 130.
   c. 84.
   d. 56.

4. Hypertension is
   a. high blood pressure.
   b. low blood pressure.
   c. nervousness.
   d. rapid pulse.

5. You have taken the blood pressure of a patient and are not sure of the reading. Your best action is to
   a. tell another nursing assistant.
   b. look up the last reading and record the same numbers.
   c. tell the nurse about your uncertainty and ask her what to do.
   d. ignore the reading and take the patient's blood pressure the next day.

6. You take Bill Walker's blood pressure and find that it is 220/160. Mr. Walker has hypertension and previously had a stroke. You know that this blood pressure reading is
   a. too high.
   b. normal for a patient with hypertension.
   c. hypotensive.
   d. too low.

7. The usual location for taking blood pressure is the
   a. carotid artery.
   b. brachial artery.
   c. radial vein.
   d. femoral vein.

8. The blood pressure taken during the resting phase of the heart cycle is
   a. systolic.
   b. diastolic.

   c. tachycardia.
   d. prehypertension.

9. Hypotension is blood pressure
   a. under 140/90.
   b. over 140/90.
   c. under 100/60.
   d. over 90/60.

10. The instrument used to take a blood pressure reading is the
    a. thermometer.
    b. aneroid dial.
    c. mercury probe.
    d. sphygmomanometer.

B. Nursing Assistant Challenge

You are assigned to take Mr. King's blood pressure at 12:00 noon. He is a very heavy man and has an IV inserted in his left arm. His blood pressure was 180/140 at 8:00 AM. Answer the following questions.

11. What effect will his size have on your selection of cuff? *bigger cuff*

12. On which arm will you apply the cuff? *right*

13. Will you report your findings? *HBP*

14. Why or why not?

UNIT **21**

Measuring Height and Weight

OBJECTIVES

After completing this unit, you will be able to:
- Spell and define terms.
- List six nursing assistant actions to ensure that height and weight measurements are accurate.
- Identify at least four types of scales and give an example of when each type is used.

- Describe the proper use of an overbed scale.
- Demonstrate the following procedure:
  - Procedure 35 Measuring Weight and Height

VOCABULARY

Learn the meaning and the correct spelling of the following words and phrases:

balance bar	centimeter (cm)	kilogram (kg)	pound (lb)
baseline	increment		

WEIGHT AND HEIGHT MEASUREMENTS

Changes in weight are often used as an indicator of the patient's condition.
- A **baseline** (original) measurement of height and weight is usually obtained when the patient is admitted. These measurements are usually noted on the Kardex.
- Weights are frequently measured when patients are given drugs (diuretics) to increase their urine output.
- Weight is an indicator of the patient's nutritional status.
- Measurements of weight and height must be accurate and recorded according to facility policy, because medications may be ordered according to the patient's size.

- Height measurements may be recorded in feet (') and inches (") or in **centimeters (cm)**.
- Weight measurements may be recorded in **pounds (lb)** or **kilograms (kg)**.

  Note: Some facilities use the metric system, so you may be recording weight in kilograms. If your facility uses this measurement system, the scales will be calibrated for the metric system. You will not be required to convert measurements from the inch and pound system to the metric system.

- The upright scale is used for ambulatory patients who can stand unattended on the platform (Figure 21-1).
- A mechanical lift with scale can be used to weigh patients who cannot stand when a wheelchair scale is not available (Figure 21-2).

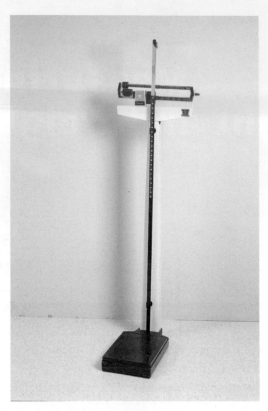

FIGURE 21-1 An upright scale is used only for patients who can stand unaided on the platform. *(© Delmar/ Cengage Learning)*

- Sling scales can be used to weigh patients whose conditions do not permit the use of a mechanical lift/scale (Figure 21-3).

- Chair scales are used to weigh patients who cannot stand long enough to be weighed, and are seated in chairs or wheelchairs (Figure 21-4).

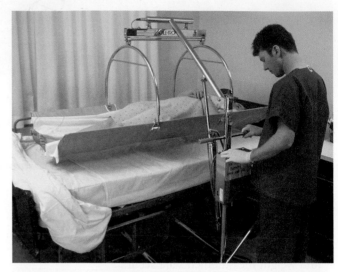

FIGURE 21-3 The sling scale is used for bedfast patients who are not ambulatory or are too heavy or difficult to move. *(© Delmar/Cengage Learning)*

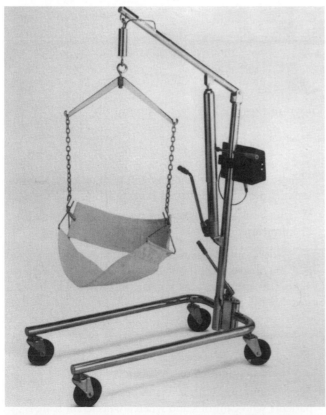

FIGURE 21-2 The scale on the mechanical lift is used when patients cannot stand and a wheelchair is not available. *(Photo courtesy Health O Meter®)*

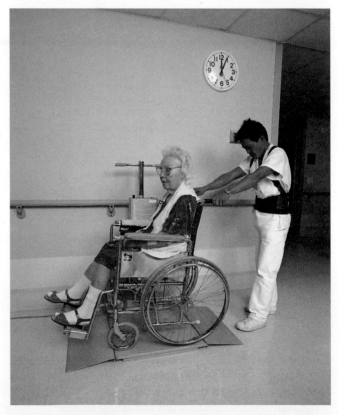

FIGURE 21-4 Electronic chair scales are used for patients who cannot stand on an upright scale. *(© Delmar/ Cengage Learning)*

Clinical Information ALERT

If the patient uses a lap tray on the wheelchair, remove the tray before weighing the patient. If the tray cannot be removed, weigh the empty wheelchair (with the tray), then subtract the combined weight from the total patient weight. Lap trays can add as much as 8 pounds to the total weight. (Refers to the type of scale pictured in Figure 21-4.) ∎

Clinical Information ALERT

Some patients have orders for daily weight. A weight gain usually suggests fluid retention. A 2-pound gain in a short time suggests that the patient is retaining an extra liter of fluid. Weight loss means that excess fluid has left the body. ∎

GUIDELINES *for*

Obtaining Accurate Weight and Height Measurements

To obtain an accurate weight measurement, you must:

- Always balance the scale before using it so the weights hang free.
- Have the patient empty his or her bladder.
- If the patient uses incontinent briefs, be sure the brief is dry before weighing.
- If the patient has an indwelling catheter, empty the bag before weighing.
- Weigh the patient at the same time of day each time.
- Have the patient wear the same type of garments each time.
- Use the same method and the same scale each time, if possible.
- If the patient has a cast, has recently had a cast removed, or has new onset edema, consult the nurse about possible weight discrepancies.

You must learn to read the scale correctly. There are two bars on the upright scale (see Figure 21-1). The **balance bar** should hang free to start.

- The lower bar indicates weights in 50-pound **increments** (amounts).
- The upper bar denotes one-quarter-pound increments (Figure 21-5).
- The even-numbered pounds are marked with numbers.
- The long line between each number indicates the odd-numbered pounds.
- Each small line indicates one-quarter pound, or 4 ounces.

The two figures are added and recorded as the person's total weight. The sum is recorded according to facility policy in either pounds or kilograms. For example:

Lower bar = 100 pounds

Upper bar = +22 pounds

Total = 122 pounds

Height is measured with the ruler attached to an upright scale or with a tape measure when the patient is in bed.

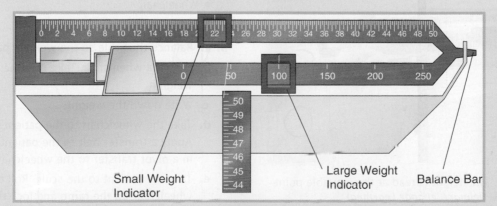

FIGURE 21-5 The upper bar indicates smaller pound weights. The weight shown on the lower bar is measured in 50-pound increments. This figure is added to the amount shown on the upper bar. (© *Delmar/Cengage Learning*)

PROCEDURE

35

MEASURING WEIGHT AND HEIGHT

Using a Standing Scale

1. Carry out initial procedure actions.

2. Assemble equipment:
   - Scale
   - Paper towels
   - Pad and pen

3. **a.** Balance the scale so the bar hangs freely on the end.

   b. Place a paper towel on the scale platform.

   c. Assist the patient to remove shoes and stand on the platform.

   d. Move the weights on the bars until they hang freely.

   e. Add the amounts on the two bars to determine the patient's weight. Write this down on your note pad or remember it (see Figure 21-5).

   f. Assist the patient to turn around, facing away from the scale.

   g. Raise the height bar until it is level with the top of the patient's head.

   h. Record the measurement in the center of the height bar (Figure 21-6).

   i. Help the patient down from the scale and assist to put on shoes, if necessary.

   j. Remove and discard the paper towel.

   k. Carry out ending procedure actions.

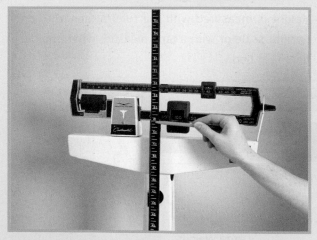

FIGURE 21-6 The height is read at the movable point of the ruler. (© *Delmar/Cengage Learning*)

Using a Chair Scale

Note: This procedure refers to a scale with a permanently mounted chair.

4. Carry out initial procedure actions.

5. Assemble equipment:
   - Chair scale
   - Wheelchair
   - Transfer belt

6. **a.** Balance the scale so the weights hang free.

   b. Apply a transfer belt to the patient and assist in a pivot transfer to the wheelchair.

   c. Take the patient in the wheelchair to the chair scale. Lock the brakes. Be sure the brakes of the chair scale are locked in place.

   d. Apply a transfer belt to the patient and assist in a pivot transfer to the chair on the scale. Instruct the patient to sit down when the chair is felt against the back of the legs. Once the patient is seated, be sure the patient's feet are on the footrest(s) of the chair.

   e. Walk behind the scale to obtain the reading.

   f. Transfer the patient back to the wheelchair.

   g. Carry out ending procedure actions.

Using a Wheelchair Scale

This procedure refers to the scale used in Figure 21-4.

7. Carry out initial procedure actions.

8. Assemble equipment:
   - Wheelchair scale
   - Wheelchair
   - Transfer belt

9. **a.** Balance the scale so the weights hang free.

   b. Obtain a wheelchair. Take it to the scale and weigh it.

   c. Write down the weight.

   d. Take the wheelchair to the patient's room. Apply a transfer belt to the patient and assist in a pivot transfer to the wheelchair.

   e. Take the patient to the scale. Roll the wheelchair up the ramp and lock the brakes.

continues

PROCEDURE 35 CONTINUED

f. Adjust the weights until the balance bar hangs freely on the end. Write down this number on your note pad.

g. Unlock the brakes and slowly guide the wheelchair down the ramp.

h. Return to the patient's room and assist the patient to transfer out of the wheelchair.

i. Subtract the weight of the empty wheelchair from the total weight of the patient and chair and record this number.

j. Carry out ending procedure actions.

Using a Bed Scale

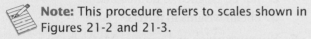 **Note:** This procedure refers to scales shown in Figures 21-2 and 21-3.

10. Carry out initial procedure actions.

11. Assemble equipment:
   - Manual or electronic bed scale or mechanical lift scale
   - Chains and straps
   - Clean sheet

12. Follow the guidelines in Procedure 20 for assisting the patient into the lift seat or sling.

13. a. Balance the scale with the canvas seat, clean sheet, chains, or straps attached. The bars should hang freely.

   b. Cover the sling with a clean sheet if the patient is undressed.

   c. Remove the sling from the scale and position the patient on the sling.

   d. Connect the straps and elevate the lift above the level of the bed. Raise the sling so the patient's body and the sling hang freely over the bed.

   e. Adjust the weights until the balance bar hangs freely on the end, or read the electronic display screen (Figure 21-7). Remember this number or write it on your note pad.

   f. Lower the patient back into the bed and remove the sling.

   g. Carry out ending procedure actions.

Measuring the Patient in Bed

14. Carry out initial procedure actions.

15. Assemble equipment:
   - Tape measure
   - Pad and pen

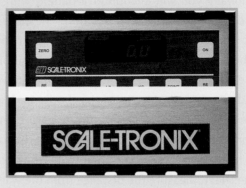

FIGURE 21-7 Press the "on" button to calibrate the scale. This will cause the reading to return to zero. *(Courtesy of Scale-Tronix, White Plains, NY)*

16. a. Position the patient in the supine position.

   b. Straighten the patient's back, arms, and legs so that she is lying as straight as possible.

   c. Straighten and tighten the sheets.

   d. Place a pencil mark on the sheet even with the patient's head.

   e. Place another pencil mark at the level of the patient's heels.

   f. Measure the distance between the two marks with a tape measure to obtain the patient's height (Figure 21-8).

   g. Carry out ending procedure actions.

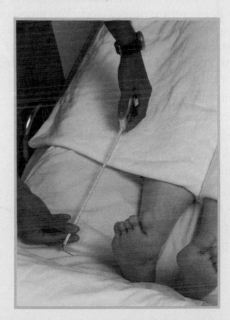

FIGURE 21-8 To find the height of the patient in bed, measure from the pencil line at the bottom of the feet to the pencil line at the top of the head. *(© Delmar/ Cengage Learning)*

Clinical Information ALERT

Occasionally you will encounter a patient who is badly contracted in the fetal position. The easiest way to measure this person is to use a tape measure when the patient is in the side-lying position. Be sure the tape measure is taut, straight, and not twisted or folded. Measure the body in two or three segments, depending on the nature and location of the contractures. Measure from the top of the head to the waist, and then write down the number. Next, measure the distance from the waist to behind the knees. Write down this number. Now measure from behind the knees to the bottoms of the heels. Write down this number. Finally, add together all of the numbers you have recorded to obtain the total height measurement. ■

REVIEW

A. Multiple Choice

Select the one best answer for each of the following.

1. Ramona Bjork is a 72-year-old patient with kidney disease. She is on fluid restriction. She goes to the dialysis center three times a week. You must take her vital signs when she returns from dialysis. The care plan states that you are to weigh her daily. Her weight on Monday is 133 pounds. On Tuesday, her weight is 140. You should
   a. inform the nurse of the weight gain.
   b. record the weight before going home.
   c. call the dialysis center and ask their advice.
   d. tell the patient she is drinking too many fluids.

2. When weighing a patient on the balance scale, you know that each marking on the lower bar represents
   a. 1 pound.
   b. 5 pounds.

   c. 25 pounds.
   d. 50 pounds.

3. You are assigned to weigh Mrs. Abrera using an electronic scale. When you plug the unit into the outlet, a spark shoots out. The digital display comes on, suggesting that the scale is working properly. You should
   a. avoid using the scale and apply a lockout tag.
   b. continue with the procedure.
   c. return the scale to the utility room.
   d. close the door in case there is a fire.

4. Your facility records all weights as metric values. This means you will
   a. use a scale set to metric values.
   b. convert pounds to centimeters.
   c. not be assigned to do weights.
   d. obtain weights in meters.

5. You must weigh and measure Mr. Volbrecht, a bedfast patient who is contracted in the fetal position. You will use a
   a. balance scale with height bar.
   b. yardstick and wheelchair scale.
   c. ruler and electronic scale.
   d. tape measure and sling scale.

6. When measuring a patient's height using the ruler bar on the balance scale, you will read the height measurement
   a. at the top of the height bar.
   b. on the lower balance beam.
   c. at the movable part of the height bar.
   d. in the center of the ruler.

7. You will calibrate the digital scale by
   a. balancing the weights.
   b. turning the scale on.
   c. standing on the platform.
   d. placing a weight on each side.

8. When using a sling scale to weigh a bedfast patient,
   a. raise the sling at least 3 feet above the bed.
   b. move the sling completely away from the bed.
   c. neither the sling nor the patient should touch the bed.
   d. hold the sling so it does not sway back and forth.

B. Nursing Assistant Challenge

Mrs. Haughn is in bed recovering from a stroke. She is unable to walk or stand. She is receiving diuretics. Her doctor wants to order some new medication that is given according to the patient's size. You are assigned to weigh and measure the height of this patient. Answer each of the following by selecting the correct answer.

9. The best way to weigh this patient is with
   a. an upright scale.
   b. an overbed scale.
   c. a wheelchair scale.
   d. a chair scale.

10. The best way to measure this patient is
    a. with a height bar.
    b. with a tape measure.

c. to ask the patient.
d. to estimate the height.

11. One reason the physician might have asked for the patient's weight is because the patient
    a. is receiving diuretics.
    b. has had a stroke.
    c. cannot stand.
    d. cannot walk.

12. The patient measures 63 inches. This may be expressed as
    a. 5 feet 6 inches.
    b. 5 feet 8 inches.
    c. 5 feet 3 inches.
    d. 6 feet 3 inches.

SECTION 7

Patient Care and Comfort Measures

UNIT 22

Admission, Transfer, and Discharge

OBJECTIVES

After completing this unit, you will be able to:
- Spell and define terms.
- List the ways the nursing assistant can help in the processes of admission, transfer, and discharge.
- List ways in which the nursing assistant can develop positive relationships with a patient's family members.

- Demonstrate the following procedures:
  - Procedure 36 Admitting the Patient
  - Procedure 37 Transferring the Patient
  - Procedure 38 Discharging the Patient

VOCABULARY

Learn the meaning and the correct spelling of the following words and phrases:

admission   baseline assessment   discharge   transfer

INTRODUCTION

The nurse is responsible for overseeing and carrying out hospital procedures and physician's orders regarding all admissions, transfers, and discharges. You will assist by carrying out the routine procedures associated with these activities.

A nursing assistant or someone from the admissions office accompanies the new patient to the unit. Someone must always escort the patient to the unit for admission. In many facilities, someone must also escort the patient from the unit at the time of discharge. Personnel must accompany patients during transfers to other units in the facility.

You can do much to make these activities easier for the patient, family, and the other staff members by:

- Having equipment and materials prepared for the activity.
- Being very observant during each activity.

- Documenting observations carefully and accurately. These make a valuable contribution to the nurse's initial **baseline assessment** of the patient's condition.
- Reporting observations to the nurse.
- Giving attention to the details of each procedure.
- Being aware of the emotional stress on patients and their families.
- Being courteous to everyone.

ADMISSION

When a person enters a health care facility, the **admission** process is often stressful to the patient, family, and friends. The first impression created is very important. The patient's perception of what is happening may be affected by illness, pain, and fear (Figure 22-1). You will be one of the first staff members the patient sees, so it is important that you be courteous, confident, and efficient. (See Procedure 36.)

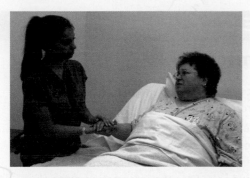

FIGURE 22-1 Treat patients and families with courtesy, respect, compassion, and understanding. Remember that admissions can be stressful for both the patient and family. First impressions are lasting ones, and you represent your facility to the patient. *(© Delmar/Cengage Learning)*

Open and prepare the unit as soon as you are notified of a new admission. If the patient will be admitted by ambulance or stretcher, elevate the bed to the highest horizontal height, and open the bed. Move furnishings, if necessary, so the stretcher can be positioned next to the bed.

When a patient is ready for admission, ask the nurse if:

- The patient requires a stretcher or wheelchair to reach the unit.

- Any special equipment, such as oxygen or an IV pole, is needed.

- There are any special instructions, such as withholding fluids or foods.

Introduce yourself and observe the patient carefully. Listen for complaints as you escort and assist the patient to the room and to bed. The nurse will assess the patient and begin a care plan. Your observations, and vital sign, height, and weight measurements, contribute to this assessment. You should also note and report your observations about unusual skin problems, pressure ulcers, patient concerns or problems, and any abnormalities. Monitor the patient's ability to transfer and ambulate.

Offer to assist in unpacking and storing the patient's belongings. Complete the personal belongings inventory, and ask the patient to sign it. Fill in all admission forms for which you are responsible, and make the patient and family as comfortable as possible.

If you must ask visitors to leave, do so in a kind and polite manner. They will be anxious to remain and see the patient settled and comfortable. Inform them where they may wait. Notify them when you have finished the admission process, so they can return.

FAMILY DYNAMICS

The family is an extension of the patient. They must make many adjustments when the patient is admitted to the hospital. This is often a very emotional time. Family members may feel relieved because the patient is getting help. They may also feel guilty for being unable to care for the loved one at home.

Communication HIGHLIGHT

There is a common expression that "first impressions are usually lasting ones." Making a good first impression on the patient and family members is important. If the first impression of the nursing assistant is negative, this may color the patient's and family's impression of all health care workers, and even the whole facility. Think about this and do your best to provide a positive, professional impression. ■

Understanding the emotions that families experience (Figure 22-2) should give you an appreciation of why making a good first impression is so important. Introduce yourself and explain your responsibilities as a nursing assistant in the care of their loved one (Figure 22-3). Introduce the patient and family to roommates and other staff members. Make them feel welcome and show that you are sincerely interested in the patient.

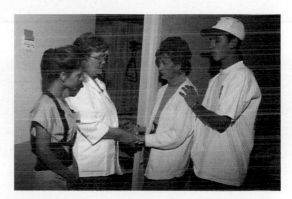

FIGURE 22-2 Families experience a wide range of emotions when a loved one is admitted to the hospital. Use good communication skills and show that you care. *(© Delmar/Cengage Learning)*

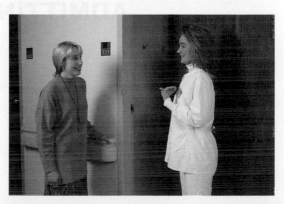

FIGURE 22-3 Make it a point to speak to family members when they visit. Treat each family member with warmth, courtesy, kindness, and respect. *(© Delmar/Cengage Learning)*

GUIDELINES *for*

Family Dynamics

know

✗ Get to know family members. Greet them warmly when they visit.

✗ Wear a name badge. Introduce yourself by name and position.

✗ Work to build a positive and trusting relationship with family members.

● Be available to talk to the family. Tell them about the patient's activities. Listen carefully to what they have to say and respond appropriately.

✗ Let the family know that you respect and support their role as their loved one's caregivers.

● Familiarize the family with facility routines and services.

● Refer questions of a medical or personal nature to the nurse.

✗ Listen to family members' suggestions, complaints, and comments. Inform the nurse of complaints or

concerns, or refer the family to the nurse, as appropriate.

● If the family has been caring for the patient at home, they often know what works best. Listen closely to family members' advice about patient care. Pass the information on to the nurse.

● Inform the nurse if a visit is stressful or tiring to a patient.

● Avoid judging the family and decisions they make. Stay out of family disagreements.

● Avoid gossiping with the family, and do not discuss facility business with family members.

● Allow the family to participate in the patient's care, if the patient does not object. However, avoid making the family feel as if they must assist with the care of the patient.

Safety ALERT

Never leave the room until the patient is safe, has the call signal in reach, and knows how to use it. ■

PROCEDURE

36

ADMITTING THE PATIENT

1. Wash hands.

2. Assemble equipment:

   ● Equipment for urine specimen collection, if needed

   ● Equipment for taking temperature

   ● Pad and pencil

   ● Patient's chart or worksheet

   ● Stethoscope

   ● Admission kit

     – water pitcher

     – glass

     – liquid soap

     – washcloth

     – towel

PROCEDURE 36 CONTINUED

- – basin
- – lotion
- – mouthwash
- Scale
- Blood pressure cuff and manometer
- Watch with second hand
- Disposable gloves (if urine specimen is required)

3. Prepare the unit for the patient by:
   a. Making sure that all necessary equipment and furniture are in their proper places and in good working order.
   b. Checking the unit for adequate lighting.
   c. Loosening the top linen at the foot of the bed. This is called a *toe pleat* (see Unit 23).
   d. Opening the bed (Figure 22-4).

4. Introduce yourself and identify the patient both by asking the name and checking the identification bracelet.

5. Ask the patient to be seated, if ambulatory.
   a. Ask the family to go to the lounge or lobby while the patient is being admitted.
   b. Introduce the patient to the other patients in the room, unless it is a private room.

6. Screen the unit to provide privacy (Figure 22-5).

7. Help the patient to undress and put on a hospital gown or night clothes from home. Care for clothing according to facility policy.

8. Check the patient's vital signs, weight, and height.

9. Help the patient get into bed. Adjust the side rails as needed.

10. Follow your facility policies for caring for valuables or sending them home.

11. Tell the patient if a urine specimen is necessary.
    a. Put on gloves and assist the patient as necessary.
    b. Allow the patient to use the bathroom, if ambulatory, or offer the bedpan or urinal.

12. Pour the patient's specimen from the bedpan or urinal into the specimen bottle. Apply the cap. Remove gloves and dispose of them according to facility policy. Be sure to label the specimen correctly (see Unit 26).

13. Complete the admission form (Figure 22-6).

14. If admission is to a long-term care facility, label clothing and complete the personal belongings inventory form according to facility policy.

15. Orient the patient to the unit.

16. Carry out ending procedure actions.

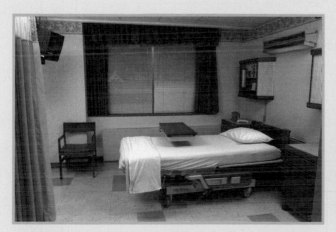

FIGURE 22-4 An open bed notifies everyone that a patient is expected. (© Delmar/Cengage Learning)

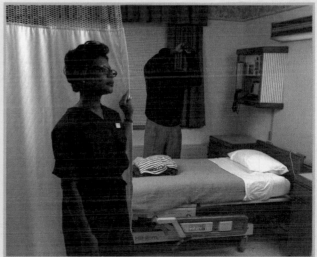

FIGURE 22-5 Provide privacy so the patient can undress. (© Delmar/Cengage Learning)

continues

PROCEDURE 36 CONTINUED

PATIENT PREFERS TO BE ADDRESSED AS:

_____

FROM: ☐ E.R.   ☐ E.C.F.   ☐ HOME   ☐ M.D.'S OFFICE

COMMUNICATES IN ENGLISH: ☐ WELL   ☐ MINIMAL

☐ INTERPRETER (NAME PERSON)   ☐ NONE

_____

MODE OF TRANSPORTATION:

☐ AMBULATORY   ☐ OTHER   **SMOKER:** ☐ Y ☐ N

☐ WHEELCHAIR   _____

☐ STRETCHER   _____

☐ NOT AT ALL   ☐ OTHER LANGUAGE (SPECIFY) _____

HOME TELEPHONE NO. ( ) _____

WORK TELEPHONE NO. ( ) _____

ORIENTATION TO ENVIRONMENT:

☐ ARMBAND CHECKED   ☐ CALL LIGHT

☐ BED CONTROL   ☐ PHONE

☐ TV CONTROL   ☐ SIDE RAIL POLICY

☐ BATH ROOM   ☐ VISITATION POLICY

☐ PERSONAL PROPERTY POLICY   ☐ SMOKING POLICY

PERSONAL BELONGINGS: (CHECK AND DESCRIBE)

☐ CLOTHING _____

☐ JEWELRY _____

☐ MONEY _____

☐ WALKER _____

☐ WHEELCHAIR _____

☐ CANE _____

☐ OTHER _____

DENTURES: **CONTACT LENSES:**

☐ UPPER   ☐ PARTIAL   ☐ HARD   ☐ LT   ☐ RT

☐ LOWER   ☐ NONE   ☐ SOFT

GLASSES: ☐ Y ☐ N   **HEARING AID:** ☐ Y ☐ N

PROSTHESIS: ☐ Y ☐ N

(DESCRIBE) _____

DISPOSITION OF VALUABLES:

☐ PATIENT

☐ HOME   GIVEN TO: _____

   RELATIONSHIP: _____

☐ PLACED
   IN SAFE _____

   (CLAIM NO.)

IN CASE OF EMERGENCY NOTIFY:

NAME: _____

RELATIONSHIP: _____

HOME TELEPHONE NO. ( ) _____

WORK TELEPHONE NO. ( ) _____

VITAL SIGNS

TEMP: _____ ☐ ORAL   ☐ RECTAL   ☐ AXILLARY

PULSE: _____ ☐ RADIAL   ☐ APICAL   RESPIRATORY
RATE _____

☐ RT

B/P: _____ ☐ LT ☐ STANDING ☐ SITTING   ☐ LYING

HEIGHT: _____ WEIGHT: _____   ☐ BEDSIDE

   ☐ STANDING

ALLERGIES:

MEDICATIONS: ☐ NONE KNOWN   FOOD: ☐ NONE KNOWN

☐ PENICILLIN   ☐ TAPE   (SHELLFISH, EGGS, MILK, ETC.)

☐ SULFA   ☐ OTHER (LIST)   _____

☐ IODINE   _____   _____

☐ ASPIRIN   _____   _____

☐ MORPHINE   _____   _____

☐ DEMEROL   _____   _____

(PRESCRIPTIVE & NON PRESCRIPTIVE)

MEDICATIONS: **DOSE/FREQUENCY**   (DATE/TIME) **LAST DOSE**

1. _____   _____   _____

2. _____   _____   _____

3. _____   _____   _____

4. _____   _____   _____

5. _____   _____   _____

6. _____   _____   _____

DISPOSITION OF MEDICATIONS:

☐ NONE BROUGHT TO HOSPITAL

☐ SENT HOME _____

   WITH _____

☐ TO PHARMACY: (LIST) _____

_____

ADMITTING DIAGNOSIS: _____

NURSE'S SIGNATURE: _____   RN/LVN   DATE _____ TIME _____

CHARTER SUBURBAN HOSPITAL
16453 SOUTH COLORADO AVENUE
PARAMOUNT, CALIFORNIA 90723
NURSING ADMISSION ASSESSMENT PAGE 1 of 6

FIGURE 22-6 Recording accurate and complete admission information is an important contribution to the nursing assessment. (© Delmar/Cengage Learning)

TRANSFER

It may be necessary for the patient to be moved to another unit. Preparations for the transfer will be handled by the nurse, but you may be asked to assist (see Procedure 37).

The **transfer** may be the patient's own preference, or may be done because a change in the patient's condition requires a different type of care. It may be temporary or permanent. If it is permanent, the patient is discharged from one unit, then admitted to another. Be positive and supportive. Recognize that the patient may be very anxious.

PROCEDURE

37

TRANSFERRING THE PATIENT

1. Find out which unit the patient will be transferred to. Check to see that it is ready.

2. Learn from the nurse in charge the method of transfer. Get the necessary vehicle (wheelchair, stretcher, or patient's own bed).

3. Check to see if any equipment is to be transferred with the patient.

4. Carry out initial procedure actions.

5. Explain to the patient what you are doing.

6. Gather all the patient's belongings together.

   a. Place disposables in a paper bag to transport with you.

   b. Check against personal inventory list.

7. Assist the patient to put on robe and slippers, if permitted. Assist the patient into wheelchair or stretcher, as directed. The entire bed is often used. Make sure the side rails are up during transport.

8. Obtain from the nurse:

   • Patient's chart
   • Nursing care plan
   • Medications
   • Paper bag

9. Transport the patient and belongings to the new unit (Figure 22-7). Use all precautions related to safe transport.

10. Give medications, the nursing care plan, and the chart to the nurse in charge of the new unit.

11. Introduce the patient to staff. Proceed to the patient's room.

12. Assist staff in helping the patient into bed, if needed.

13. Before leaving the unit, carry out ending procedure actions.

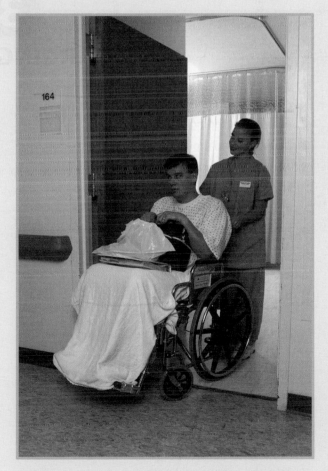

FIGURE 22-7 Transfer the patient calmly and efficiently. Never leave the patient unattended. (© Delmar/ Cengage Learning)

Safety ALERT

Never leave the patient, the records, or medications unattended. ■

DISCHARGE

In recent years, the cost of health care has increased steadily. A government program known as *diagnosis-related groups* (*DRGs*) was introduced to control hospital costs. Hospitals are paid a fixed amount of money for the care of an individual who has a particular condition or disease that is covered by a DRG.

If the hospital can provide the needed care and **discharge** the patient early, the hospital saves money and may keep the difference between the actual expenses and the DRG payment. If the patient requires a longer stay, the hospital absorbs the additional cost. (These standards apply only to patients whose care is being paid for by the federal government, such as Medicare patients.)

DRGs were developed for Medicare patients, but they are used today by all insurance companies to determine how many hospital days they will pay for. This has resulted in sicker patients being discharged from acute care facilities sooner.

The discharge procedure is usually simple if the patient is going to another facility. The social worker and nurse relay information to the receiving facility. The patient and his or her belongings are sent to the new facility. Discharge to the patient's home is more complicated and requires a number of actions called *discharge planning*.

The discharge, or authorized release, of a patient requires a written order from the physician. If a patient plans to leave without an order, inform the nurse.

PROCEDURE

38

DISCHARGING THE PATIENT

1. Check to be sure the physician has written a discharge order. If not, check with the nurse before proceeding.

2. Carry out initial procedure actions.

3. Assemble equipment:
   - Wheelchair
   - Cart to transport items (Figure 22-8)

4. Help the patient to dress, if necessary.

5. Collect the patient's personal belongings.
   a. Pack, if necessary.
   b. Check valuables against the admission list according to facility policy.
   c. Check the closet and bedside stand to be sure the patient has not forgotten anything.
   d. Check to see if medications or other equipment are to be sent home.
   e. Verify that the patient has received discharge instructions.

6. Help the patient into a wheelchair.

7. Take the patient to the discharge entrance of the facility.
   a. Help the patient to transfer safely into the vehicle.
   b. Be gracious as you say goodbye.

8. Return the wheelchair.

9. Return to the patient unit.
   a. Strip the bed. Dispose of linen according to facility policy.
   b. Clean and replace equipment used in patient care.

10. Wash your hands.

11. Record the discharge in accordance with facility policy.

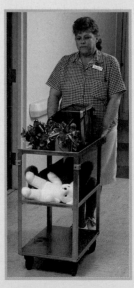

FIGURE 22-8 Use a cart to transfer the patient's belongings, to avoid injury to your back. (© *Delmar/ Cengage Learning*)

REVIEW

A. Multiple Choice

Select the one best answer for each of the following.

1. The assistant can facilitate the admission procedure by
   a. preparing equipment after the patient arrives on the unit.
   b. letting the nurse make all the observations.
   c. giving attention to the details of the procedure.
   d. recognizing that the admission causes staff anxiety.

2. When working with the newly admitted patient's family, you should
   a. treat them with courtesy.
   b. send them home.
   c. let the nurse deal with them.
   d. ask them to help with the admission.

3. Part of the admission procedure includes
   a. securing a stool specimen.
   b. obtaining a sputum specimen.
   c. showing the patient that you are efficient.
   d. measuring vital signs.

4. Valuables that accompany the patient to her unit should be
   a. taken away.
   b. cared for according to policy.
   c. left in the bedside stand.
   d. tucked under the pillow for safety.

5. When a patient is transferred, you should always include his
   a. personal belongings.
   b. bed.
   c. pillow.
   d. blood pressure cuffs.

B. Nursing Assistant Challenge

Mrs. Leon is being admitted because her emphysema is making it very difficult for her to breathe. She is accompanied by her husband and both are obviously nervous. The next morning, her condition worsens. She is moved to the intensive respiratory care unit. Answer the following questions yes or no.

6. ___NO___ The anxiety of the patient and family is not natural.

7. ___Yes___ You should answer questions about facility routines during admission.

8. ___NO___ When taking vital signs, you should use an oral thermometer.

9. ___Yes___ When Mrs. Leon is transferred, take all of her personal articles with her.

10. ___Yes___ One way to prepare the unit for admission might include checking for the need for oxygen.

11. ___NO___ You should turn Mrs. Leon's oxygen up to at least 6 liters to assist with her breathing.

UNIT **23**

Bedmaking

OBJECTIVES

After completing this unit, you will be able to:
- Spell and define terms.
- Operate each type of bed.
- Properly handle clean and soiled linens.

- Demonstrate the following procedures:
  - Procedure 39 Making a Closed Bed
  - Procedure 40 Opening the Closed Bed
  - Procedure 41 Making an Occupied Bed
  - Procedure 42 Making the Surgical Bed

VOCABULARY

Learn the meaning and the correct spelling of the following words and phrases:

box (square) corner	electric bed	low bed	open bed
closed bed	gatch bed	mitered corner	toe pleat

INTRODUCTION

The room, especially the bed, is the patient's home while he or she is in the health care facility. A well-made bed offers both comfort and safety. It is an extremely important contribution to the well-being of the patient. Review the guidelines for maintaining medical asepsis in Unit 13. These apply to making the bed, handling clean and soiled linen, and handling other supplies in patient units.

OPERATION AND USES OF BEDS IN HEALTH CARE FACILITIES

The types of beds and the methods used to operate them may vary in different health care facilities, but the basic

principles of bedmaking are the same. The most common beds are the:

- **Gatch bed**—a stationary bed about 26 inches high. These beds may be operated manually by turning the cranks. Most hospitals have eliminated these beds, but some long-term care facilities and clients receiving home care continue to use them.
- **Electric bed**—a bed that can be raised or lowered; the knee and head areas can also be adjusted. It is operated electrically (Figure 23-1). You will be using this bed most often.
- **Low bed**—low beds (Figure 23-2) are commonly used in health care facilities for patients who are at risk of falls, for whom use of side rails is not desirable. The bed frame is 4 to 6 inches from the floor to the top of the frame deck.

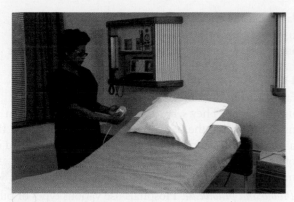

FIGURE 23-1 The typical hospital bed is electronically operated. The head and foot can be adjusted for patient comfort. The height of the bed can be raised, making it easier to give care. (© *Delmar/Cengage Learning*)

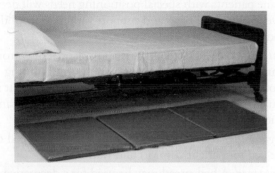

FIGURE 23-2 Low beds are often used for patients who are at high risk for falls. Organize the bedmaking procedure carefully to prevent back injury. (*Courtesy of Skil-Care Corporation, Yonkers, NY, (800) 431–2972*)

Other types of beds are available for the treatment of patients with certain medical conditions, such as multiple or advanced pressure ulcers, skin surgery and some skin conditions, burns, and intractable pain. Your facility will teach you how to operate the special beds used on your unit.

OSHA ALERT

Elevating the bed to a working height that is comfortable for you takes a minute, but it is one of the most important things you can do to protect your back. Stay on one side of the bed until it is completely made before moving to the other side. This helps organize your time and conserves energy. Avoid moving quickly. Studies have shown that rapid motion increases the risk of injury. To reduce stress on your low back, remove soiled linen a few pieces at a time, rather than in a large bundle all at once. Keep your spine straight and use good body mechanics. Make beds with a partner, if possible. ■

GUIDELINES *for*
Making the Bed

- Use good body mechanics at all times to prevent back injury.
- Work on one side of the bed at a time to complete removal of soiled linen and placement of clean linen.
- Make sure the bottom sheet and draw sheet (if used) are smooth and unwrinkled (wrinkles in bed linens can lead to discomfort and skin breakdown, especially for patients who must remain in bed).
- Follow the care plan for positioning the head and foot of the bed, the number of pillows to be used, and the use of pillows for positioning.

GUIDELINES *for*
Low Beds

Caring for and making the low bed is very similar to making a regular hospital bed. However, certain adaptations must be made to reduce your risk of injury. You should:

- Mentally plan and prepare yourself for the procedure.
- Use good body mechanics.
- Organize your work to reduce the total number of motions required to complete the task.
- Make sure you have everything you need before entering the room.
- Elevate the bed, if possible.
- Place linen and needed items on the patient's chair or within close reach. Stack them in the order of use.
- Maintain a neutral posture and bend from the legs, not the waist. Avoid twisting.
- You may squat, sit, or kneel on the plastic mat next to the bed if doing so is easier for you and helps keep your spine straight.
- Slowly remove the bed linen several pieces at a time. Roll the soiled side inward. Avoid trying to remove all the linen in one bundle. The weight of the linen and your posture increase the risk of back injury.
- Make one side of the bed at a time. This is faster, more efficient, and conserves energy.
- Use a fitted bottom sheet to reduce the number of movements necessary for making the bed, thereby lowering the risk of back strain.

Correct operation of any bed or equipment is important for patient safety. Never try to operate any bed or equipment with a patient in it without first practicing and gaining security and skill in the procedures. Although different types of hospital beds may be similar in design, the operating instructions vary. For safety, always follow the manufacturers' directions.

BEDMAKING

Bed linen is always changed when soiled. It is routinely changed:

- Daily in the acute care facility.
- Two or three times a week in long-term care facilities.

Residents in long-term care may prefer to use their own pillows, blankets, and spreads.

Supplies for Bedmaking

You will need to gather supplies for making a bed. The supplies will vary slightly, depending on the type of bedmaking procedure you will be using. Gather and stack them in the order of use, so that the item used first is on top and the item used last is on the bottom. Bring only needed linen to the room. To do a complete linen change, you will need:

- *Mattress pad*, if used by the facility. A mattress pad is a heavy, quilted cotton pad. Mattress pads may be either flat or fitted to the mattress.
- Two sheets. In some facilities, two large flat sheets are used to make each bed. Many facilities use a flat sheet on top and a fitted sheet on bottom.
- *Linen draw sheet*, or half sheet, if used by the facility. This sheet may be used with or without a protective plastic or rubber draw sheet underneath.
- *Incontinent pad*, *underpad*, or *bed protector*. These terms are often used interchangeably to describe soft, absorbent pads. Disposable incontinent pads consist of layers of soft paper with a plastic backing. These pads may be called by their brand name, such as Chux. The pads are

large, usually about 30 to 36 inches square. They are used to protect the bed linen for patients who are incontinent, use the bedpan or urinal when in bed, or have heavy drainage from a wound or surgical site. Heavy, absorbent cotton pads are also used in many facilities. The reusable cotton pads are about 36 to 42 inches square. They serve a dual purpose and are often used for moving the patient in place of a lifting sheet. If a patient is incontinent, the disposable or reusable pad is often the only item that has to be changed, which is more efficient for staff and economical for the facility.

- *Pillow and pillowcase.* Hospitals use various types of pillows. Many are disposable, and are sent home with the patient or discarded. Some are reusable. The reusable pillows are usually covered with a plastic pillow protector. The pillow is always covered with a linen pillowcase. Some patients with special positioning needs will need several pillows to prop and support various areas of the body for alignment and comfort.
- *Bath blanket.* A bath blanket is a soft flannel or cotton blanket that is used for modesty and warmth during procedures in which the patient's body is exposed. It is usually folded and stored in the closet or bedside stand when not in use.
- *Regular blanket.* A thermal cotton blanket is applied to the bed for patient comfort and warmth.
- *Bedspread.* A bedspread may be used for a decorative touch and to give the room a neat appearance.

Occasionally, facilities use other items, such as *bed boards*, to meet special patient needs. Bed boards are placed between the mattress and bed frame to offer extra-firm support to the patient's back. Bed cradles (Unit 25) may be used to keep the weight of the linen off the patient's skin. A *footboard* (Unit 25) may also be applied to the foot of the bed for patients who have special positioning needs or are at risk of contractures.

The Closed Bed

The **closed bed** is made following discharge of a patient and after the unit is cleaned (terminal cleaning). It remains closed until a new patient is admitted. Details are important. The same procedure is followed when making an unoccupied bed, but the bed is opened as a final step when a patient is to occupy it shortly.

PROCEDURE

39

MAKING A CLOSED BED

1. Wash your hands and assemble equipment:

   - 2 pillowcases
   - Pillow
   - Spread
   - Blankets, as needed
   - 2 large sheets (90" × 108") (substitute one fitted sheet, if used)
   - Cotton draw sheet or half sheet (if used; a cotton incontinent pad may be used instead of a draw sheet, according to facility policy)
   - Plastic or rubber draw sheet (if used in your facility)
   - Mattress pad and cover, if mattress is not plastic-treated

   Note: Mattresses that are treated with plastic do not require a moisture-proof sheet or cotton half sheet (draw sheet). In some cases, the half sheet is used as a lifter to assist in moving the patient. It is sometimes used simply to keep the bottom sheet clean. Some facilities use fitted bottom sheets. If your facility does so, use a fitted sheet in place of one of the large flat sheets.

2. Elevate the bed to a comfortable working height in the horizontal position. Put the side rails down. Lock the wheels so the bed will not roll. Place a chair at the side of the bed.

3. Arrange the linen on the chair in the order in which it is to be used.

4. Position the mattress to the head of the bed by grasping the mattress handles (or the edge of the mattress, if no handles are present). Pull the mattress up to the head of the bed.

5. You will work entirely from one side of the bed until that side is completed. Then go to the other side of the bed. This conserves time and energy.

6. Place the mattress pad even with the top of the mattress and unfold it.

7. Place the bottom sheet on the bed and unfold it, seam side down and wide hem at the top. The small hem should be brought to the foot of the mattress (Figure 23-3). The center fold should be at the center of the bed. If a fitted bottom sheet is used, fit it smoothly around one corner (Figure 23-4).

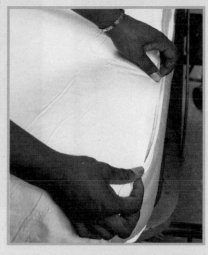

FIGURE 23-3 Place the flat bottom sheet even with the end of the mattress at the foot of the bed. *(© Delmar/Cengage Learning)*

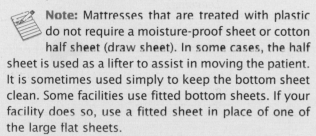

FIGURE 23-4 If a fitted bottom sheet is used, pull and smooth it around the corner. *(© Delmar/Cengage Learning)*

8. Tuck 12 to 18 inches of sheet smoothly over the head of the mattress (Figures 23-5A to C).

9. Make a **mitered corner** (Figure 23-6). The square corner, preferred by some facilities, is made in a way similar to the mitered corner.

10. Tuck in the sheet on one side, keeping the sheet straight. Work from the head to the foot of the bed. If using a fitted sheet, adjust it over the head and bottom ends of the mattress.

11. If used, place the plastic draw sheet and half sheet with upper edge about 14 inches from the head of the mattress and tuck under one side. Be sure that the half sheet covers the plastic sheet. Alternately,

continues

PROCEDURE 39 CONTINUED

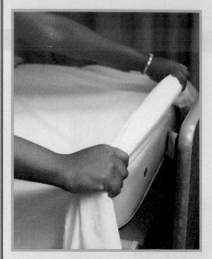

FIGURE 23-5A Gather about 12 to 18 inches of the top sheet at the bottom of the bed. *(© Delmar/ Cengage Learning)*

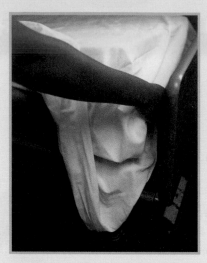

FIGURE 23-5B Face the foot of the bed and lift the mattress with your near hand. *(© Delmar/ Cengage Learning)*

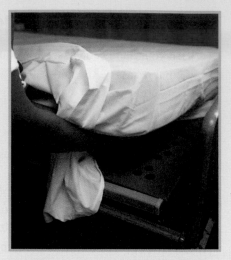

FIGURE 23-5C Bring the sheet smoothly over the end of the mattress with your opposite hand. *(© Delmar/Cengage Learning)*

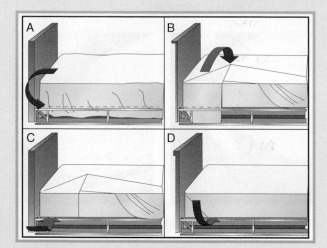

FIGURE 23-6 Making a mitered corner. A. The sheet is hanging loose at the side of the bed. B. Pick up the sheet about 12 inches from the end of the bed to form a triangle. C. Tuck the sheet in at the end of the bed. Pick up the triangle and place your other hand at the edge of the bed near the end to hold the edge of the sheet in place. Bring the triangle over the edge of the mattress and tuck it smoothly under the mattress. Tuck in the rest of the sheet along the side of the mattress. Make sure the sheet is wrinkle-free. *(© Delmar/Cengage Learning)*

a reusable or disposable underpad may be used. The sheet or pad should cover the area from below the patient's shoulders to below the hips.

12. Unfold and place the top sheet on the bed, seam up, top hem even with the upper edge of the mattress and the center fold in the center of the bed.

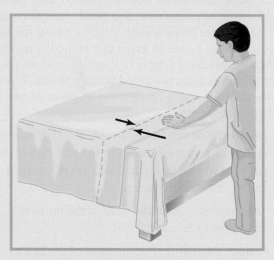

FIGURE 23-7 The toe pleat provides space for movement of the feet. For bedfast patients, the extra space reduces the risk of contractures and pressure ulcers. The extra space is much more comfortable for all patients. *(© Delmar/Cengage Learning)*

13. Spread the blanket over the top sheet and foot of the mattress. Keep the blanket centered.

14. Make a **toe pleat** by folding the top linen over 2 to 3 inches at the end of the bed (Figure 23-7). The toe pleat provides extra space and keeps the linen from pulling the feet downward. This is more comfortable for the patient and reduces the risk of contractures.

15. Tuck the top sheet and blanket under the mattress at the foot of the bed as far as the

PROCEDURE 39 CONTINUED

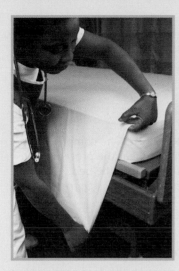

FIGURE 23-8A Make the square (box) corner following the steps shown in Figures 23-6A to 23-6C. Then, holding the corner with your left hand, grasp the bottom of the sheet and pull it straight down until the fold is even with the edge of the mattress. *(© Delmar/Cengage Learning)*

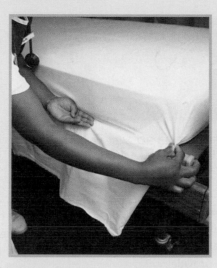

FIGURE 23-8B Holding the square corner in place, tuck the remaining sheet under the mattress. *(© Delmar/Cengage Learning)*

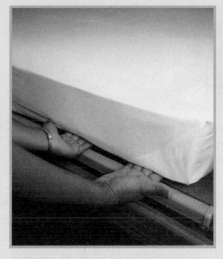

FIGURE 23-8C The finished square corner should look like this. *(© Delmar/Cengage Learning)*

center only. Make a **box (square) corner** (Figures 23-8A to 23-8C).

16. Place the spread with its top hem even with the head of the mattress. Unfold the spread to the foot of the bed.

17. Tuck the spread under the mattress at the foot of the bed and miter the corner. Sometimes the spread may be placed directly on top of the sheet. Rather than tucking the sheet, blanket, and/or spread under the end of the mattress separately and forming separate corners, all of the covers may be tucked under at the same time and one corner formed (Figures 23-9A to 23-9E).

18. Go to the other side of the bed. Fanfold the top covers to the center of the bed so you can work with the lower sheets and pad.

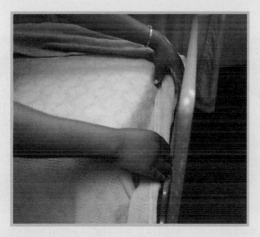

FIGURE 23-9A Gather the top sheet and bedspread together. Smooth evenly over the end of the mattress. *(© Delmar/Cengage Learning)*

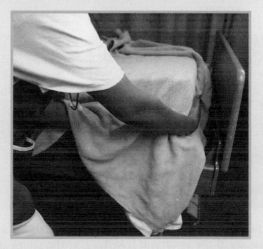

FIGURE 23-9B Tuck the sheet and spread under the mattress together. *(© Delmar/Cengage Learning)*

continues

PROCEDURE 39 CONTINUED

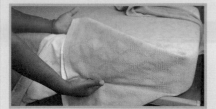

FIGURE 23-9C Continue as with the procedure for a mitered corner. *(© Delmar/Cengage Learning)*

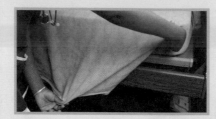

FIGURE 23-9D Slide your finger to the end to make a smooth edge. *(© Delmar/Cengage Learning)*

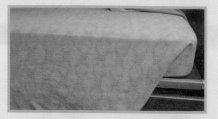

FIGURE 23-9E The completed top bedding. Repeat the procedure on the other side of the bed. *(© Delmar/Cengage Learning)*

19. Tuck the bottom sheet under the head of the mattress and miter the corner. Working from top to bottom, smooth out all wrinkles and tighten these sheets as much as possible to provide comfort. (Adjust a fitted bottom sheet smoothly and securely around the mattress corners.)

20. Grasp the protective draw sheet (if used) and cotton draw sheet in the center. Tuck these sheets tightly under the mattress.

21. Tuck in the top sheet and blanket at the foot of the bed and miter the corner.

22. Fold the top sheet back over the blanket, making an 8-inch cuff at the head of the bed.

23. Tuck in the spread at the foot of the bed and miter the corner. Bring the top of the spread to the head of the mattress.

24. Insert the pillow into a pillowcase:

    a. Place your hands in the clean case, freeing the corners.

    b. Grasp the center of the end seam with a hand outside the case and turn the case back over your hand (Figure 23-10A).

    c. Grasp the pillow through the case at the center of one end. Pull the case over the pillow with your free hand (Figures 23-10B and 23-10C). (Do not allow the pillow to touch your uniform.)

    d. Adjust the corners of the pillow to fit in the corners of the case.

25. Place the pillow at the head of the bed with the open end away from the door.

26. Lower the bed to the lowest horizontal position.

27. Arrange the room as follows:

    a. Replace the bedside table parallel to the bed. Place the chair in its assigned location.

    b. Place the overbed table over the foot of the bed opposite the chair.

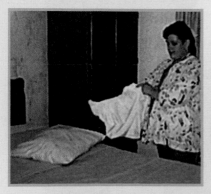

FIGURE 23-10A Grasp the pillowcase at the seam and fold it back and over your wrist, inside out. *(© Delmar/Cengage Learning)*

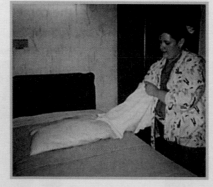

FIGURE 23-10B Grab the end of the pillow in the center with your pillowcase-covered hand. *(© Delmar/Cengage Learning)*

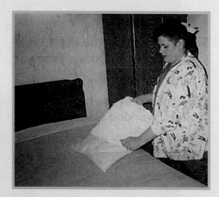

FIGURE 23-10C Unfold and smooth the pillowcase over the pillow. *(© Delmar/Cengage Learning)*

PROCEDURE 39 CONTINUED

c. Place the signal cord within easy reach of the patient.

d. Leave the side rails down.

e. Check for possible safety hazards.

28. Leave the unit neat and tidy.

29. Wash your hands.

30. Report completion of the task to the nurse.

PROCEDURE

OPENING THE CLOSED BED

1. Wash your hands.

2. Raise the bed to a comfortable working height in the horizontal position. Move the overbed table to one side.

3. Lock the bed wheels.

4. Loosen the top bedding.

5. Facing the head of the bed, grasp the top sheet and spread and fanfold the top bedding to the foot of the bed.

6. Return the bed to the lowest horizontal position. Place the overbed table over the foot of the bed.

7. Place the call bell near the pillow or within easy reach. It should be visible and within reach of the patient at all times.

8. Leave the unit neat and tidy.

9. Wash your hands.

10. Report completion of the task to the nurse.

The Unoccupied Bed

Beds are often made while patients are out of the room or up in a shower or chair. Follow the procedure for making a closed bed, but then fanfold the top bedding three-fourths of the way down. This "opens" the bed and makes it easier for the patient to get into it.

The Open Bed

The **open bed** is like a sign saying "welcome" to the new patient (Figure 23-11). It also shows that the unit has been prepared. (See Procedure 40.) In long-term care facilities, the bed is not opened unless the resident is going to bed soon.

The Occupied Bed

Unless the patient is permitted out of bed by physician's order, the bed is made with the patient in it.

(See Procedure 41.) Bedmaking usually follows the bed bath, while the patient is covered with a bath blanket. It may, however, be done any time it would add to the patient's comfort.

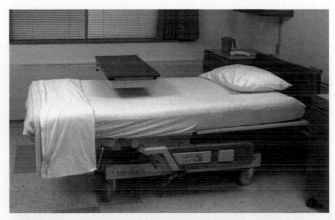

FIGURE 23-11 Open the closed bed by drawing the bedding to the foot of the bed and fanfolding it. (© Delmar/Cengage Learning)

Infection Control ALERT

Wear gloves when removing bed linen that is wet or soiled. Place the soiled linen in a plastic bag or linen hamper. Avoid contaminating environmental surfaces with gloves that have handled soiled linen. Remove one glove, if necessary. Follow facility policy for disinfecting the mattress. Allow it to dry. Discard your gloves and wash your hands. This is an important step. The used gloves will contaminate clean linen. Gloves are not necessary when handling clean linen. Cracks in the mattress are a potential source of odors and contamination. Report cracks in a mattress to the proper person in your facility. ■

The Surgical Bed

The surgical bed provides a safe, warm environment to receive the postsurgical patient. It is made so that movement from stretcher to bed can be done with maximum safety and minimum effort. For this reason, the bed should be left open and at stretcher height. (See Procedure 42.)

Obtain the equipment needed to monitor vital signs; make sure that it is in place and ready for use. Be alert for the patient's return so you can help with the transfer from stretcher to bed.

Safety ALERT

Never turn your back on the patient or leave the bedside when the bed is in the high position and the side rail is down. ■

PROCEDURE

MAKING AN OCCUPIED BED

1. Carry out initial procedure actions.

2. Assemble equipment:
   - Disposable gloves (if linens are soiled with blood, body fluids, secretions, or excretions)
   - Cotton draw sheet, turning sheet, or incontinent pad for selected patients
   - 2 large flat sheets (or one large flat sheet and one fitted bottom sheet)
   - 2 pillowcases
   - Laundry hamper

3. Place the bedside chair at the foot of the bed.

4. Arrange the clean linen on the chair in the order in which it is to be used.

5. The bed should be flat, with wheels locked, unless otherwise indicated. Raise the bed to a working horizontal height. Lower the side rail on your side of the bed.

6. If the bed linens are soiled with blood or other body fluids, wash your hands and put on disposable gloves.

7. Loosen the bedclothes on your side by lifting the edge of the mattress with one hand and drawing the bedclothes out with the other. Never shake the linen. This spreads germs.

8. Put the side rail up and go to the opposite side of the bed.

9. Adjust the mattress to the head of the bed (Figure 23-12). Get help, if necessary.

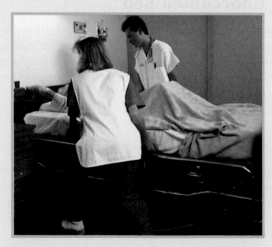

FIGURE 23-12 The patient grasps the head of the bed and pushes in with the heels while two nursing assistants pull the mattress to the head of the bed. (© Delmar/Cengage Learning)

PROCEDURE 41 CONTINUED

10. Remove the top covers except for the top sheet, one at a time. Fold them to the bottom of the bed. Pick them up in the center. Place them over the back of chair if they are to be reused.

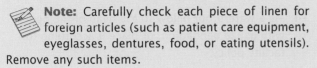 **Note:** Carefully check each piece of linen for foreign articles (such as patient care equipment, eyeglasses, dentures, food, or eating utensils). Remove any such items.

11. Place the clean sheet or bath blanket over the top sheet. Have the patient hold the top edge of the clean sheet if able. If the patient is unable to help, tuck the sheet beneath the patient's shoulder.

12. Slide the soiled sheet out, from top to bottom. Put it in a hamper or plastic bag.

13. Ask the patient to move to the side of the bed toward you. Assist if necessary. Move one pillow with the patient and remove other pillows. Pull up the side rail. (Alternatively, you may ask the patient to turn toward the opposite side of the bed, holding onto the raised side rail. You would then fanfold the sheet, as in Step 14, but there would be no need to go to the other side of the bed.)

14. Go to the other side of the bed. Fanfold the soiled cotton draw sheet, if used, and bottom sheet close to the patient (Figure 23-13).

15. Straighten the mattress pad. If the bottom sheet is to be changed, place a clean sheet on the bed so that the narrow hem comes to the edge of the mattress at the foot. The seamed side of the hem is toward the bed. The lengthwise center

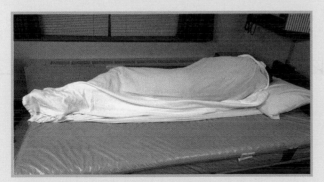

FIGURE 23-13 Fanfold the soiled bottom sheet to the center of the bed as close to the patient as possible. Note that the bottom linen is flat and the patient is positioned to the far side of the bed with the rail up. (© Delmar/Cengage Learning)

fold of the sheet is at the center of the bed. Fanfold the opposite side of the sheet close to the patient.

16. Tuck the top of the sheet under the head of the mattress.

17. Make a mitered corner.

18. Tuck the side of the sheet under the mattress, working toward the foot of the bed.

19. Position a fresh draw sheet, if used. Tuck it under the mattress.

20. Ask or assist the patient to roll toward you, over the fanfolded linen. Move the pillow with the patient.

21. Raise the side rails. Test for security.

22. Go to the other side of the bed. Lower the side rail. Remove the soiled linen by rolling the edges inward. *Keep soiled linen away from your uniform.* Placed soiled linen in the hamper or plastic bag. (Raise the side rail if leaving the bedside.)

23. Remove gloves, if worn, and discard according to facility policy.

24. Wash your hands.

25. Pull the clean bottom sheet into place. Tuck it under the mattress at the head of the bed. Make a mitered corner.

26. Pull gently to eliminate wrinkles. Then tuck the side of the sheet under the mattress, working from top to bottom.

27. Pull the draw sheet smoothly into place. Tuck it firmly under the mattress.

28. Place the top sheet over the patient. Remove the bath blanket.

29. Complete the bedmaking as for an unoccupied bed. To reduce pressure on toes, make a toe pleat or grasp the top bedding over the toes and pull straight up. Some patients prefer not to have the blanket and top sheet or spread tucked in.

30. Assist the patient to turn on his or her back. Place a clean pillowcase on the pillow that is not being used. Replace that pillow. Change the other pillowcase.

31. Carry out ending procedure actions.

PROCEDURE

42

MAKING THE SURGICAL BED

1. Wash your hands.

2. Check assignment for unit location.

3. Assemble equipment:
   - Disposable gloves (if linens are soiled with blood or body fluids)
   - Articles for basic bed
   - One extra draw sheet
   - Bath blanket for warmth
   - One protective (rubber or plastic) draw sheet (if used in facility) or incontinent pad
   - Roll of one-inch gauze bandage

4. Lock the bed.

5. Apply gloves if linen is wet or soiled with blood or body fluids.

6. Strip and discard used linen.

7. Remove gloves and discard according to facility policy.

8. Wash your hands.

9. Make the bottom foundation bed (Steps 1–11 in Procedure 39). Repeat on the opposite side of the bed.

10. Place a protective draw sheet or bed protector, if used, over the head of the mattress sheet. Cover with a cotton draw sheet. Miter the corners and tuck them in on the sides.

11. Place the top sheet, blanket, and spread in the usual manner. Do not tuck them in.

12. Fold the linen back at the foot of the bed even with the edge of the mattress.

13. Fanfold the upper covers and top sheet to the far side of the bed (Figure 23-14).

14. Tie a waterproof pillow to the head of the bed with gauze bandaging, or place it according to facility policy.

15. Arrange the bed so there is adequate room to position a stretcher next to it. Leave the bed locked and at the same height as a stretcher.

16. Check the unit for obvious hazards.

17. Leave the room neat and tidy.

18. Wash your hands.

19. Report completion of the task to the nurse.

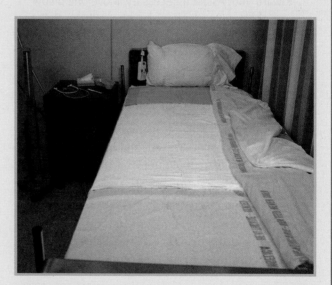

FIGURE 23-14 Prepare the surgical bed by fanfolding the covers to the far side of the bed. Raise the bed to stretcher height. (© *Delmar/Cengage Learning*)

REVIEW

A. Multiple Choice

Select the one best answer for each of the following.

1. Loosening the top bedding at the foot of the bed is done
   a. to improve the appearance of the bed.
   b. in unoccupied beds.
   c. as folds in the bottom sheet.
   d. to reduce pressure on the feet.

2. When making an unoccupied bed, make the
   a. entire bottom first.
   b. far side of the bottom and top first.
   c. near side of the entire bed first.
   d. far side of the bottom first.

3. Before making an unoccupied bed,
   a. elevate it to a comfortable working height.
   b. keep the bed at the lowest horizontal height.
   c. raise the head portion.
   d. raise the side rails on the opposite side.

4. Before making any bed, always
   a. raise the side rails.
   b. lower the bed to the lowest horizontal height.
   c. lock the bed wheels.
   d. raise the head of the bed.

5. Sheets should be smoothly tucked in over the head of the mattress
   a. 5 to 7 inches.
   b. 12 to 18 inches.
   c. 20 to 24 inches.
   d. 26 to 30 inches.

6. If a draw sheet or lift sheet is used, it should be placed so that it covers the area under the patient's
   a. head and shoulders.
   b. heels and lower legs.
   c. buttocks only.
   d. shoulders to buttocks.

7. When placing the case on the pillow,
   a. tuck it under your chin.
   b. lay the pillow on the chair.
   c. pull the case over while grasping the pillow with the opposite hand.
   d. lay the pillow on the bedside stand.

8. When opening a closed bed,
   a. fanfold top bedding to the foot.
   b. loosen all top bedding.
   c. leave the bed at its highest horizontal height.
   d. raise the head of the bed.

9. The top bedding in a ~~surgical bed~~ is *Fan Folded, untucked.*
   a. untucked and draped.
   b. tucked in on two sides.
   c. untucked and fanfolded.
   d. made without a blanket.

10. A common element in all bedmaking is
    a. fanfolding the linen.
    b. leaving the unit neat and tidy. *neat tidy.*
    c. leaving the bed in the high position.
    d. using the same linen and equipment.

11. When making a low bed, the nursing assistant should
    a. bend from the waist.
    b. sit on the floor.
    c. kneel, sit, or squat on a mat.
    d. position the bed in the low position.

B. Nursing Assistant Challenge

12. You are assigned to make a closed bed. You have washed your hands and assembled the following equipment: pillow, blanket, spread, mattress pad, and mattress cover. What else will you need?

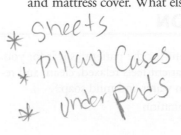

* Sheets
* Pillow Cases
* under pads

UNIT 24

Patient Bathing

OBJECTIVES

After completing this unit, you will be able to:
- Spell and define terms.
- Describe the safety precautions for patient bathing.
- List the purposes of bathing patients.
- Demonstrate the following procedures:
  - Procedure 43 Assisting with the Tub Bath or Shower
  - Procedure 44 Bed Bath or Waterless Bed Bath (Bag Bath)

- Procedure 45 Changing the Patient's Gown
- Procedure 46 Partial Bath
- Procedure 47 Female Perineal Care
- Procedure 48 Male Perineal Care
- Procedure 49 Hand and Fingernail Care
- Procedure 50 Bed Shampoo
- Procedure 51 Dressing and Undressing the Patient

VOCABULARY

Learn the meaning and the correct spelling of the following words and phrases:

axilla	cuticle	perineal care	pubic
bag bath	genitalia	perineum	waterless bathing

INTRODUCTION

A daily bath is as important for the patient as it is for you. Following the bath, the patient feels relaxed, clean, and refreshed. A bath with warm water and mild soap:
- Removes dirt and perspiration
- Increases circulation
- Provides mild exercise
- Provides an opportunity for close observation

You will be able to see firsthand how the patient's condition is improving, declining, or changing. These observations are valuable aids to accurate nursing assessments.

With the physician's permission, the patient may be allowed to take regular tub baths or showers. Some patients will be bathed in bed.

During bathing, special attention should be given to skin areas that touch, such as:
- Between the legs
- Under the arms
- Under the breasts
- Under the scrotum
- Between the buttocks
- Around the anus
- For obese people, under folds of skin or fat

Gently sponge and pat these areas dry. Avoid the use of talcum or corn starch unless requested by the patient or listed on the care plan. If these products are requested by the patient, use them sparingly. Avoid shaking powder or spraying deodorant near patients who have respiratory disorders.

WATERLESS BATH

Some facilities are taking a new approach to bathing, called **waterless bathing**. It may also be called **bag bath**. The bathing procedure is similar to that for the bed bath. The only equipment needed is a package of pre-moistened, disposable washcloths (Figure 24-1). Each package contains washcloths moistened with a no-rinse cleansing solution that does not require drying. The kits are available with either eight cloths or four cloths, depending on the purpose of the bath. The washcloths can be warmed in the microwave or special product warmer (Figure 24-2), or used at room temperature. Use caution when using the microwave, which may heat unevenly. Monitor for hot spots.

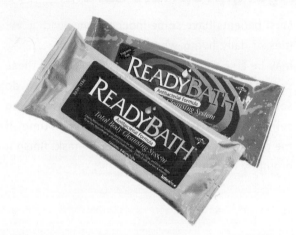

FIGURE 24-1 Waterless bathing has become popular for its comfort and convenience. Although the product is more costly than more conventional methods of bathing, the time savings make it worthwhile. Bag bath contains a no-rinse cleanser and does not contain soap, so it is gentle on patients' skin. *(Courtesy of Medline Industries, Inc. (800) MEDLINE)*

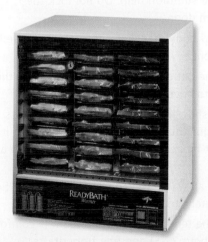

FIGURE 24-2 The waterless bathing system may be used at room temperature, or warmed for comfort. Use the product warmer, if available, because heating the cloths in the microwave increases the risk for uneven heating and burns. *(Courtesy of Medline Industries, Inc. (800) MEDLINE)*

Infection Control ALERT

Waterless bathing products are designed to be used for one bath. The package may be resealed if not all of the cloths are used. Date the open package and discard it in 48 to 72 hours, if not used. Follow facility policy for discarding unused cloths. Avoid flushing them down the toilet. A plastic bag at the bedside works well for cloth disposal. ■

This product can be used by the nursing assistant to bathe a person or by the patient to self-bathe. Giving a complete bath with the kit takes approximately 8 to 10 minutes. The washcloths are very gentle on the skin.

WHIRLPOOL BATH

The most stimulating form of bathing is a therapeutic bath that is given in a whirlpool tub (Figure 24-3). The whirlpool benefits patients because:

- The temperature of the water remains constant.
- The movement of the water stimulates circulation.
- Warm, circulating water is relaxing and invigorating.
- It provides the value of whirlpool activity with cleansing.

Care of the hair, teeth, and nails usually follows the bath procedure, but may be carried out as independent procedures. Range-of-motion exercises frequently follow bathing.

*[handwritten margin note: * Therapeutic * temperature constant]*

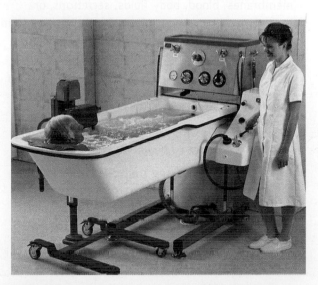

FIGURE 24-3 The water in the whirlpool circulates, maintaining a constant temperature and stimulating circulation. *(Courtesy of Arjo-Century, Inc.)*

Culture ALERT

A patient may prefer to receive personal care from someone of the same sex. Honor these requests, whenever possible, and do not be offended that the request was made. In some cultures, a male cannot even be in the same room with a female unless she is covered from head to foot. ■

PATIENT BATHING

Nursing assistants are frequently assigned to bathe patients. Follow the guidelines and the procedures for bathing carefully to ensure patient comfort and safety.

Safety ALERT

Make sure a chair is available next to the tub or shower in case the patient needs to sit quickly. Turn the hot water on last and off first to prevent injury. ■

Safety Measures for Special Treatments

Patients receiving special treatments, such as an IV, feeding tube, drainage tube, or oxygen can be bathed, but need special care. When bathing and moving these patients:

- Be careful to avoid stress on the tubes.
- Do not turn off, modify the flow of solution, or disconnect medical devices.
- Never lower an IV or tube feeding container below the level of the infusion site.
- Avoid raising a drainage bag above the insertion site.

Age-Appropriate Care ALERT

Most patients have some independence with activities of daily living when they are at home. They may be able to continue doing all or part of these skills. Organize your work so that you can do something else while the patient is performing self-care. This makes good use of your time. If the patient is unable to complete the task, finish it promptly without complaint. ■

GUIDELINES *for*

Patient Bathing

- Apply the principles of standard precautions if there may be contact with open lesions, mucous membranes, blood, body fluids, secretions, or excretions. Change your gloves before moving from one part of the body to another area in which the skin is open or mucous membranes are present.
- Make sure the shower or tub is cleaned before and after each use (Figure 24-4).
- Check that all safety aids, such as hand rails, shower chairs, and tub seats/benches are present and in proper working order.
- Transport patients to and from the tub room and carry out bathing procedures as efficiently as possible.
- Make sure the patient's body is covered during transport.

- If a patient falls or feels faint during bathing, do not leave him alone. Use the emergency call button to summon help. Do not lock the bathroom door.
- Use good body mechanics to protect yourself and the patient.
- Assist the patient with transfers related to the bath. Be sure to have enough help.
- Using a shower chair prevents patient stress and fatigue, but it must be secured so that it does not move as the patient transfers into and out of it.
- Wipe up all water spilled or dripped on the floor immediately, to prevent falls.
- Adjust the temperature so the room is comfortably warm (about 72°F) and free from drafts.

continues

GUIDELINES *continued*

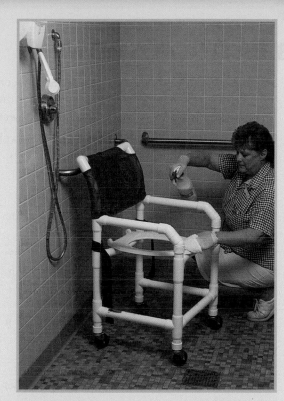

FIGURE 24-4 Clean the tub or shower chair before and after use. Wipe all areas, including the hand rails. *(Stock image)*

- Cover the patient with a bath blanket during a bed bath, and for modesty and warmth after the tub bath, whirlpool, or shower.
- Drape the patient's genital area with a bath towel for modesty during a tub bath, whirlpool, or shower.
- The temperature of the water for a shower, tub bath, or bed bath should be maintained at about 105°F. Water that is cooler than approximately 97°F may be too cool. Use a bath thermometer to check the temperature of the water. If no bath thermometer is available, check the temperature with your elbow.
- Observe the patient's skin for any changes or irregularities. Note any reddened areas. Report anything unusual.
- If you will be using liquid soap from a wall-mounted dispenser, dispense soap into a small cup for use at the bedside. Pour the liquid soap onto the washcloth. Do not pour it directly into the water.

- If your facility uses refillable liquid soap bottles, be sure each patient has a bottle labeled with his or her name for his or her use only.
- Once a washcloth or towel has been used below the waist, avoid using it above the waist.
- Place the hand-held shower spray on the hook when not in use. Do not let it hang down or touch the floor, which is always considered dirty.

Additional Guidelines for Giving a Whirlpool Bath

- Check with the nurse before giving a whirlpool to a patient who is confused, or who has an infection, surgical incision, or pressure ulcer.
- The water temperature in the whirlpool is set at 97°F because the temperature in the tub remains constant. (Use common sense; if the tub is steaming, the water is probably too hot. Use a thermometer to check the water temperature.) The constant movement of water keeps the patient warm and stimulates circulation.
- Always fasten the safety belt when moving a patient into or out of a whirlpool tub with a hydraulic lift seat. Keep the belt fastened throughout the procedure. If the patient is frightened of the lift, explain the procedure and reassure him or her.
- Use low-suds or no-suds products that are designed for whirlpool use. Never pour liquid soap or shampoo into the whirlpool tub. A tiny bit will result in an abundance of suds. If a suds problem occurs, rub a bar of soap against the walls of the tub to reduce the bubbles.
- The whirlpool provides a cleansing action. However, if you will be assisting the patient with bathing, apply the principles of standard precautions.
- The jets in some whirlpool tubs have the potential to harbor dangerous pathogens. Follow cleansing directions and run the disinfectant through the jets for the correct length of time.
- When the bath is completed, raise the lift seat out of the soapy water and rinse with the hose, using comfortably warm water.

PROCEDURE

43

ASSISTING WITH THE TUB BATH OR SHOWER

1. Carry out initial procedure actions.

2. Assemble equipment:
   - Disposable gloves
   - Liquid soap
   - Washcloth(s)
   - 2–3 bath towels
   - Bath blanket
   - Bath lotion
   - Deodorant
   - Chair or stool beside shower or tub
   - Bath or shower chair, as needed
   - Patient's gown, robe, and slippers
   - Bath mat

3. Take the supplies to the bathroom. Prepare the bathroom for the patient. Make sure the tub is clean.

4. Fill the tub half full of water at 105°F or adjust the shower flow. If a bath thermometer is available, check the water temperature. If a bath thermometer is not available, test the water with your elbow. The water should feel comfortably warm.

5. Help the patient put on a robe and slippers. Escort the patient to the bathroom. Completely cover the patient when going to or from the bath or shower.

6. Help the patient undress. Give the patient a towel to wrap around the waist.

7. Position a shower chair in tub or shower, if needed (Figure 24-5).

8. Assist the patient into the tub or shower. For the patient's safety, the bottom of the tub and the shower floor are covered with a nonskid surface.

9. Put on disposable gloves if the patient has open skin lesions.

10. Encourage the patient to wash his or her body. Assist in washing as needed.

11. Wash the patient's back. Observe the skin for signs of redness or breaks. See Unit 35 for information on caring for pressure sores or other skin lesions.

12. The patient may wash the **genitalia** (external reproductive organs), if able.
   - If the patient is not able to wash the genitalia, then you will also perform this part of the bath.

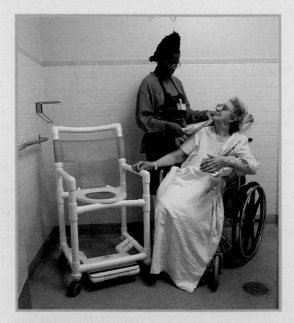

FIGURE 24-5 The shower chair is used to enable the patient to bathe safely. Lock the wheels during transfers. *(Stock image)*

PROCEDURE 43 CONTINUED

Apply disposable gloves before bathing the genital area.

- After washing the genitalia, remove gloves and discard them according to facility policy.
- Wash your hands.
- After washing the genitalia, avoid using the same washcloth, towel, and gloves elsewhere on the body. If further bathing or touching is necessary, apply new gloves and use different linen.

13. If the patient shows any signs of weakness:
    - Get help. Use the call button.
    - Remove the plug and let the water drain.
    - Turn the water off.
    - Allow the patient to rest until feeling better before making any attempt to assist the patient out of the tub or shower.
    - Keep the patient covered with a bath blanket to avoid chilling.

14. If the patient wants a shampoo and you have permission to do so:
    - Ask the patient to hold a washcloth over the eyes.

- Pour a small amount of water on hair (enough to wet hair thoroughly).
- Use a small amount of shampoo to lather hair.
- Massage scalp gently.
- Rinse hair with warm water.
- Repeat lathering, massaging, and rinsing, if necessary.
- Towel hair dry.

15. Hold the bath blanket around the patient as he or she steps out of the tub or shower. The patient may choose to remove the wet towel from under the bath blanket.

16. Assist the patient to dry, apply deodorant, dress, and return to the unit.

17. Escort the patient back to his or her unit. Return supplies to the patient's unit.

18. Carry out ending procedure actions.

19. Return to the bath or shower room. Put on gloves and clean and disinfect the tub, shower chair, and hand rails.

20. Discard soiled linen.

21. Wash your hands.

Tips: Using a bath blanket and towels to drape the patient is essential during bathing and personal care procedures, even if the room is completely private. Being exposed is uncomfortable for most people. Draping the patient properly provides a sense of dignity, reduces feelings of vulnerability, and protects the patient's modesty and self-esteem. Do not omit this important step for any patient, regardless of his or her age.

Towel Bath

The towel bath procedure has become popular for bathing patients with dementia who become agitated by a tub or shower bath. Creating a comfortable environment is an important part of the procedure. The room may be darkened, with soothing music and pleasant aromas. Bathing is done with a prepared kit using no-rinse skin cleanser. Two washcloths, two hand towels, one large towel, and two bath blankets are needed. Cover the patient completely with a warm bath blanket, if possible.

Use the call signal to ask another assistant to warm additional blankets, if necessary.

Prepare the bathing kit in advance, and bring it to the room in a large plastic bag. Cover the patient with a bath blanket and gradually undress him or her. Apply warm, moist towels from the kit, one at a time, over a large area of the patient's body. Apply the towels in a sequence that is not upsetting to the patient, such as beginning with the feet and lower legs. Use the towels to massage and cleanse the skin. Rinsing and drying are not necessary, because the no-rinse cleanser evaporates quickly when the towels are removed. Speak with the patient in a calm, soothing manner during the bath. Avoid rushing. Replace the warm bath blankets and towels to keep the patient comfortable.

The goal of the towel bath is to keep the patient clean and odor-free, while avoiding anxiety and stress. Personalize the procedure to the patient's response to make it as pleasurable as possible, while respecting his or her autonomy. Despite being a more creative method of bathing, it is not more work and is not more time-consuming.

PROCEDURE

44

BED BATH OR WATERLESS BED BATH (BAG BATH)

Note: Apply the principles of standard precautions if the patient has draining wounds, nonintact skin, or if contact with blood, body fluids, mucous membranes, secretions, or excretions is likely.

1. Carry out initial procedure actions.

2. Assemble equipment:
   - Disposable gloves
   - Bed linen
   - Bath blanket
   - Laundry bag or hamper
   - Bath basin
   - Bath thermometer
   - Soap and soap dish, or liquid soap
   - Washcloths
   - Face towel
   - 2 bath towels
   - Bag bath product kit of 8 cloths, if a waterless product will be used
   - Plastic bag to discard bag bath cloths
   - Hospital gown or patient's night clothes
   - Lotion
   - Equipment for oral hygiene
   - Nail brush, emery board, and orangewood stick (if needed)
   - Deodorant
   - Brush and comb
   - Bedpan and cover or urinal
   - Paper towel or protector

3. Close the windows and door to prevent chilling the patient.

4. Close the privacy curtain.

5. Put clean towels and linen on a chair in the order of use. Place a laundry bag or hamper nearby.

6. Offer the bedpan or urinal. If the patient wants to use the bedpan or urinal, put on gloves. Empty and clean the bedpan or urinal before proceeding with the bath. Remove gloves and discard according to facility policy. Wash your hands.

7. Lower the head of the bed and the side rail on the side where you are working.

8. Loosen the top bedclothes. Remove and fold the blanket and spread and place them over the back of the chair.

9. Place a bath blanket over the top sheet (Figure 24-6) and slide the sheet down and out from under the bath blanket. Place the sheet in a laundry hamper.

10. Leave one pillow under the patient's head. Place the other pillows on a chair.

11. Remove the patient's night wear and place it in a laundry hamper. (Consult the nurse if the patient has an IV.)

12. Fill a bath basin two-thirds full with water at 105°F. Use a bath thermometer, if available, to be sure of the proper temperature.

13. Assist the patient to move to the side of the bed nearest you.

14. Fold a face towel over the upper edge of the bath blanket to keep the blanket dry. Put on gloves.

15. Form a mitt by folding a washcloth around your hand (Figure 24-7 shows a mitt being made on a gloved hand).
    a. Wet the washcloth.
    b. Wash the patient's eyes, using separate corners of the cloth for each eye.
    c. Wipe from inside to outside corner (Figure 24-8).

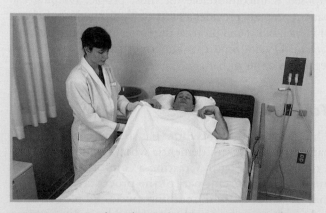

FIGURE 24-6 Replace the top bedding with a bath blanket by covering the bedding with the bath blanket, then pulling the bedding out from underneath while the patient holds the blanket in place. (© Delmar/Cengage Learning)

PROCEDURE 44 CONTINUED

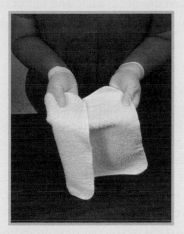
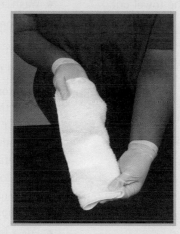
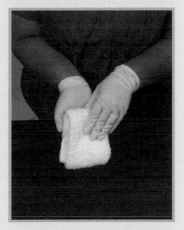

FIGURE 24-7 To make a mitt over a gloved hand, wrap the washcloth in thirds around one hand. Then bring the free end over the palm and tuck in the end. The thumb is free to hold the washcloth in place. *(© Delmar/Cengage Learning)*

   d. Do not use soap near eyes.

   e. After you have washed the eyes, remove gloves and discard according to facility policy.

   f. Do not use soap on the face unless the patient requests it.

16. Rinse the washcloth and apply soap if the patient desires. Squeeze out excess water. Do not leave soap in water.

17. Wash and rinse the patient's face, ears, and neck well. Use a towel to dry.

18. Expose the patient's far arm. Protect the bed with a bath towel placed underneath the arm.

   a. Wash, rinse, and pat dry arm and hand.

   b. Be sure the **axilla** (armpit) is clean and dry.

   c. Repeat for other arm (Figure 24-9).

   d. Apply deodorant if the patient requests it.

19. Care for hands and nails as necessary. Follow the guidelines in Procedure 49. Check with the nurse or care plan for special instructions.

20. Discard used bath water and refill the basin two-thirds full with water at 105°F.

21. Put a bath towel over the patient's chest. Then fold the blanket to the waist. Under the towel:

   a. Wash, rinse, and pat dry chest.

   b. Rinse and dry folds under the breasts of a female patient carefully to avoid irritating the skin.

22. Fold the bath blanket down to the **pubic** area (location of external genitalia). Wash, rinse, and pat dry abdomen. Fold the bath blanket up to

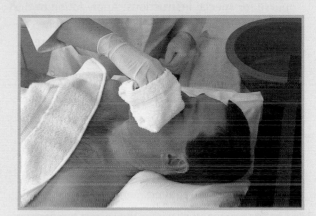

FIGURE 24-8 Avoid soap in the eye area. Wipe from the inner corner to the outer corner. Turn the washcloth before moving to the other eye. *(© Delmar/Cengage Learning)*

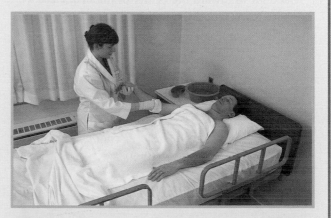

FIGURE 24-9 Place the towel under the patient's arm. Support the arm as you wash it. *(© Delmar/Cengage Learning)*

continues

Don't use soap on their body.

Give them (phin) to chose

PROCEDURE 44 CONTINUED

cover the abdomen and chest. Slide the towel out from under the bath blanket.

23. Ask the patient to flex the far knee, if possible. Fold the bath blanket up to expose the thigh, leg, and foot. Protect the bed with a bath towel.

    a. Put the bath basin on the towel.

    b. Place the patient's foot in the basin.

    c. Wash and rinse the leg and foot (Figure 24-10).

24. Lift the leg and move the basin to the other side of the bed. Dry the leg and foot. Dry well between the toes.

25. Repeat for the other leg and foot. Take the basin off the bed before drying the leg and foot.

26. Care for toenails as necessary. Check with the nurse for special instructions. Apply lotion to the feet of a patient with dry skin. Do not apply lotion between the toes, as this keeps the area moist and promotes fungal growth.

    • Do not attempt to cut thickened nails.

    • File nails straight across.

    • Do not round edges.

    • Do not push back the **cuticle**, because it is easily injured and infected.

    • If the patient is diabetic, inform the nurse if toenail care is required.

27. Change water and check for the correct temperature with a bath thermometer. Change the water any time it becomes cold or too soapy.

28. Help the patient turn on the side away from you and move toward the center of the bed. Place a bath towel lengthwise next to the patient's back.

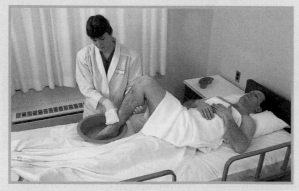

FIGURE 24-10 Support the leg and place the foot in the basin. (© Delmar/Cengage Learning)

• Wash, rinse, and dry neck, back, and buttocks.

• Use long, firm strokes when washing the back.

29. Give a backrub with lotion (see Unit 25).

30. Help the patient to turn on the back.

31. Place a towel under the buttocks and upper legs. Change the water and check the temperature. Provide a washcloth, soap, basin, and bath towel and ask the person to complete the bath by washing the genitalia. Assist if necessary. If the patient cannot complete the procedure, finish the bath. Patients may be reluctant to admit that they need help. Apply gloves when washing the genital area.

    • For a female patient, wash and rinse from front to back, drying carefully.

    • For a male patient, carefully wash, rinse, and dry the penis, scrotum, and groin area. If the patient is not circumcised, gently push the foreskin back and carefully wash and dry the penis. Then gently pull the foreskin down to its original position.

32. When using this procedure for the waterless bath (bag bath), apply the same rules for draping the patient. Use a new washcloth for each area of the body, washing in this order:

    a. Face and neck

    b. Far arm and hand

    c. Near arm and hand

    d. Chest and abdomen

    e. Far leg and foot

    f. Near leg and foot

    g. Back and buttocks

    h. Perineum

33. Remove gloves and discard according to facility policy.

34. Carry out range-of-motion exercises as ordered (see Unit 37 for these procedures).

35. Cover the pillow with a towel. Comb or brush the patient's hair. Oral hygiene is usually given at this time (see Unit 25).

36. Discard towels and washcloth in a laundry hamper.

37. Provide a clean gown. Apply the gown over the bath blanket, then tuck it underneath, or remove the blanket if done.

38. Clean and replace equipment according to facility policy.

If not Comfortable

PROCEDURE 44 CONTINUED

39. Put clean washcloth and towels in the bedside stand, or hang according to facility policy.

40. Change the bed linen, following the procedure for making an occupied bed. Replace and discard soiled linen in a laundry bag or hamper.

41. Remove and discard disposable gloves according to facility policy. Wash your hands.

42. Raise the side rails, if required.

43. Carry out ending procedure actions.

PROCEDURE

OBRA

CHANGING THE PATIENT'S GOWN

Note: Apply the principles of standard precautions if the patient has draining wounds or nonintact skin, or if contact with mucous membranes, blood, body fluids, secretions, or excretions is likely.

1. Carry out initial procedure actions.

2. Assemble equipment:
- Disposable gloves
- Bath blanket
- Clean gown
- Laundry bag or hamper

3. Place a bath blanket over the top sheet. Pull the sheet down and slide it out from under the bath blanket.

4. Loosen the gown from the patient's neck.

5. Slip the gown down the arms.

6. Make sure the patient is covered by a bath blanket (Figure 24-11).

Note: This procedure is to be used only when the patient has an IV that is NOT run through an electric pump. If the patient is wearing a gown that snaps at the shoulder, you may remove it without touching the IV bag, pump, or tubing. If the patient is wearing a nonsnap gown, call the nurse for assistance. Never disconnect the tubing from the insertion site or pump.

7. For a patient wearing a regular gown (nonsnap):

  a. Remove the gown from the arm without the IV and bring the gown across the patient's chest to the other arm.

  b. Place a clean gown over the patient's chest.

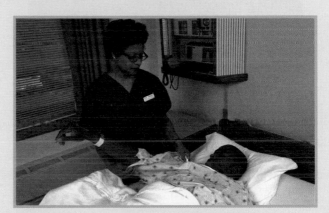

FIGURE 24-11 Keeping the patient covered with the bath blanket, remove the patient's gown. *(© Delmar/ Cengage Learning)*

  c. On the arm with the IV, gather the gown in one hand so there is no pull or pressure on the IV line (Figure 24-12A), and slowly draw the gown over the tips of the patient's fingers.

  d. With your free hand, lift the IV off the standard and slip the gown over the bag of fluid (Figure 24-12B), removing the gown from the patient's body. *Never lower the bag of fluid below the patient's arm.*

  e. Slip the sleeve of a clean gown over the bag of fluid and tubing, then up the patient's arm.

  f. Replace the bag of fluid on the IV standard.

  g. Remove the soiled gown and place it at the end of the bed. Finish putting the clean gown on the patient's other arm. Secure the neck ties.

  h. Place the soiled gown in a laundry hamper.

  i. Make sure the IV is dripping at the required rate and that the tubing is not kinked or twisted.

continues

PROCEDURE 45 CONTINUED

8. If the patient has a weak or paralyzed arm, always undress the patient in the following manner:

   a. Untie the gown and remove the back sides of the gown from underneath the patient.

   b. Remove the gown from the stronger arm first.

   c. Drape the gown across the chest and slide the gown down over the weak arm.

   d. Gently lift the weak arm and slip the gown over the patient's hand.

   e. Reverse the procedure to apply a clean gown. Put the gown over the weaker arm first.

9. Pull the sheet up over the bath blanket. Remove the bath blanket.

10. Carry out ending procedure actions.

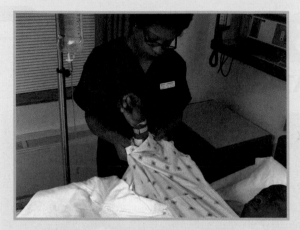

FIGURE 24-12A Gather the gown material in one hand so there is no traction on the IV line. Slowly draw the gown over the tips of the patient's fingers. (© Delmar/ Cengage Learning)

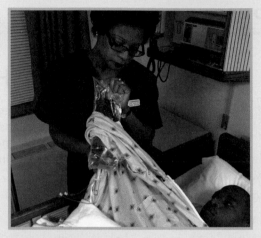

FIGURE 24-12B With your free hand, lift the IV off the standard and slip the gown over the bag of fluid. (© Delmar/Cengage Learning)

Difficult SITUATIONS

Bathing can upset patients who have Alzheimer's disease and other types of dementia. Increased motor activity and a change in tone of voice are early signs of distress. The patient may perceive being disrobed and having the body handled as a form of sexual assault. As the anxiety worsens, he or she may scream and fight. Bathing becomes a source of stress for both the patient and nursing assistant. The patient's aggressive behavior is a way of telling you that he or she cannot tolerate this method of bathing. The behavior is a means of asking you to find a better way of doing it. Consider a different method of bathing, such as using a bag bath or towel bath. Bathing should never be traumatic to a patient. Being flexible and considerate of patients' needs improves their quality of life, reduces stress, and saves time for the nursing assistant. ■

Difficult SITUATIONS

Bathing patients who have dementia requires the use of many nursing assistant skills, including communication, problem solving, and creativity. Strive to make the bath pleasant and comforting, dignified, patient-centered, and based on the patient's individual needs, instead of being a routine ritual of nursing assistant practice. ■

Whatever you can't do am care to assist you. you can't force them

PROCEDURE

46

PARTIAL BATH

1. Carry out initial procedure actions.

2. Assemble equipment:
   - Disposable gloves
   - Bed linen
   - Bath blanket
   - Bath thermometer
   - Soap and soap dish or liquid soap
   - Washcloth
   - Face towel
   - Bath towel
   - Bag bath product instead of bathing supplies, if this will be used
   - Gown and robe
   - Laundry bag or hamper
   - Bath basin
   - Lotion
   - Equipment for oral hygiene
   - Nail brush, emery board, and orangewood stick
   - Brush, comb, and deodorant
   - Bedpan or urinal and cover
   - Paper towels or protector

   Note: A bag bath product may be used, if approved by facility policy. Apply the principles of standard precautions if the patient has draining wounds or nonintact skin, or if contact with blood, body fluids, mucous membranes, secretions, or excretions is likely.

3. Close windows and door and turn off fans to prevent chilling the patient.

4. Put the towels and linen on the chair in the order of use. Make sure a laundry bag or hamper is available.

5. Put on disposable gloves.

6. Offer the bedpan or urinal (see Unit 26). Empty and clean it before proceeding with the bath. Remove gloves and discard according to facility policy. Wash your hands.

7. Elevate the head of the bed, if permitted, to a comfortable position.

8. Loosen the top bedclothes. Remove and fold the blanket and spread and place them over the back of the chair. Place a bath blanket over the top sheet. Slide the top sheet down and out from under the bath blanket.

9. Leave one pillow under the patient's head. Place the other pillow on the chair.

10. Assist the patient to remove the gown. Place the gown in the laundry hamper. Make sure the patient is covered with a bath blanket.

11. Place paper towels or a bed protector on the overbed table.

12. Fill a bath basin two-thirds full with water at 105°F. Place the basin on the overbed table.

13. Push the overbed table comfortably close to the patient.

14. Place towels, washcloth, and soap on the overbed table within easy reach.

15. Instruct the patient to wash as much as she is able and tell her that you will return to complete the bath.

16. Place the call bell within easy reach. Ask the patient to signal when ready.

17. Wash hands and leave the unit.

18. Wash hands and return to the unit when the patient signals. Put on a new pair of gloves.

19. Change the bath water. Finish the bath by washing those areas the patient could not reach. Make sure the face, hands, axillae, buttocks, back, and genitals are washed and dried.

20. Remove gloves and discard according to facility policy.

21. Wash your hands.

22. Give a backrub with lotion.

23. Assist the patient in applying deodorant and a fresh gown.

24. Cover the pillow with a towel. Comb or brush the patient's hair. Assist with oral hygiene, if needed (see Unit 25).

25. Clean and replace equipment according to facility policy.

26. Put a clean washcloth and towels in the bedside stand, or hang according to facility policy.

27. Change the bed linen, following the procedure for making an occupied bed. Put soiled linen in the laundry hamper.

28. Carry out ending procedure actions.

PERINEAL CARE

The **perineum** is the area between the legs. In females, it is the area between the vagina and the anus. In males, it is the area between the scrotum and the anus.

Perineal care may be performed as part of general bathing or as a separate procedure, as needed. **Perineal care** means washing the area that includes the genitals and anus (see Procedures 47 and 48). Always wear gloves and use standard precautions when caring for the perineal area.

Tips: If the patient has been incontinent, remove the wet pad or linen and replace with a dry pad before beginning perineal care. Remove excess stool with toilet tissue. Patients who need assistance with perineal care and those who become incontinent may feel guilty and embarrassed. Avoid showing disgust. Be sensitive to the patient's feelings.

Clinical Information ALERT

Urine and stool are very damaging to the skin. The effects of the excretions cause skin damage (similar to a rash or chemical burn) and skin breakdown. The damage to the skin worsens with the length of exposure to the substances. ∎

Infection Control ALERT

Providing perineal care is one of the most important procedures you will perform as a nursing assistant. Always apply the principles of standard precautions. Remember that there are mucous membranes in the genital area. If you are wearing gloves, change them before beginning care. Using proper technique is critical because of the high risk of contamination and infection. Avoid scrubbing back and forth. Always wipe from clean to dirty with a single wipe, then turn or discard the cloth, according to facility policy.

Guidelines for female perineal care vary with the institution. In some facilities, you will be instructed to clean the center first, then each side. In others, you will clean the sides of the genitalia first, then the center. Know and follow your facility policies. Discard your gloves properly and avoid contaminating environmental surfaces with your used gloves. ∎

PROCEDURE

FEMALE PERINEAL CARE

Note: The guidelines and sequence for this procedure vary slightly from state to state, and from one facility to the next. Your instructor will inform you if the sequence in your state or facility differs from the procedure listed here. Know and follow the required sequence for your state and facility policies.

1. Carry out initial procedure actions.

2. Assemble equipment:
   - Disposable gloves
   - Bath blanket or top sheet
   - Bedpan and cover
   - Liquid soap
   - Basin
   - Bath thermometer
   - Bed protector
   - Washcloth and towel
   - Plastic bag(s), if needed to discard linen or trash
   - Laundry barrel or hamper

3. Lower the side rail on the side where you will be working. Be sure the opposite side rail is up and secure.

4. Remove the bedspread and blanket. Fold and place them on the back of the chair.

5. Position the patient on her back. Cover with a bath blanket and fanfold the sheet to the foot of the bed.

6. Put on disposable gloves. Fill a basin with water at 105°F.

PROCEDURE **47** CONTINUED

7. Place a bed protector under the patient's buttocks.

8. Offer the bedpan to the patient.

   a. If used and the patient is on intake and output, record the amount.

   b. Empty and clean the bedpan before continuing with the procedure.

   c. Remove gloves and discard according to facility policy.

   d. Wash your hands and put on a new pair of gloves.

9. Position the bath blanket so that only the area between the legs is exposed.

10. Ask the patient to separate her legs and flex her knees.

    Note: If the patient is unable to spread her legs and flex her knees, turn the patient on her side with the legs flexed. This position provides easy access to the perineal area.

11. Wet the washcloth, make a mitt, and apply a small amount of liquid soap.

    Note: Heavy soap application may be difficult to rinse off completely. Soap residue is irritating.

12. Separate the labia with one gloved hand. Keep the labia separated as much as possible during the procedure. Avoid placing your fingers on an area after washing it. Turn the washcloth so you are using a clean section each time you move to a new area. Use a second washcloth, if necessary. You may need several washcloths to perform the procedure without contamination. (Some facilities require a second, clean washcloth for rinsing; the used cloth is not put back into the water basin). If a urinary catheter is present, hold the tubing securely to one side and support against the leg to avoid unnecessary movement or traction on the catheter. In some facilities, the proximal catheter is washed as part of perineal care. Keep the tubing and drainage bag below the level of the bladder.

    - With the other gloved hand, wash the center of the labia, using a single downward stroke from top to bottom.
    - Turn the washcloth to a clean area.
    - Wash the far side of the labia, using a single downward stroke from top to bottom (Figure 24-13A).

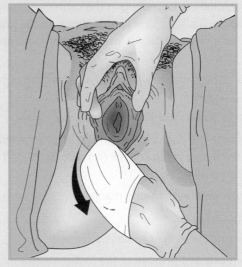

FIGURE 24-13A Spread the vulva with one hand. With the washcloth in the other hand, start in the front and stroke downward along the outer labia. *(© Delmar/ Cengage Learning)*

- Turn the washcloth to a clean area.
- Wash the near labia, using a single downward stroke from top to bottom.
- Continue to alternate from side to side, working outward to the thighs, using the same technique. Turn the washcloth or use a new washcloth, if necessary, so that a fresh section is used to cleanse each area.
- If a urinary catheter is present, wash, rinse, and dry the perineal area surrounding the urinary meatus and catheter. Change the washcloth. Beginning at the urinary meatus, wash down the catheter approximately 3 to 4 inches. Use a single downward stroke. Do not rub back and forth. Rinse and dry in the same direction. Hold the catheter firmly to avoid pulling and traction. After washing the catheter, continue with perineal care.
- Rinse the area from top to bottom with the washcloth. Avoid rubbing back and forth. Rinse in the same sequence, beginning in the center and moving outward from side to side. Turn the washcloth so a clean surface is used for each downward stroke.
- Gently pat the area dry with a towel. Avoid rubbing back and forth. Dry in the same

continues

PROCEDURE 47 CONTINUED

sequence, beginning in the center and moving outward from side to side. Position the towel so a clean surface is used for each downward stroke.

13. Turn the patient away from you. Flex the upper leg slightly.

14. Make a mitt, wet it, and apply soap lightly.

15. Expose the anal area. Wash the area, stroking from perineum to coccyx (front to back) (Figure 24-13B).

16. Rinse well in the same manner.

17. Dry carefully.

18. Return the patient to her back.

19. Remove and dispose of the bed protector according to facility policy.

20. Cover the patient with a sheet or bath blanket.

21. Remove and dispose of gloves according to facility policy. Wash your hands.

22. Remove, fold, and store the bath blanket according to facility policy.

23. Replace the top covers, tuck them under the mattress, and make mitered corners. (Some patients prefer that the top covers not be tucked in.)

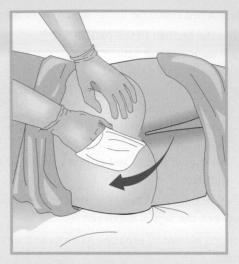

FIGURE 24-13B With one hand, lift up on the buttocks to expose the anal area. Wipe from the perineum back toward the anus. *(© Delmar/Cengage Learning)*

24. Put up the side rail, if required.

25. Put on gloves. Empty the water. Clean equipment and dispose of or store it, according to facility policy.

26. Remove gloves and discard according to facility policy. Wash your hands.

27. Carry out ending procedure actions.

Clinical Information ALERT

Be gentle when cleansing patients after incontinent episodes. Scrubbing produces extra friction. The excretions are irritating to the skin, and vigorous scrubbing is abrasive, increasing the risk of infection and skin breakdown. ▪

Infection Control ALERT

When giving perineal care, wash from the most clean area to the least clean. Turn the cloth frequently and rinse well. Avoid using the washcloth, towel, and gloves elsewhere on the body. If further bathing or touching is necessary, apply new gloves and use different linen. Some patients may have orders for barrier cream or another product following perineal care. If you will be applying barrier cream, remove your gloves, wash your hands, and apply new gloves. Your gloves become contaminated during the perineal care procedure, and you must use new (clean) gloves to apply barrier cream. Avoid contaminating the jar or tube of cream with your used gloves. ▪

PROCEDURE

48

MALE PERINEAL CARE

📝 **Note:** The guidelines and sequence for this procedure vary slightly from state to state, and from one facility to the next. Your instructor will inform you if the sequence in your state or facility differs from the procedure listed here. Know and follow the required sequence for your state and facility policies.

1. Carry out initial procedure actions.

2. Assemble equipment:
   - Disposable gloves
   - Bath blanket
   - Bath thermometer
   - Urinal and cover or bedpan and cover
   - Soap, washcloth, and towel
   - Plastic bag
   - Bed protector or bath towel
   - Ordered solution (if other than water)
   - Basin
   - Laundry hamper

3. Fill a basin with warm water at approximately 105°F.

4. Lower the side rail on the side where you will be working.

5. Fanfold the blanket and spread to the foot of the bed. Remove, fold, and place them on the back of the chair.

6. Cover the patient with a bath blanket and fanfold the sheet to the foot of the bed.

7. Put on disposable gloves.

8. Place a bed protector under the patient's buttocks.

9. Offer the bedpan or urinal.
   - If used and the patient is on intake and output, record the amount.
   - Empty and clean the bedpan or urinal before continuing with the procedure.
   - Remove gloves and discard according to facility policy.
   - Wash your hands and put on a new pair of gloves.

10. Have the patient flex and separate his knees.

📝 **Note:** If the patient is unable to spread his legs and flex the knees, the perineal area can be washed with the patient on his side with the legs flexed. This position provides easy access to the perineal area.

11. Draw the bath blanket upward to expose the perineal area only.

12. Make a mitt with a washcloth and apply a small amount of soap.

📝 **Note:** Heavy soap application may be difficult to rinse off completely. Soap residue is irritating.

13. Grasp the penis gently with one hand and wash. Begin at the meatus and wash in a circular motion (Figure 24-14A). If a urinary catheter is present, hold the tubing securely to one side and support it against the leg to avoid unnecessary movement or traction on the catheter. Keep the tubing and drainage bag below the level of the bladder.

14. If the patient is not circumcised, draw the foreskin back (Figure 24-14B). Be sure the entire penis is washed. Rinse thoroughly.

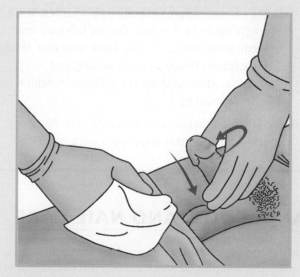

FIGURE 24-14A Grasp the penis gently with one hand. With the other, wipe in a circular motion, beginning with the urinary meatus, working outward over the glans (head of the penis). Continue to wash down the penis and the rest of the perineal area, including the scrotum, using downward strokes and working outward to the thighs. (© Delmar/Cengage Learning)

continues

PROCEDURE 48 CONTINUED

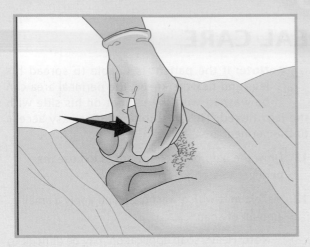

FIGURE 24-14B If the patient is not circumcised, gently push the foreskin back so the glans can be washed. Once the penis is washed and dried, return the foreskin to its normal position. *(© Delmar/Cengage Learning)*

15. Continue to wash down the penis and the rest of the perineal area, including the scrotum, using downward strokes and working outward to the thighs. Lift the scrotum and wash the perineum.

   - If a urinary catheter is present, wash, rinse, and dry the perineal area surrounding the urinary meatus and catheter. Change the washcloth. Beginning at the urinary meatus, wash down the catheter approximately 3 to 4 inches. Use a single downward stroke. Do not rub back and forth. Rinse and dry in the same direction. Hold the catheter firmly to avoid pulling and traction. After washing the catheter, continue with perineal care.

16. Rinse the washcloth and remake a mitt. Rinse the urethral and perineal areas well, working in the same direction until the entire area is clean and soap-free.

17. Dry the washed area with a towel. Reposition the foreskin if necessary.

18. Turn the patient away from you. Flex his upper leg slightly if permitted.

19. Make a mitt, wet it, and apply soap lightly.

20. Expose the anal area. Wash the area, stroking from perineum to coccyx.

21. Rinse well in the same manner.

22. Dry carefully.

23. Return the patient to his back.

24. Remove and dispose of the bed protector according to facility policy.

25. Cover the patient with a sheet.

26. Remove and dispose of gloves according to facility policy. Wash your hands.

27. Remove, fold, and store the bath blanket, according to facility policy.

28. Replace the top covers, tuck them under the mattress, and make mitered corners. (Some patients prefer that the top covers not be tucked in.)

29. Put up the side rail, if required.

30. Put on gloves. Empty the water. Clean equipment and dispose of or store it, according to facility policy.

31. Remove gloves and discard according to facility policy. Wash your hands.

32. Carry out ending procedure actions.

HAND, FOOT, AND NAIL CARE

Many patients are unable to care for their own nails and extremities. You will provide this care, or assist the patient to do these tasks, as needed. Nail care is often combined with bathing.

Infection Control ALERT

In many facilities, nursing assistants are not permitted to clip nails. However, some facilities permit assistants to perform nail care on nondiabetic patients. Be aware that the clippers are a potential source of infection, especially of *Streptococcus A*, which is called the "flesh-eating strep." Make sure you disinfect clippers and any other reusable items thoroughly after each use. ■

GUIDELINES *for*

Providing Hand, Foot, and Nail Care

- Know and follow your facility policy for who is allowed to clip and clean nails. Use clippers or nail scissors only if you are permitted to do so according to state law and facility policies. Do not use regular scissors.

- Cleaning and trimming nails is easier immediately after the nails have been soaked or bathed.

- Avoid the use of nail files and other sharp objects for cleaning nails. An orange stick is a disposable, pointed, wooden stick that can be safely used.

- When trimming nails, be very careful not to accidentally clip or damage the skin surrounding the nail.

- If you observe any abnormalities, such as redness, cracking, or signs of infection, by the fingernails or toenails, report it to the nurse.

- Clip nails straight across, then round the edges with an emery board.

- Push the cuticles back with a washcloth or the dull end of the orange stick.

- Dry the feet well. Carefully dry between each toe and inspect for red or cracked areas. Moisture promotes fungal growth and skin breakdown, which can lead to more serious complications.

- Lotion may be applied to the hands or feet if the skin is dry. Do not apply lotion between the toes.

PROCEDURE

OBRA DVD

HAND AND FINGERNAIL CARE

Note: Check with the nurse and nursing care plan to learn if this procedure is permitted for the patient or if it is to be modified because of the patient's condition. Use clippers and sharp instruments only if you are permitted to do so according to state law and facility policies.

This procedure can be carried out independently, or can be modified and added to the bath procedure.

1. Carry out initial procedure actions.

2. Assemble equipment:
   - Basin
   - Bath thermometer
   - Soap
   - Bath towel and washcloth
   - Lotion
   - Plastic protector
   - Nail clippers
   - Emery board
   - Orangewood stick
   - Nail polish (optional)

3. Elevate the head of the bed, if permitted, and adjust the overbed table in front of the patient. Assist the patient to transfer to a chair and position the overbed table waist-high across the patient's lap.

4. Place a plastic protector on the overbed table.

5. Fill a basin with warm water at approximately 105°F, using the bath thermometer to test the temperature. Place the basin on the overbed table.

6. Place the patient's hands in the basin and soak for approximately 5 minutes. Cover the basin with a towel to help retain heat. Add warm water if necessary. Remove the patient's hands before adding water.

7. Wash the patient's hands. Push cuticles back gently with a washcloth or an orangewood stick (Figure 24-15A). (A cream may be used to soften the cuticles first.) Use a soft brush or orangewood stick to clean under nails. (Check with the nurse before using an orangewood stick on a person with diabetes.)

8. Dry the patient's hands with a towel.

continues

PROCEDURE 49 CONTINUED

9. Use nail clippers to cut fingernails straight across, if permitted (Figure 24-15B).
   - Do not cut below the tips of the fingers.
   - Keep nail clippings on the protector to be discarded.
10. Shape and smooth the fingernails with an emery board (Figure 24-15C). Apply polish to nails if the patient desires.

11. Pour a small amount of lotion in your palms and gently smooth it on the patient's hands.
12. Empty the water from the basin. Gather equipment. Clean and store it according to facility policy.
13. Return the overbed table to the foot of the bed. If the patient has been sitting up for the procedure, assist the patient to get into bed.
14. Carry out ending procedure actions.

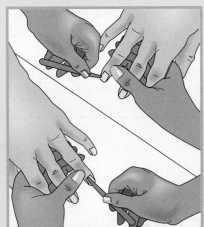

FIGURE 24-15A Gently push the cuticles back with a washcloth or orangewood stick, if permitted. (© Delmar/Cengage Learning)

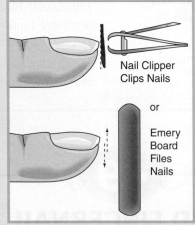

Nail Clipper Clips Nails

or

Emery Board Files Nails

FIGURE 24-15B Clip the nails straight across. (© Delmar/Cengage Learning)

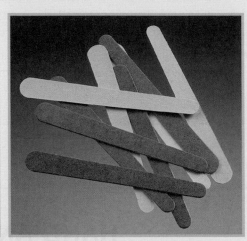

FIGURE 24-15C Round the edges with an emery board. (Courtesy of Medline Industries, Inc. (800) MEDLINE)

SHAMPOOING THE HAIR

Many patients are unable to care for their hair. You will provide this care, or assist the patient to do these tasks, as needed. For some patients, a shampoo may be combined with the bath.

Clinical Information ALERT

In some facilities, a doctor's order is needed for a shampoo. If permitted, you may wash the hair as part of the tub bath or shower. Offer the patient a washcloth or towel to hold over the face while washing and rinsing the hair. This procedure is done in bed for patients who are on complete bedrest. Some facilities use dry chemical shampoos that are brushed out. No-rinse shampoos are also available for bedfast patients. ■

Difficult SITUATIONS

Like bathing, washing a cognitively impaired person's hair under running water can be a cause of great stress and anxiety. Consider using a bed shampoo tray, an inflatable shampoo basin, or a shampoo cap or dry shampoo product. ■

PROCEDURE

50

BED SHAMPOO

1. Carry out initial procedure actions.

2. Assemble equipment needed:
   - Shampoo tray
   - Shampoo
   - Washcloths
   - 3 bath towels
   - Bath blanket
   - Bath thermometer
   - Pitcher of water (105°F)
   - Safety pin
   - 2 bed protectors
   - Waterproof covering for pillow
   - Large bucket to collect used water
   - Hair dryer, if available (portable)
   - Hairbrush and comb
   - Small empty pitcher or cup
   - Larger pitcher of water (105°F)—use if additional water is needed
   - Plastic bag or container for soiled linen

3. Place a large, empty basin or bucket on the floor under the spout of the shampoo tray.

4. Arrange on the bedside stand, within easy reach (Figure 24-16A):
   - Large pitcher of water (105°F)
   - Washcloth
   - 2 bath towels
   - Shampoo
   - Small pitcher of water (105°F)

5. Replace the top bedding with a bath blanket.

6. Ask the patient to move to the side of the bed nearest you. Assist as needed.

7. Replace the pillowcase with a waterproof covering.

8. Cover the head of the bed with a bed protector. Be sure it goes well under the patient's shoulders.

9. Loosen neck ties of the gown.

10. Place a towel under the patient's head and shoulders. Brush hair, working tangles out carefully.

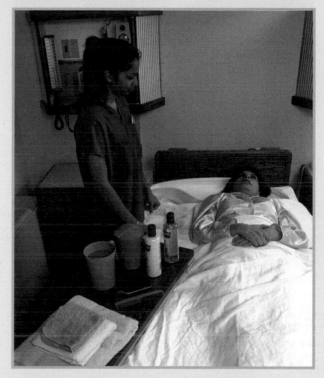

FIGURE 24-16A Assemble equipment. (© Delmar/ Cengage Learning)

11. Bring the towel down around the patient's neck and shoulders and pin it. Position the pillow under the shoulders so that the patient's head is tilted slightly backward.

12. Raise the bed to a good working height.

13. Raise the patient's head slightly and position the shampoo tray (Figure 24-16B) so that the drain is over the edge of the bed directly above the basin or bucket.

14. Give the patient a washcloth to cover the eyes (Figure 24-16C).

15. Recheck the temperature of water in the basin.

16. Using the small pitcher (Figure 24-16D), pour a small amount of water over hair until thoroughly wet. Use one hand to help direct the flow away from the patient's face and ears.

17. Apply a small amount of shampoo, working up a lather (Figure 24-16E). Work from scalp to hair ends.

continues

PROCEDURE 50 CONTINUED

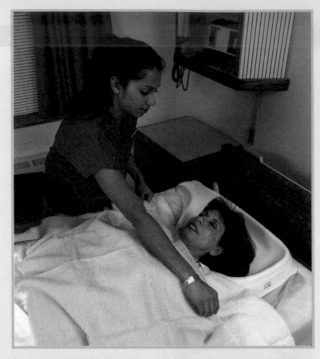

FIGURE 24-16B Position the patient with the head on the shampoo tray. Protect the patient with a towel and the bed with a protector. *(© Delmar/Cengage Learning)*

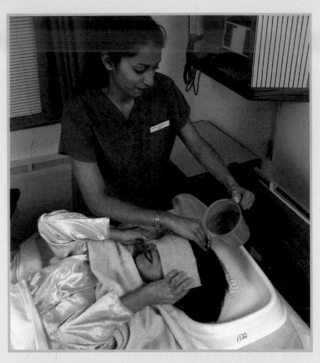

FIGURE 24-16D Wet the hair by slowly pouring warm water. *(© Delmar/Cengage Learning)*

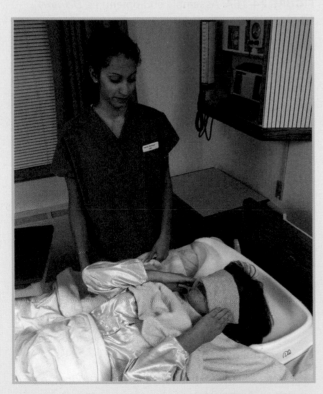

FIGURE 24-16C Give the patient a folded washcloth to protect the eyes. *(© Delmar/Cengage Learning)*

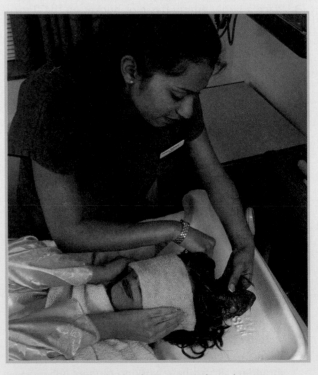

FIGURE 24-16E Apply shampoo and work it into a lather, using your fingertips. *(© Delmar/Cengage Learning)*

PROCEDURE 50 CONTINUED

18. Massage the scalp with your fingertips. Do not use your fingernails.

19. Rinse thoroughly, pouring from hairline to hair tips. Direct the flow into the drain. Use water from the pitcher if needed, but be sure to check the water temperature before using it.

20. Repeat lathering and rinsing (Steps 16–19).

21. Lift the patient's head. Remove the tray and bed protector. Adjust the pillow and slip a dry bath towel underneath the head.

22. Place the tray on the basin. Wrap hair in a towel. Be sure to dry face, neck, and ears as needed.

23. Dry hair with the towel. If available and not otherwise contraindicated, use a portable hair dryer to complete the drying process. Brushing the hair as you blow-dry helps the hair to dry. Keep the dryer moving and not too close to the head.

24. Comb hair appropriately. Remove the protective pillow cover. Replace with a cloth cover.

25. Replace the bedding and remove the bath blanket.

26. Help the patient to assume a comfortable position. Lower the bed to the lowest horizontal position. Leave the call bell within reach.

27. Allow the patient to rest undisturbed. The length of this procedure may tire the patient.

28. Empty the water from the collection basin.

29. Carry out ending procedure actions.

The Waterless Shampoo

Various waterless preparations are available for washing the hair of patients whose hair cannot be shampooed by other methods. Shampoo caps (Figure 24-17) are a popular alternative for washing the hair of bedfast patients. These are most comfortable if they are warmed in the product warmer, or in a microwave for 30 seconds or less. If the microwave is used, feel the outside of the cap by pressing the various areas against your forearm to make sure there are no hot spots. Place the cap on the patient's head, then rub gently for 1 to 2 minutes for short hair and 4 to 5 minutes for long hair. Remove the cap; then towel-dry and comb the hair. Shampoo caps contain a no-rinse product that reduces tangling and does not leave residue like some dry chemical products.

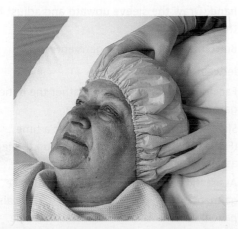

FIGURE 24-17 Shampoo caps simplify the hair-washing procedure for bedfast patients, and require no rinsing. Conditioners in the product leave the hair soft and reduce the incidence of tangling. (*Courtesy of Medline Industries, Inc. (800) MEDLINE*)

DRESSING A PATIENT

Patients in hospitals generally wear hospital gowns because they are in bed most of the time. However, some patients prefer to wear their own nightgowns or pajamas and will need assistance in dressing. Patients in the rehabilitation unit and those who participate in some special programs may be up and fully dressed each day. You may also need to assist patients to dress when they are discharged from the hospital. It is usually easier to help patients dress while they are still in bed.

GUIDELINES *for*

Dressing and Undressing Patients

The patient who requires help in dressing may wish to sit in a chair with clothing placed nearby. You can help by:

- Allowing the patient to choose the clothing to be put on.

- Encouraging the patient to do as much as he or she is able.

- Being prepared to assist with shoes and stockings even for patients who can do much themselves. Bending over to adjust shoes and stockings can result in dizziness and loss of balance.

- Putting clothing on the weak or paralyzed side first.

- Removing clothing from the unaffected or strongest side first.

PROCEDURE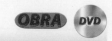

51

DRESSING AND UNDRESSING THE PATIENT

1. Carry out initial procedure actions.

2. Select clothing and arrange in order of application. Encourage the patient to select clothes, if able.

3. Cover the patient with a bath blanket and fanfold top bedclothes to the foot of the bed.

4. Elevate the head of the bed to sitting position.

5. Assist the patient to a comfortable sitting position.

6. Remove night clothing, keeping the patient covered with the bath blanket. Remove from strong side first. Place night clothes in a laundry bag or hamper or fold them to be taken home.

7. If the patient wears a bra, slip the straps over the patient's hands (weak side first), move the straps up her arms, and position them on her shoulders. Adjust the breasts in the bra cups. Then assist the patient to lean forward and hook the bra in back.

8. For an undershirt, or any garment that slips on over the head:

   a. Gather the undershirt and place it over the patient's head (Figure 24-18A).

   b. Grasp the patient's hand and guide it through the armhole by reaching into the armhole from the outside.

   c. Repeat the procedure with the opposite arm.

   d. Assist the patient to lean forward, and adjust the undershirt so it is smooth over the upper body.

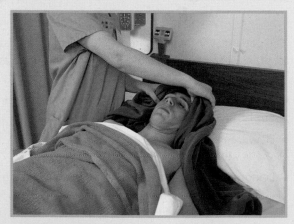

FIGURE 24-18A Gather the garment and pull it over the patient's head. (© Delmar/Cengage Learning)

9. Alternate procedure for slipover garments:

    Note: A garment must be large enough or made of stretchy fabric for this procedure.

   a. Place the garment front side down on the patient's lap, with the bottom opening facing the patient.

   b. Put the patient's hands into the bottom of the garment and, one at a time, into the sleeve holes.

   c. Pull the sleeves up as far as possible on the patient's arms and pull the hands through at the wrist if it is a long-sleeved garment. The garment should now be high on the patient's chest.

   d. Gather the back up with your hand and slip the garment over the patient's head.

   e. Smooth the garment down and position it comfortably about the patient's body. Adjust sleeves and shoulders as needed.

10. Shirts or dresses that fasten in the front:

    a. Insert your hand through the sleeve and grasp the patient's hand. Draw the sleeve over your hand and the patient's.

    b. Adjust the sleeve at the shoulder.

    c. Assist the patient to sit forward. Arrange clothing across the patient's back.

    d. Gather the sleeve on the opposite side by slipping your hand in from the outside.

    e. Grasp the patient's wrist and pull the sleeve of the garment over your hand and the patient's hand. Draw the sleeve upward and adjust it at the shoulder.

    f. Button, zip, or snap the garment.

11. Underwear or pants:

    a. Facing the foot of the bed, gather the patient's garment from waist to leg hole.

    b. Slip the garment over one foot at a time (Figure 24-18B). Pull the garment up the legs as high as possible.

    c. Assist the patient to raise the hips. Draw the garment over the buttocks and up to the waist. If patient cannot raise the buttocks, assist the

PROCEDURE 51 CONTINUED

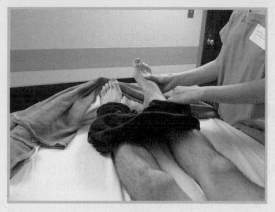

FIGURE 24-18B Slip pants over feet and lower legs. *(© Delmar/Cengage Learning)*

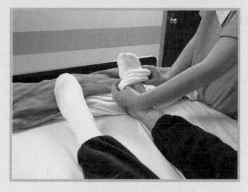

FIGURE 24-18D Adjust socks smoothly over toes. Leave about 1/4 inch of space between the ends of the toes and the toe of the stocking, to prevent pulling and pressure. *(© Delmar/Cengage Learning)*

patient to roll first to one side, as you pull up the garment, and then the other side (Figure 24-18C). Adjust the garment until comfortable.

   d. Fasten the garment, if required.

12. Socks or knee-high (or thigh-high) stockings:

   a. Roll a sock or stocking with the heel in back and place it over the patient's toes (Figure 24-18D).

   b. Draw the sock up over the foot and adjust until smooth. Pull stockings smoothly up to knee or thigh.

   c. Repeat for other foot.

13. Pantyhose:

   a. Gather pantyhose and adjust over toes and feet. Draw up legs as high as possible.

   b. Draw over hips as described in step 11c. Adjust until comfortable at waist.

14. Shoes:

   a. Slip shoe on, using a shoe horn if necessary. Open laces of shoes completely so the foot can easily slip into the shoe (Figure 24-18E).

   b. Be sure the shoe is fastened securely (Velcro tabs or ties). If the shoes tie, be sure that the shoelaces do not drag on the floor. The shoes should be tight enough so they do not slip off the patient's feet but not so tight that circulation is impaired.

   c. Shoes should be appropriate to the floor surface.

15. To undress, reverse order of steps.

16. Carry out ending procedure actions.

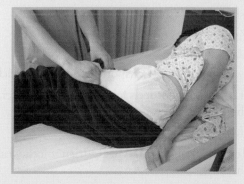

FIGURE 24-18C Have the patient roll onto the strong side first, then pull pants over hip. Then roll the patient to the other side and pull up pants. Adjust for comfort. *(© Delmar/Cengage Learning)*

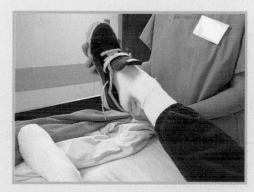

FIGURE 24-18E Open the shoelaces completely and slip the foot into the shoe. *(© Delmar/Cengage Learning)*

REVIEW

A. Multiple Choice

Select the one best answer for each of the following.

1. The room temperature during the bath procedure should be about
   a. 62°F.
   b. 68°F.
   c. 72°F.
   d. 86°F.

2. When providing perineal care to a female patient,
   a. wash from the front to the back.
   b. wash the genitals from side to side.
   c. wipe from back to front.
   d. scrub back and forth vigorously.

3. Bath water temperature should be approximately
   a. 105°F.
   b. 90°F.
   c. 80°F.
   d. 120°F.

4. When giving hand and nail care, the hands should be soaked for approximately
   a. 1 hour.
   b. 1/2 hour.
   c. 20 minutes.
   d. 5 minutes.

5. When a patient takes a bath, the bathroom door should
   a. not be locked.
   b. be left wide open.
   c. be locked for privacy.
   d. be left partially open.

6. The temperature in the whirlpool tub should be set at
   a. 110°F.
   b. 90°F.
   c. 105°F.
   d. 97°F.

7. The towel bath is an effective method of bathing patients
   a. who need to use a bag bath.
   b. who need perineal care.

c. with dementia.
d. who need a partial bath.

8. You are assigned to do perineal care on Mr. Yarbrough, a patient with a catheter. You will
   a. ask the nurse to care for the catheter.
   b. hold the tubing securely to one side.
   c. avoid washing near the catheter.
   d. scrub up and down the catheter.

9. You must dress Mr. Luna, a patient whose right side is paralyzed as a result of a stroke. You will
   a. dress the patient's right arm first.
   b. select pullover clothing.
   c. dress the patient's left arm first.
   d. remove pants on the right side first.

10. When giving a patient a whirlpool,
    a. pour liquid soap into the water.
    b. wet the patient's hair in the tub water.
    c. never shampoo the hair in the whirlpool.
    d. cover the patient's genitals with a towel.

B. Nursing Assistant Challenge

Mr. Rodriguez is taking a shower before going home. He had bowel surgery four days ago. Answer the following about his care by selecting the correct word.

11. The person responsible for the cleanliness of the shower is the ___NA___.
    (patient) (nursing assistant)

12. The patient ___should___ be assisted into and out of the shower.
    (should not) (should)

13. You can protect the patient from fatigue by ___wheelchair___ to the shower.
    (walking slowly) (transporting him by wheelchair)

14. If Mr. Rodriguez feels faint during his shower, you should turn the water ___off___.
    (to cold) (off)

15. To prevent chilling if Mr. Rodriguez feels weak, you should _____.
    (turn on the warm water) (wrap him in a bath blanket)

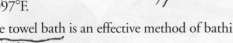

UNIT 25

General Comfort Measures

OBJECTIVES

After completing this unit, you will be able to:
- Spell and define terms.
- Discuss the reasons for early morning and bedtime care.
- List the purposes of oral hygiene.
- Identify patients who require frequent oral hygiene.
- Explain nursing assistant responsibilities for a patient's dentures.
- State the purpose of backrubs.
- Describe safety precautions when shaving a patient.
- Describe the importance of hair care.

- Explain the use of comfort devices.
- Demonstrate the following procedures:
  - Procedure 52 Assisting the Patient to Floss and Brush Teeth
  - Procedure 53 Providing Mouth Care for an Unresponsive Patient
  - Procedure 54 Caring for Dentures
  - Procedure 55 Backrub
  - Procedure 56 Shaving a Male Patient
  - Procedure 57 Daily Hair Care

VOCABULARY

Learn the meaning and the correct spelling of the following words and phrases:

AM care	caries	footboard	oral hygiene
anticoagulants	dentures	halitosis	PM care
bridging	foot drop		

INTRODUCTION

The procedures in this chapter contribute to patients' general comfort and feelings of well-being.

AM CARE AND PM CARE

Early morning (AM) care prepares the patient for a day of activities and PM (bedtime) care prepares the patient for a night of rest. Each provides an opportunity for the patient to meet elimination needs and to be refreshed. When assisting with these procedures, you have an opportunity to closely observe each patient's condition and to interact supportively.

AM Care

Early morning or AM **care** helps to set the tone for the entire day. If the patient is refreshed and comfortable before

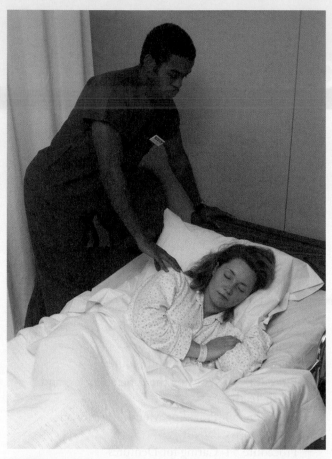

FIGURE 25-1 Early AM care. Wake the patient by saying the patient's name, then gently touching the arm, if necessary. (© Delmar/Cengage Learning)

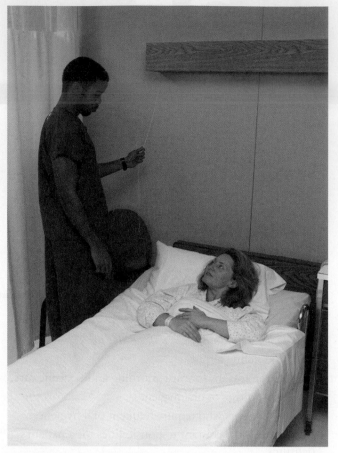

FIGURE 25-2 Turn off the light when the patient is settled and comfortable. (© Delmar/Cengage Learning)

eating breakfast, the day is off to a good start. The nursing assistant provides AM care by:

- Awakening the patient gently before breakfast by saying the patient's name, and gently touching the arm, if necessary (Figure 25-1).
- Giving the patient the opportunity to use the bathroom, if permitted, or to use the bedpan or urinal.
- Helping the patient to wash hands and face.

The patient is not awakened early if he or she is:

- Going to surgery
- Having tests and cannot eat breakfast

PM Care

The care given to the patient just before bedtime is similar to that given in the early morning. Bedtime care is called **PM care** (or HS care). The nursing assistant gives PM care:

- In a quiet, unrushed manner that will help prepare the patient for sleep (Figure 25-2)
- Before sleeping medication is given by the nurse

Other routine procedures that may be carried out during AM and PM care include:

- Measuring vital signs

- Giving a backrub
- Providing mouth and hair care

ORAL HYGIENE

Oral hygiene is care of the mouth and teeth. (Refer to Procedures 52 to 54.)

- Offer and assist patients with routine oral hygiene (including brushing and flossing the teeth) at least three times a day.
- Allow and encourage patients to do as much as possible for themselves.
- *Special oral hygiene* is the cleansing of the mouth of the unresponsive or dependent patient using commercially prepared lemon and glycerin swabs, sponge applicators, or other preparations.

Patients requiring more frequent oral hygiene include those who are:

- Unconscious
- Vomiting
- Experiencing a high temperature
- Receiving certain medications
- Dehydrated

Infection Control ALERT

A clean mouth contains about 100 million bacteria. If the teeth are not regularly brushed, these bacteria can multiply quickly. They will move to other areas, including the pharynx, sinuses, larynx, and lungs. In patients with dysphagia (Unit 28), small amounts of oral fluid are aspirated frequently and rapidly. Even healthy adults occasionally aspirate small amounts of saliva during deep sleep, increasing the risk of pneumonia. However, they usually do not get sick because they brush their teeth regularly and have healthy immune systems. ■

- Breathing through the mouth
- Receiving oxygen
- Receiving tube feeding
- Using tubes in the mouth or nose (such as an endotracheal tube)
- Dying

Infection Control ALERT

Store the patient's toothbrush in a clean area such as the emesis basin. It may also be covered and stored away from other items, such as the hairbrush. ■

Infection Control ALERT

Apply the principles of standard precautions when selecting protective equipment for assisting with dental procedures. Always wear gloves. If there is a chance of spraying or splashing of oral secretions, you will need a gown, gloves, mask, and eye protection. ■

Proper cleansing of the teeth and mouth helps:
- Prevent tooth decay (**caries**)
- Eliminate bad breath (**halitosis**)
- Contribute to the patient's comfort

PROCEDURE

ASSISTING THE PATIENT TO FLOSS AND BRUSH TEETH

1. Carry out initial procedure actions.
2. Assemble equipment:
   - Disposable gloves and face mask
   - Toothbrush
   - Toothpaste
   - Dental floss
   - Mouthwash solution in cup
   - Emesis basin
   - Bath towel
   - Straw
   - Tissues
   - Cup of fresh water
   - Plastic bag
   - Bed protector

3. Raise the head of the bed so that the patient may sit up, if condition permits.
4. Lower the side rails and position the overbed table across the patient's lap.
5. Cover the table with a protector and place equipment on the table.
6. Place a bath towel over the patient's gown and bedcovers.
7. Be prepared to help as the patient brushes and flosses teeth.
8. Pour water over the toothbrush and put toothpaste on the brush.
9. Put on disposable gloves. A face mask and eye protection may be used.

continues

PROCEDURE 52 CONTINUED

10. Brush teeth as follows (Figures 25-3A to 25-3E):
    a. Insert the toothbrush into the mouth with bristles pointing downward.
    b. Turn the toothbrush with bristles toward teeth.
    c. Brush all tooth surfaces with a back-and-forth motion using short strokes.
    d. Use the "toe" end of the brush to clean the inner surfaces of the front teeth, using a gentle up-and-down motion.
    e. Brush the front of the tongue gently, if tolerated by the patient. Avoid the back of the tongue, as this may cause gagging and coughing.

11. Give the patient water in a cup to rinse the mouth. Use a straw, if necessary. Turn the

patient's head to one side, with the emesis basin near the chin, for return of fluid.

12. Repeat steps 10 and 11 as necessary.

13. To floss the patient's teeth:
    a. Select a piece of dental floss about 12 inches long. Wrap the end of the floss around your gloved middle fingers, leaving the center area free (Figure 25-4).
    b. Ask the patient to open the mouth. Gently insert the floss between each tooth down to, but not into, the gum line.
    c. Ask the patient to rinse the mouth using the emesis basin.

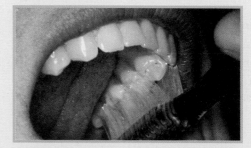

FIGURE 25-3C Scrub the chewing surfaces of the teeth. *(© Delmar/Cengage Learning)*

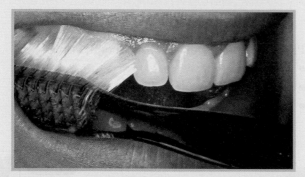

FIGURE 25-3A Brush teeth in the direction they grow and across the chewing surfaces. (Toothbrushing photos and descriptions compliments of the American Dental Association.) Place the head of the toothbrush beside the teeth, with the bristle tips at a 45° angle against the gumline. Move the brush back and forth in short strokes several times, using a gentle scrubbing motion. Brush the outer surfaces of each tooth, upper and lower, keeping the bristles angled against the gumline. *(© Delmar/ Cengage Learning)*

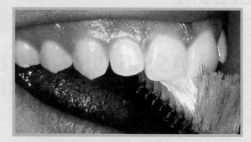

FIGURE 25-3D To clean the inside surfaces of the front teeth, tilt the brush vertically and make several gentle up-and-down strokes with the "toe" (front part) of the brush. *(© Delmar/Cengage Learning)*

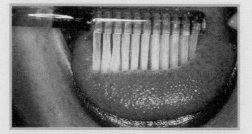

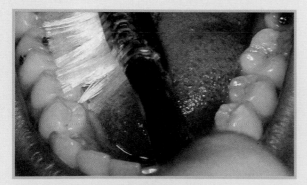

FIGURE 25-3B Use the same method on the inside surfaces of all the teeth, still using short back-and-forth strokes. *(© Delmar/Cengage Learning)*

FIGURE 25-3E Brushing the patient's tongue will help freshen breath and clean the mouth by removing bacteria. *(© Delmar/Cengage Learning)*

PROCEDURE 52 CONTINUED

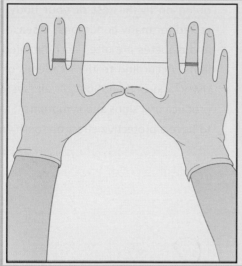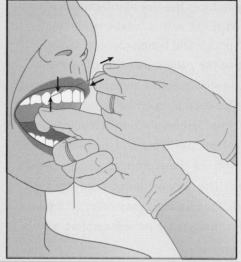

FIGURE 25-4 Floss is wrapped around the middle fingers (left). The proper method of using the floss to clean between the teeth (right). *(© Delmar/Cengage Learning)*

14. Offer the patient mouthwash. Dilute the mouthwash if the patient wishes.

15. Remove the basin. Wipe the patient's mouth and chin with tissue. Discard the tissue in a paper bag.

16. Remove the towel.

17. Rinse the toothbrush with water.

18. Remove and dispose of gloves and mask according to facility policy.

19. Carry out ending procedure actions.

Culture ALERT

Many individuals have tongue piercings for fashion or cultural reasons. Many risks accompany this practice. Inform the nurse promptly if a patient with a tongue piercing has pain, bleeding, increased flow of saliva, swelling, or signs of infection in the mouth. Swelling of the tongue can become severe, closing off the airway. ▪

Clinical Information ALERT

The mouth produces between 700 and 1800 mL of saliva a day. Saliva is needed for tasting and digesting food. When a patient breathes from the mouth or uses oxygen, the mouth becomes very dry. However, the area between the gums and cheek will stay moist even with a mouth breather unless patient is dehydrated. ▪

DENTURES

Some patients have full sets of dentures. Other patients have partial plates that are removable, but attach by small metal clips to existing teeth. Partial plates should be given the same care as full dentures. **Dentures** are artificial teeth that are removable. They must be cleaned daily. The patient may feel embarrassed about wearing dentures and may dislike being seen after the dentures have been removed. Always provide privacy when dentures are removed and cleaned. (See Procedure 54.)

Tooth brush Clean Place
＊   ＊

Infection Control ALERT

Studies have shown that providing thorough, regular oral hygiene reduces the risk of infection in elderly persons and those with a weakened immune system. Avoid sponge and lemon-glycerin swabs if there is a risk that the patient may bite off or swallow the swab. Lemon-glycerin swabs are drying, and should not be used frequently. Some patients complain that the lemon-glycerin combination makes them feel thirsty. (This is a problem, because patients who use these products usually cannot eat or drink.) The sponge-tipped products are more refreshing. The physician may order an artificial saliva product to increase patient comfort. ■

Clinical Information ALERT

The mouth provides a useful window into what is going on in the rest of your body. Saliva can be tested for many conditions. Diseases such as AIDS and diabetes are often accompanied by oral problems. According to the Academy of General Dentistry, more than 90% of all systemic diseases produce oral signs and symptoms. Saliva is believed to have a protective effect on tooth enamel. ■

PROCEDURE

PROVIDING MOUTH CARE FOR AN UNRESPONSIVE PATIENT

Note: Special oral hygiene is provided when the patient is unresponsive or cannot participate actively in such care.

1. Carry out initial procedure actions.

2. Assemble equipment:
   - Disposable gloves
   - Sponge applicators (such as Toothettes®) or lemon-glycerin applicators
   - Cotton swabs
   - Emesis basin
   - 2 bath towels
   - Plastic bag
   - Tissues
   - Tongue depressor
   - Water-based lubricant for lips
   - Laundry hamper

3. Put on gloves.

4. Cover pillow with a towel. If the patient is able to sit up, elevate the head of the bed. If the patient is unable or not permitted to sit up, turn the patient's head to one side and slightly forward so any excess fluid will not run down the throat. Cover the patient's upper chest with a towel. Place an emesis basin under the patient's chin.

5. Gently pull down on the chin to open the mouth, or open the mouth gently with a tongue depressor.

6. Using moistened sponge applicators or lemon-glycerin swabs, wipe gums, teeth, tongue, and inside of mouth (Figure 25-5).

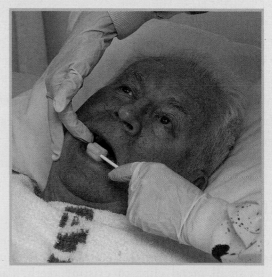

FIGURE 25-5 Using premoistened applicators, wipe gums, teeth, and tongue. (© Delmar/Cengage Learning)

PROCEDURE 53 CONTINUED

7. Discard used applicators in a plastic bag.

8. Wipe the patient's face with tissue, as needed.

9. Using cotton swabs, apply lubricant to the patient's lips. Place used applicators in a plastic bag.

10. Remove towels. Clean and replace equipment.

11. Remove and dispose of gloves properly. Wash your hands.

12. Carry out ending procedure actions.

Age-Appropriate Care ALERT

Elderly patients and those who use oxygen or breathe through the mouth often experience dry mouth and reduced saliva production. This may also occur as a side effect of medications. Related complaints are burning or sore throat, difficulty in swallowing, hoarseness, and dry nasal passages. Saliva is needed to help break down food for digestion. It also neutralizes acids in the mouth caused by plaque. Artificial saliva products are available, as are medicated oral rinses, gum, and lozenges. Inform the nurse if the patient experiences problems with saliva production. ■

Denture Care

Denture care includes:

• Handling dentures carefully to prevent damage.

• Cleaning and brushing dentures daily under cool running water. Soaking does not eliminate the need for brushing. Avoid hot water when caring for dentures.

• Rinsing dentures well before brushing under running water. Do not rinse them in standing water in the sink.

• Brushing the tissues and gums daily, even if the person has no teeth. Use a soft-bristled brush to improve circulation and remove oral debris.

• Cleaning and checking the person's mouth for signs of irritation.

• Checking the patient's lips for cracking and dryness, and applying cream, petroleum jelly, or glycerin to lips to avoid excessive dryness.

• Storing dentures in a safe place when they are out of the patient's mouth, such as in the drawer of the bedside stand in a container labeled with the patient's name (Figure 25-6).

• Changing the soaking solution and washing the denture cup with soap and water daily. Rinse well.

If you must place items such as the toothbrush, toothpaste, or dentures on the counter, put them on a clean paper towel. Never place them in the sink or an unprotected countertop.

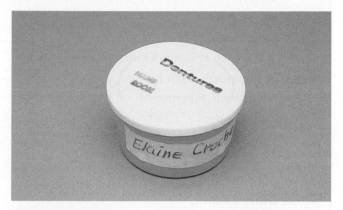

FIGURE 25-6 Dentures are stored in a cup labeled with the patient's name. The dentures are usually kept covered with water. (© Delmar/Cengage Learning)

Safety ALERT

Remove dentures from a comatose patient to prevent accidental airway obstruction by the denture. Remove dentures from patients preoperatively to prevent potential damage to the dentures and accidental airway obstruction during surgery. ■

Age-Appropriate Care ALERT

Dentures are made to fit tightly. Natural aging changes in the bones and gums causes the shape of the mouth to change over time. If dentures are loose or fit poorly, it is probably because of aging changes. Loose dentures can cause sores in the mouth, and in the worst case can cause choking. Denture adhesives can be used temporarily to help keep dentures in place, but the patient will need to be referred to a dentist. Inform the nurse if a patient has problems with ill-fitting dentures. ■

PROCEDURE

CARING FOR DENTURES

1. Carry out initial procedure actions.

2. Assemble equipment:
   - Disposable gloves
   - Tissues
   - Emesis basin
   - Tongue depressor
   - Toothbrush or denture brush (Figure 25-7)
   - Toothpaste or tooth powder
   - Mouthwash, if permitted
   - Cup of water
   - Straw
   - Gauze squares
   - Applicators
   - Denture cup

3. Apply disposable gloves.

4. Allow the patient to clean the dentures, if able. If the patient cannot, hand the person a tissue and ask her to remove the dentures. Assist if necessary.

   a. To remove upper dentures, grasp firmly, ease them downward and then forward, then remove from the mouth (Figure 25-8).

   b. To remove lower dentures, grasp the dentures firmly, ease them upward and then forward, and remove from the mouth.

5. Place the dentures in a denture cup padded with gauze squares. Take them to the bathroom or utility room.

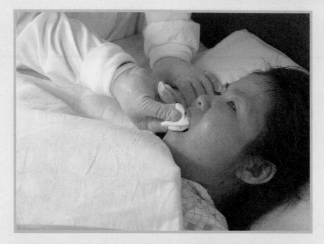

FIGURE 25-8 Grasp the upper dentures firmly with gauze-covered fingers to prevent slipping. Ease down and forward to remove. (© Delmar/Cengage Learning)

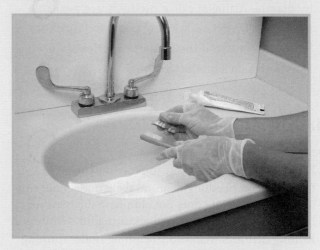

FIGURE 25-9 Brush dentures until all surfaces are clean. (© Delmar/Cengage Learning)

6. Place a paper towel or washcloth in the sink to protect the dentures (Figure 25-9). Fill the sink half full with cool water. The combination of water and towel protects the dentures if they are accidentally dropped in the sink.

7. Dentures may be soaked in a solution with a cleansing tablet before brushing, if desired.

8. Wet the dentures by rinsing under cool water.

9. Put toothpaste or tooth powder on a brush. Hold the dentures and brush until all surfaces are clean.

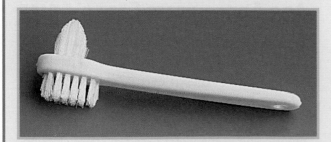

FIGURE 25-7 The denture brush has a smaller head than a toothbrush. The back side has a smaller tuft of bristles that works well for cleaning between teeth and in areas that are otherwise difficult to reach. (Courtesy of Medline Industries, Inc. (800) MEDLINE)

PROCEDURE **54** CONTINUED

10. Rinse the dentures thoroughly under cool running water. Never use hot water. Rinse the denture cup.

11. Place fresh gauze squares in the denture cup with clean, cool water.

12. Place the dentures in the gauze-lined cup and return to the bedside.

13. Assist the person to rinse her mouth with mouthwash or water, as desired. Gently hold the mouth open with a tongue depressor. Clean the gums and tongue with applicators moistened with mouthwash, sponge swabs, or a soft toothbrush.

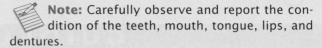 **Note:** Carefully observe and report the condition of the teeth, mouth, tongue, lips, and dentures.

14. Use a paper towel or gauze to hand wet dentures to the patient. If the patient is able, she can remove the dentures from the cup. Insert them for the patient if necessary, upper denture first.

15. Clean and replace equipment.

16. Remove and dispose of gloves according to facility policy.

17. Carry out ending procedure actions.

Safety ALERT

Health care workers have known for years that denture cleaning tablets can cause serious injury to a confused or pediatric patient, if swallowed. The fizzing, foaming action of the tablet causes burns of the mucous membranes in the mouth, throat, esophagus, and stomach. In 2005, new information was published about the ingestion and systemic absorption of denture adhesive paste. Zinc is used in the paste as a bonding agent and odor blocker. It is not always listed on the label. Ingestion of denture paste poses a risk of zinc toxicity, although the potential for harm is not known at this time, and further research is needed. Keep all denture cleaners and paste preparations out of the hands of confused and pediatric patients, as well as others (such as a suicidal patient) who may ingest them. ■

BACKRUBS

When properly given, backrubs can be:
- Stimulating to the patient's circulation
- A major aid in preventing skin breakdown (*pressure ulcers*)
- Soothing and comforting
- Refreshing and relaxing

Keep your nails short to prevent injury to the patient. The backrub provides a good opportunity for you to observe the condition of the patient's skin. Report all observations to the nurse. Look for:
- Reddened areas that do not blanch (whiten) when pressed
- Open areas or other skin abnormalities
- Condition of skin over bony prominences

Lotion is used to reduce friction during the back massage. Warm the lotion under warm water at the sink, by floating it in the warm bath water, or by applying it to your palm and rubbing your hands together. Long, smooth strokes are relaxing. Short, circular strokes tend to be more stimulating. Avoid massaging red areas over bony prominences. Rub the skin for 3 to 5 minutes until lotion is absorbed.

Difficult SITUATIONS

For many years, backrubs were almost a sacred part of routine nursing care. Over time, we have become much more dependent on technology. When we are busy or staffing is short, it seems as if there is no time to give backrubs. Yet, calming the agitated patient who cannot sleep is time-consuming; the pregnant mother with a backache may use the call signal frequently; the patient with spasticity just cannot get into a comfortable position. You may find that taking a few minutes to give a backrub will save you a great deal of time in caring for your patients. ■

A good backrub is comforting and relaxing. Agitated patients often calm down. Uncomfortable patients become more comfortable and demand less attention. Do not omit this important part of nursing care that pays such large dividends in patient comfort and satisfaction. In the long run, it may even make your job easier.

GUIDELINES *for*

Applying Lotion to the Patient's Skin

- Patients who are elderly and those with very dry, fragile skin will benefit from an application of lotion several times a day to keep skin supple and more resistant to injury.

- Check with the care plan and nurse before massaging the backs of patients who have an extensive skin condition, those who have had recent back surgery, and those who have blood clots, heart, or lung disorders.

- Each facility has a house lotion that is used for skin care. It is usually alcohol-free.

- Applying lotion immediately after the bath helps hold moisture in the skin. This is a good time to apply lotion to dry areas of skin, such as the patient's hands, elbows, and heels.

- Always use smooth, light strokes.

- Never rub red areas that may be stage I pressure ulcers.

- Avoid massaging the legs. If lotion is needed for dry skin, gently pat it on. Massage can cause complications related to blood clots.

- You may apply lotion to the feet, but avoid putting lotion between the toes.

PROCEDURE

OBRA **DVD**

55

BACKRUB

1. Carry out initial procedure actions.

2. Assemble equipment:
   - Disposable gloves
   - Basin of water (105°F)
   - Washcloth
   - Bath towel
   - Soap and lotion

3. Put up the far side rail.

4. Place the lotion in a basin of water to warm (Figure 25-10).

5. Put on disposable gloves if the patient has open lesions.

6. Turn the patient on the side with the back toward you.

7. Expose and wash the back; dry carefully. This step is not necessary if the backrub is given after a bath.

8. Pour a small amount of lotion into one hand and warm it in the palm of your hand. Cold lotion may be very uncomfortable for the patient.

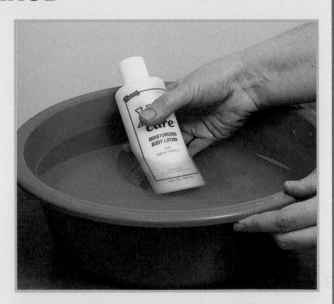

FIGURE 25-10 Cool lotion causes an unpleasant sensation on the patient's back and may cause chilling. Warming the lotion in water for several minutes will make it more comfortable for the patient. (© *Delmar/Cengage Learning*)

PROCEDURE 55 CONTINUED

9. Apply the lotion to the patient's skin and rub with gentle but firm strokes (Figure 25-11). Do not rub red areas. Report these to the nurse, if noted.

10. Begin at the base of the spine:

    a. With long, soothing strokes, rub up the center of the back, around the shoulders, and down the sides of the back and buttocks (Figure 25-12A).

    b. Repeat the previous step four times, using long, soothing upward strokes and a circular motion on the downstroke (Figure 25-12B).

    c. Repeat, but on the downward stroke rub in small circular motions with the palm of your hand. Include areas over the coccyx (base of the spine) (Figure 25-12C).

    d. Repeat long, soothing strokes (Figure 25-12A) on muscles for 3 to 5 minutes, or until all lotion is absorbed.

    e. Straighten and tighten the bottom sheet and draw sheet.

11. Change the patient's gown, if necessary.

12. Remove gloves if used. Discard according to facility policy and wash your hands.

13. Replace equipment.

14. Carry out ending procedure actions.

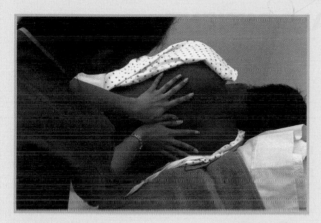

FIGURE 25-11 Use long, smooth, firm strokes to apply lotion. (© Delmar/Cengage Learning)

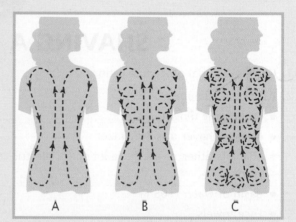

FIGURE 25-12 Strokes to be used during the backrub: A. soothing strokes; B. circular movement; C. passive movement. (© Delmar/Cengage Learning)

DAILY SHAVING

Daily shaving is part of the self-care routine of most men. It should not be neglected in a health care facility. When patients are unable to shave themselves, it is your responsibility. Older women often have an increase in the growth and coarseness of hairs on the chin and upper lip. Many women find this distressing. Tweezers can be used to remove some of the hairs, but a more permanent method is to have the hairs removed professionally with an electric needle. Some women may require a shave. In some facilities nursing assistants are not permitted to shave female patients. Be sure to check your facility's policy.

Infection Control ALERT

Shaving may be done with an electric razor that is the patient's personal property. Such a razor is used for one patient only and cleaned according to manufacturer's directions after each use. Cleaning involves brushing the razor heads with a small brush designed for this purpose. Remove all hair from the head of the razor. Some men may spray the head with razor lubricating spray after cleaning. Many electric razors must be recharged periodically. Electric razors are expensive. Handle the razor carefully and avoid dropping it. Wearing gloves is usually not necessary when an electric razor is used. ■

GUIDELINES *for*
Safety in Shaving

- Use the patient's own shaving equipment if possible. For safety, use an electric razor or rotary razor.
- If the patient is receiving **anticoagulants** (medications that thin the blood and increase the risk of bleeding), check with the nurse for the proper procedure.

- If oxygen is being used, it may be possible to discontinue it during this procedure. Consult the nurse and follow hospital policy.
- The patient may use a preshave or aftershave product as desired. Keep these products out of the hands of patients who may swallow them.

PROCEDURE

56

SHAVING A MALE PATIENT

1. Carry out initial procedure actions.

2. Assemble equipment:
   - Disposable gloves
   - Electric shaver or safety razor
   - Shaving lather, or preshave lotion for electric razor
   - Basin of water (105°F)
   - Face towels
   - Mirror
   - Washcloth
   - Aftershave lotion

3. Raise the head of the bed. Place equipment on the overbed table.

4. Put on gloves if a safety razor is used.

5. Place one face towel across the patient's chest and one under his head.

6. Moisten face and apply lather (or preshave lotion).

7. Starting in front of one ear:
   a. Hold the skin taut and bring the razor down over the cheek toward the chin (Figure 25-13).
   b. Repeat until lather on the cheek is removed and the area has been shaved. Rinse frequently.
   c. Repeat on the other cheek.
   d. Use firm, short strokes. Shave in the direction of hair growth.
   e. Rinse the razor frequently.

8. Ask the patient to tighten his upper lip. Shave from the nose to the upper lip in short, downward strokes.

9. Ask the patient to tighten his chin. Shave the chin in downward strokes.

10. Assist the patient to tip his head back.

11. Lather the neck area and stroke up toward the chin. Rinse and repeat until all lather is removed.

12. Wash the patient's face and neck and dry thoroughly.

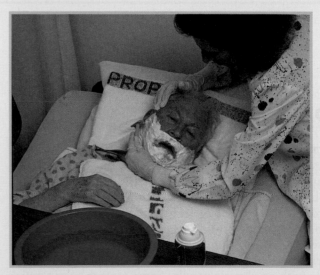

FIGURE 25-13 Shaving is part of the daily routine for most men. (© *Delmar/Cengage Learning*)

PROCEDURE 56 CONTINUED

13. Apply aftershave lotion if desired.

14. If the skin is nicked, apply a small piece of tissue and hold pressure directly over the area with your gloved hand. Report the injury to the nurse.

15. Clean and replace equipment. Discard the safety razor in the sharps container. Remove

the head of an electric razor and clean it with a razor brush. Charge and store the electric razor.

16. Remove and dispose of gloves according to facility policy.

17. Carry out ending procedure actions.

DAILY HAIR CARE

Daily care of the hair, for both male and female patients, is usually performed after the patient's bed bath.

The hair should be combed and brushed each morning. Tangles can be loosened by sectioning the hair with a comb or brush, working with one section at a time. Grasp the hair near the scalp to reduce pulling (Figure 25-14). Start combing or brushing tangles out, starting at the ends and working toward the scalp. Braiding long hair helps to reduce tangles. Tangles can be reduced in wiry, dry hair by using conditioner and keeping the hair short or in braids.

Tips: Avoid braiding a patient's hair tightly, because it can be uncomfortable. Secure the braids with hair ties. Avoid rubber bands, if possible. Place the hair ties so the patient does not end up lying on them, which is uncomfortable. If the hair is very tangled, applying a small amount of alcohol, conditioner, hair grease, or oil to the tangle will make it easier to remove. A mixture of vinegar and water will also work, but the smell is unpleasant, and the hair may have to be washed to remove the odor after the tangle is removed.

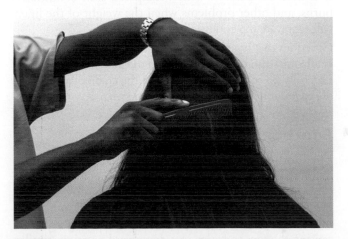

FIGURE 25-14 To remove tangles from long hair, divide the hair into sections. Work with one section at a time. Hold the hair near the scalp to reduce pulling and start combing at the end of the hair, working up toward the scalp. *(© Delmar/Cengage Learning)*

Difficult SITUATIONS

Hair is important to everyone's self-esteem and appearance. Some diseases and medications cause hair loss. Some cause changes to the volume and texture of hair. Some medications cause hair to become dry and brittle. Patients who have problems with their hair may become anxious or angry because the appearance of the hair affects their self-esteem. If the patient is experiencing problems with hair, treat it gently. Use products such as baby shampoo and conditioner. Use tepid water. Pat the hair dry rather than rubbing it with a towel. Use a wide-toothed comb to style the hair gently. Avoid using rubber bands, which may worsen the problem. Assist the patient to wear a scarf or turban, if desired. ■

Procedure 57 assumes that the patient is a female. Hair care for a male is very similar, however, so the procedure can easily be adapted.

Care of African American Patients' Hair

African American patients have special hair-care needs. With these patients, hair texture can vary from soft and silky to coarse and thick. Patients with coarse hair need special care to prevent damage, tangling, and breaking. Asking the patient or family how to care for the hair is not offensive. In fact, it shows that you care about meeting the patient's needs.

In general, avoid using hair products designed for Caucasian persons. Most of these are designed to eliminate oil. Eliminating the oil from the hair is one of the worst things to do when caring for African Americans' hair. Use products marketed specifically for black hair. In

PROCEDURE

OBRA DVD

57

DAILY HAIR CARE

1. Carry out initial procedure actions.

2. Assemble equipment:
   - Towel
   - Comb and brush

3. Ask the patient to move to the side of the bed nearest you; or the patient may sit in a chair if permitted. If the patient is sitting up, put a towel around her shoulders.

4. Cover the pillow with a towel.

5. Part or section the hair and comb with one hand between the scalp and the ends of the hair.

6. Brush carefully and thoroughly.

7. Have the patient turn so that you can comb and brush the hair on the back of her head. If the hair is tangled, work section by section to detangle it, beginning near the ends and working toward the scalp.

8. Complete the brushing and arrange the hair attractively. Braid long hair to prevent repeated tangling. Allow the patient to choose the style, if able.

9. Clean and replace equipment according to facility policy.

10. Carry out ending procedure actions.

many cases, the patient or family will provide a product that they know works for them. Wash the hair once every week or two, as specified on the care plan, and according to the patient's preference. Washing more often than this dries the hair and causes breakage. If a special shampoo is not available, use baby shampoo. Wash the hair using the guidelines in Procedure 57. Use a detangling conditioner according to product directions.

After washing the hair, gently towel it dry. Cover the patient's shoulders with a dry towel. Use a wide-toothed comb or pick to comb through the damp hair. Be gentle and patient. It may take time to work through the tangles.

African Americans need additional oil on the hair at all times. Some patients use products they refer to as hair "grease." If the patient does not have a product preference, apply baby oil *to the scalp, not the hair*. Then, using a soft brush, brush from the scalp to the ends of the hair until all the hairs are covered with oil. You may need to apply this heavily. If it is too oily, wipe the excess with a towel. If you use enough, the hair will appear shiny.

The patient's hair can be braided while damp. Run the wide-toothed comb through the hair to remove tangles, following the guidelines in Procedure 57. Gently twist the hair and apply an elastic or cloth-covered hair tie. Avoid using rubber bands, which break and damage the hair. If a rubber band must be used, apply hair grease or baby oil liberally to your fingers. Roll the rubber band around in the hair grease until it is well coated, then apply it to the hair. Style the hair in a pony tail, then section and braid it. When you get to the end, apply more grease. Wrap the ends around a barrette and snap it shut, or use a hair tie or grease-coated rubber band.

COMFORT DEVICES

The physician, nurse, or physical therapist orders comfort devices such as bed cradles, footboards, and pillows. These devices are designed to relieve pressure on specific areas or to help maintain body position.

Bed Cradle

A bed cradle (Figures 25-15A and 25-15B) prevents the weight of the bedclothes from falling on some part of the body. It can be used therapeutically or as a comfort device. It is used for persons with widespread skin conditions, burns, and other problems when the weight of the linen will aggravate the condition.

Coverings that maintain some degree of warmth within the cradle may also be needed to keep the patient comfortable. Carefully position the limbs within the cradle. Pad the cradle edges, if necessary, to prevent injury.

Footboard or Footrest

The **footboard** or footrest is a device placed between the mattress and bed to keep the feet at right angles to the legs (natural standing position). A footboard is always padded. It is used to prevent a type of contracture called **foot drop**. In foot drop, the muscle in the calf of the leg tightens, causing the toes to freeze in a downward position, similar to the position of a woman wearing a high-heeled shoe. Foot drop may develop when the patient must remain in bed for a long period of time. Even a brief period in bed is

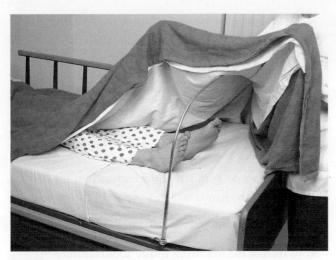

FIGURE 25-15A A bed cradle keeps the sheet and blanket from putting pressure on the feet. (© Delmar/ Cengage Learning)

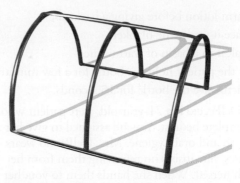

FIGURE 25-15B A wide cradle is used for patients with skin conditions such as burns or widespread lesions. The wide cradle supports the weight of heavy bedding and relieves pressure from a larger area of skin surface. (© Delmar/Cengage Learning)

sufficient to cause a degree of foot drop that makes walking difficult and painful. If a footboard is not available, a pillow folded lengthwise may be placed against the foot of the bed to serve the same purpose. Some facilities use special tennis shoes or soft boots to prevent foot drop in bedfast patients who are at risk for contractures.

Pillows

Pillows and other props can be used for comfort and to maintain alignment. For directions on positioning patients, refer to Unit 15.

Pillows are also used to relieve pressure in such a way that spaces are left for specific areas (Figure 25-16). This technique is called **bridging**. Bridging elevates an area of the body off the surface of the bed. It is useful for patients who have healing pressure ulcers. Bridging is commonly used for the sacrum, hips, heels, and ankles. No special equipment is necessary. Facilities may use a combination of pillows, foam props, and folded or rolled bath blankets to support an area.

Bed Boards

Bed boards are used when a person has a back ache, or the mattress sags. Two types of bed boards are used. One type consists of two pieces of plywood covered with vinyl. One

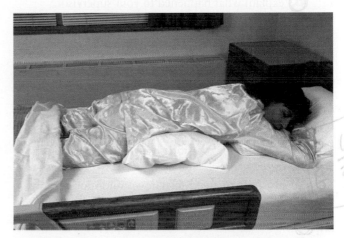

FIGURE 25-16 The patient is positioned on her abdomen and pillows are used to form a bridge, preventing pressure on her breasts. (© Delmar/Cengage Learning)

piece is placed under the mattress at the head of the bed, and the other at the foot of the bed. This enables the patient to elevate the head of the bed. The knee area of the bed cannot be elevated.

The second type rolls up like a bamboo curtain. It is made of many pieces of plywood that are approximately 1½ to 2 inches wide. The plywood is covered with vinyl, with a seam between each board. This type of bed board is quite flexible. When it is used, the patient can raise both the head and knee areas of the bed.

REVIEW

A. Multiple Choice

Select the one best answer for each of the following.

1. Which of the following patients should be given special mouth care?

   a. Mrs. Strong, who can brush her own teeth
   b. Mr. Lieberman, who drinks water ad lib
   c. Ms. Mendoza, who has a broken leg
   d. Mr. Zimmerman, who has a nasogastric tube

2. To warm lotion before giving a backrub,
   a. place it under the blanket.
   b. soak it in a basin of warm water.
   c. let the patient hold the bottle for a few minutes.
   d. microwave the bottle for 15 seconds.

3. Mrs. DelPeccio is a 71-year-old, alert patient who is on complete bedrest. You are assigned to give her a bed bath and oral hygiene. Mrs. DelPeccio wears dentures. She insists on removing them from her mouth herself. When she hands them to you, her hand bumps the overbed table and the dentures fall to the floor, breaking in half. She begins yelling that you are careless and that you broke her dentures. You should
   a. tell everyone that the patient is confused.
   b. explain what happened to your supervisor.
   c. glue the dentures together.
   d. tell the patient it was her fault.

4. When brushing a patient's teeth, the best technique includes
   a. inserting the toothbrush with the bristles down.
   b. scrubbing the outer surface well and avoiding the sensitive inner surface.
   c. inserting the toothbrush with bristles facing the teeth.
   d. brushing the teeth in a downward motion only.

5. Backrubs are given
   a. routinely as a comfort measure.
   b. before use of the bedpan.
   c. if you have time.
   d. only for patients with red areas.

6. Mr. Corazion's hands shake because of his illness. He is able to wash his face and upper body. You finish the rest of his bath. It is time to shave the patient. He uses a safety razor and shaving cream and wants to shave himself. When Mr. Corazion begins to shave his cheek, his hand is shaking badly. He seems embarrassed. You should
   a. leave the room so that the patient is not embarrassed.
   b. ask Mr. Corazion if he would like you to shave him.
   c. tell Mr. Corazion not to shave until he buys an electric razor.
   d. tell the patient that he must grow a beard and mustache.

7. Mrs. Chlebowy is a 77-year-old, comatose patient. She is fed by tube because she cannot eat. You are assigned to do special oral hygiene for this patient. You should do all of the following except
   a. turn the patient's head to the side when doing mouth care.

   b. explain what you are going to do even though the patient may not hear you.
   c. use a toothbrush and toothpaste, scrubbing the teeth and gums vigorously.
   d. observe the patient's mouth for signs of irritation.

8. Which of the following should be done when giving a partial bath to Mrs. DePalma?
   a. Take her to the shower room to give the partial bath.
   b. Let her do as much of the bath as possible.
   c. Wash the hands and feet as part of the procedure.
   d. Avoid giving peri care, as this is not part of the procedure.

9. Which of the following is true about dentures?
   a. Dentures should be cleaned while in the patient's mouth.
   b. Dentures should be removed when eating.
   c. Dentures are expensive and can break if dropped.
   d. Only the nurse should handle the patient's dentures.

10. The oral hygiene procedure includes
    a. a complete bed bath and linen change.
    b. cleaning of the mouth, teeth, and gums.
    c. helping the patient ambulate.
    d. cleansing the perineal area.

11. You are assigned to care for Mrs. Grossbeck. She cannot walk and spends much of her time in a wheelchair, but she can use her hands and arms well. What is the best way for you to help her brush her teeth?
    a. Set her up in the bathroom so she can brush her teeth.
    b. Brush her teeth for her when she is up in the wheelchair.
    c. Get the nurse to help her brush her teeth.
    d. Tell her she must brush her teeth before going to bed.

B. Nursing Assistant Challenge

Your patient, Mrs. Ubanan, has a history of heavy smoking and breathes through her mouth. She has plastic dentures and her care plan indicates that she needs assistance with denture care. Answer the following questions regarding this patient.

12. State two reasons why special oral hygiene has been ordered for Mrs. Ubanan.

13. Where are the dentures stored when not in use?

14. Should the dentures be kept dry or wet?

15. Should you wear gloves when removing her dentures?

16. Will you clean the dentures in cool or hot water?

Principles of Nutrition, Hydration, and Elimination

UNIT 26

Urinary Elimination

OBJECTIVES

After completing this unit, you will be able to:

- Spell and define terms.
- Identify aging changes of the urinary system.
- List some common diseases of the urinary system.
- Identify signs and symptoms of the urinary system that the nursing assistant must observe and report.
- Describe nursing assistant actions related to the care of patients with urinary system diseases and conditions.
- Demonstrate the following procedures:
  - Procedure 58 Assisting with the Bedpan
  - Procedure 59 Assisting with the Urinal
  - Procedure 60 Assisting with Use of the Bedside Commode
  - Procedure 61 Collecting a Routine Urine Specimen
  - Procedure 62 Collecting a Clean-Catch Urine Specimen
  - Procedure 63 Collecting a 24-Hour Urine Specimen
  - Procedure 64 Collecting a Urine Specimen from an Infant
  - Procedure 65 Giving Indwelling Catheter Care
  - Procedure 66 Emptying a Urinary Drainage Unit
  - Procedure 67 Collecting a Urine Specimen through a Drainage Port
  - Procedure 68 Disconnecting the Urinary Catheter
  - Procedure 69 Applying a Condom for Urinary Drainage
  - Procedure 70 Connecting a Catheter to a Leg Bag
  - Procedure 71 Emptying a Leg Bag

VOCABULARY

Learn the meaning and the correct spelling of the following words and phrases:

catheter	emesis	intake and output (I&O)	renal colic
condom catheter	excretes	kidney	renal failure
cystitis	fluid balance	lithotripsy	retention catheter
dehydration	Foley catheter	nephritis	suprapubic catheter
dialysis	force fluids	oliguria	urinalysis
diaphoresis	graduate	port	urinary incontinence
diuresis	hematuria	prostate gland	voids
dysuria	hydronephrosis	push fluids	
edema	indwelling catheter	renal calculi	

INTRODUCTION

The urinary system consists of the **kidneys**, ureters, bladder, and urethra. The functions that this system performs are vital to the body. It:

- Excretes liquid wastes
- Manages blood chemistry
- Manages fluid balance

AGING CHANGES IN THE URINARY SYSTEM

The urinary system plays a major role in maintaining fluid balance in the body. Aging changes in the urinary system include:

- Bladder capacity decreases, increasing the frequency of urination
- Kidney function increases at rest, causing the aging person to have to get up during the night to urinate
- Bladder muscles weaken, causing leaking of urine or inadequate emptying of the bladder
- The prostate gland frequently enlarges, causing frequency of urination, dribbling, urinary obstruction, and urinary retention. (The **prostate gland** is a tubular gland that encircles the urethra just below the bladder, in the male.)

COMMON CONDITIONS

Infection and inflammation are the most common conditions of the urinary system. These problems can result in permanent damage to the kidneys. Complications

Clinical Information ALERT

An average human drinks about 16,000 gallons of water in a lifetime. The human body is about 66% water. Death will result if you lose 12% of your body fluids. An average person urinates 6 times per day. The yellow color of urine is caused by pigment derived from bile. About 440 gallons of blood flow through the kidneys each day. If all the renal tubules were laid end to end, they would measure about 66 yards. ■

TABLE 26-1 COMMON CONDITIONS RELATED TO THE URINARY SYSTEM

Cystitis	Inflammation of the urinary bladder
Dialysis	The process of removing wastes from the blood with a hemodialysis machine, commonly called an artificial kidney
Dysuria	Pain or burning on urination
Hematuria	Blood in the urine
Hydronephrosis	A condition resulting from too much fluid on the kidney
Lithotripsy	A procedure that uses sound waves to crush kidney stones
Nephritis	Inflammation of the kidney
Oliguria	Decreased urine production
Renal calculi	Kidney stones
Renal colic	Severe renal pain
Urinary incontinence	Loss of control over urination

can lead to acute or chronic renal failure. Common conditions affecting the urinary system are listed in Table 26-1.

Signs and symptoms of genitourinary disorders that should be reported to the nurse are listed in Table 26-2.

Renal Failure

Renal failure is the inability of the kidneys to maintain fluid and electrolyte balance, excrete waste products, and regulate essential body functions. Dehydration and inadequate fluid intake together are a major contributing cause of renal failure in elderly persons. The average adult requires at least 1-½ liters of fluid each day to maintain kidney function.

The kidneys filter the blood. When the amount of circulating fluid decreases, the kidneys do not function correctly. Filtration of wastes decreases. Waste products

TABLE 26-2 SIGNS AND SYMPTOMS OF GENITOURINARY DISORDERS THAT SHOULD BE REPORTED TO THE NURSE IMMEDIATELY

- Urinary output too low
- Oral intake too low
- Urinary output greatly exceeds fluid intake
- Fluid intake and output not balanced
- Fluid intake exceeds fluid restriction
- Signs of dehydration, including low fluid intake; low output of dark urine with strong odor; weight loss; dry skin; dry mucous membranes of the lips, mouth, tongue, eyes; drowsiness; confusion
- Edema; obvious fluid retention in tissues, particularly face, fingers, legs, ankles, feet
- Abnormal appearance of urine: dark, concentrated, red, cloudy
- Unusual substances in urine: blood, pus, particles, sediment
- Complaints of difficulty urinating
- Foul-smelling urine
- Complaints of pain, burning, urgency, frequency, pain in lower back
- Frequent urination of small amounts
- Sudden-onset incontinence
- Sudden weight loss or gain
- Respiratory distress
- Changes in mental status
- Complaints of inability to empty bladder, or inability to empty bladder completely

accumulate in the bloodstream. Without adequate fluid, the kidneys continue to filter wastes, but the rate of filtration is slow, so waste products are reabsorbed into the blood instead of being excreted in the urine.

Renal failure can occur in patients of any age. Two types of renal failure are acute and chronic. Patients with *acute renal failure* (ARF) have a sudden, rapid decrease in renal function. This condition can sometimes be reversed if it is identified promptly and the cause is corrected. *Chronic renal failure* (CRF) is characterized by progressive and irreversible damage. It usually develops over a long period of time.

Renal Dialysis

When the kidneys fail, end-stage renal disease (ESRD) develops. In this condition, the kidneys perform at less than 10% of the necessary function. Many complications develop throughout the body. High blood pressure and weight gain occur. Mechanical dialysis (Figure 26-1) is used to remove wastes from the blood. Some persons with ESRD are placed on a waiting list for a kidney transplant, if they qualify.

Patients with renal failure are usually on strict intake and output monitoring. Their fluid intake is restricted and carefully measured. Nursing and dietary staff must coordinate the fluids they give. You will monitor blood pressure frequently. Daily weights will be ordered. Some foods will be limited or restricted. Patients receiving dialysis usually have tubing permanently placed in the arm to make it easier to connect to the dialysis machine (Figures 26-2A and 26-2B). Never use this arm to measure

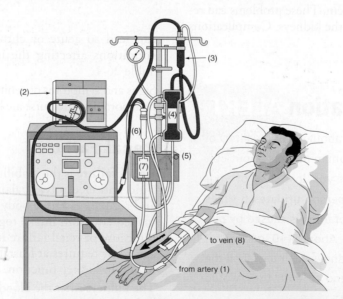

FIGURE 26-1 Hemodialysis is done through the graft or fistula. Most commonly, the patient is fully dressed and sits in a reclining chair during dialysis. Occasionally, it is done at the bedside of an unstable patient.
(© Delmar/Cengage Learning)

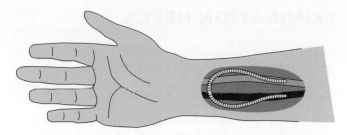

Ends of natural or synthetic graft sutured
into an artery and a vein.

FIGURE 26-2A The arteriovenous fistula.
(© Delmar/Cengage Learning)

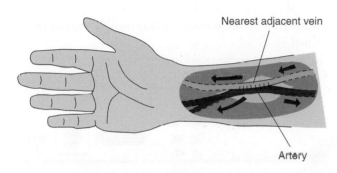

Nearest adjacent vein

Artery

Edges of incision in artery and vein are
sutured together to form a common opening.

FIGURE 26-2B The arteriovenous vein graft.
(© Delmar/Cengage Learning)

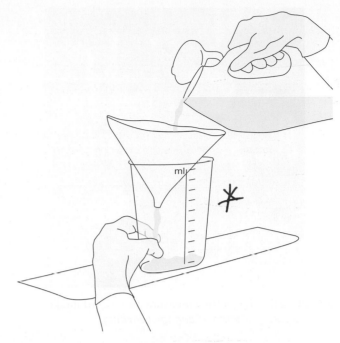

FIGURE 26-3 When the physician writes an order to
strain urine, each voiding is poured through filter paper
to retrieve kidney stones. *(© Delmar/Cengage Learning)*

- When it is impossible for the patient to pass the stones,
surgery may be necessary. Sometimes the stones can be
reached and removed only through a surgical incision or
other surgical procedure.

blood pressure. The only means of eliminating the need
for dialysis is to have a kidney transplant.

Renal Calculi

kidney stone.

<u>Renal calculi</u> are kidney stones. They can cause obstruc-
tions when they become lodged in the urinary passageways. There may be no sign of renal calculi until some
obstruction develops; then pain is sudden and intense.
Stones may be passed in the urine, causing **hematuria**
(blood in the urine).

The goal of treatment is to relieve the blockage and
eliminate the stones.

- Encouraging fluids increases urine output. This helps to
move the stones along the urinary tract.

- All urine must be strained through gauze or filter
paper, which is inspected for stones before the urine
is discarded (Figure 26-3). Stones that are found
can be analyzed. With information from the stones,
the diet can sometimes be changed to make the formation of stones less likely.

RESPONSIBILITIES OF THE NURSING ASSISTANT

The care of patients with diseases of the urinary system
varies with the condition. Be sure you understand the orders for each patient in your assignment. Orders regarding
positioning, drainage, fluid intake, dietary restrictions,
weight measurement, monitoring of vital signs, other special monitoring, specimen collection, and patient activity
will be listed on the care plan.

Some important measures that apply to urinary patients in
your care are:

- Straining the urine if a stone is suspected in the kidneys
or bladder.

- Assisting with urination, collecting urine samples, and
straining urine for stones.

- Knowing the proper steps to take for encouraging
fluid intake (forcing fluids) and for limiting
fluids.

- Carefully monitoring fluid intake and output
(Figure 26-4), weight, and vital signs.

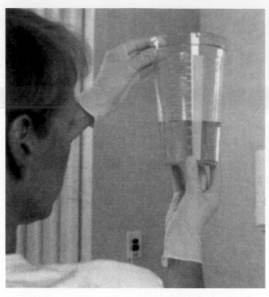

FIGURE 26-4 Accurately measure and record intake and output. *(© Delmar/Cengage Learning)*

ELIMINATION NEEDS

Regular elimination of body wastes is essential for good health. Patients who are confined to bed rely on you to help them with this task. You should know that:

- A urinal is used by bedfast male patients when they need to urinate. A bedpan is used by female patients to void when they are confined to bed.
- A regular bowel movement (which is the discharge of solid waste from the body) is also important to a patient's health. This solid waste is called *feces* or *stool* (see Unit 27).
- Both male and female patients use a bedpan for elimination of solid waste when confined to bed.
- Many patients are sensitive about using a bedpan or urinal.
- Bedpans are very uncomfortable.

PROCEDURE

OBRA DVD

58

ASSISTING WITH THE BEDPAN

1. Carry out initial procedure actions.

2. Assemble equipment:
   - Disposable gloves
   - Bedpan and cover
   - Bed protector
   - Plastic protector or pad for chair
   - Bath blanket
   - Plastic bag for trash, if needed

3. Lower the head of the bed, if necessary.

4. Put on gloves.

5. Take the bedpan and toilet tissue from the bedside stand.
   - Place a protector on the chair. Place the bedpan (Figure 26-5) on it.
   - Never place a bedpan on the bedside stand or overbed table.
   - Put the remainder of the articles on the bedside table.

6. Place the bedpan cover at the foot of the bed.

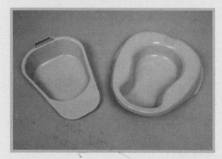

Figure 26-5 Orthopedic (fracture) bedpan (left) and regular bedpan (right). *(© Delmar/Cengage Learning)*

 Note: Never carry or allow a used bedpan to sit uncovered. If a bedpan cover is not available, cover the bedpan with a towel, bed protector, pillowcase, newspaper, plastic bag, or paper towels.

7. Cover the patient with a bath blanket. Fold the top bedcovers back at a right angle. Raise the patient's gown.

8. Ask the patient to flex the knees and rest weight on the heels, if able.

PROCEDURE **58** CONTINUED

9. Help the patient to raise the buttocks by:
   - Putting one hand under the small of the patient's back and lifting gently and slowly with that hand.
   - With the other hand, place a bed protector under the hips. Place the bedpan under the patient's hips, on the bed protector.
   - The pan may also be placed by rolling the patient to one side, positioning the bedpan against the buttocks, and rolling the patient back onto the pan (Figure 26-6A). Check to be sure the bedpan is positioned properly.
   - Alternatively, if a trapeze is in place over the bed, place the bedpan under the patient as the patient lifts self using the trapeze (Figure 26-6B).
   - The patient's buttocks should rest on the rounded shelf of the regular bedpan.
   - The narrow end should face the foot of the bed. If a fracture pan is being used, the narrow end is positioned under the patient's buttocks, with the handle facing the foot of the bed.

10. Replace the top bedcovers. Raise the head of the bed to a comfortable height. Remove your gloves and dispose of them properly.

11. Make sure the toilet paper and signal cord are within easy reach. Leave the patient alone unless contraindicated.

12. Wash your hands.

 Note: If a specimen is to be taken or the patient's output is being monitored, provide a small plastic bag. Instruct the patient to discard used toilet tissue in the bag.

13. Watch for the patient's signal.

14. Answer the patient's call signal immediately. Wash your hands and put on disposable gloves.

15. Fold the top bedcovers back so that the patient remains covered only with the bath blanket.

16. Remove the bedpan from under the patient.
   - Ask the patient to flex the knees and rest weight on the heels. Place one hand under the small of the patient's back and lift gently to help raise the buttocks off the bedpan. Take the bedpan with the other hand. Cover it and place it on the chair.
   - If the patient is unable to raise the buttocks, roll the patient off the pan to the side and remove the pan. Lift and move carefully. Hold the pan firmly with one hand (Figure 26-6C).
   - Many patients have difficulty cleaning adequately after using the bedpan. You may need to clean and dry the patient yourself.

17. If the bed protector is wet, change it. Provide perineal care.
   - Discard used toilet tissue in the bedpan unless a specimen is to be collected.
   - Cover the bedpan again.
   - Cleanse the patient with warm water and soap, if necessary.

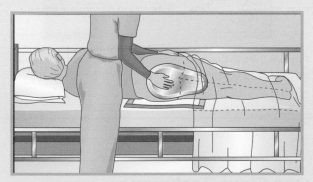

Figure 26-6A Roll the patient away from you. Provide support by placing one hand on the hip. Position the bedpan with the other hand, then roll the patient back onto the bedpan. *(© Delmar/Cengage Learning)*

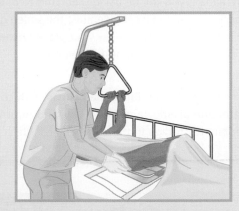

Figure 26-6B The patient assists by lifting with the trapeze as the nursing assistant places the bedpan. Support the small of the patient's back with one hand when the patient pulls up on the trapeze. *(© Delmar/Cengage Learning)*

continues

PROCEDURE 58 CONTINUED

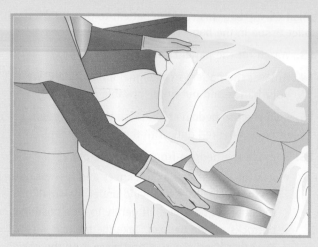

Figure 26-6C Hold the bedpan securely while the patient turns to the side. *(© Delmar/Cengage Learning)*

18. Replace the bedclothes, changing linen as necessary.

19. Cover the patient with the top bedding and remove the bath blanket.

20. Take the covered bedpan to the bathroom or utility room and observe its contents. Measure, if required. Some facilities use bedpans with self-fitting lids (Figure 26-6D). If no lid or bedpan cover is available, use a bed protector (Figure 26-6E), a plastic or paper bag, or a piece of newspaper as a cover. Wear a glove on the hand you use to carry the bedpan. Do not wear a soiled glove on the opposite hand if you will be using that hand to open doors or turn on faucets. Remove the soiled glove or hold a paper towel under your gloved hand to prevent contamination of the environment.

21. Empty the bedpan.

22. Turn on the faucet. Rinse the bedpan with cold water and disinfectant. Rinse, dry, and return the bedpan to storage in the patient's bedside stand.

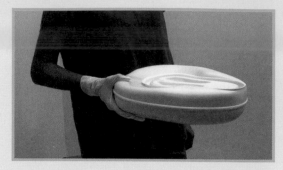

Figure 26-6D Always cover the full bedpan when carrying it. This bedpan has a lid that fits securely. *(© Delmar/Cengage Learning)*

23. Remove your gloves and dispose of them properly. Wash your hands.

24. Assist the patient to wash hands and freshen up after the procedure. An antiseptic hand rub or alcohol product may be used, if desired.

25. Carry out ending procedure actions.

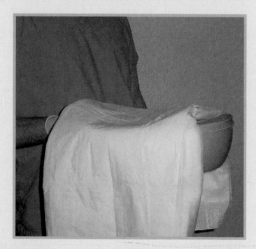

Figure 26-6E If a lid is not available, use a disposable underpad to cover the bedpan. *(© Delmar/Cengage Learning)*

Culture ALERT

Females from some cultures may prefer to do their own perineal care with soap and water (or water only) after toileting. Some use toilet tissue; others prefer peri care with water instead of using tissue. ∎

One-Glove Technique

Wear gloves on both hands when removing the bedpan or urinal. When you have successfully removed the bedpan, take off a glove from one hand. Carry the used glove in your gloved hand under the contaminated item. Use the ungloved hand to open doors and turn on faucets. By using this method, you avoid contaminating the environment with your gloves.

PROCEDURE

59

ASSISTING WITH THE URINAL

1. Carry out initial procedure actions.

2. Assemble equipment:
   - Urinal (Figure 26-7)
   - Disposable gloves

3. Put on gloves. Hand the urinal to the patient or lift the top bedcovers and place the urinal underneath so the patient can grasp the handle. Instruct the patient to place his penis in the urinal opening. If he cannot do this, place the penis in the opening.

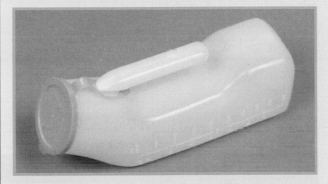

Figure 26-7 A male urinal with a snap-on lid.
(© Delmar/Cengage Learning)

4. Remove your gloves and dispose of them properly. Wash your hands. Make sure the signal cord is within easy reach. Leave the patient alone if possible. Watch for his signal.

5. Answer the patient's signal immediately. Wash your hands.

6. Put on gloves. Ask the patient to hand the urinal to you. Cover it. Rearrange the bedclothes if necessary.

7. Cover the urinal and take it to the bathroom or utility room. Observe the contents. Measure, if required. Do not empty the urinal if you observe anything unusual (such as blood). Save abnormal contents for the nurse's inspection.

8. Empty the urinal. Rinse it with cold water and clean it with warm soapy water. Rinse, dry, and cover the urinal and replace it in the bedside stand. Remove your gloves and dispose of them properly. Wash your hands.

9. Assist the patient to wash hands. An antiseptic hand rub or alcohol product may be used, if desired.

10. Carry out ending procedure actions.

PROCEDURE

60

ASSISTING WITH USE OF THE BEDSIDE COMMODE

1. Carry out initial procedure actions.

2. Assemble equipment:
   - Disposable gloves
   - Portable commode
   - Toilet tissue
   - Bath blanket

3. Position the commode beside the bed, facing the head. Lock the commode wheels and open the lid. Be sure a container is in place under the seat.

4. If the bed and side rails are elevated, lower the side rail nearest you and lower the bed to the lowest horizontal position. Lock bed wheels.

5. Put on gloves.

6. Assist the patient to a sitting position. Swing the patient's legs over the edge of the bed.

7. Assist the patient to put on a robe and slippers. Assist the patient to stand. If needed, use a transfer belt.

8. Support the patient with hands on either side of the transfer belt. Remember to use proper body mechanics. Pivot the patient and lower her to the commode.

9. Cover the patient's legs with a bath blanket.

continues

PROCEDURE 60 CONTINUED

10. Leave the call bell and toilet tissue within reach.

11. Remove your gloves and discard them according to facility policy. Wash your hands.

12. When the patient signals, return promptly. Wash your hands and put on gloves.

13. Remove the bath blanket. Assist the patient to stand.

14. Cleanse the anus and/or perineum if the patient is unable to do so.

15. Allow the patient to wash and dry her hands. Remove your gloves and dispose of them according to facility policy. Wash your hands.

16. Assist the patient to return to bed. Adjust bedding and pillows for comfort.

17. Leave the signal cord within easy reach.

18. Put on gloves.

19. Remove the container from the commode and cover it. Close the commode lid.

20. Take the container to the bathroom. Note its contents and measure them if required.

21. Empty and clean the container. Replace it in the commode. Remove and dispose of gloves properly.

22. Put the commode in its proper place.

23. Carry out ending procedure actions.

Infection Control ALERT

When caring for patients in a room with two or more beds, label the bedpans and urinals with each patient's name. Use the labeled bedpan and urinal only for the named patient. After cleaning the bedpan or urinal, store it properly in the bedside stand or according to facility policy. Do not leave uncovered bedpans and urinals on the floor or in the bathroom. ■

Age-Appropriate Care ALERT

Incontinence is up to five times more common in persons over the age of 50 than in younger adults. However, *incontinence is not a normal aging change.* ■

URINARY INCONTINENCE

Urinary incontinence (loss of control of urination) may be due to one or a combination of factors. It is not unusual to have more than one factor causing the problem. Urinary incontinence may be temporary or permanent, due to a physical or mental condition, or due to physical inability to reach the bathroom on time.

GUIDELINES *for*

Caring for the Patient with Incontinence

Nursing assistant responsibilities include:

- Assisting patients who need help to toilet regularly.

- Answering call lights promptly.

- Always being courteous and patient when assisting with toileting procedures.

- Maintaining a positive attitude when changing soiled garments and bed linen.

- Performing regular perineal care and being sure the patient's skin is clean and dry.

- Regularly checking the skin for signs of irritation.

- Giving special attention to patients who are confused or forgetful, because they may be unable to clearly state their need for assistance.

- Changing wet or soiled linen immediately.

- Helping with procedures to maintain continence.

- Assisting with an incontinence management or bowel and bladder retraining program, if ordered (see Unit 28).

FLUID BALANCE

Fluid balance is the balance between liquid intake and liquid output. Because two-thirds of the body's weight consists of water, under normal conditions there must be a balance between the amount of fluid taken into the body and the amount lost. This balance usually takes care of itself, but additional monitoring is required for patients who have conditions of the urinary system.

The metric system is used for fluid measurements: milliliters (mL) or cubic centimeters (cc). A mL and a cc are the same amount. Table 26-3 compares U.S. customary liquid and metric measurements.

cc and mL same

Intake

Most adults take in approximately 2½ to 3 quarts (2,500 to 3,000 mL) of fluid daily in liquids; foods such as fruits and vegetables; and artificially, such as by physician-ordered intravenous infusions or tube feedings.

Most adults should consume at least 600 to 800 mL of fluid during each eight-hour shift. Because a patient sleeps during most of the night shift, additional fluids must be provided during waking hours to keep the body in balance. Excessive fluid retention in the tissue is called **edema**. Inadequate fluid intake results in **dehydration**, which is a lack of sufficient fluid in body tissues. Some medications and disease conditions may change the amounts of fluid the patient is allowed to have.

Output

Typical output equals about 2½ quarts daily, in the form of:
- Urine, 1½ quarts (1,500 mL)
- Perspiration
- Moisture exhaled from the lungs
- Moisture lost from the bowel as bowel movements

Excessive fluid loss also results in dehydration. This usually occurs through diarrhea, vomiting, excessive urine output (**diuresis**), excessive perspiration (**diaphoresis**), and wound drainage or blood loss.

Recording Intake and Output

An accurate recording of **intake and output (I&O)**, or fluid taken in and given off by the body, is basic to the care of many patients. Intake and output records are kept when specifically ordered by the physician or registered nurse.

Some patients' care plans will have a notation instructing you to increase their oral fluid intake. This is called **push fluids** or **force fluids**. *Forcing fluids* is an old term that is not quite accurate. You should never actually force patients to consume water or other beverages. "Force fluids" really means that you must encourage the patient to drink each time you are in the room. If the patient will not drink water, provide other beverages that the patient likes, if possible. Such a patient will be on intake and output monitoring.

In some situations (such as with patients who are in renal failure or on dialysis), the physician may order a fluid restriction. This means that the fluids the patient takes in are limited to a certain amount each day. Nursing and dietary must share this amount. The care plan will list the total amount of fluid the patient should consume on your shift. This patient will be on intake and output. Check the I&O worksheet before giving the patient a drink, because other staff may have given fluids, such as the nurse during medication administration.

Fluid intake and output are calculated by measuring and recording the fluids the patient takes in and the fluids the patient **excretes** (eliminates from the body) (Table 26-4). When a patient is on intake monitoring, an estimate of fluids consumed is made and recorded. This is done by:
- Knowing what each liquid container holds when full. For example:
  - Coffee/tea cup, 8 oz = 240 mL
  - Water carafe, 16 oz = 480 mL
  - Foam cup, 8 oz = 240 mL
  - Plastic water glass, 8 oz = 240 mL

Standard Precaution

Emesis: vomiting

TABLE 26-3 COMPARISON OF U.S. CUSTOMARY AND METRIC MEASUREMENTS

U.S. Customary Units	Metric Units
1 minim	0.06 milliliter (mL)
16 minims	1 mL (1 cc)
1 ounce	30 mL (30 cc)
1 pint	500 mL (500 cc)
1 quart	1,000 mL (1,000 cc, 1 liter)

TABLE 26-4 COMPUTING INTAKE AND OUTPUT

Intake		Output	
By mouth	2,000 mL	Urine	1,500 mL
IV	1,500 mL	Vomitus	500 mL
		Drainage	600 mL
Total	3,500 mL	**Total**	2,600 mL

- Soup bowl, 6 oz = 180 mL
- Jello, 1 serving = 120 mL
- Ice chips, full 4 oz glass = 120 mL
- Estimating how much is gone from the container (what the patient drank)
- Converting this to mL

Example: A water glass holds 240 mL when filled. The patient drinks ¾ of the glass of water: ¾ of 240 mL = 180 mL. Intake is recorded as 180 mL.

You must calculate and record patient intake of all liquids, including water, juices, soda, coffee, tea, milk, and soup. Foods that melt at room temperature, such as ice cream, sherbet, and gelatin (Jello), are also recorded.

 Note: Container sizes vary from one facility to the next. Each facility should have a chart that tells you what each size of glass, cup, and bowl holds when full.

Fluids taken by mouth, through intravenous infusion, or through gastric feeding are recorded separately (Figure 26-8). At the end of each 8-hour shift and the end of 24 hours, the figures are totaled.

Fluid output amount is obtained by measuring *all* fluids excreted from the body. This includes urine, **emesis** (vomitus), and drainage from body cavities, such as gastric drainage. A container called a **graduate** is marked in mL or cc. To accurately measure the patient's output, pour the substance into a graduate. Urine and any other excretions are recorded separately. When patients are incontinent, the bed protectors or disposable briefs may be weighed to estimate the urinary output.

Date Amount	Time	Method of Adm.	Solution	Intake amounts Rec'd	Time	Output Urine Amount	Others	
							Kind	
7/16	0700	PO	water	120 mL		500 mL		
	0830	PO	coffee	240 mL				
			or. ju.	120 mL				
	1030	PO	cran.ju.	120 mL				
	1100					300 mL		
	1230	PO	tea	240 mL				
	1400	PO	water	150 mL				
Shift Totals	1500			990 mL		800 mL		
	1530	PO	gelatin	120 mL				
	1700	PO	tea	120 mL				
			soup	180 mL				
	2000					512 mL		
	2045						vomitus	500 mL
	2205						vomitus	90 mL
Shift Totals	2300			420 mL		512 mL		590 mL
	2345						vomitus	80 mL
	0130	IV	D/W	500 mL				
	0315			400 mL				
Shift Totals	0700			500 mL		400 mL		80 mL
24 Hour Totals				1910 mL		1712 mL	vomitus	670 mL

FIGURE 26-8 Sample intake and output record. (*© Delmar/Cengage Learning*)

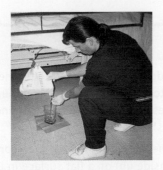

FIGURE 26-9 The nursing assistant uses the principles of standard precautions to collect urinary drainage. Measure the urinary output in the graduate pitcher, and record the total amount on the intake and output record. (© *Delmar/Cengage Learning*)

> **Note:** Standard precautions must be followed when measuring any body excretion. Gloves are required for measuring all forms of output (Figure 26-9).

CHANGING WATER

Water is essential to life. Regular provision of fresh water is an important nursing assistant responsibility. Check the care plans to learn whether patients are allowed ice or tap water and if water consumption is to be encouraged. A patient should drink 6 to 8 glasses of liquid every 24 hours, unless the patient is NPO (nothing by mouth) or is on fluid restriction. Give special attention to confused patients, patients who may not be able to reach a source of water, and older patients.

DIAGNOSTIC TESTS

You will assist with procedures and collect specimens used to diagnose problems of the urinary tract. These include several kinds of urine specimens.

Infection Control ALERT

Avoid contaminating the ice chest or ice scoop when filling pitchers and passing fresh drinking water. Keep the ice scoop covered when not in use. The handle is contaminated and should not touch the clean ice supply. Avoid filling the pitcher over the source of clean ice. If ice hits the rim of the pitcher and drops back into the clean ice supply, the whole supply is contaminated. Do not allow the scoop to touch the pitcher. Always keep water pitchers covered at the bedside. If more than one patient shares the room, make sure each pitcher and cup are labeled with a single patient's name. To reduce the potential for infection, some facilities are now giving patients a bottle of water each shift, and upon request, rather than filling a carafe. If ice is requested, staff provides it in a plastic bag or disposable cup with a lid. ■

Routine Urine Specimen

The properties of the urine provide a great deal of information about the function of the body. **Urinalysis**—an analysis of the urine—is the most common laboratory test. The specimen is usually obtained when the patient first **voids** (urinates) in the morning. Transport the specimen to the laboratory promptly or refrigerate it until delivery can be made.

Catheterized Urine Specimen

When a urine specimen is needed that is free of contamination from organisms found in areas near the urinary meatus (opening), the specimen may be collected by

PROCEDURE

COLLECTING A ROUTINE URINE SPECIMEN

1. Carry out initial procedure actions.

2. Assemble equipment:
   - Disposable gloves
   - Bedpan/urinal with cover or specimen container for use in toilet
   - Bed protector
   - Toilet tissue
   - Small plastic bag
   - Specimen container and cover
   - Completed label

continues

PROCEDURE 61 CONTINUED

- Graduate pitcher
- Laboratory requisition slip, properly filled out
- Biohazard specimen transport bag

3. Completely fill out the label of the specimen container.

4. Wash your hands and put on disposable gloves.

5. If the patient cannot ambulate, offer the bedpan or urinal.

6. Instruct the patient not to discard toilet tissue in the container with the urine. Provide a small plastic bag in which to place the soiled tissue.

7. After the patient has voided, cover the urinal or bedpan and place it on the bed protector on the chair. Assist the patient with cleansing, if needed.

8. If the patient can ambulate to the bathroom, place a specimen collector in the toilet.

9. Assist the patient to the bathroom. Ask the patient to void into the specimen collector. Remind the patient to discard toilet tissue in the plastic bag.

10. Provide privacy.

11. Put on gloves. Remove the specimen collector from the toilet. If the patient is on I&O, note the amount of urine (Figure 26-10). If the patient

used a bedpan or urinal, pour the urine into a graduate to measure it. Note the amount. Remove your gloves and discard them according to facility policy. Wash your hands.

12. Remove the cap from the specimen container, and place it (inside up) on a flat surface in the bathroom or utility room. Do not touch the inside of the cap or container.

13. Put on gloves. Carefully pour about 120 mL of urine into the specimen container from the collector (Figure 26-11).

14. Remove and discard gloves according to facility policy.

15. Wash your hands.

16. Place the cap on the specimen container. Do not contaminate the outside of the container. Attach the completed label to the container (Figure 26-12). Place the specimen container in a biohazard specimen transport bag and attach a laboratory requisition slip (Figure 26-13).

17. Assist the patient with handwashing and comfort measures, if needed.

18. Carry out ending procedure actions.

19. Follow facility policy for transporting the specimen to the laboratory.

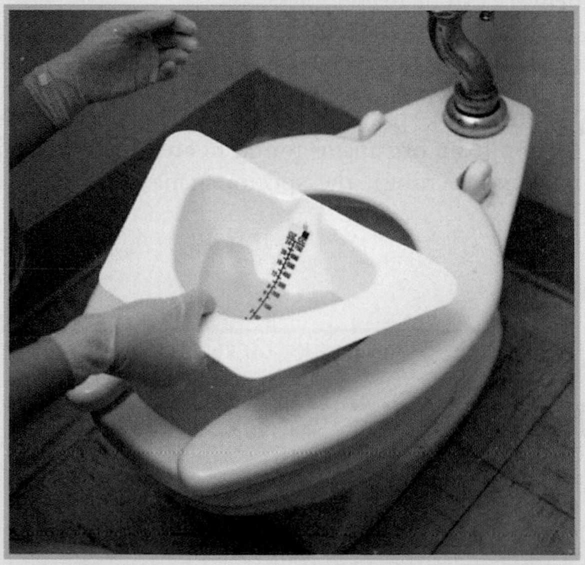

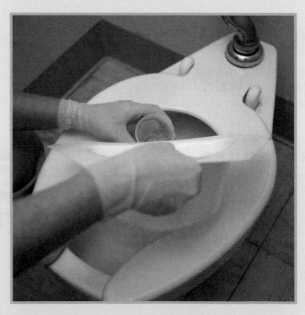

FIGURE 26-10 Remove the collection device. Note the total amount if the patient is on I&O. (© Delmar/Cengage Learning)

FIGURE 26-11 Carefully pour the specimen into the container. (© Delmar/Cengage Learning)

PROCEDURE 61 CONTINUED

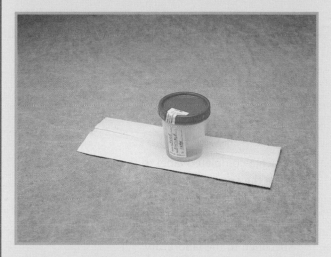

FIGURE 26-12 After placing the cap on the container, apply the label. *(© Delmar/Cengage Learning)*

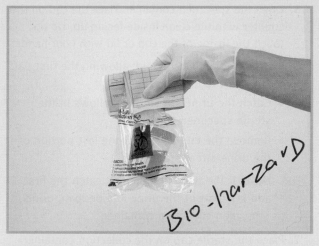

Bio-harzard

FIGURE 26-13 The properly labeled container is placed in a transport bag with the laboratory requisition attached. *(© Delmar/Cengage Learning)*

indwelling: balloon

PROCEDURE

62

COLLECTING A CLEAN-CATCH URINE SPECIMEN

1. Carry out initial procedure actions.

2. Assemble equipment:
   - Disposable gloves
   - Small plastic bag
   - Sterile specimen container and cover
   - Completed label for container
   - Gauze squares or cotton
   - Antiseptic solution
   - Laboratory requisition slip, properly filled out
   - Biohazard specimen transport bag

3. Wash your hands and put on disposable gloves.

4. Wash the patient's genital area properly or instruct the patient to do so. If the area is soiled due to incontinence, perform perineal care.

   a. *For female patients:*
      - Hold the outer folds of the vulva (folds are also called *labia* or *lips*) open with one

hand. Using the cotton and antiseptic solution, cleanse the innermost area (meatus or urinary opening) of the labia from front to back. Discard the cotton. Pick up another cotton ball and cleanse the far side of the labia from front to back. Discard the cotton. Pick up another cotton ball and cleanse the near side of the labia from front to back. Discard the cotton in the plastic bag.

   - Keep the labia separated throughout the procedure so that the folds do not fall back and cover the meatus.

   b. *For male patients:*
      - Using the cotton and the antiseptic solution, cleanse the tip of the penis. Begin at the meatus, working outward and using a circular motion. Wash the remainder of the penis using downward strokes.
      - Discard the cotton in the plastic bag.

continues

PROCEDURE 62 CONTINUED

5. Open the specimen container. Place the cap on the counter with the clean inside facing up. Do not touch the inside of the cup or lid with your hands.

6. Instruct the patient to void, allowing the first part of the urine to escape. Then:
   - Catch the urine stream that follows in the sterile specimen container.
   - Remove the cup and allow the last portion of the urine stream to escape.

   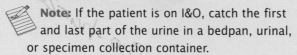

   Note: If the patient is on I&O, catch the first and last part of the urine in a bedpan, urinal, or specimen collection container.

7. Place the sterile cap on the collection container immediately to prevent contamination of the specimen.

8. With the cap securely tightened, wash and dry the outside of the specimen container.

9. Remove and dispose of gloves according to facility policy.

10. Assist the patient with handwashing and comfort measures, if needed.

11. Wash your hands.

12. Attach a completed label to the container and place the specimen in the transport bag.

13. Carry out ending procedure actions.

14. Follow facility policy for transporting the specimen to the laboratory.

---

inserting a sterile tube (**catheter**). The nurse will perform this procedure.

Twenty-Four-Hour Specimens

When a 24-hour urine specimen is ordered, all urine excreted in a 24-hour period is collected and saved. When this specimen is ordered, the patient will begin the 24-hour collection period with an empty bladder.

Age-Appropriate Care ALERT

The pediatric urine collection device should not be used for children with diaper rash, inflamed or broken skin, or those who are allergic to adhesive tape. If a clean specimen is needed, another option may be to place several sterile cotton balls directly over the external urinary meatus, inside the diaper. After the child has voided, collect the cotton and squeeze the urine into a specimen cup (with your gloved hands). ■

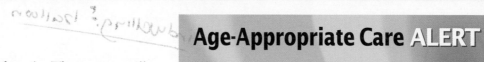

GUIDELINES *for*

Collecting 24-Hour Urine Specimens

For a 24-hour urine collection, nursing assistant responsibilities include:

- Asking the patient to void. Discard this urine and note the time. The bladder must be empty when the test begins.

- Saving all urine for the next 24 hours, including urine voided as the test time finishes.

- Providing a plastic bag for tissue disposal. Instruct the patient to avoid dropping tissue into the specimen.

- Saving all urine in a large, carefully labeled container that is supplied by the laboratory and may contain a preservative. Pack the container in ice and refresh the ice whenever necessary as the ice melts.

- Informing the nurse if a specimen becomes contaminated with stool or toilet tissue, or if you or the patient forget to save a specimen. The test will be discontinued and restarted for a new 24-hour period.

PROCEDURE

63

COLLECTING A 24-HOUR URINE SPECIMEN

1. Carry out initial procedure actions.

2. Assemble equipment:
   - Disposable gloves
   - 24-hour specimen container (supplied by health care facility)
   - Bedpan, urinal, or commode, or specimen collector for toilet
   - Plastic bag
   - Sign for patient's bed
   - Biohazard bag
   - Completed label for the container

3. Explain the procedure to the patient and note the importance of saving all urine passed for the next 24 hours.

4. Place the specimen collection container in the bathroom in a pan of ice (Figures 26-14A and 26-14B). The ice will keep the specimen cool for 24 hours.

5. Put on disposable gloves

6. Allow the patient to void.
   a. Assist with the bedpan or urinal as needed.
   b. Measure the amount of urine passed if the patient is on I&O.
   c. Discard the urine specimen.
   d. Note the date and time of voiding. This time will mark the start of the 24-hour collection.

7. Place a sign on the patient's bed to alert other health care team members that a 24-hour urine specimen is being collected. (The sign may read: *Save all urine—24-hour specimen.*)

8. From this time on, for a period of 24 hours, all urine voided is added to the specimen container (Figure 26-14C). The container is kept on ice. Check facility policy regarding handling of the specimen container.

9. Instruct the patient not to discard toilet tissue into the specimen collection container. Provide small plastic bags for this purpose.

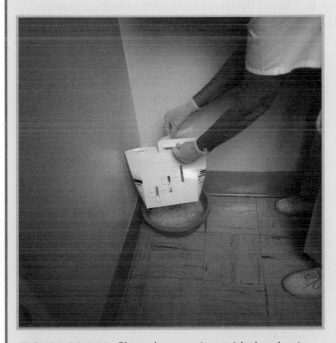

FIGURE 26-14A Close the container with the plastic fastener. Place the 24 hour specimen container in the patient's bathroom in a pan of ice. (© *Delmar/Cengage Learning*)

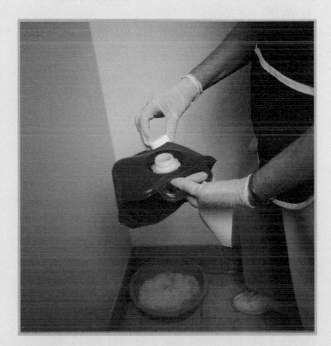

FIGURE 26-14B Some facilities use plastic containers for collecting a 24-hour specimen. (© *Delmar/Cengage Learning*)

continues

PROCEDURE 63 CONTINUED

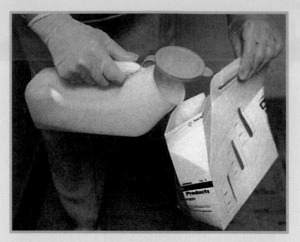

FIGURE 26-14C Open the mouth of the container wide to avoid spilling the specimen. (© *Delmar/Cengage Learning*)

10. At the end of the 24-hour period, apply gloves, and ask the patient to void one more time. Add this last specimen to the container.

11. Remove the sign from the patient's bed. Check the container label for accuracy and completeness. Attach the appropriate requisition slip.

12. Remove and discard gloves according to facility policy.

13. Place the specimen in a protective biohazard bag for transport.

14. Carry out ending procedure actions.

15. Clean and replace all equipment used, according to facility policy.

16. Follow facility policy for transporting the specimen to the laboratory.

PROCEDURE

64

COLLECTING A URINE SPECIMEN FROM AN INFANT

1. Wash your hands.

2. Assemble supplies:
   - Disposable gloves (at least 2 pair)
   - Soap and water, or cleanser used by facility
   - Cotton balls or washcloth to cleanse perineum
   - Towel
   - Clean diaper
   - Bed protector
   - Plastic bag
   - Pediatric urine collection bag
   - Syringe to withdraw specimen from collection bag, if this is facility policy
   - Urine specimen cup
   - Completed label
   - Transport bag

3. Remove the infant's diaper.

4. Wash the perineum with soap and water. Make sure to remove powder or ointment.

5. Rinse the perineum and dry well.

6. Discard the used diaper, cotton balls, and other used supplies in the plastic bag.

7. Apply the urine collection bag by removing the paper backing to expose the adhesive and positioning the center of the hole in the bag over the external urinary meatus in a female, or over the penis in a male.

8. Gently press the bag in place to seal the adhesive.

9. Reapply the diaper, leaving the bag unfolded. In some facilities, the bag is pulled through to the outside of the diaper, or a hole is cut in the diaper so the bag can be pulled through to the outside.

10. Remove gloves and discard them in the plastic bag.

11. Wash your hands.

12. Remove the collection device immediately after the child voids.

13. Place the collection device on a bed protector or other clean area. Put the bag down and position

PROCEDURE 64 CONTINUED

the hole in the center carefully to avoid spilling the contents.

14. Cleanse the infant's perineum and apply a clean diaper.

15. Leave the infant in a position of comfort and safety.

16. Open the specimen collection cup. Place the lid on the table, with the clean inner side facing up. Avoid touching the inside of the lid or specimen container.

17. Carefully pour the specimen into the collection container, or withdraw it with a syringe (with no needle attached) and gently push the plunger to move the specimen to the cup. Some facilities cap the syringe and send it to the lab as is. Follow your facility policy for specimen handling.

18. Apply the lid to the specimen cup. Place the cup in the transport bag.

19. Carry out ending procedure actions.

URINARY DRAINAGE

Some patients will have a catheter for urinary drainage.

- Urine is drained from the bladder through a tube called a *catheter.*
- French catheters or straight catheters (Figure 26-15A) are hollow tubes. They are usually made of soft rubber or plastic. These catheters are used to drain the bladder. They do not remain in the bladder.
- **Foley catheters** (Figure 26-15B) have a balloon surrounding the neck. The balloon is inflated after the catheter is introduced into the bladder. This is known as an **indwelling** or **retention catheter**.
- A **suprapubic catheter** (Figure 26-16) is inserted surgically through the abdominal wall directly into the bladder.
- A **condom catheter** is an external catheter used on males. It is applied over the penis and attached to drainage tubing.

The insertion of a catheter is a sterile procedure. It is performed by the nurse or advanced care provider. Closed

Infection Control ALERT

Catheters are used only as a treatment of last resort because of the risk of complications. As many as 28,000 patients die each year in the United States because of catheter-related infections. Careful handling and attention to technique when caring for and emptying the catheter will reduce the risk of infection. ■

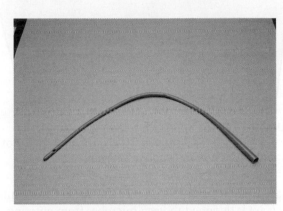

FIGURE 26-15A A straight catheter is inserted to collect a specimen, then removed. (© Delmar/Cengage Learning)

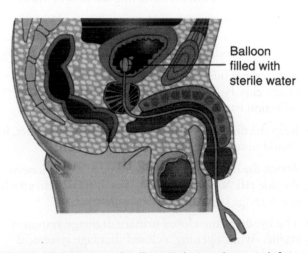

Balloon filled with sterile water

FIGURE 26-15B An indwelling (Foley) catheter is left in place to empty the bladder. The balloon is inflated with sterile water to hold the catheter in place. (© Delmar/Cengage Learning)

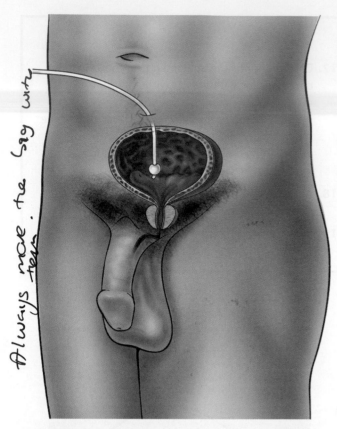

Always move the bag with tem. (handwritten note)

FIGURE 26-16 The suprapubic catheter is surgically inserted through the abdominal wall. The urethra is not functional. *(© Delmar/Cengage Learning)*

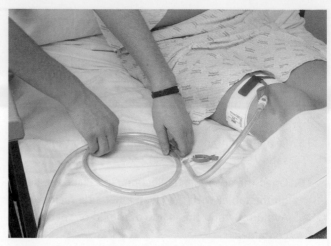

FIGURE 26-17 A Velcro strap is used to fasten the catheter to the leg. Coil the tubing on the bed. These measures prevent the catheter from moving and accidentally being pulled out during movement or transfers. *(© Delmar/Cengage Learning)*

urinary drainage systems protect the patient from infection. Care is designed to keep microbes from entering the closed system.

- Avoid traction on the catheter during patient care. Apply a catheter strap or similar device to the leg to secure the catheter (Figure 26-17). Position the catheter on the top side of the leg to avoid obstructing the flow of urine.

- Know the position of the catheter at all times. Use care when lifting, moving, and transferring patients to avoid accidentally dislodging the catheter by pulling on the tubing.

- Attach the tubing to the bed with a rubber band and plastic clip. Position it so there is a direct drop to the collection bag.

- Keep the drainage bag below the level of the bladder. It should never touch the floor.

- Attach the drainage bag to the frame of the bed, never the side rail. When the person is in a wheelchair, attach the drainage bag to the frame of the chair.

- The inside of the closed urinary drainage system is sterile. Avoid opening a closed drainage system, if possible.

- Measure the amount of drainage in the collection bag at the end of each shift, and record the information on the I&O sheet.

- In certain medical conditions, the physician will order an hourly output measurement. In this situation, a catheter drainage bag with a *urimeter* (Figure 26-18) will be used. The urine drains into the small chamber. You will obtain the reading from the marks on the plastic, then empty the chamber into the bag every hour and inform the nurse of the output measurement.

- Check the entire drainage setup at the beginning and end of your shift.

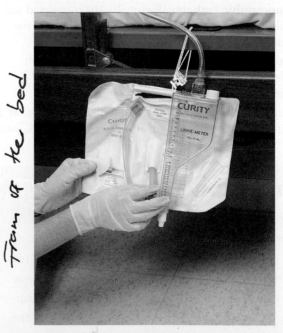

From of the bed (handwritten note)

FIGURE 26-18 The drainage bag with a urimeter is used when the physician orders hourly output measurements. *(© Delmar/Cengage Learning)*

Difficult SITUATIONS

Unless the patient is on a fluid restriction, encourage the catheterized patient to drink fluids each time you are in the room. Increasing fluid intake to 2,500 mL a day is best. The increased fluid prevents sediment formation and flushes the catheter. Check the level of urine in the drainage bag each time you are in the room. Empty the bag if it is full and document the output. ∎

- Monitor the level of urine in the drainage bag.
- Notify the nurse if redness, irritation, drainage, crusting, or open areas are present at the catheter insertion site, or if the patient complains of pain, burning, or tenderness, or has other signs or symptoms of urinary tract infection.

Catheter Care

Wash the area around the urinary meatus daily with a solution approved by your facility, or with soap and water. This care is called **indwelling catheter** *care*. Indwelling catheter care may be performed during routine morning care, as part of perineal care, or as a separate procedure.

PROCEDURE

GIVING INDWELLING CATHETER CARE

1. Carry out initial procedure actions.

2. Assemble equipment:
   - Disposable gloves
   - Bed protector
   - Bath blanket
   - Plastic bag for disposables
   - Daily catheter care kit (if available)
   - Washcloth, towel, basin, and soap if kit is unavailable
   - Antiseptic solution
   - Sterile applicators
   - Tape or Velcro strap

3. Raise the bed to a comfortable working height. Be sure the opposite side rail is up and secure. Position the patient on the back, with legs separated and knees bent, if permitted.

4. Cover the patient with a bath blanket and fanfold bedding to the foot of the bed.

5. Place a bed protector underneath the patient.

6. Position a bath blanket so that only the genitals will be exposed.

7. Arrange a catheter care kit on the overbed table. Open the kit. Place the open bag at the foot of the bed.

8. Wash your hands. Put on gloves and draw the drape or bath blanket back.

   a. *For the male patient:*
      - Gently grasp the penis and draw the foreskin back, if not circumcised (Figure 26-19).

- Using a new applicator dipped in antiseptic solution for each stroke, cleanse the glans from the meatus toward the shaft for approximately 4 inches.
- After each stroke, discard the applicator in a plastic bag.
- **Alternate action:** Clean around the catheter first and then around the meatus and glans. Wash with soap and water, using a circular motion. Dry in the same manner.

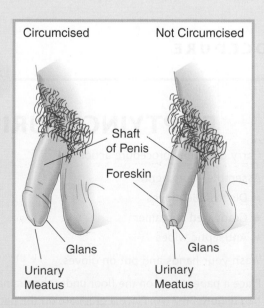

FIGURE 26-19 Comparison of circumcised and uncircumcised penis. (© *Delmar/Cengage Learning*)

continues

PROCEDURE 65 CONTINUED

Make sure to return the foreskin (if not circumcised) to its proper position.

b. *For the female patient:*

- Separate the labia.
- Using a new applicator dipped in antiseptic for each stroke, cleanse from front to back. Begin at the center, then cleanse each side.
- After each stroke, discard the applicator in a plastic bag.
- Clean the catheter down about 4 inches.
- Dry carefully.

10. Remove your gloves and discard them in the plastic bag. Wash your hands.

11. Check the catheter to be sure it is secured properly to the leg. Readjust the Velcro strap for slack, if needed. If a Velcro strap or adhesive device is not available, use tape (Figure 26-20) or an adhesive tube holder that sticks to the leg.

12. Be sure the tubing is coiled on the bed so it hangs straight down into the drainage container. Empty the bag and measure the contents, if necessary. Be sure that the tubing and drainage bag do not touch the floor.

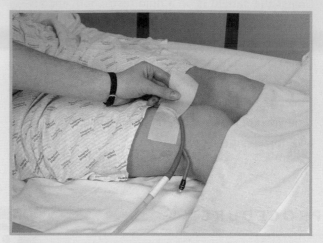

FIGURE 26-20 The catheter tubing may be taped to the thigh or attached using an adhesive tube holder. The nurse may instruct you to tape the catheter to the abdomen in male patients. (*© Delmar/Cengage Learning*)

13. Replace bedding and remove the bath blanket.

14. Fold the bath blanket and store, or put it in the linen hamper.

15. Lower the bed. Adjust side rails for safety.

16. Carry out ending procedure actions.

PROCEDURE

66

EMPTYING A URINARY DRAINAGE UNIT

1. Carry out initial procedure actions.

2. Assemble equipment:
- Disposable gloves
- Graduated container
- Antiseptic wipes

3. Wash your hands and put on gloves.

4. Place a paper towel on the floor under the drainage bag (Figure 26-21A). Place a graduate on the paper towel under the drain of the collection bag.

5. Remove the drain from the holder (Figure 26-21B) and open the drain. Allow the urine to drain into the graduate, using aseptic technique. Do not allow the tip of the tubing to touch the sides of the graduate.

6. Close the drain and replace it in the holder. If accidental contamination occurs, wipe the drain tip with an antiseptic wipe before returning it to the holder. (In some facilities, this is done each time the drain is open and closed.) Discard the used antiseptic wipes in a plastic bag.

PROCEDURE **66** CONTINUED

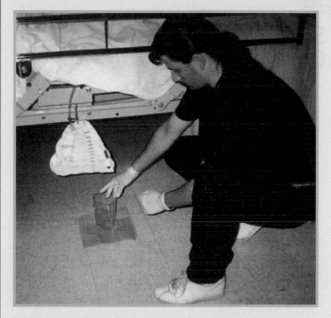

FIGURE 26-21A Place a paper towel on the floor.
(© Delmar/Cengage Learning)

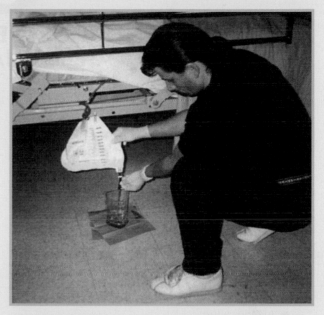

FIGURE 26-21B Center the graduate under the drainage spout. If you accidentally touch the spout with your fingers or the edge of the graduate, wipe it with an alcohol sponge before returning it to the drainage bag.
(© Delmar/Cengage Learning)

7. Check the position of the drainage tube.

8. Pick up the paper towel, touching the top surface only, and discard it.

9. Take the graduate to the bathroom, check the amount, and empty it.

10. Wash and dry the graduate and store it according to facility policy.

11. Record the amount of urine and note its character.

12. Remove your gloves and discard them according to facility policy.

13. Carry out ending procedure actions.

Collecting a Specimen from a Closed Urinary Drainage System

At some time, it may be necessary to collect a fresh specimen of urine when the patient is on a closed urinary drainage system. Keep in mind that the:

- Urine sample must be fresh. This means that the specimen must be taken directly from the catheter.

- The procedure used is determined by the type of catheter that is in place. If the catheter has a **port** (opening) for fluid withdrawal, follow Procedure 67. Be very conscientious with your technique, to avoid introducing pathogens into the system.

Infection Control ALERT

Select a sterile specimen collection cup when obtaining a urine specimen from a patient with a catheter. Avoid touching the inside of the cup and the lid with your hands. Place the lid with the clean, inner side up on the table. If you have clamped the catheter to collect the specimen, remove the clamp before leaving the room, or urine will back up into the patient's bladder. ■

PROCEDURE

67

COLLECTING A URINE SPECIMEN THROUGH A DRAINAGE PORT

1. Carry out initial procedure actions.

2. Assemble equipment:
   - Disposable gloves
   - Tube clamp
   - Laboratory requisition
   - Completed label
   - Emesis basin
   - 10-mL syringe
   - Specimen cup and lid
   - 21-gauge or 22-gauge needle
   - Sharps container
   - Alcohol wipe
   - Bed protector
   - Biohazard specimen transport bag

3. Go to the bedside half an hour before the sample is to be collected.

4. Clamp the drainage tube.

5. Wash your hands. Return to the bedside after 30 minutes.

6. Put on gloves.

7. Place a bed protector on the bed and place an emesis basin on the bed protector under the catheter drainage port.

8. Wipe the drainage port with an alcohol wipe (Figure 26-22).

9. Carefully remove the cap on the syringe. Do not contaminate the tip.

10. Attach the needle carefully. Do not contaminate the needle tip.

11. Open the package with the specimen container. Remove the lid and lay it, inside up, on the bedside stand. Do not touch the inside of the cup or the lid with your hands.

12. Insert the needle into the port and withdraw the specimen (Figure 26-23).

13. Carefully withdraw the needle.

14. Wipe the port with the alcohol wipe.

15. Transfer the urine sample to the specimen container (Figure 26-24).

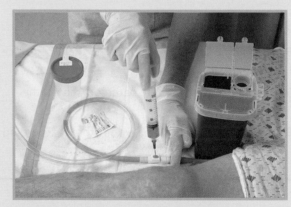

FIGURE 26-23 Draw the specimen into the needle. (© Delmar/Cengage Learning)

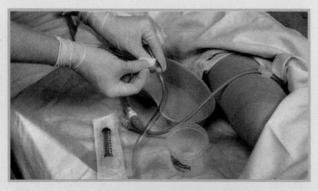

FIGURE 26-22 Wipe the port with an antiseptic wipe or alcohol sponge. (© Delmar/Cengage Learning)

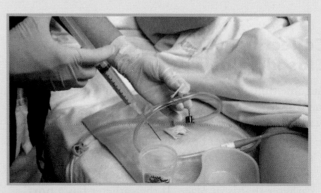

FIGURE 26-24 Transfer the specimen to the container. (© Delmar/Cengage Learning)

PROCEDURE 67 CONTINUED

16. Handling the lid by the top only, cover the container.

17. Do not recap the needle. Do not detach the needle from the syringe. Discard the needle and syringe into the sharps' container at the bedside.

18. Remove your gloves and discard them according to facility policy. Wash your hands.

19. Remove the catheter clamp.

20. Complete the information on the label and put the label on the container. Compare the label to the requisition to be sure that the information is complete and accurate.

21. Place the specimen container in a biohazard transport bag, seal the bag, and attach the completed laboratory requisition (Figure 26-25).

22. Carry out ending procedure actions.

23. Follow instructions for care and transport of the specimen.

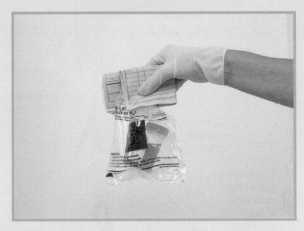

FIGURE 26-25 Place the specimen in the biohazard transport bag, seal the bag, and attach the laboratory requisition. (© Delmar/Cengage Learning)

External Drainage Systems (Male)

External urinary drainage systems are preferred for male patients who require long periods of urinary drainage. Because the catheter is placed externally, the risk of infection is lower. A condom catheter (sometimes called a "Texas catheter") is applied to the penis. An external drainage bag is attached to the catheter. The catheter is held in place by an adhesive inside the condom, or a strip that is wrapped in a spiral around the outside of the catheter (see Procedure 69). Complications, ranging from minor irritation to circulatory impairment, can occur if the external adhesive strip encircles the penis. The catheter should extend about an inch beyond the tip of the penis.

Urine may be collected in a regular drainage bag that hangs from the bed, or a smaller bag attached to the patient's leg. The condom is removed every 24 hours and the penis is washed and dried. Once removed, the used condom is discarded and a new catheter applied.

Disconnecting the Catheter

Maintaining the closed urinary drainage system is preferable, but at times disconnecting the catheter may

Difficult SITUATIONS

Inspect the condom catheter periodically to make sure it is not twisted, which causes urine to collect inside the catheter. As the urine accumulates, the catheter will expand until it eventually comes off. ∎

be necessary. If sterile caps and plugs are available, use them. If not, protect the disconnected ends with sterile gauze sponges.

Carefully follow the procedure for disconnecting the catheter. The catheter is hollow, so it creates a high risk for infection. There are several sites where pathogens can enter the drainage system (Figure 26-26):

- Urinary meatus, where the catheter is inserted
- Connection between the catheter and the drainage tube
- Connection between the drainage bag and the drainage tubing
- Opening used to empty the drainage bag

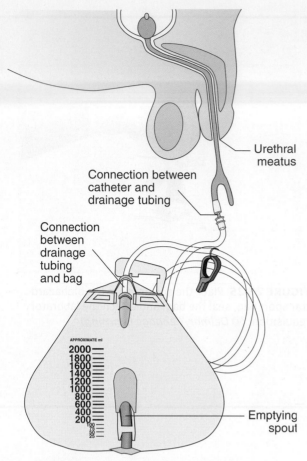

FIGURE 26-26 Handle the closed drainage system carefully to avoid accidental contamination of these areas. (© Delmar/Cengage Learning)

Leg Bag Drainage

Some patients use the smaller leg bag (Figure 26-27) for modesty when out of bed. Because the bag attaches to the upper thigh, it is not visible under clothing. The leg bag is fastened to the leg with Velcro or elastic straps. This bag is smaller than a regular drainage bag, so it must be emptied more often. Never use the leg bag when the person is in bed. Connect the catheter to a regular drainage bag.

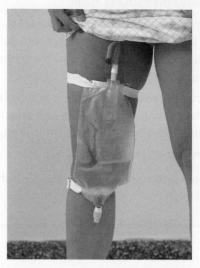

FIGURE 26-27 The leg bag is held in place by adjustable straps. The bag is smaller than a bed collection bag and must be emptied more often. (© Delmar/Cengage Learning)

PROCEDURE

DISCONNECTING THE URINARY CATHETER

1. Carry out initial procedure actions.

2. Assemble equipment:
   - Disposable gloves
   - Antiseptic wipes
   - Gauze sponges
   - Sterile caps/plugs
   - Clamps

3. Wash your hands and put on gloves.

4. Clamp the catheter. Open packages, if needed.

5. Disconnect the catheter and drainage tubing. Hold the ends to prevent them from touching anything. If accidental contamination occurs, wipe the ends with antiseptic wipes before inserting the plug or placing the cap. Dispose of used antiseptic wipes in a plastic bag.

6. Insert a sterile plug in the end of the catheter. Place a sterile cap over the exposed end of the drainage tube (Figure 26-28).

PROCEDURE 68 CONTINUED

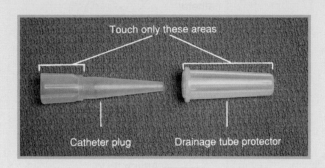

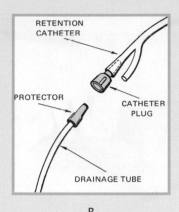

A   B

FIGURE 26-28 A. Sterile catheter plug and protective cap. B. Plug and protective cap in place. *(© Delmar/Cengage Learning)*

7. Secure the drainage tube to the bed frame so that the tube will not touch the floor.

8. Remove and dispose of gloves according to facility policy. Wash your hands.

9. Carry out ending procedure actions.

Note: Reverse the procedure to reconnect the catheter. If you find an unprotected, disconnected tube in the bed or on the floor, *do not reconnect it. Report it at once.*

PROCEDURE

69

APPLYING A CONDOM FOR URINARY DRAINAGE

1. Carry out initial procedure actions.

2. Assemble equipment:

- Disposable gloves
- Basin of warm water
- Washcloth
- Towel
- Condom with drainage tip
- Bed protector
- Bath blanket
- Towel

3. Arrange equipment on the overbed table.

4. Raise the bed to a comfortable working height. Be sure the opposite side rail is up and secure for safety.

5. Lower the side rail on the side where you will be working.

6. Cover the patient with a bath blanket and fanfold bedding to the foot of the bed.

7. Wash your hands and put on gloves.

8. Place a bed protector under the patient's hips.

9. Adjust the bath blanket to expose the genitals only.

10. Carefully wash and dry the penis. Observe for signs of irritation. Check to see if the condom has a "ready stick" surface.

11. Place the condom at the top of the penis and roll toward the base of the penis. Leave an inch between the tip and the end of the penis (Figure 26-29). If the patient is not circumcised, be sure that the foreskin is in normal position.

12. Spiral-wrap the tape provided to secure it to the penis (Figure 26-30).

continues

PROCEDURE 69 CONTINUED

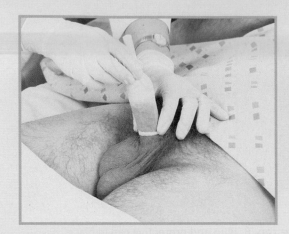

FIGURE 26-29 Leave room between the glans penis and the drainage tip on the condom to prevent irritation and allow sufficient space for drainage. Roll the condom down to the base of the penis.
(© Delmar/Cengage Learning)

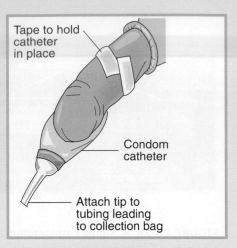

FIGURE 26-30 Correctly applied and secured condom catheter ready to be attached to the drainage tubing.
(© Delmar/Cengage Learning)

13. Connect the condom to the collection bag.

14. Remove your gloves and discard them according to facility policy.

15. Wash your hands.

16. Adjust bedding and remove the bath blanket. Fold the bath blanket and store it in the room, or place it in the laundry hamper.

17. Lower the bed. Adjust the side rails for safety.

18. Carry out ending procedure actions.

19. To change the catheter, remove the adhesive strip and roll the condom back over the tip of the penis. Discard it in a plastic bag.

  a. Observe the skin on the penis for redness, irritation, swelling, and open areas. If noted, inform the nurse before applying a new condom catheter.

  b. After a catheter has been removed, it is not reapplied. A new catheter is used each time.

  c. Provide perineal care before applying another external catheter.

PROCEDURE

70

CONNECTING A CATHETER TO A LEG BAG

 Note: Always check with the care plan or nurse before using a leg bag.

1. Carry out initial procedure actions.

2. Assemble equipment:
   • Disposable gloves
   • Antiseptic wipes

• Leg bag and tubing
• Emesis basin
• Bed protector
• Sterile cap/plug
• Clamp

3. Wash your hands and put on gloves.

PROCEDURE 70 CONTINUED

4. Place a bed protector under the connection between the catheter and the drainage tube.

5. Clamp the catheter.

6. Disconnect the catheter and drainage tubing. Hold the ends to prevent them from touching anything.

7. Insert a sterile plug in the end of the catheter. Place a sterile cap over the exposed end of the drainage tube.

 Note: If accidental contamination occurs, wipe the area with antiseptic wipes before inserting a sterile plug or replacing a sterile cap over the exposed end of the drainage tubing. Discard used antiseptic wipes in a plastic bag.

8. Secure the drainage tube to the bed frame.

9. Remove the catheter plug.

10. Insert the end of the leg bag tubing into the catheter (Figure 26-31).

11. Release the catheter clamp.

12. Secure the leg bag to the leg. Avoid tension on the tubing. There must be a straight drop from the catheter to the drainage bag. Check for leakage.

13. Remove the bed protector and discard it.

14. Remove your gloves and discard them according to facility policy. Wash your hands.

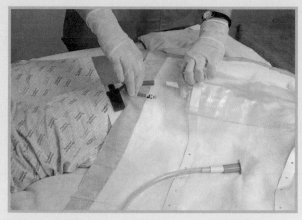

FIGURE 26-31 Carefully connect the catheter to the leg bag. Avoid touching anything against the end of the catheter. The drainage tubing on the bed bag is covered with a sterile cap that is left in place until it is reconnected to the catheter. *(© Delmar/Cengage Learning)*

15. Assist the patient to get out of bed, if needed. The leg bag and bed drainage bag are disinfected or discarded in the biohazardous waste container, according to facility policy.

16. Carry out ending procedure actions.

Note: To reconnect the regular drainage bag, reverse this procedure.

PROCEDURE

71

EMPTYING A LEG BAG

1. Carry out initial procedure actions.

2. Assemble equipment:
   - Disposable gloves
   - Antiseptic wipes
   - Emesis basin
   - Graduate pitcher
   - Paper towels

3. Position the patient safely.

4. Wash your hands and put on gloves.

5. Release the straps holding the leg bag and move the bag away from the leg.

6. Place a paper towel on the floor under the drainage outlet.

7. Place a graduate on the paper towel.

8. Remove the cap on the distal end, being careful not to touch the tip. Drain the collected urine into the graduate. Do not put the cap down and do

continues

PROCEDURE 71 CONTINUED

not touch the inside of the cap. If accidental contamination occurs, wipe with antiseptic wipes before replacing the cap. Discard used wipes in a plastic bag.

9. Wipe the drainage outlet with an antiseptic wipe and replace the cap.

10. Refasten the straps to secure the drainage bag to the leg.

11. Make sure the patient is comfortable and safe.

12. Discard the paper towel.

13. Measure the urine and note the amount, if required.

14. Discard the urine. Clean and store the graduate.

15. Remove your gloves and discard them according to facility policy.

16. Carry out ending procedure actions.

ABDOMINAL DRAINAGE

People with some conditions must use a catheter all the time. Some wear a device called an abdominal urine bag ("belly bag," Figure 26-32) at home. The bag is changed every three to four weeks during home use. If a person is admitted with an abdominal bag, it may be left in place unless the physician orders another drainage system.

The abdominal drainage bag has a soft backing and may be worn 24 hours a day. It is worn at the waist, under the clothing, and is held in place with a belt. A valve prevents backflow of urine into the bladder. Empty the bag by twisting the drainage tube. Consult the nurse before using any substitute bag that you are not familiar with. Become familiar with the instructions for the bags used in your facility.

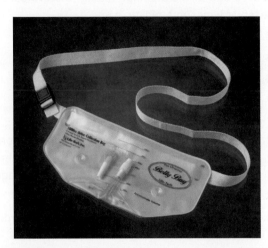

FIGURE 26-32 The disposable abdominal drainage bag is removed and a new bag applied after 3 to 4 weeks of home use. Users of this bag say it is superior to other types of drainage systems. *(Courtesy of Medline Industries, Inc., (800) MEDLINE)*

REVIEW

A. Multiple Choice

Select the one best answer for each of the following.

1. The urinary system
   a. is an extension of the endocrine system.
   b. filters solid waste from the body.
   c. manages blood chemistry.
   d. regulates blood sugar and potassium.

2. The purpose of straining (filtering) urine is to
   a. identify signs and symptoms of infection.
   b. detect kidney or bladder stones.
   c. ensure that wastes are removed.
   d. monitor the urine concentration.

3. A major factor contributing to renal failure in elderly persons is
   a. edema.
   b. dehydration.
   c. tachycardia.
   d. sodium in the diet.

4. Renal failure
   a. can occur in persons of any age.
   b. always develops slowly.
   c. is always reversible.
   d. affects only the urinary system.

5. The inside of the closed urinary drainage system is
   a. clean.
   b. soiled.
   c. contaminated.
   d. sterile.

6. Aging changes to the urinary system include
   a. urine production increases gradually.
   b. kidney function increases at night.
   c. the prostate gland shrinks.
   d. the bladder stretches.

7. A belly bag
   a. is used only with a condom catheter.
   b. always increases the risk of infection.
   c. must be changed daily.
   d. may be worn 24 hours a day.

8. Before urine withdrawal, the port of a closed urinary drainage system should be cleaned with
   a. soap and water.
   b. a paper towel.
   c. an alcohol pad. ✓
   d. a sterile 4 × 4 gauze pad.

9. A suprapubic catheter is inserted through the
   a. urethra.
   b. abdomen.
   c. ureter.
   d. kidney.

10. The average person excretes
    a. 20 to 40 mL urine per hour.
    b. 30 to 60 mL urine per hour.
    c. 50 to 80 mL urine per hour.
    d. 80 to 110 mL urine per hour.

     30-60

11. Signs and symptoms to report when a patient has a urinary disorder include
    a. hunger.
    b. thirst.
    c. temperature elevation.
    d. voiding every 3 to 4 hours.

12. Indwelling catheter care is
    a. a licensed nurse responsibility.
    b. performed during AM care.
    c. safely omitted when the patient is in bed.
    d. performed twice a week.

B. Nursing Assistant Challenge

Mr. Starkman is 68 years of age. An external urinary condom is to be applied. Answer the following regarding his care while the condom is being applied.

13. You should wear gloves to apply the condom.
    yes
    (yes) (no)

14. The condom should be applied by _____ of the penis.
    (pulling it up toward the tip) (rolling it down toward the base)

15. When applying the condom, you should _____ space between the drainage tip and the glans of the penis.
    (leave) (not leave) avoid irritation

Gastrointestinal Elimination

OBJECTIVES

After completing this unit, you will be able to:

- Spell and define terms.
- Describe aging changes of the gastrointestinal system.
- Describe some common disorders of the gastrointestinal system.
- Describe nursing assistant actions related to the care of patients with disorders of the gastrointestinal system.
- List signs and symptoms the nursing assistant should observe for and report.

- Demonstrate the following procedures:
- Procedure 72 Collecting a Stool Specimen
- Procedure 73 Testing Stool for Occult Blood
- Procedure 74 Giving a Soap-Solution Enema
- Procedure 75 Giving a Commercially Prepared Enema
- Procedure 76 Inserting a Rectal Suppository
- Procedure 77 Giving Routine Stoma Care

VOCABULARY

Learn the meaning and the correct spelling of the following words and phrases:

abdominal distention	constipation	hernia	suppository
appliance	diarrhea	ileostomy	ulcer
bile	diverticulitis	ostomy	ulcerative colitis
cholecystectomy	enema	peristalsis	urgency
cholecystitis	fecal impaction	rectal prolapse	
cholelithiasis	fecal material	stoma	
colostomy	flatus	stool	

INTRODUCTION

The digestive tract extends from the mouth to the anus. It receives the help of the teeth, tongue, salivary glands, liver, gallbladder, and pancreas in breaking food into simpler substances. The body uses these substances as a source of nutrition and eliminates unused portions as waste.

CHANGES IN DIGESTIVE SYSTEM FUNCTION ASSOCIATED WITH AGING AND DISEASE

Changes in digestive system function may be caused by aging, disease, surgery, diet, and medications. Lack of privacy may also affect the patient's ability to have a

Clinical Information ALERT

The average U.S. resident eats more than 50 tons of food in his or her lifetime. Food remains in the stomach (where digestion begins) for about 3 to 4 hours. The stomach can stretch to 50 times its empty size and holds about a gallon (4 liters). A healthy person releases 3.5 oz. of gas in a single emission, or about 17 oz. (about a pint) each day. Most gas comes from swallowed air and fermentation of undigested food. ■

Constipation.

bowel movement. When people age, the colon slows down, causing slower food absorption and elimination. Aging changes in the digestive system include:

- Taste buds are lost, beginning with sweet and salt. This helps explain why some elderly persons put a great deal of sugar and salt on their food. To a younger person with intact taste buds, the amount used may seem excessive.
- Saliva production in the mouth decreases, interfering with digestion of starch, causing problems with swallowing, and increasing the potential for tooth decay.
- The gag reflex in the throat is less effective, increasing the risk of choking.
- Movement of food into the stomach through the esophagus is slower.
- The stomach takes longer to empty into the small intestine, so food remains there longer.
- Fewer digestive enzymes are present in the stomach, causing indigestion and slower absorption of fat.
- Movement of the food mass through the large intestine is slower, resulting in constipation.

Other factors affecting bowel function are:

- Bedrest
- Inactivity
- Inadequate exercise
- Inability to chew foods properly
- Loose or missing teeth
- Inadequate fluid intake
- Stress
- Change in environment
- Change in diet
- A diet that does not contain enough fiber, fruits, or vegetables

REPORTING OBSERVATIONS RELATED TO BOWEL ELIMINATION

You will observe the amount, color, odor, character, and consistency of the patient's bowel movement. Save the stool for the nurse to assess if these observations are abnormal, or if there is blood, mucus, parasites, or food particles (except corn and raisins) in the stool. Other signs and symptoms of gastrointestinal problems are listed in Table 27-1.

TABLE 27-1 SIGNS AND SYMPTOMS OF GASTROINTESTINAL DISORDERS THAT SHOULD BE REPORTED TO THE NURSE IMMEDIATELY

- Sores or ulcers inside the mouth
- Difficulty chewing or swallowing food
- Unusual or abnormal appearance of feces
- Blood, mucus, parasites, or other unusual substances in stool
- Unusual color of feces
- Hard stool, difficulty passing stool
- Dry or pasty looking stool
- Extremely small or extremely large stool
- Loose, watery stool
- Complaints of pain, constipation, diarrhea, bleeding
- Frequent belching
- Changes in appetite
- Excessive thirst
- Fruity smell to breath
- Complaints of indigestion
- Excessive gas (flatus)
- Nausea, vomiting
- Choking
- Abdominal pain
- Abdominal distention (swelling)
- Oral or rectal bleeding
- Vomitus, stool, or drainage from a nasogastric tube that looks like coffee grounds

COMMON CONDITIONS OF THE GASTROINTESTINAL SYSTEM

The tube-like mucous membrane structure of the digestive canal is prone to many medical problems. An **ulcer** (sore or tissue breakdown) can occur anywhere along the digestive tract. Common places are the:

- Colon—**ulcerative colitis**. In colitis, malnutrition and dehydration are brought about by loss of fluids

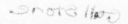

in frequent, watery, foul-smelling stools containing mucus and pus.

* Stomach—gastric ulcer.
* Duodenum—duodenal ulcer.

Patients with gastric or duodenal ulcers have periodic burning pain about 2 hours after eating. Most patients improve when they are placed on a diet in which foods that cause distress are not served. Medications are given to neutralize the acids in the stomach, and to decrease anxiety. Some ulcers respond to antibiotic treatment.

Gastroesophageal Reflux Disease

Gastroesophageal reflux disease (GERD) is a backflow of stomach contents into the esophagus. This condition commonly described as having "heartburn," which is painful and irritating. Over time, the acids in the stomach cause erosion of the walls of the esophagus. Everyone has occasional heartburn. People with GERD have this problem much of the time. Treatment involves elevating the head of the bed, modifying one's lifestyle, and eliminating irritating food and beverages. For some people, sleeping on the side is also effective.

Hernias

A **hernia** results when a structure such as the intestine pushes through a weakened area in a normally restraining wall. The danger of such abnormal protrusions is that some of the protruding tissue can become trapped in the weakened area. Circulation then becomes limited so that the tissue is in danger of dying. Hernias are usually repaired surgically.

Frequent sites of herniation are:

* Groin area (inguinal hernia)
* Near the umbilicus (umbilical hernia)
* Through a poorly healed incision (incisional hernia)
* Through the diaphragm (hiatal hernia)

Gallbladder Conditions

Two common conditions affecting the gallbladder are:

* Cholecystitis—an inflammation of the gallbladder.
* Cholelithiasis—the formation of stones in the gallbladder. The stones may obstruct the flow of **bile** (fluid that aids digestion), giving rise to signs and symptoms such as:
  - Indigestion
  - Pain

- Jaundice (yellow discoloration of the skin and whites of the eyes)

Cholecystitis and cholelithiasis may be treated by:

* Low-fat diet.
* Surgery to remove the gallbladder and stones. This surgical procedure is called a **cholecystectomy**.
* Laser therapy to break up the stones.

Drains are often placed in the operative areas. Initially, large amounts of yellowish-green drainage may be expected. In addition to routine postoperative care:

* Position the patient in a semi-Fowler's position
* Do not disturb drains
* If you notice fresh blood on the dressing, increased jaundice, or dark urine, report it immediately to the nurse

PROBLEMS RELATED TO THE LOWER BOWEL

The frequency of bowel elimination varies with the individual. Some people have more than one bowel movement (BM) a day, but others have a BM every two or three days. **Fecal material** (solid body waste, bowel movement, BM, **stool**) is normally brown, but the color can be affected by certain foods, medications, and diseases. If stool passes through the colon too slowly, the fecal material becomes hard, dry, or sticky and pasty in consistency. This is referred to as **constipation**. Certain foods, medications, infections, and diseases can cause constipation and diarrhea.

Gas forms as foods move through the gastrointestinal tract by **peristalsis**. "Passing flatus" or flatulence are medical terms for expelling gas. Gas accumulates in the intestine if it is not passed, causing the abdomen to appear large and bloated. This is called **abdominal distention**, and is an important observation to report to the nurse. Abdominal distention may also be caused by some medical conditions, constipation, and urinary retention.

Fecal Impaction

Inform the nurse if a patient complains of constipation, has not had a bowel movement in more than three days, strains, or passes hard, marble-like stools. **Fecal impaction** (Figure 27-1) is the most serious form of constipation. It is caused by retention of stool in the rectum, where water is absorbed. Over time, the stool becomes hard and dry. The patient cannot pass it. The dried waste irritates the bowel. Mucus dissolves the hard, outer part of the mass. The rectum becomes so

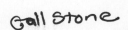
Gall Stone

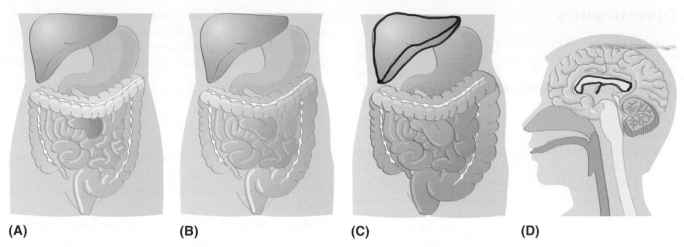

(A)   **(B)**   **(C)**   **(D)**

FIGURE 27-1 Progression of a fecal impaction, a life-threatening condition: A. A fecal impaction blocks the rectum. The rectum and sigmoid colon become enlarged. B. The colon continues to enlarge. C. Fecal material fills the colon. Digested and undigested food back up into the small intestines and stomach. The patient has signs and symptoms of acute illness, including lethargy, distention, constipation, and dull, cramping pain. D. The entire system is full, and the patient vomits fecal material. The feces are commonly aspirated into the lungs. (© Delmar/Cengage Learning)

full that fluid escapes around the impaction and is eliminated from the rectum as diarrhea. The patient may complain of:

- Abdominal or rectal pain
- Nausea
- Loss of appetite
- Feeling the need to have a bowel movement, but being unable to do so
- Bladder leakage as a result of pressure from stool in the rectum

Other signs and symptoms of impaction are passing excessive flatus, abdominal distention, frequent urination with inability to empty the bladder, and leaking around the catheter. The patient may be mentally confused, have a fever, and pass liquid stool that is often mistaken for diarrhea.

Fecal impaction is a very serious condition that is treated by manual removal of the mass by the nurse. Laxatives and enemas may also be used. Observe patients' bowel elimination closely, and document according to facility policy. Alert the nurse if a patient has not had a BM for three days.

Diarrhea

The bowel movement is normally soft and formed. If it passes through the colon too quickly, it is loose and watery when it is expelled. Multiple watery stools is called **diarrhea**. When this occurs, the need to defecate is urgent. The person may expel stool involuntarily because the pressure is very strong. He or she

may also experience flatulence, abdominal pain, and cramping.

Diarrhea can cause dehydration and other serious problems if untreated. Most facilities have a standard definition of diarrhea, such as having three or more loose stools within a defined period of time. One loose stool is not diarrhea. When reporting loose stools to the nurse, be objective. Report the color, odor, consistency, character, amount, and frequency of stools. Also report patient complaints of pain or other discomfort.

Infection Control ALERT

C. difficile (see Unit 12) finds its way to workers' hands when they touch feces or contaminated surfaces. This pathogen and its spores can survive under fingernails, in skin folds, and on jewelry. *C. difficile* is then spread to the worker and patients by direct and indirect contact. Workers' hands may pick up and leave the pathogen in bathrooms, and on faucets, countertops, door handles, clean linen, side rails, call buttons, and toilets. Remember not to use alcohol-based hand cleaner if the patient has infectious diarrhea suspected of being caused by a pathogen such as *C. difficile* that is spread by spores. ■

Diverticulitis

Diverticulitis is an inflammation of small sacs protruding from the wall of the colon. This causes stagnation of fecal material, fever, chills, nausea, vomiting, pain, bloating, and sometimes bleeding. The patient may experience constipation or diarrhea. The condition may result in bowel obstruction or perforation. Treatment involves avoiding problem foods and making lifestyle modifications. Many patients respond to antibiotics. Some patients are placed on a liquid diet to give the bowel a rest. The diet is increased gradually, and the patient is encouraged to eat foods that are high in fiber. The patient should avoid junk food, corn, nuts, and highly processed food. Drinking plenty of water will also help ensure that the stool stays soft and passes quickly.

Bowel Incontinence

Bowel incontinence is involuntary passage of feces from the anus. It is not as common as urinary incontinence. It has many causes, including trauma, neurological diseases, and inability to reach the toilet on time. Fecal material is very irritating, and causes skin breakdown. Cleanse the patient promptly after each incontinence. Be professional, compassionate, and understanding when assisting with bowel elimination and incontinence. Patients with bowel incontinence may be placed on a bowel retraining or incontinence management program.

Prolapsed Rectum

The rectum is securely attached to the pelvis with muscles and ligaments. The attachment holds the rectum firmly in place. Problems associated with age, childbirth, large hemorrhoids, and chronic constipation can cause these muscles and ligaments to loosen, stretch, and weaken over time. The attachment of the rectum to the body also becomes weaker. When this occurs, the rectum may *prolapse*, or fall out of place, so it protrudes from the anus. A **rectal prolapse** is the condition that occurs when a large portion of the rectum protrudes from the body. In the early stages, the rectum may intermittently protrude and retract, but over time the rectum will protrude permanently. Inform the nurse promptly if a section of intestine protrudes from the anus.

Reducing the need to strain during bowel movements is a preventive and corrective treatment for rectal prolapse. High-fiber foods, stool softeners, suppositories, and enemas may be ordered for elimination. Surgery is often necessary to reattach and secure the rectum. The nursing assistant should:

- Give suppositories and enemas as ordered
- Encourage intake of high-fiber foods
- Encourage fluid intake
- Inform the nurse if the patient has large hemorrhoids, loose stools, constipation, or rectal pain, or strains to have a bowel movement.

ASSISTING WITH BOWEL ELIMINATION

Always apply the principles of standard precautions when assisting with elimination. Avoid contaminating environmental surfaces with your gloves. If an adult must wear a protective garment to contain incontinence, avoid calling the garment a "diaper," which is an offensive, demeaning term. Use another term, such as brief, adult brief, or clothing protector, or call the garment by the product name, such as Depends®.

Clinical Information ALERT

Moisture from urinary and fecal incontinence increases the risk of friction and shearing on the skin. Continued exposure to moisture weakens the skin and reduces its protective function. Enzymes that normally break down food during digestion pass through the digestive system in feces. They also break down the skin during prolonged exposure to stool. Studies have shown that fecal incontinence is a contributing factor to more than half of all pressure ulcers in the torso and buttock area. ■

Communication HIGHLIGHT

Bowel activity is a normal body function. Be tactful and do not show disgust in your facial expressions when assisting with elimination. Accurate documentation is essential. The nurse depends on your documentation to identify and treat problems related to bowel elimination. ■

GUIDELINES *for*
Assisting Patients with Bowel Elimination

- Apply the principles of standard precautions.
- Encourage patients to consume an adequate amount of fluid. Fluid intake is as important for bowel elimination as it is for urinary elimination.
- Encourage patients to eat a well-balanced diet.
- Encourage patients to chew food well. Cut it into small pieces if necessary.
- If you observe that a patient has not eaten fiber foods, fruits, or vegetables, offer a substitute. The dietitian may visit the patient to discuss likes and dislikes and ensure that the patient will eat the foods served.
- Assist with exercise and activity, as allowed and tolerated.
- Assist patients with regular toileting; provide privacy and allow adequate time for elimination.

- Place patients in a sitting position, if allowed, for bowel elimination.
- Use a bath blanket to cover a patient who is using the bedpan or commode, for dignity, modesty, privacy, and warmth.
- Leave the call signal and toilet tissue within reach and respond to the call signal immediately.
- Provide perineal care as needed.
- Assist patients with handwashing after elimination.
- Monitor bowel elimination.
- Record bowel movements on the flow sheet and report irregularities. If a patient is independent, ask each day if she has had a bowel movement.

SPECIAL DIAGNOSTIC TESTS USING STOOL SPECIMENS

A *stool specimen* is a sample of fecal material collected in a special container. The specimen is sent to the laboratory for examination.

Occult Blood

Occult blood is a small amount of blood in the stool that is not visible to the eye because the color of the stool disguises it. Special chemicals will identify the presence of occult blood.

PROCEDURE

72

COLLECTING A STOOL SPECIMEN

1. Carry out initial procedure actions.
2. Assemble equipment:
   - Disposable gloves
   - Bedpan and cover or collection container
   - Specimen container and cover
   - Biohazard specimen transport bag
   - Completed label
   - Toilet tissue
   - Tongue depressors
   - Basin
3. Wash your hands and apply gloves.
4. Uncover the container that was used to collect the bowel movement (bedpan, commode receptacle, or toilet insert). If the patient is

incontinent of feces, use tongue depressors to obtain a specimen from bed linens, the adult brief, or protective padding.

5. Assist the patient with handwashing, if needed.
6. Take the container to the bathroom. Use tongue blades to remove a teaspoon from each part of the specimen and place it in a specimen container (Figure 27-2). Do not contaminate the outside of the container or the cover.
7. Empty the collection container into the toilet, then clean or discard the container. If the patient was incontinent, dispose of the soiled brief or padding as biohazardous waste.
8. Remove and discard gloves according to facility policy.

continues

PROCEDURE 72 CONTINUED

9. Wash your hands.

10. Cover the specimen container tightly and attach the completed label. Place the container in a biohazard transport bag.

11. Take or send the specimen to the laboratory promptly.

12. Carry out ending procedure actions.

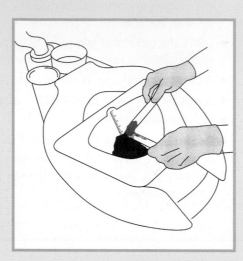
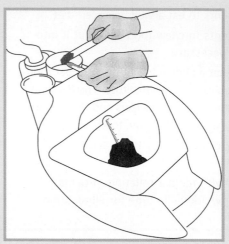

FIGURE 27-2 Use tongue blades to transfer the specimen from the collection device to the specimen cup. (© Delmar/Cengage Learning)

30 – 60 seconds

PROCEDURE 73

TESTING STOOL FOR OCCULT BLOOD

1. Wash your hands and assemble equipment:

   - Disposable gloves
   - Bedpan with fresh specimen
   - Hemoccult® slide packet with developer
   - Tongue blade
   - Paper towel

2. Place the paper towel on a flat surface and open the flap of the Hemoccult® packet, exposing the guaiac paper.

3. Put on gloves.

4. Using a tongue blade, take a small sample of feces and smear it on the paper area marked *A* (Figure 27-3A).

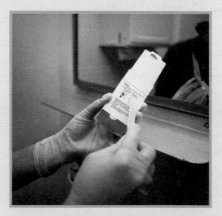

FIGURE 27-3A A small stool specimen is placed on a special area of the card for an occult blood test. (© Delmar/Cengage Learning)

PROCEDURE **73** CONTINUED

5. Repeat the procedure, taking the fecal sample from a different part of the specimen and making a smear in area *B*.

6. Close the tab and turn the packet over.

7. Open the back tab.

8. Apply two drops of Hemoccult® developer directly over each smear (Figure 27-3B). Time the reaction.

9. Read the results 30 to 60 seconds later.

10. A blue discoloration around the perimeter indicates that blood is present.

11. Dispose of the specimen.

12. Clean the bedpan and dispose of the paper towel, packet, and tongue blade in the biohazardous waste.

13. Remove and dispose of gloves. Wash your hands.

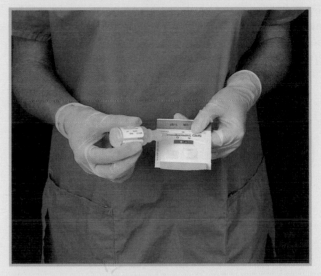

FIGURE 27-3B Apply drops of Hemoccult® developer on the exposed guaiac paper. (© *Delmar/Cengage Learning*)

ENEMAS

A cleansing **enema** is the introduction of fluid into the rectum to remove feces and **flatus** (gas) from the colon and rectum. (Refer to Procedures 74 and 75.)

The enema fluid creates a feeling of urgency in the patient's bowel. **Urgency is the term used to describe the need to empty the bowel.** Solutions are expelled a short time after they are given.

*before bath
before breakfast*

GUIDELINES *for*
Giving Enemas

- Apply the principles of standard precautions. Avoid contaminating the environment with your gloves.

- Administer an enema only upon the direction of a licensed nurse.

- If the patient is to get up to expel the enema, make sure the bathroom will be available before giving the enema.

- Give the enema before the patient's bath or before breakfast, if possible.

- Do not give an enema within an hour following a meal.

- Consult the care plan or the nurse for the amount and type of solution to use, and any special instructions.

Position

The best position for the patient to receive an enema is in the left Sims' position (Figure 27-4). Fluid flows into the bowel more easily when the patient is in this position. The enema may have to be administered with the patient on the bedpan in the supine position with knees flexed and separated, if necessary. Avoid administering an enema to a patient in a sitting position, such as on the toilet. The solution will not flow high into the colon if the patient is seated. It will force the rectum to enlarge, causing rapid expulsion of the fluid.

Disposable Enema Units

Disposable enema sets are usually used. The units are simple to use and save time.

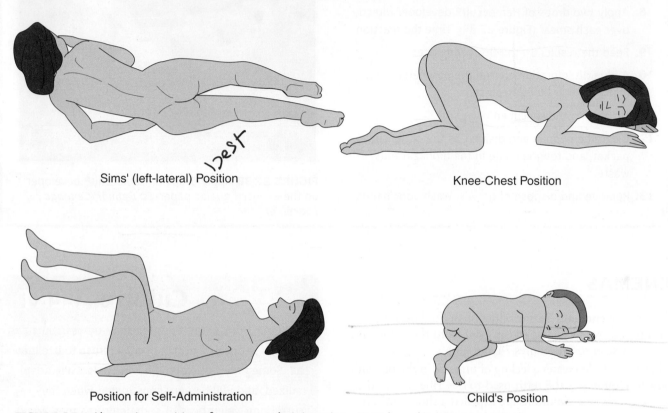

Sims' (left-lateral) Position

Knee-Chest Position

Position for Self-Administration

Child's Position

FIGURE 27-4 Alternative positions for enema administration. (© Delmar/Cengage Learning)

PROCEDURE

74

GIVING A SOAP-SOLUTION ENEMA

1. Carry out initial procedure actions.

2. Assemble equipment:

   • Disposable gloves

   • Disposable enema equipment, consisting of a plastic container, tubing with rectal tube, clamp, and lubricant (equipment is commercially available as a kit)

   • Bedpan and cover

   • Bed protector

   • Toilet tissue

   • Bath blanket

   • Castile soap packet

   • Towel, soap, basin

PROCEDURE 74 CONTINUED

3. In the utility room:

    a. Connect the tubing to the solution container (Figure 27-5A).

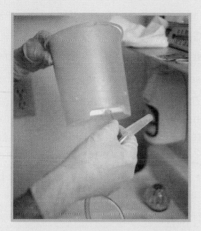

FIGURE 27-5A Attach the tubing to the container. *(© Delmar/Cengage Learning)*

    b. Adjust the clamp on the tubing and snap it shut (Figure 27-5B).

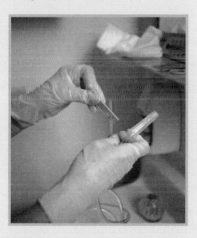

FIGURE 27-5B Slip the clamp over the tubing. *(© Delmar/Cengage Learning)*

    c. Fill the container with warm water (105°F) to the 1,000-mL line (500 mL for children) (Figures 27-5C and 27-5D).

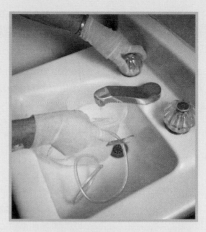

FIGURE 27-5C Fill the container with warm water. *(© Delmar/Cengage Learning)*

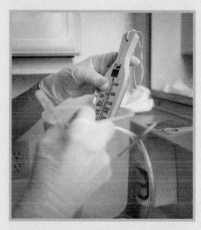

FIGURE 27-5D Use a bath thermometer to make sure the temperature is about 105°F. *(© Delmar/Cengage Learning)*

    d. Open the packet of liquid soap and put the soap in the water (Figure 27-5E).

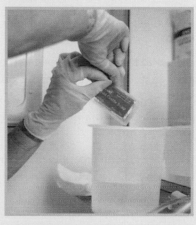

FIGURE 27-5E Add soap from the packet. *(© Delmar/Cengage Learning)*

continues

PROCEDURE 74 CONTINUED

e. Using the tip of the tubing, stir the solution or rotate the bag to mix the soap. (Mix gently and avoid shaking to prevent suds from forming.)

f. Run a small amount of solution through the tube to eliminate air and warm the tube (Figure 27-5F). Clamp the tubing (Figure 27-5G).

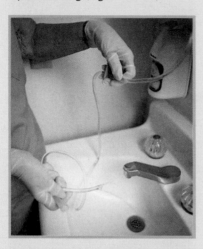

FIGURE 27-5F Run a small amount of water through the tubing to expel air. (© Delmar/Cengage Learning)

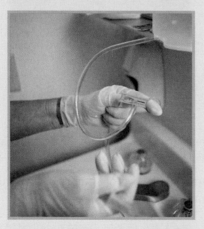

FIGURE 27-5G Clamp the tubing. (© Delmar/Cengage Learning)

4. Place a chair at the foot of the bed and cover it with a bed protector. Place the bedpan on it.

5. Elevate the bed to a comfortable working height. Be sure the opposite side rail is up and secure for safety.

6. Cover the patient with a bath blanket and fanfold linen to the foot of the bed.

7. Wash your hands and put on gloves.

8. Place a bed protector under the patient's buttocks.

9. Help the patient turn on the left side and flex the knees.

10. Place the container of solution on the chair so the tubing will reach the patient.

11. Adjust the bath blanket to expose the anal area.

12. Expose the anus by raising the upper buttock.

13. Lubricate the tip of the tube. The patient should breathe deeply and bear down as the tube is inserted, to relax the anal sphincter. Insert the tube 2 to 4 inches into the anus.

14. Never force the tube. If the tube cannot be inserted easily, get help. There may be a tumor or a mass of feces blocking the bowel.

15. Open the clamp and raise the container 12 inches above the level of the anus so that the fluid flows in slowly (Figure 27-5H).

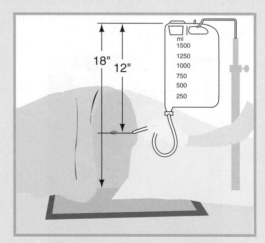

FIGURE 27-5H Raise the container above the anus so the flow of fluid is unobstructed. (© Delmar/Cengage Learning)

• Ask the patient to take deep breaths to relax the abdomen.

• If the patient complains of cramping, clamp the tube and wait until the cramping stops. Then open the tubing to continue the fluid flow.

16. Clamp the tubing before the container is completely empty.

17. Tell the patient to hold his breath while the upper buttock is raised and the tube is gently withdrawn.

PROCEDURE 74 CONTINUED

18. Wrap the tubing in a paper towel. Put it in the disposable container.

19. Instruct the patient to hold the solution for 20 minutes, or as long as possible. Place the call signal within reach. Return promptly when the person signals.

    OR

    Place the patient on a bedpan or assist him to the bathroom so he can expel the enema immediately.

20. Remove one or both gloves to avoid contamination. Use an ungloved hand to raise the head of the bed to a comfortable height if the patient is on the bedpan. Raise the side rail for safety if needed.

21. Provide privacy. Place the signal cord near the patient's hand, but check on the patient every 5 minutes. If the patient is in the bathroom, stay nearby. Caution the patient not to flush the toilet.

22. Discard disposable materials in the biohazardous waste.

23. Remove and discard your gloves. Wash your hands.

24. Return promptly when the patient signals. Put on fresh gloves.

25. Remove the bedpan. Place it on a bed protector on the chair and cover it.

26. Assist the patient with hygiene if necessary.

27. Remove the bed protector and discard according to facility policy.

28. Remove your gloves and wash your hands.

29. Replace the top bedding and remove the bath blanket.

30. Put on gloves. Take the bedpan to the bathroom. Dispose of contents or, using a paper towel, flush the toilet.

31. Remove and discard gloves.

32. Wash your hands.

33. Air the room and leave the room in order.

34. Unscreen the unit.

35. Clean and replace all other equipment used.

36. Carry out ending procedure actions.

Giving a Commercially Prepared Enema

Commercially prepared enemas are convenient to administer and more comfortable for the patient. The enema may be either an oil-retention enema or a phosphate enema and may be followed by a cleansing (soap-solution) enema.

- The solution is pre-measured and ready to use.
- The phosphosoda enema draws fluid from the body to stimulate peristalsis. This causes water to be drawn into the lower bowel, making the stool softer and easier to pass than a large, hard, constipated stool.
- The oil-retention enema solution lubricates and softens the feces, making them easier to expel.
- The enema contains 4 ounces of solution. A small amount will remain in the container when you have finished.
- The tip of the container is prelubricated.

PROCEDURE

GIVING A COMMERCIALLY PREPARED ENEMA

 Note: Be sure this is a nursing assistant procedure in your facility.

 Note: Use this procedure when giving an oil-retention or a phosphosoda enema.

1. Carry out initial procedure actions.

2. Assemble equipment:
   - Disposable gloves
   - Disposable prepackaged enema

continues

PROCEDURE 75 CONTINUED

- Bedpan and cover
- Bed protector

3. Open the package and remove the enema solution. Follow the nurse's instructions for warming the solution container in warm water.

4. Lower the head of the bed to a horizontal position and elevate the bed to a comfortable working height. Raise the side rail on the opposite side of the bed for safety.

5. Put on gloves.

6. Place a bedpan and cover on the chair close at hand.

7. Cover the patient with a bath blanket and fanfold linen to the foot of the bed.

8. Place a bed protector under the patient.

9. Assist the patient to turn to the left side and flex the right leg.

10. Expose only the patient's buttocks by drawing the bedding upward in one hand.

11. Remove the cover from the enema tip (Figure 27-6). Gently squeeze to make sure the tip is patent (open).

12. Separate the buttocks, exposing the anus, and ask the patient to breathe deeply and bear down slightly.

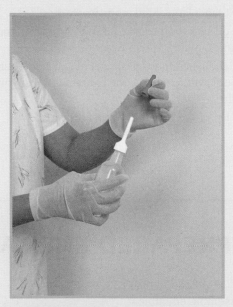

FIGURE 27-6 Remove the cover from the prelubricated tip of the container. *(© Delmar/Cengage Learning)*

13. Insert the lubricated enema tip 2 inches into the rectum.

14. Gently squeeze and roll the container until the solution is administered (Figure 27-7). A small amount will remain in the container. Avoid releasing pressure on the container, or the solution will return.

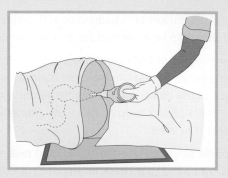

FIGURE 27-7 Squeeze the bottle from the bottom. A small amount of fluid will remain in the container. *(© Delmar/Cengage Learning)*

15. Remove the tip from the patient and place the container in the box. Encourage the patient to hold the solution for 20 minutes or as long as possible.

16. Remove gloves. Wash your hands. Discard the gloves and enema container in the biohazard waste.

17. Provide privacy. Give the patient the call signal and toilet tissue. Leave the room.

18. Return promptly when the person signals. When the patient feels the urge to defecate, lower the bed and assist to the bathroom or commode, or position on the bedpan.

19. Raise the head of the bed to a comfortable height if the patient is using a bedpan.

20. Place the signal cord near the patient's hand, but check on the person every 5 minutes. Raise the side rail for safety if the bed is left in high position. If the patient is in the bathroom, stay nearby. Caution the patient not to flush the toilet.

21. Return promptly when the patient signals. Wash your hands. Lower the nearest side rail, if it is up. Put on gloves.

22. Remove the bedpan and place it on the bed protector covering the chair. Observe the contents, then cover the bedpan.

PROCEDURE 75 CONTINUED

23. Assist the person with hygiene if necessary.

24. If the patient has used a commode or toilet:

  a. Clean the anal area, if required.

  b. Observe the contents of the commode or toilet.

  c. Flush the toilet using a paper towel, or cover the commode.

  d. Remove your gloves and discard them according to facility policy. Assist the patient into bed.

25. Put on gloves. Take the bedpan or commode container and equipment to the bathroom. Dispose of contents.

26. Remove and dispose of gloves properly. Wash your hands.

27. Return equipment. Leave the side rails down, unless needed for safety, and leave the bed in low position.

28. Carry out ending procedure actions.

GUIDELINES *for*

Inserting a Rectal Tube and Flatus Bag

The rectal tube is used to relieve flatus (gas) in the bowel. Inserting the tube provides a passageway for the gas to escape. Assist the patient as follows.

- Accept the expulsion of gas as a natural body function. Do not contribute to the patient's embarrassment.

- Use flatus-reducing procedures when ordered.

- Insert a rectal tube with flatus bag if ordered. (Be certain that you are permitted to do this in your facility.) The tube may be used once in a 24-hour period for no more than 20 minutes.

- Check the amount of abdominal distention (stretching).

- Relief may occur as soon as the tube is inserted.

- Question the patient about the degree of relief.

RECTAL SUPPOSITORIES

Rectal **suppositories** are used to stimulate bowel evacuation or to administer medication. Medicinal suppositories must be inserted by the nurse. You may be asked to insert the type of suppository that softens stool and promotes elimination. (See Procedure 76.) Be sure this is a nursing assistant function. The suppository must be placed beyond the rectal sphincter (circular muscle that controls the anal opening) and against the bowel wall so it can melt and lubricate the rectum.

PROCEDURE

76

INSERTING A RECTAL SUPPOSITORY

 Note: Be sure this is a nursing assistant procedure in your facility.

1. Carry out initial procedure actions.

2. Assemble equipment:

- Disposable gloves
- Suppository as ordered

- Toilet tissue
- Bedpan and cover, if needed
- Lubricant
- Bed protector

3. Cover the patient with a bath blanket and fanfold linen to the foot of the bed.

continues

PROCEDURE 76 CONTINUED

4. Wash your hands and put on gloves.

5. Place a bed protector under the patient's hips.

6. Help the patient turn on the left side and flex the right leg.

7. Unwrap the suppository.

8. Expose only the patient's buttocks by drawing the bedding upward in one hand.

9. With your left hand, separate the patient's buttocks, exposing the anus.

10. Apply a small amount of lubricant to the anus and suppository. Gently insert the suppository about 2 inches beyond the anal sphincter (Figure 27-8).

11. Encourage the patient to take deep breaths and relax (until the need to defecate is felt in 5 to 20 minutes).

12. Remove your gloves and discard them properly. Wash your hands.

13. Adjust the bedding and help the patient to assume a comfortable position.

14. Place the signal cord near the patient's hand, but check on the patient every 5 minutes. Return promptly when the patient signals.

15. Wash your hands and put on gloves.

16. Assist the patient to the bathroom or commode, or position the patient on a bedpan.

17. Provide privacy. Once the patient is finished, assist with hygiene if necessary.

18. Observe results and note any unusual characteristics of the stool. If stool is abnormal, save it and inform the nurse.

19. Discard the stool, clean equipment, and store reusable items.

20. Remove and discard gloves. Wash your hands.

21. Carry out ending procedure actions.

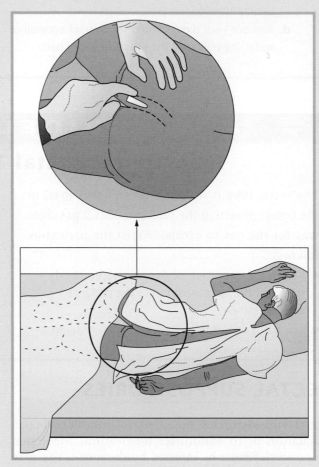

FIGURE 27-8 Lubricate the anus and insert the suppository beyond the sphincter muscle.
(© Delmar/Cengage Learning)

OSTOMIES

The surgical removal of a section of diseased bowel requires the creation of an artificial opening (**ostomy**) in the abdominal wall for elimination of solid waste and flatus.

Care of the Patient Who Has a Colostomy

When the colon is brought through the abdominal wall, the opening is called a **colostomy**. The mouth of the opening is called a **stoma** (Figure 27-9). The ostomy may

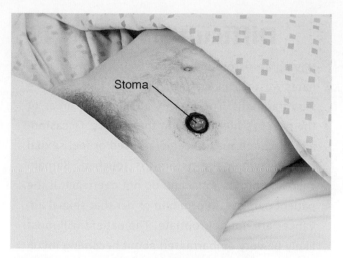

FIGURE 27-9 Typical colostomy stoma. (© Delmar/Cengage Learning)

be temporary or permanent. The location of the ostomy (Figure 27-10) determines if the feces are formed, soft and mushy, semiliquid, or liquid.

The person with a colostomy does not have normal sphincter control, and cannot voluntarily control bowel emptying. If the colostomy is located in the part of the bowel where stool is formed, regular elimination may be established. Liquid to mushy fecal drainage from a stoma is collected in a disposable drainage pouch, called an **appliance**, that is attached over the stoma. (Refer to Procedure 77.) Proper stoma care is required to maintain healthy tissue, because the area around the opening comes into contact with liquid or semiliquid stool. A person with a stoma may have problems with leakage, odor control, and skin irritation. Keep the area clean and dry, and provide stoma care when needed.

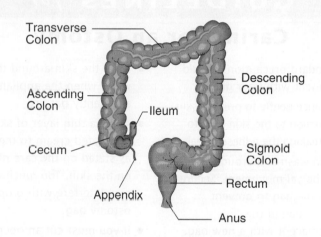

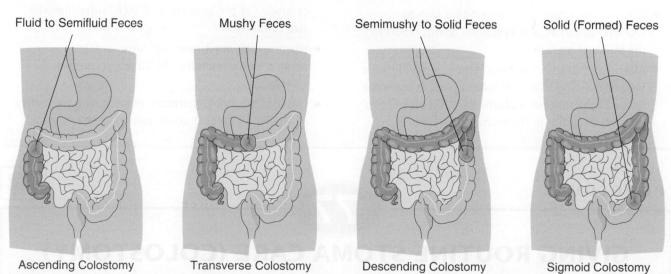

FIGURE 27-10 The location of the ostomy determines the character of the feces. (© Delmar/Cengage Learning)

Difficult SITUATIONS

The two-piece system has an outer ring that snaps onto the pouch. An improper fit can injure the stoma. The ring must not fit so tightly that it squeezes the stoma. Read the directions and make sure you understand how to use the type of device you have. ■

Difficult SITUATIONS

Having an ostomy alters the way a patient eliminates waste. This alteration of body image can be very traumatic. The ostomy affects many areas of the patient's life, including the sex life. Occasionally, a patient may become aroused or feel sexual pleasure when the ostomy is touched. Remain calm and professional and do not overreact. If the patient persists, inform him or her that sexual advances are not appropriate. The patient will most likely be very embarrassed about becoming involuntarily sexually aroused. ■

GUIDELINES *for*
Caring for an Ostomy

- Apply the principles of standard precautions. Avoid contaminating the environment with your gloves.
- Remove and apply the appliance gently to prevent skin irritation. Applying gentle traction to the skin next to the appliance is helpful in breaking the adhesive seal.
- Empty the reusable bag and wash it thoroughly with soap and water after each bowel movement. Secure the clamp at the bottom of the bag to prevent leaking. Discard a disposable bag in the biohazardous waste and replace it with a new bag.
- Observe the stoma and surrounding skin for redness, irritation, and skin breakdown; report to the nurse, if present.
- After the appliance has been removed, gently wipe the surrounding skin with toilet tissue. Discard the tissue in the toilet or a plastic bag. If a plastic bag is used, discard it in the biohazardous waste.

- Wash the skin around the stoma with mild soap and water when the appliance is removed. Rinse well and gently pat dry.
- Apply a thin layer of skin barrier, lubricant, or medicated cream to the area surrounding the stoma as stated on the care plan. Avoid caking products on the skin. Too much of any skin care product may interfere with proper sealing of the fresh ostomy bag.
- If you must cut an opening into the appliance, carefully cut the area about ⅛ inch larger than the size of the stoma.
- When reapplying a new appliance, seal the entire area surrounding the stoma, to prevent leaking.
- Observe the color, character, amount, and frequency of stools, and report abnormalities to the nurse.

PROCEDURE

GIVING ROUTINE STOMA CARE (COLOSTOMY)

1. Carry out initial procedure actions.
2. Assemble equipment:
   - Disposable gloves
   - Washcloth and towel
   - Basin of warm water
   - Bed protectors

PROCEDURE 77 CONTINUED

- Bath blanket
- Disposable colostomy bag and belt
- Bedpan
- Skin lotion as directed
- Prescribed solvent and dropper
- Cleansing agent
- Adhesive wafer
- 4 × 4 gauze square
- Toilet tissue
- Plastic bag

3. Cover the patient with a bath blanket. Fanfold the top bedding to the foot of the bed.

4. Wash your hands and put on gloves.

5. Place a bed protector under the patient's hips.

6. Place a bedpan and cover on a bed protector on the chair.

7. Remove the soiled disposable stoma bag (appliance) and place it in the bedpan or a plastic bag—note the amount and type of drainage.

8. Remove the belt that holds the stoma bag and save it, if clean.

9. Gently clean the area around the stoma with toilet tissue to remove feces and drainage (Figure 27-11A). Dispose of used tissue in the bedpan or plastic bag.

10. Gently wash the area around the stoma with soap and water. Rinse thoroughly and pat dry.

11. If ordered, apply barrier cream lightly around the stoma.

12. Position a clean belt around the patient. Inspect the skin under the belt for signs of irritation.

13. If it was necessary to remove the adhesive wafer, use the guide to stoma size to select the proper replacement wafer size (Figure 27-11B).

14. Replace the adhesive wafer (Figure 27-11C). Apply a clean ostomy bag over the stoma and secure the belt.

15. Remove and discard the bed protector. Check to be sure the bottom bedding is not wet. Change it if necessary.

16. Remove your gloves and discard them according to facility policy. Wash your hands.

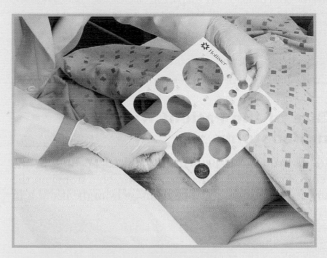

FIGURE 27-11B Check the stoma size to make sure the correct size barrier is used. (© Delmar/Cengage Learning)

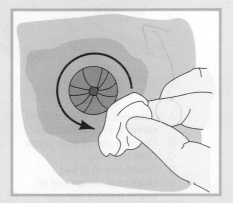

FIGURE 27-11A The area around the stoma is cleansed gently, then dried before a new appliance is applied. (© Delmar/Cengage Learning)

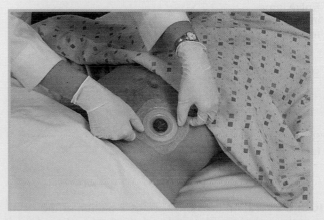

FIGURE 27-11C Apply a new barrier adhesive wafer around the stoma. (© Delmar/Cengage Learning)

continues

PROCEDURE 77 CONTINUED

17. Replace the bath blanket with the top bedding, and make the patient comfortable. Assist with hygiene if necessary.

18. Using a paper towel to protect your hands, gather and cover the soiled materials and bedpan

or plastic bag. Take them to the utility room and discard them in the biohazardous waste.

19. Empty, wash, dry, and store the bedpan.

20. Carry out ending procedure actions.

Difficult SITUATIONS

Most ostomy appliances are odor-free. If odor control is a problem, consult the nurse. Commercial products are available to eliminate odors in the bag. Leave a small amount of air in the bag when changing it, to allow stool to fall to the bottom. ■

liquid form and contains digestive enzymes that are irritating to the skin. Excellent skin care is necessary.

The licensed nurse cares for the patient with a new ileostomy. Routine care may be given by nursing assistants. It is important that the ring fit the stoma well, so that leakage does not occur. This is true for both the disposable and reusable types of appliances (Figure 27-13). The procedure for caring for a person with an ileostomy is in the Online Companion to this book.

Care of the Patient Who Has an Ileostomy

An **ileostomy** is a permanent artificial opening in the ileum (Figure 27-12) that drains through a stoma on the surface of the abdomen. The drainage from the ileum is in

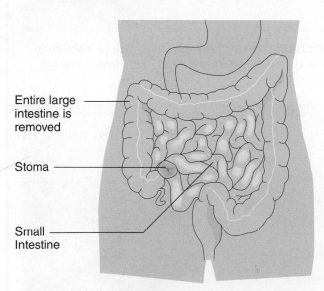

Entire large intestine is removed

Stoma

Small Intestine

FIGURE 27-12 An ileostomy brings a section of the ileum through the abdominal wall. (© Delmar/Cengage Learning)

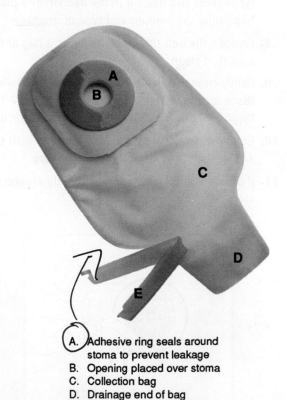

A. Adhesive ring seals around stoma to prevent leakage
B. Opening placed over stoma
C. Collection bag
D. Drainage end of bag
E. Secures drainage end of bag to prevent leakage

FIGURE 27-13 Stoma protector and collection bag. (Courtesy of Hollister, Inc., Libertyville, Illinois.)

REVIEW

A. Multiple Choice

Select the one best answer for each of the following.

1. Enemas are given
   a. after the patient showers.
   b. at bedtime.
   c. before diagnostic testing. *(circled)*
   d. after surgery.

2. The oil-retention enema is usually
   a. preceded by a soap-solution enema.
   b. retained for 1 hour.
   c. followed by a soap-solution enema. *(circled)*
   d. given in the semi-Fowler's position.

3. Urgency is a term that means
   a. inability to have a BM.
   b. need to eliminate. *(circled)*
   c. pain from flatus.
   d. need to vomit.

4. Diarrhea is defined as
   a. one watery, loose stool.
   b. 6 or more loose stools.
   c. 10 or more loose stools.
   d. multiple, watery stools. *(circled)*

5. Occult blood is
   a. easily seen in the patient's stools.
   b. hidden blood that you cannot see. *(circled)*
   c. always black, tarry, and pasty.
   d. seen only when a person vomits.

6. The reaction time for a Hemoccult® test is
   a. 2 to 4 seconds.
   b. 30 to 60 seconds. *(circled)* ✓
   c. 2 to 3 minutes.
   d. 90 to 120 seconds.

7. During routine care, the area around a colostomy should
   a. be cleaned with an alcohol sponge. *(crossed out)*
   b. be covered with petroleum jelly.
   c. be washed with soap and water. *(circled)*
   d. be cleaned with an antiseptic.

8. An aging change in the digestive system results in
   a. a decrease in the amount of formed stool in the bowel movement.
   b. slower movement of food through the large intestine, resulting in constipation. *(circled)*

   c. an increase in digestive enzymes, causing irritable bowel and other uncomfortable conditions.
   d. faster movement of food through the large intestine, resulting in diarrhea.

9. You are giving routine stoma care to a patient with a colostomy and find the area surrounding the stoma red and irritated. You should
   a. complete the procedure.
   b. clean the area with alcohol.
   c. apply powder and attach the ostomy bag.
   d. cover the area and notify the nurse. *(circled)*

10. Fecal impaction
    a. is the most serious form of constipation. *(circled)*
    b. results from rapid movement of stool.
    c. is a complication of persistent diarrhea.
    d. has no identifiable signs and symptoms.

11. When giving a soap-suds enema,
    a. position the patient in the sitting position.
    b. insert the tubing 2 to 4 inches into the rectum. *(circled)*
    c. the water temperature should be 90°F.
    d. put the soap in the enema container first.

12. A rectal tube may be inserted
    a. every 2 hours.
    b. whenever necessary. *(circled)*
    c. once every 24 hours.
    d. 3 times daily.

B. Nursing Assistant Challenge

Mrs. Knight, who is 60 years old, was in an accident and received a broken right leg and two broken wrists. She has a long-standing colostomy, but because of her injuries cannot provide her own colostomy care. Answer the following questions about her care.

13. Will you need to wear gloves to give her colostomy care? *yes*

14. What will you use to remove feces from around the stoma? *toilet paper — soap/water*

15. What will happen if you apply lotion around the stoma? *It's not going to stick*

16. How will the ostomy bag be held in place? *adhesive*

17. What are the three major problems associated with having a stoma?
    inflammation
    discomfort

UNIT 28

Nutritional Needs and Diet Modifications

OBJECTIVES

After completing this unit, you will be able to:

- Spell and define terms.
- Define normal nutrition.
- List the essential nutrients.
- Name the six groups listed on the food pyramid.
- Identify the basic facility diets and describe each.
- State the purpose of calorie counts and food intake studies.

- Describe general care for the patient with dysphagia and swallowing problems.
- List types of alternative nutrition.
- Demonstrate the following procedures:
  - Procedure 78 Serving Meal Trays
  - Procedure 79 Feeding the Dependent Patient

VOCABULARY

Learn the meaning and the correct spelling of the following words and phrases:

amino acids	essential nutrients	minerals	protein
carbohydrates	fats	nasogastric (NG) feeding	pureed diet
cellulose	full liquid diet	nourishments	soft diet
central venous catheter (CVC)	gastrostomy feeding	nutrients	supplement
	hyperalimentation	nutrition	therapeutic diets
clear liquid diet	intravenous infusion (IV)	percutaneous endoscopic gastrostomy (PEG)	total parenteral nutrition (TPN)
digestion	jejunostomy tube (J-tube)		
dysphagia	mechanical soft	peripheral intravenous central catheter (PICC)	vitamins
enteral feeding	mechanically altered		

INTRODUCTION

Nutrition is the process by which the body takes in food for growth and repair and uses it to maintain health.

NORMAL NUTRITION

The mouth is the beginning of the digestive tract. **Digestion** is the process of breaking down foods into simple substances that can be used by body cells for nourishment. These substances are called **essential nutrients**.

Essential Nutrients

To be well nourished, we must eat foods that:

- Supply heat and energy
- Build and repair body tissues
- Regulate body functions

These foods are called **nutrients**. The six nutrients essential to health are protein, carbohydrates, fats, vitamins, minerals, and water.

Protein Protein is an essential nutrient that is present in every body cell. It is the only nutrient that can make new cells and rebuild tissue. Proteins are made of small building blocks called **amino acids**. The body can manufacture some of the amino acids, but not all of them.

Carbohydrates and fats **Carbohydrates** and **fats** are called "energy foods" because the body uses them to produce heat and energy. When a person eats more energy foods than the body needs, the remainder is stored as fat. Foods that contain the greatest amount of carbohydrates come from plants (Figure 28 1). Carbohydrates also supply the body with fiber or roughage (**cellulose**), which is important to bowel regularity.

Vitamins and minerals Vitamins regulate body processes. They help promote growth and strengthen resistance to disease. Fat-soluble vitamins do not dissolve easily in water. They can be stored in the body. Vitamins A, D, E, and K are fat-soluble vitamins. Vitamins B and C are water soluble. They dissolve in water, and are lost during cooking. These substances are not stored in large amounts in the body, so deficiencies in water-soluble vitamins are more common.

Minerals help to build body tissues, especially the bones and teeth. They also regulate the chemistry of body fluids such as the blood and digestive juices. Minerals needed in the daily diet include:

- Calcium
- Copper
- Iodine
- Iron
- Phosphorus
- Potassium

Vitamins and minerals are present, in varying amounts, in many different foods. The best way to be sure that you are getting enough vitamins and minerals is to include a wide variety of foods in your daily diet.

Water Water is an essential nutrient that is necessary to life. A person can live only a few days without water.

The Food Groups and the USDA Food Guide Pyramid

The U.S. Department of Agriculture (USDA) studies nutrition and issues guidelines for balanced food intake. Figure 28-2 shows the USDA Food Guide Pyramid. The food pyramid is designed to be individualized by each person to maintain a healthy weight. The food pyramid contains 12 intake levels, ranging from 1,000 calories per day to 3,200 calories per day. To determine your personal pyramid recommendations, visit http://www.mypyramid.gov.

The food categories listed in the pyramid are the:

- Grains group
- Vegetables group (Figure 28-3)
- Fruits group (Figure 28-4)
- Oils group (Figure 28-5)
- Milk group (Figure 28-6)
- Meat and beans group

Healthful fats Healthful fats, such as those found in fish, olive oil, and nuts, are permitted. The FDA advises consumers to limit sugars and saturated fats such as butter and margarine.

Discretionary calories Each person needs a certain number of calories each day for proper body function and for energy. *Essential calories* are those required to meet your nutrient needs. If you select foods that are low in fat and sugar, you may not use up your entire calorie allocation, so you would be able to take in extra calories. These are *discretionary calories.* For most people, the discretionary calorie allowance is very small (between 100 and 300 calories daily).

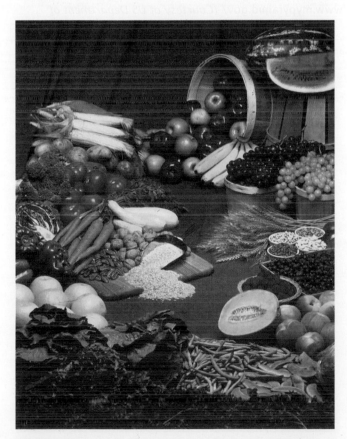

FIGURE 28-1 Fruits, vegetables, grains, and some dairy products are good sources of carbohydrates. *(Courtesy of Agricultural Research Service, USDA)*

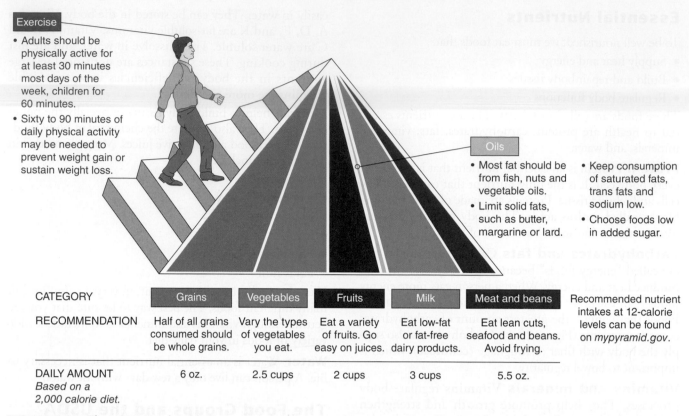

Exercise

- Adults should be physically active for at least 30 minutes most days of the week, children for 60 minutes.
- Sixty to 90 minutes of daily physical activity may be needed to prevent weight gain or sustain weight loss.

Oils

- Most fat should be from fish, nuts and vegetable oils.
- Limit solid fats, such as butter, margarine or lard.

- Keep consumption of saturated fats, trans fats and sodium low.
- Choose foods low in added sugar.

CATEGORY	Grains	Vegetables	Fruits	Milk	Meat and beans	Recommended nutrient intakes at 12-calorie levels can be found on *mypyramid.gov*.
RECOMMENDATION	Half of all grains consumed should be whole grains.	Vary the types of vegetables you eat.	Eat a variety of fruits. Go easy on juices.	Eat low-fat or fat-free dairy products.	Eat lean cuts, seafood and beans. Avoid frying.	
DAILY AMOUNT *Based on a 2,000 calorie diet.*	6 oz.	2.5 cups	2 cups	3 cups	5.5 oz.	

FIGURE 28-2 The USDA Food Guide Pyramid serves as a guide to menu planning. Each person should personalize the pyramid to meet individual needs. This may be done at http://www.mypyramid.gov/ *(Courtesy of US Department of Agriculture)*

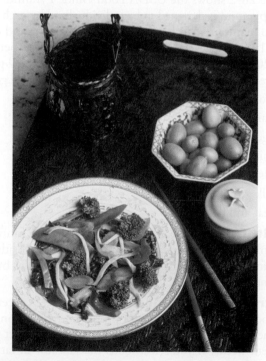

FIGURE 28-3 The traditional Chinese diet is a good source of vegetables. Chinese food has become very popular in the United States. Dishes containing many vegetables are among the most healthful of the many types of Chinese dishes. *(Stock image)*

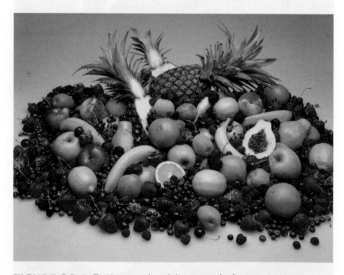

FIGURE 28-4 Fruits are healthy, good alternatives to snacks that are high in sugar. *(Stock image)*

BASIC FACILITY DIETS

The food you serve to patients will be prepared by the dietary department (Figure 28-7). It includes the essential nutrients. Sometimes very strict dietary control is needed.

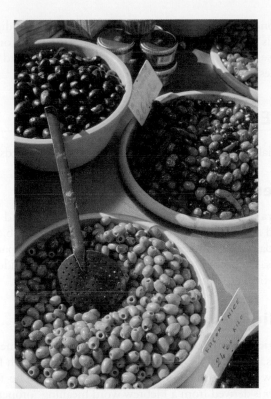

FIGURE 28-5 Mediterranean food is prepared with various types of olives and oils. *(Stock image)*

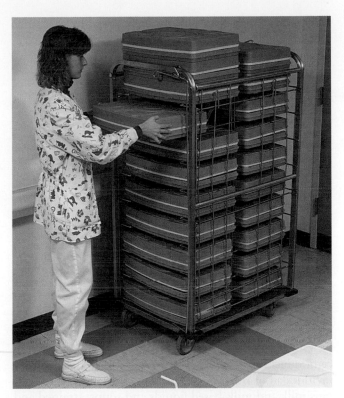

FIGURE 28-7 Patient diets are prepared in the dietary department and transported to the units in containers designed to maintain the temperature. *(© Delmar/ Cengage Learning)*

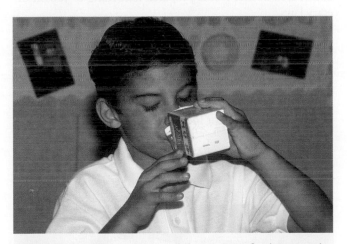

FIGURE 28-6 Milk is an excellent source of calcium and phosphorus. These minerals are essential for growth and development of bones and teeth. *(© Delmar/Cengage Learning)*

Health care facilities have many types of diets. Four common diets are:

- Regular or house, sometimes called a general diet
- Full liquid
- Clear liquid
- Soft

Patients are given a progression of diets after surgery, beginning with ice chips and sips of water. When the patient tolerates the diet at one level, he or she is advanced to the next level.

Regular Diet

The regular or house diet is a normal or general diet that is based on the food pyramid. The regular diet includes a wide variety of foods. In the hospital, the diet has a lower calorie count, because inactive patients do not require as many calories as they would at home. In many health care facilities, patients may select foods from a menu. This may be called a *selective diet.*

Liquid Diets

Clear liquid diet A **clear liquid diet** (Figure 28-8) is a temporary diet, because it consists of water and carbohydrates for energy but is inadequate for full nutrition. When a clear liquid food item is held up to the light, you can see through it. Foods that become liquid at room temperature (such as popsicles and gelatin) are also included. The liquids on this diet do not irritate, cause gas, or encourage bowel movements (*defecation*). Feedings are given every two, three, or four hours. One purpose of the diet is to replace fluids that may have been lost by vomiting or diarrhea.

Full liquid diet The **full liquid diet** supplies some nourishment. It is also considered a temporary diet because

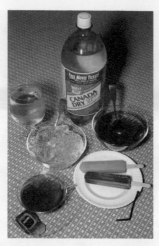

FIGURE 28-8 Items on a clear liquid diet include only liquids you can see through. (© Delmar/Cengage Learning)

it is not nutritionally complete. However, it may be used for longer periods of time than the clear liquid diet. Six to eight ounces are usually given every 2 to 3 hours. The diet includes all of the foods allowed on the clear liquid diet, plus milk and milk-based liquids and soups, strained and blenderized soups, yogurt, and ice cream.

Soft Diet

The **soft diet** usually follows the full liquid diet. This diet nourishes the body, but between-meal feedings may be given to increase the calorie count. Foods allowed on the soft diet are low in residue, unseasoned or only mildly

seasoned, and prepared in a manner that is easy to digest. Foods on this diet have a soft texture, such as cottage cheese, fish, chicken, some types of cooked fruits and vegetables, and crackers. Fried foods are not served.

SPECIAL DIETS

Special diets are planned to meet specific patient needs.

Therapeutic Diets

Therapeutic diets are planned by the dietitian and prepared according to a patient's individual health problems. Standard diets can be changed to conform to special patient needs. Commonly prescribed therapeutic diets include the diabetic diet, sodium-restricted diet, and low-fat diet.

Religious Restrictions

Religious practice requires changes in diet for some patients. For example, persons of the Orthodox Jewish faith follow strict kosher food laws (Figure 28-9). The term *kosher* is derived from a Hebrew word meaning "proper" or "pure." The kosher dietary rules apply to the type of food eaten, the kinds of foods combined in one meal, food preparation, and how an animal is killed. Any food can be considered kosher if it is prepared according to Jewish dietary laws.

- Shellfish and non-kosher meats such as pork are prohibited.
- There are strict rules regarding the sequence in which milk products and meat may be consumed.
- Certain fishes, such as tuna and salmon, are permitted.
- The utensils used for food preparation are not used for other food items.

Some other cultural and religious restrictions are summarized in Table 28-1.

Clinical Information ALERT

Hospital food is the subject of many jokes. For example, a person jokes that the food at the hospital is better than the food at a local restaurant. Hospitals receive more complaints about food than anything else. Studies have shown that up to a third of the food served each day is not touched. Many facilities are now employing gourmet chefs and providing a more diverse menu. Medical and nutritional professionals recognize that good-tasting, culturally appropriate food served at the correct temperature is well accepted by patients. Attractive presentation is also important, because "we eat with our eyes." This means that if food looks good, we are more likely to eat it. Another bonus is the cost savings realized because of reduced waste. ∎

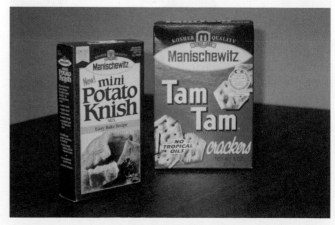

FIGURE 28-9 Persons of the Orthodox Jewish faith eat only kosher foods, which require special preparation. (© Delmar/Cengage Learning)

TABLE 28-1 CULTURAL AND RELIGIOUS DIETARY PRACTICES

					Restricted Food			
Faith	Coffee	Tea	Alcohol	Pork/Pork Products	Caffeine-Containing Foods	Dairy Products	All Meats
Christian Science	●	●	●				
Roman Catholic							1 hour before communion, Ash Wednesday, Good Friday
Latter Day Saints (Mormons)	●	●	●		●		
Seventh Day Adventist	●	●	●	●	●		●
Some Baptist	●	●	●				
Greek Orthodox (on fast days)						●	Fasting from meat and dairy products on Wed./Fri. during Lent and other holy days
Jewish Orthodox				● (also shellfish)		Certain holy days	Forbids the serving of milk and milk products with meat; regulates food preparation; forbids cooking on the Sabbath
Muslim, Islamic			●	●			Fasting during Ramadan during day, feasting at night
Hindu							Some are vegetarians
Buddhist							Meat must be blessed and killed in special ways; some sects are vegetarians

The Diabetic Diet

Proper diet is essential to the well-being of the person with diabetes mellitus. A proper diet may be all that is needed to control the disease. Usually, however, the food intake is balanced by the administration of medications (Figure 28-10). Pay close attention to the patient's food intake and appetite.

Sodium-Restricted Diet

Sodium-restricted diets may be ordered for patients with chronic kidney and heart disease. Sodium-restricted diets are some of the most difficult diets to follow. The average American consumes 2 to 6 grams of sodium in food each day. Much of the sodium comes from processed foods.

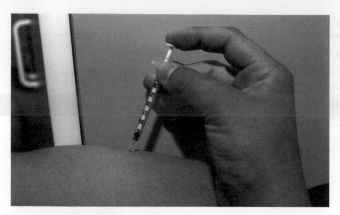

FIGURE 28-10 Many diabetics self-administer insulin injections one or more times each day for blood sugar control. Approximately 15.7 million people (5.9% of the U.S. population) have diabetes. An estimated 5.4 million people are not aware that they have the disease. Each day approximately 2,200 new cases of diabetes are diagnosed. Diabetes is a chronic disease that cannot be cured, but can be controlled through a combination of diet, exercise, and medications. The risk of complications is high if the condition is not diagnosed and medically managed. (© Delmar/Cengage Learning)

About 10 percent of dietary sodium comes from natural food content. Table salt is a major source of discretionary sodium in the diet. The National Institutes of Health (NIH) recommends that adults limit their sodium intake to 2,400 mg (about 2½ grams) per day.

The physician may order several different levels of sodium restriction. These are listed in Table 28-2, in order of most to least salt content. The order includes sodium that occurs naturally in some foods and sodium used in food preparation, as well as free salt added to foods at the table.

Clinical Information ALERT

For many years, calorie counts were used when ordering the diet for diabetic patients. The trend has moved to more relaxed diets that are better accepted and will control blood sugar without being overly restrictive. These are often called *liberal* or *liberalized* diets. For example, the "no concentrated sweets" diet restricts sources of free sugar, heavy syrups in fruit, and cakes, pies, and sweetened desserts. The *consistent-carbohydrate diabetes meal plan* does not measure calories. Instead, it focuses on maintaining a consistent carbohydrate content. The dietitian may make further adjustments for each patient to meet medical and cultural needs. ∎

TABLE 28-2 SODIUM-RESTRICTED DIETS

Type of Low-Sodium Diet	Amount of Sodium
No added salt (limited salt used in cooking, no salt added at meals)	3 to 4 grams daily
2 grams sodium	2 grams daily
1 gram sodium	1 gram daily
500-mg sodium	½ gram daily

Some foods naturally contain relatively large amounts of sodium: pork, ham, bacon, potato chips, pretzels, other similar snack foods, saltine crackers, pickles, olives, processed meats, some canned vegetables and soups, and some soda pop. These foods may be restricted for this diet.

Calorie-Restricted Diet

Calorie-restricted diets are ordered for patients who are overweight. The dietitian plans the diet to meet nutritional needs, considering the patient's energy output, overall nutrition, and weight goal.

Low-Fat/Low-Cholesterol Diet

Low-fat/low-cholesterol diets are ordered for patients with heart, blood vessel, liver, or gallbladder disease. Fats are limited and calories are balanced by increasing proteins and carbohydrates. Foods are baked, roasted, or broiled.

Mechanically Altered Diets

Any diet may be **mechanically altered**. This means that the consistency and texture are modified, making the food easier to chew and swallow. The **mechanical soft** diet (Figure 28-11) is served to patients who have no

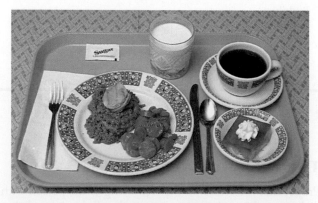

FIGURE 28-11 The mechanical soft diet is blenderized so foods are the consistency of ground beef. Soft foods, such as bread and cooked carrots, are easily chewed and so are not blended. (© Delmar/Cengage Learning)

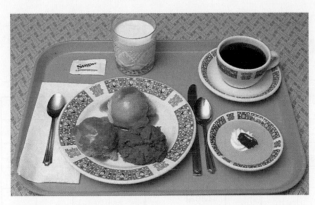

FIGURE 28-12 The pureed diet is given to patients who have difficulty swallowing. Food should have a consistency firm enough to support a plastic spoon in an upright position. Attention is given to attractive appearance so food is not runny and does not resemble baby food. *(© Delmar/Cengage Learning)*

teeth, or those with dental problems. Meats and hard foods are ground to the consistency of hamburger. Soft items, such as bread, are not ground. The **pureed diet** (Figure 28-12) is blended with gravy or liquid until it is the consistency of pudding. This diet is used for patients who have difficulty swallowing. Pureed foods should not be watery. Properly prepared food items will support a plastic spoon in the upright position.

Supplements and Nourishments

Many patients receive a nutritional **supplement** or between-meal nourishments. They are given to make up for nutritional deficiencies, but are not nutritionally complete and are not meal substitutes. They are very filling,

and should never be given with meals or immediately before mealtime. Supplements have a definite therapeutic value and meet specific medical needs. They come in a variety of flavors, and may be liquid or any easily digestible form, such as pudding. They usually taste best when served cold. Supplements are expensive and should not be wasted!

Nourishments and snacks are substantial food items given between meals to increase nutrient intake. They are planned and ordered by the facility dietitian and include foods such as milkshakes, instant breakfast, sandwiches, and pudding.

Nourishments are given between meals. Serving snacks, nourishments, and supplements is an important nursing assistant responsibility. *Snacks* may be planned and regularly given, or unplanned upon patient request.

CALORIE COUNTS AND FOOD INTAKE STUDIES

The physician or dietitian may order intake studies for patients who have special nutritional needs. The patient's intake is carefully recorded for a period of time, usually three days. The dietitian will analyze the documentation for nutritional adequacy and number of calories consumed. He or she then uses the information to plan a diet to meet the patient's medical needs. At the end of each meal, you will accurately record the patient's food intake on the form (Figure 28-13). You will also record all snacks, liquid nutritional beverages, and food items brought from home. Completing a food intake study requires a team effort, good communication, and accurate documentation.

GUIDELINES *for*

Serving Supplements, Nourishments, and Snacks

- Wash your hands.
- Check the nourishment list for each patient for any limitations or special dietary instructions.
- Check to be sure everything you need is on the unit.
- Prepare the items, if necessary. For example, some milkshakes are frozen when they are sent to the unit. They must be thawed, but are served cold, so must not be left out too long.
- Deliver items to patient rooms. Leave a napkin and straw (if needed) with each food or beverage item served.
- Allow patients to select the nourishment or flavors whenever possible.

- Open cartons, provide straws, pour liquids, and remove wrappers, as needed.
- Assist those who are unable to take their nourishment alone.
- Return to pick up used dishes and discard trash after the patients have finished.
- Assist with wiping faces and hands, if needed.
- Note the percentage that each patient consumed.
- Record intake and output (I&O) on the worksheet, if required.
- Inform the nurse if a patient expresses a preference or dislike for a certain product or flavor, or if a patient refuses a supplement.

Diet _____

CALORIE/PROTEIN SUMMARY

PATIENT _____   ROOM # _____

DAY 1					DAY 2					DAY 3				
DATE ___/___/___					DATE ___/___/___					DATE ___/___/___				
	% 0–25	% 25–50	% 50–75	% 75–100		% 0–25	% 25–50	% 50–75	% 75–100		% 0–25	% 25–50	% 50–75	% 75–100
Breakfast					**Breakfast**					**Breakfast**				
Meat					Meat					Meat				
Milk					Milk					Milk				
Fruit					Fruit					Fruit				
Starch					Starch					Starch				
Fat					Fat					Fat				
Other					Other					Other				
AM Supp.					AM Supp.					AM Supp.				
Noon Meal					**Noon Meal**					**Noon Meal**				
Meat					Meat					Meat				
Milk					Milk					Milk				
Juice					Juice					Juice				
Starch					Starch					Starch				
Vegetable					Vegetable					Vegetable				
Bread					Bread					Bread				
Fat					Fat					Fat				
Dessert					Dessert					Dessert				
Other					Other					Other				
PM Supp.					PM Supp.					PM Supp.				
Evening Meal					**Evening Meal**					**Evening Meal**				
Meat					Meat					Meat				
Milk					Milk					Milk				
Juice					Juice					Juice				
Starch					Starch					Starch				
Vegetable					Vegetable					Vegetable				
Bread					Bread					Bread				
Fat					Fat					Fat				
Dessert					Dessert					Dessert				
Other					Other					Other				
PM Supp.					PM Supp.					PM Supp.				
Total Kcal					**Total Kcal**					**Total Kcal**				
Total Pro					**Total Pro**					**Total Pro**				
Avg.for 3 days Kcal:								**Avg.Protein for 3 days:**						

PLEASE RETURN COMPLETED FORM TO NUTRITION CARE MANAGER

FIGURE 28-13 The calorie count provides an accurate picture of the patient's calorie and nutrient intake over a three-day period. The registered dietitian analyzes the information and uses it to make adjustments in the patient's diet and nutritional plan of care. *(© Delmar/Cengage Learning)*

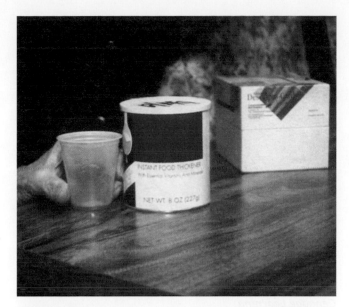

FIGURE 28-14 Food thickener is used to change the texture and consistency of liquids to prevent aspiration. (© Delmar/Cengage Learning)

DYSPHAGIA – difficult Swallow

Some patients have **dysphagia**, or difficulty swallowing food and liquids. This condition is common in patients who have had a stroke, but may also occur with other conditions, such as neurological diseases, cancer of the neck or esophagus, and dementia. People who take medications that cause sedation or reduce saliva production are also at risk of dysphagia. Patients with dysphagia are at high risk of developing malnutrition, dehydration, aspiration, and pneumonia. Consultation with a speech language pathologist and diagnostic tests for dysphagia may be necessary.

The dietitian works closely with the speech language pathologist to ensure that the patient's needs are met. Food thickeners (Figure 28-14) may be ordered to slow the movement of fluid through the esophagus. These powdered products are mixed into beverages to make swallowing easier and prevent aspiration. The care plan will specify the type and amount of thickener to use, and special exercises and approaches to use when assisting patients with meals.

PREVENTION OF FOODBORNE ILLNESS

Hot foods and beverages must be served hot and cold foods and beverages served cold. Food tastes best when it is served at the proper temperature. Imagine how a scrambled egg or cup of black coffee tastes when it is ice cold, or a popsicle or ice cream tastes when it is warm. Food acceptance is only one concern. Many of the pathogens implicated in "food poisoning" have the potential to cause serious illness and

death. Foodborne illness is often spread through the common-vehicle method of contamination (Unit 12).

Nursing personnel must ensure that patients' trays are served and dependent patients are fed when food is the proper temperature. The temperature danger zone is fairly narrow (Figure 28-15). Foods served in the danger zone are potentially hazardous and have an increased risk for pathogen growth. Hot foods must be served at 140°F or above, and cold foods must be 40°F or below. Although the food is hot when it leaves the kitchen, waiting on elevators and maneuvering in hallways is time-consuming. You may be surprised to learn that hot foods have already cooled to 140°F to 150°F by the time they are delivered to your unit. Food trays must be served promptly because the food will continue to cool quickly.

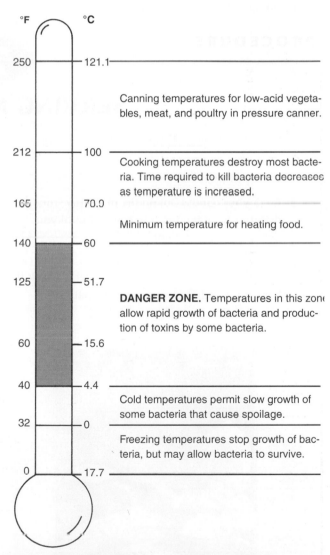

FIGURE 28-15 Temperatures of food for control of pathogens. The danger zone is very close to the average serving temperature, so the temperature of food trays must be carefully maintained. Food should be served promptly upon arrival on the unit. (© Delmar/Cengage Learning)

ASSISTING PATIENTS WITH MEALS

Eating should be an enjoyable experience. (See Procedures 78 and 79.) Prepare the patient for the meal tray before it arrives by:

- Offering the bedpan or helping the patient to the bathroom.
- Assist with repositioning, comfort, and hygiene measures, if needed.
- Raising the head of the bed, or transferring the patient into a chair, if permitted.
- Removing unpleasant sights and smells.
- Clearing the overbed table.
- Placing a towel or protector under the patient's chin (Figure 28-16). Avoid calling this item a bib, which is demeaning to adults.

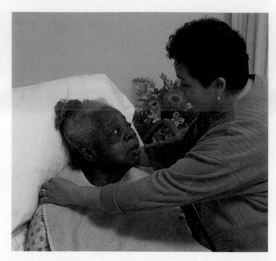

FIGURE 28-16 Place a towel or garment protector over the patient. Avoid calling this item a bib. (© Delmar/ Cengage Learning)

PROCEDURE

SERVING MEAL TRAYS

1. Carry out initial procedure actions.

2. Assemble equipment:
   - Tray of food

3. Wash your hands. Obtain the meal tray from the dietary cart. Keep the tray covered until you deliver it to the patient.

4. Check the items on the tray with the dietary card and be sure the food items are correct. Check the name on the diet card against the patient's identification band (Figure 28-17A).

5. Place the tray on the overbed table. Remove the lid on the main dish and arrange food in a convenient manner. Be sure the patient can reach the food. Avoid placing the overbed table over the top of a raised side rail. Doing this causes the food to be at shoulder height, which is difficult to cut and reach.

6. Assist with food preparation as needed (Figure 28-17B).

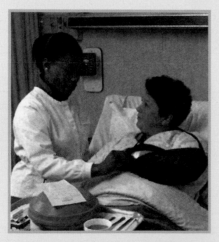

FIGURE 28-17A Check the patient's identification band against the tray card. (© Delmar/Cengage Learning)

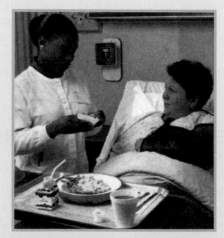

FIGURE 28-17B Assist with food preparation as needed. (© Delmar/Cengage Learning)

PROCEDURE 78 CONTINUED

7. Remove the tray as soon as the patient is finished. Note the patient's meal intake.

8. Record fluids on the I&O worksheet, if necessary.

9. Position the overbed table so it is within reach.

10. Assist the patient with repositioning, comfort, and hygiene measures, if needed.

11. Return the tray to the food cart. Do not put it in the cart if clean trays have not been served. Document the patient's food intake on the clipboard or designated area.

12. Carry out ending procedure actions.

When you have served the tray and after you have washed your hands, assist the patient as needed by:

- Opening straws, removing lids, opening prepackaged items
- Cutting meat
- Seasoning food, if the patient desires
- Pouring liquids
- Buttering bread
- Arranging the tray as if items were on the face of a clock (Figure 28-18) if the patient cannot see
- Providing food substitutes, if needed

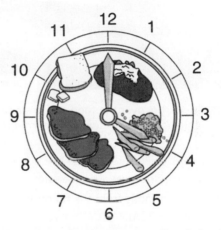

FIGURE 28-18 Describe the location of each food item compared with the positions on the face of a clock. *(© Delmar/Cengage Learning)*

PROCEDURE

OBRA DVD

FEEDING THE DEPENDENT PATIENT

1. Carry out initial procedure actions.

2. Assemble equipment:
   - Tray of food

3. Prepare the patient for the meal, as noted in Procedure 78.

4. Wash your hands. Obtain the meal tray from the dietary cart. Keep the tray covered until you deliver it to the patient.

5. Check the diet with the dietary card and be sure the diet is correct. Check the name on the diet card against the patient's identification band.

6. Place the tray on the overbed table (Figure 28-19).

7. Remove lids and wrappers, butter bread, and cut meat. Season the food, if the patient desires. Do not pour a hot beverage until the patient is ready for it.

8. Open straws and provide one for each liquid, or use a cup. Thick fluids are more easily controlled by using a straw. Use adaptive devices as indicated on the care plan.

9. Sit down so you are at the patient's eye level.

continues

PROCEDURE 79 CONTINUED

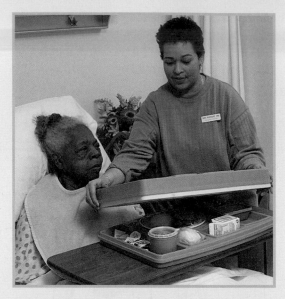

FIGURE 28-19 Uncover the food and arrange it on the overbed table. (© Delmar/Cengage Learning)

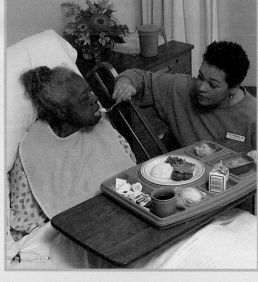

FIGURE 28-20A Give solid foods from the tip of the spoon. (© Delmar/Cengage Learning)

10. Holding the spoon at a right angle:
    - Give solid foods from the tip of the spoon (Figure 28-20A).
    - Alternate solids and liquids.
    - Inform or show the patient what kind of food you are giving.
    - Ask the patient in what order she would like the food.
    - If the patient has had a stroke, direct food to the unaffected side. Monitor the cheek on the affected side to be sure no food residue remains. Monitor the patient's ability to swallow.
    - Test hot food temperatures by dropping a small amount on the inside of your wrist (Figure 28-20B).
    - If the food is too hot, let it sit for a few minutes to cool. Never blow on the patient's food to cool it.
    - Never taste the patient's food.
    - Avoid making the patient feel rushed.
11. Allow the patient to assist to the extent that she is able.
12. Use a napkin to wipe the patient's mouth as often as necessary.

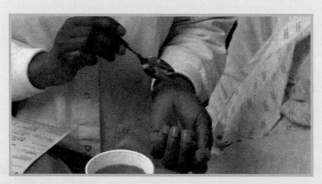

FIGURE 28-20B Check the temperature of food and beverages by placing a drop on your wrist or forearm. (© Delmar/Cengage Learning)

13. Remove the tray as soon as the patient is finished. Note the patient's meal intake.
14. Record fluids on the I&O worksheet, if necessary.
15. Push the overbed table out of the way.
16. Assist the patient with repositioning, comfort, and hygiene measures, if needed.
17. Return the tray to the food cart. Do not put it in the cart if clean trays have not been served. Document the patient's food intake on the clipboard or other designated area.
18. Carry out ending procedure actions.

Mealtime Assistance for Patients Who Have Swallowing Problems

In general:

- Position the patient as upright as possible.
- The head should face forward, with the neck flexed forward slightly.
- Reduce distractions during the meal.
- Limit conversation. The patient should focus on eating and avoid talking.

Prompt or feed the patient slowly, offering small bites. Remind the patient to chew the food well.

Mealtime Assistance for Patients Who Have Swallowing Problems

The speech therapist will recommend techniques for safety and preventing aspiration. He or she may order special positions and exercises. The care plan will list directions, such as reminding the patient to tuck the chin in when swallowing. The chin tuck changes the position of the airway, reducing the risk of aspiration in some types of dysphagia. However, it increases the risk with other types. Dysphagia care is highly individualized and many team members work to ensure that the patient's needs are safely met. The speech therapist will work closely with staff members who feed the patient.

DOCUMENTING MEAL INTAKE

Each facility has a policy and procedure for documenting each patient's meal intake. A clipboard is commonly used to record meal intake. The clipboard is usually on top of the cart where used trays are returned. The information is later transferred to the patient's chart. Keep the documented information confidential. Cover the worksheet with a piece of paper when not in use.

Many different methods are used for documenting meal intake. In many facilities, staff calculates the percentage of each meal the patients consume. Wait until each patient has finished eating before calculating meal intake. Documenting appetite means more than eyeballing the food tray and estimating how much of the food was eaten. Instead, you must document the percentage of the significant food items on the tray. Some facilities use fractions to record the amount of the food consumed. Some write "good," "fair," or "poor." Some facilities record the percentage of each

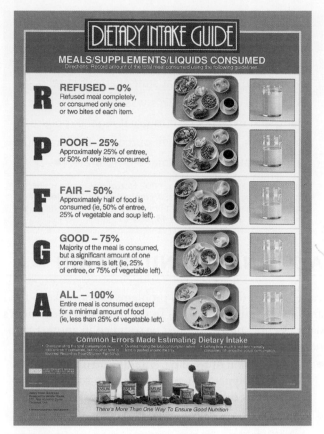

FIGURE 28-21 Accurate documentation of meal intake is an important nursing assistant responsibility. *(Photo used with permission of Ross Products Division, Abbott Laboratories, Columbus, Ohio)*

individual food item. Others estimate and document a percentage of the total meal (Figure 28-21). Inform the nurse if a patient eats less than 75% of the meal, or offer a substitute, according to facility policy. Other signs and symptoms of nutritional problems are listed in Table 28-3.

TABLE 28-3 SIGNS AND SYMPTOMS OF NUTRITIONAL PROBLEMS THAT SHOULD BE REPORTED TO THE NURSE IMMEDIATELY

- Increase or decrease in food (caloric) intake
- Increase or decrease in body weight
- Diabetic patients who do not eat all their food, or who eat more than allowed on diet
- Patients on restricted diets who do not adhere to their diet
- Refusal to accept meal, supplement, or snack
- Refusal to accept food substitute for meat or vegetable
- Meal intake of less than 50% (or 75%, according to facility policy)

ALTERNATIVE NUTRITION

Patients with some medical problems cannot take in food and fluids in the usual way. To maintain life, the patient's daily essential nutrients must be supplied in another manner. This may be done by:

- Administration of **total parenteral nutrition (TPN)** (also called **hyperalimentation**), which is a form of **intravenous infusion (IV)**, or by
- **Enteral feedings** (tubes inserted into the digestive tract).

Intravenous Therapy

Intravenous (IV) therapy refers to solutions administered directly into a vein. The IV usually consists of a single bag of solution connected to tubing with a needle or small catheter on the end. The IV tubing is usually threaded through an intravenous controller or pump that regulates the flow of solution. These devices fasten to the IV standard and operate by electricity. Most automatically switch to battery mode in the event of a power failure. Inform the nurse if the alarm on the pump sounds.

Take care to prevent dislodging the IV when you are moving the patient. The bag of IV fluid must always be above the level of the needle insertion site.

Central Venous Catheters

IV therapy can also be administered through a **central venous catheter (CVC)**. A special catheter is inserted into a vein near the patient's collar bone. The catheter tip ends in or near the heart chamber. CV therapy is used to administer medications or to provide total parenteral nutrition.

Peripheral Intravenous Central Catheter Line

A **peripheral intravenous central catheter** or **PICC** line consists of a catheter that is inserted into a peripheral vein and threaded upward through the vein to the jugular or subclavian vein. It is used to administer medications or to provide total parenteral nutrition.

Total Parenteral Nutrition

TPN is a technique in which concentrated nutrients are introduced into a large vein.

Enteral Feedings

Enteral feedings may be administered by a tube that is:

- Inserted through the nose and into the stomach (**nasogastric** or **NG feeding**) (Figure 28-22A).
- Inserted surgically through the abdominal skin and into the stomach (**gastrostomy feeding**) (Figure 28-22B). A similar surgical procedure is called a **percutaneous endoscopic gastrostomy (PEG)**. Nursing assistant care is the same for any gastric tube.

The **jejunostomy tube (J-tube)** (Figure 28-22C) is a long, small-bore tube that is threaded through the GI tract until the tip reaches the small intestine. This is a long-term feeding tube for patients who do not have a stomach, and those in whom recurrent formula aspiration is a problem.

Patients with gastric tubes are given specially prepared formula solutions containing all the nutrients required by the body. The container of solution is hung from an IV

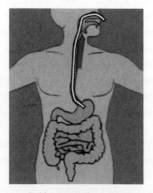
A. Nasogastric route

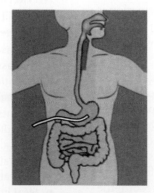
B. Gastrostomy route

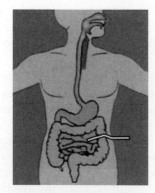
C. Jejunostomy route

FIGURE 28-22 Common methods of enteral feeding: A. nasogastric (NG) tube B. gastrostomy (G) tube C. jejunostomy (J) tube. *(© Delmar/Cengage Learning)*

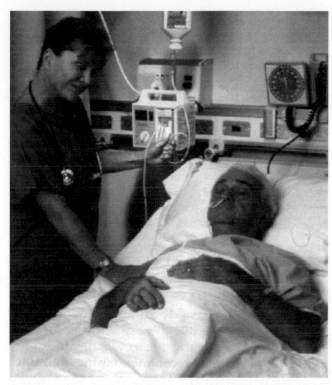

FIGURE 28-23 Enteral feedings are usually administered through a mechanical pump. *(Photo used with permission of Ross Products Division, Abbott Laboratories, Columbus, Ohio)*

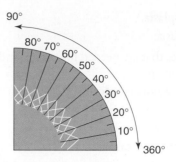

FIGURE 28-24 Elevate the head of the bed at least 30° to 45°, or as specified on the care plan, during feeding and for at least an hour after the feeding is completed. *(© Delmar/Cengage Learning)*

(intravenous) pole and is usually attached to a device that automatically controls the administration (Figure 28-23).

When caring for a person with tube feedings, you need to:

- Keep the head of the bed elevated 30° to 45° (Figure 28-24) during feeding and for 60 minutes after feeding.
- Monitor the skin on the hips and buttocks frequently, as this position increases pressure and the risk of skin breakdown.
- Check the taping of tubes. If tape is loose, pulls, or is causing skin irritation, inform the nurse.
- Report any coughing, choking, nausea, or vomiting immediately.
- Be sure the tubing is not obstructed or bent.
- Provide frequent mouth care. Patients with an NG tube will also need nasal care.

Safety ALERT

Most patients receiving tube feedings are NPO, but some are also permitted to have food or liquids orally. Verify the orders for that patient before giving food or fluids. Be sure that the head of the bed is elevated whenever the feeding is running and for at least 60 minutes after the tube feeding has finished. ■

Safety ALERT

Know the location of the tube at all times and avoid pulling on it. Serious complications can occur if a feeding tube is dislodged. ■

REVIEW

A. Multiple Choice

Select the one best answer for each of the following.

1. Feeding the patient through a nasogastric tube is known as a/an
   a. intravenous infusion.
   b. gastrostomy feeding.
   c. enteral feeding.
   d. hyperalimentation.

2. A condition that makes swallowing food and fluids difficult is
   a. dysphagia.
   b. aphasia.

c. dysplasia.

d. aplasia.

3. Calories that are needed for energy and body function are

　a. discretionary calories.

　b. calorie nutrients.

　c. essential calories.

　d. supportive calories.

4. Water is a/an

　a. vitamin.

　b. essential nutrient.

　c. mineral.

　d. discretionary calorie.

5. The diet that is most difficult for patients to adhere to is the

　a. low-sodium diet.

　b. full liquid diet.

　c. selective diet.

　d. house diet.

6. Supplemental nourishments might include

　a. hot fudge sundaes.

　b. mashed potatoes.

　c. scrambled eggs.

　d. high-protein drinks.

7. Nutritional supplements are given

　a. for a specific therapeutic purpose.

　b. when a patient refuses a meal.

　c. on request when a patient is hungry.

　d. immediately before or with a meal.

8. Mrs. Li ate approximately half of her meal tray. The nursing assistant must inform the nurse promptly if the patient is on a

　a. low-salt diet.

　b. calorie-restricted diet.

　c. diabetic diet.

　d. house diet.

Insuline

9. One nutrient is called nature's building block because of its importance to body growth and repair. This nutrient is a

　a. protein.

　b. carbohydrate.

　c. vitamin.

　d. vegetable.

10. Fats, such as those that are found in fish, olive oil, and nuts,

　a. cause narrowing of the arteries.

　b. must be limited to once a week.

　c. are in the dairy food group.

　d. are healthful and recommended.

B. Nursing Assistant Challenge

Mrs. Davenport is one of your assigned patients. She is 72 years old, is on a 1,500-calorie diabetic diet, and is a member of the Seventh Day Adventist Church. She also has Parkinson's disease with tremors of her hands, and occasionally has trouble swallowing. Mrs. Davenport sometimes eats food brought in by family and friends that is not on the 1,500-calorie diet. Consider Mrs. Davenport's care and answer the following questions.

11. Discuss safety issues that you need to think about when Mrs. Davenport is eating.　*Sugar*

12. Are there conflicts between the ordered diet and the dietary restrictions of her church? If so, what are the conflicts and how might they be resolved?

13. Do you anticipate that Mrs. Davenport will have any problems feeding herself? If so, what are those problems, and what can you do to help her eat independently?　*Tremors*

14. Discuss the issues of residents' or patients' rights that may arise because of the conflict between the patient's desire to eat more food than ordered and foods different from what the physician has prescribed.

SECTION 9

Caring for Patients with Special Needs

OBJECTIVES

After completing this unit, you will be able to:

- Spell and define terms.
- Describe the concerns of patients who are about to have surgery.
- Identify the three main components of perioperative care and list the nursing assistant responsibilities for each.
- Describe nursing assistant actions and observations related to the care of perioperative patients.
- Prepare the unit for the patient's return from the operating room.
- Give routine postoperative care.
- Recognize reportable observations of patients in the postoperative period.

- Assist the patient with deep breathing and coughing.
- Identify nursing assistant responsibilities in the care of patients with wounds and drains.
- Apply elasticized stockings and pneumatic hosiery.
- Describe the effects of heat and cold applications.
- Demonstrate the following procedures:
  - Procedure 80 Assisting the Patient to Deep Breathe and Cough
  - Procedure 81 Performing Postoperative Leg Exercises
  - Procedure 82 Applying Elasticized Stockings
  - Procedure 83 Assisting with Sequential Compression Hosiery
  - Procedure 84 Assisting the Patient to Dangle

VOCABULARY

Learn the meaning and the correct spelling of the following words and phrases:

ambulation	disruption	Montgomery straps	recovery room
anesthesia	distention	NPO	sequential compression
anti-embolism hose	drainage	operative	therapy
atelectasis	dressings	orifices	singultus
bandages	embolus	perioperative	spinal
binders	general anesthetics	postanesthesia care unit	anesthesia
constrict	generalized	(PACU)	stable
dangling	hypothermia-	postoperative	surgical bed
deep vein thrombosis	hyperthermia blanket	preoperative	TED hose
(DVT)	hypoxia	prosthesis	thrombophlebitis
dilate	local anesthetics	pulmonary embolism	

INTRODUCTION

Patients facing any surgical procedure tend to be fearful. They require emotional and physical support (Figure 29-1) from the time of admission through discharge.

Surgery is often associated with anxiety, pain, and discomfort. Before surgery, the patient is given medication to promote relaxation. During surgery, anesthetics are given to prevent pain (Figure 29-2). After surgery, medications are given to reduce discomfort.

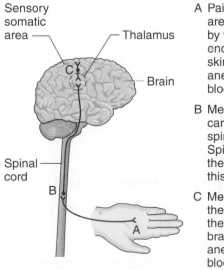

FIGURE 29-1 Patients and family members need support during the preoperative period. (© Delmar/Cengage Learning)

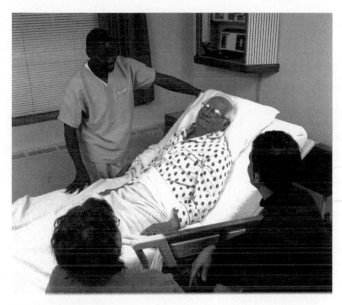

Sensory somatic area

Thalamus

Brain

Spinal cord

B

A

C

A Pain messages are picked up by free nerve endings in the skin. Local anesthetic blocks this.

B Message is carried into the spinal cord. Spinal anesthetic blocks this.

C Message is then carried to the cortex of the brain. General anesthetic blocks this.

FIGURE 29-2 Anesthetics will block pain impulses at points A, B, or C. (© Delmar/Cengage Learning)

ANESTHESIA

Anesthesia is given to prevent pain, to relax muscles, and to induce forgetfulness. **General anesthetics** cause the patient to become unconscious and block reception of pain in the brain. **Local anesthetics** induce loss of feeling in a specific area of the body. **Spinal anesthesia** is used for some surgeries. The patient will be unable to feel or move the legs after surgery. Special monitoring is required.

SURGICAL CARE

Care of the surgical patient (**perioperative**) can be divided into three parts:

- **Preoperative** (before surgery)
- **Operative** (in the operating room)
- **Postoperative** (after surgery)

Physical Preparation

The nursing assistant's responsibilities begin when the person is admitted. If the patient is in the facility the evening before surgery, part of the surgical preparation may be done then. The patient will be placed on **NPO** (nothing by mouth) orders after midnight. Remove the water pitcher from the room and post an NPO notice over the bed, on the door, on the patient's chart, and on the Kardex.

The surgical prep area You may be assigned to prepare the patient's skin before surgery. Hair removal was routine for many years. The current trend is to avoid shaving whenever possible. In many facilities, preoperative shaving requires a physician's order. Hair may be removed with clippers if it is especially thick. Studies have shown that shaved patients develop more infections than unshaved patients. You may be instructed to wash and prepare the operative area. This area will be larger than the surgical incision area (Figure 29-3).

Immediate preoperative care Approximately one hour before surgery, the nurse will give additional medication. You will be instructed to elevate the side rails. Do not let the patient get up alone after the medication is given.

Safety ALERT

All personnel involved in perioperative care must be alert to make sure that the correct surgery is done on the correct patient, on the correct site. There is no room for error in this situation! ■

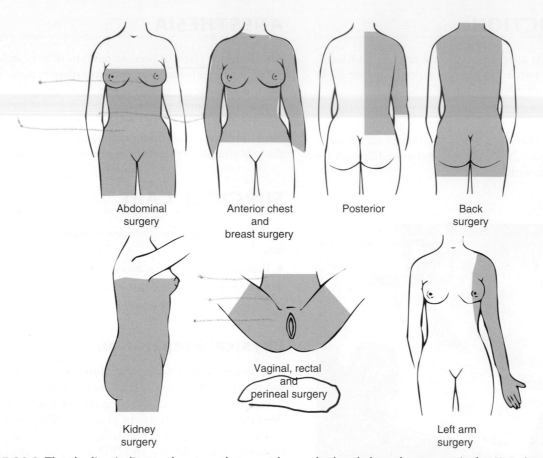

Abdominal surgery

Anterior chest and breast surgery

Posterior

Back surgery

Vaginal, rectal and perineal surgery

Kidney surgery

Left arm surgery

FIGURE 29-3 The shading indicates the areas that must be washed and shaved preoperatively. (© Delmar/Cengage Learning)

Make sure the call signal is within reach. You may be asked to:

- Take and record vital signs (Figure 29-4) (see Section 6).
- Remove dentures and any other **prosthesis** (artificial part), such as a hearing aid contact lenses, or glasses. Store these items appropriately.
- Remove nail polish, makeup, hairpins, and jewelry. You may be permitted to tape a plain wedding band in place. However, metal on the patient's body interferes with an

instrument used in some surgeries, and could result in serious burns. Check with the nurse before taping a ring.

- Dress the patient in a gown and cover the hair with a surgical cap.
- Assist the patient to void and measure the urine, if ordered. Drain the catheter, if present, and record.
- Keep the room quiet and comfortable.
- Move furnishings to one side to make room for a stretcher.
- Elevate the bed to stretcher height and assist in transferring the patient from the bed to the stretcher and, after surgery, from the stretcher to the bed. Review Procedure 19 in Unit 16.
- Complete the surgical checklist, if this is your responsibility.

During the Operative Period

While the patient is in the operating room, prepare the room for his or her return.

- Prepare the **surgical bed** (Unit 23).
- Remove everything from the top of the bedside stand except an emesis basin, tissues, tongue depressors, equipment to check vital signs, and a pen and paper.
- Obtain needed equipment, such as oxygen, IV poles, or suction.
- Watch for the return of your patient from surgery.

FIGURE 29-4 Taking vital signs is an important part of preoperative care. (© Delmar/Cengage Learning)

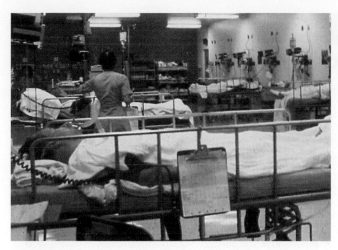

FIGURE 29-5 Postanesthesia care unit (PACU)—the unit where the patient wakes up from anesthesia after surgery. *(Courtesy of Memorial Medical Center of Long Beach, CA)*

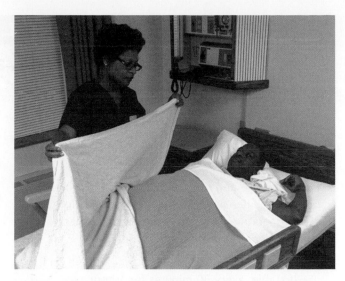

FIGURE 29-6 Patients may be cold after surgery. Cover them to prevent chilling. Use warmed blankets, if available. *(© Delmar/Cengage Learning)*

Postoperative Care

During the immediate postoperative period, the patient recovers from anesthesia. For this period, the patient is placed in a special area called the **recovery room** (Figure 29-5). The recovery room is located next to the operating room and is sometimes called the **postanesthesia care unit (PACU)**.

When the patient's condition is stabilized, the patient is returned to the unit. Upon the patient's return from the recovery room, you should:

- Identify the patient
- Assist in the transfer from stretcher to bed (see Unit 16)
- Inform the nurse if you cannot arouse the patient
- Check with the nurse for special instructions
- Notify the nurse if the patient's temperature is below 97°F.
- Have an extra blanket available—patients often feel cold upon return (Figure 29-6).

Safety ALERT

Anesthesia reduces body temperature. Keep the patient warm. If the patient's temperature is below 97°F, inform the nurse promptly. ∎

Nursing assistant observations related to the care of postoperative patients that require immediate reporting are listed in Table 29-1.

Observe the patient carefully, especially during the first 24 hours, for complications. You will assist with postoperative exercises, such as:

- Deep breathing and coughing
- Leg exercises

Safety ALERT

Patients receive many drugs before and during surgery. Some can alter the patient's mental status. They are excreted from the body slowly. The patient may sleep soundly upon return to the unit. Keep the side rails up and follow all safety precautions until the patient is fully awake and the nurse instructs you that side rails are no longer necessary. Do not leave liquids at the bedside until the nurse instructs you that it is safe to do so. Check on the patient regularly. ∎

TABLE 29-1 POSTOPERATIVE OBSERVATION AND REPORTING

- Decreased responsiveness or unresponsiveness
- Change in the level of responsiveness
- Increased restlessness accompanied by complaints of thirst
- Changes in blood pressure
- Weak, rapid, or irregular pulse
- Changes in temperature
- Changes in respiratory rate
- Difficulty breathing; labored or noisy respirations
- Nausea or vomiting
- Complaints of pain
- Increased drainage, wet or saturated dressings
- Active bleeding
- Coughing or choking

GUIDELINES *for*

Postoperative Care

- Apply the principles of standard precautions.
- Take vital signs upon the patient's arrival (Figure 29-7) and every 15 minutes for four readings. The patient's temperature is not taken at this time.
- Count pulse and respiration for one full minute. Most facilities have specified frequencies for taking postoperative vital signs; the frequency decreases if the patient is **stable**. For example:
  - every 15 minutes for 1 hour
  - if stable, every 30 minutes for 1 hour
  - if stable, every hour for 2 hours
  - if stable, every 4 hours for 24 hours

- Monitor the patient's level of consciousness (drowsy, unresponsive, alert) each time you check the vital signs.
- Ask the patient if he or she is having pain each time you check the vital signs. Inform the nurse if pain is present (Figure 29-8).
- Check dressings for amount and type of any **drainage**.
- Check IV solution for flow rate. Monitor other tubes.
- Encourage the patient to breathe deeply, cough, and move in bed. Change the patient's position at least every 2 hours.
- Turn the patient's head to one side and support if vomiting. Assist with oral care after vomiting. Note the type and amount of vomitus and record on the output worksheet.
- Measure and record the first postoperative voiding. Inform the nurse.

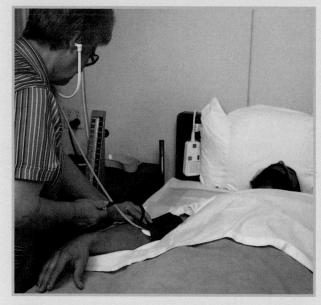

FIGURE 29-7 Check the vital signs regularly until they are stable. (© *Delmar/Cengage Learning*)

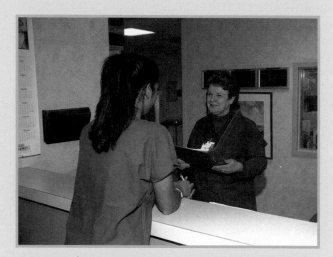

FIGURE 29-8 Report complaints of pain or discomfort to the nurse. (© *Delmar/Cengage Learning*)

Safety ALERT

Some patients are very sensitive and will not let anyone see them unless their dentures are in the mouth. Be sure they do not insert their dentures before they are fully awake. Remove dentures from an unconscious or comatose patient to prevent accidental airway obstruction by the denture. ■

SURGICAL WOUNDS

Patients often return from surgery with a variety of tubes and drains in place.

- Some tubes may deliver materials into the patient. Examples are oxygen tubes or intravenous tubes.
- Other tubes may have been placed in the patient to provide drainage from wounds or body cavities. Examples are drains in the incision or urinary catheters.

Managing Wounds with Drains

Drains remove fluids that have collected below the skin. The drain exits the skin through a small incision, and may be sutured in place. Some drains are hollow, and empty directly to the outside of the body. Others are connected closed containers, and must be emptied. Care of the device varies with physician orders and the type of drain used. Wound drains are considered sterile, and are usually managed by the nurse.

Use sterile technique when assisting with drains. Consider the drain as a portal of entry through which pathogens can enter the body. Always apply the principles of standard precautions.

Drains are used to remove body fluids, such as blood, pus, serous drainage, or gastric contents before or after surgery. The drainage outlet may be a:

- Catheter
- T-tube
- Jackson-Pratt (J-P)® or Hemovac® drain
- Penrose drain
- Cigarette drain

Special precautions in the care of patients with drains include:

- Always wear gloves if contact with drainage from the tube is likely.
- Learn the type, purpose, and location of each tube.
- Check drainage for character and amount.
- Check for obstructions to the tube system.
- Check flow rate of infusions from intravenous lines.
- Keep **orifices** (body openings) clear of secretions and discharge.
- Never disconnect tubes or raise drainage bottles above the level of the drainage site.
- Never lower infusion bottles below the level of the infusion site.
- Never put stress on the tubes when moving the patient or giving care.
- Monitor levels of infusions and report to the nurse before they run out.
- Report any signs of leakage or disconnected tubes immediately.
- Report pain, discoloration, or swelling at sites of drainage and infusion.
- Check with the nurse before changing or reinforcing a dressing.

Use sterile technique whenever you manipulate or empty a tube or drain or change a dressing. Be sure this is a permitted nursing assistant procedure in your facility.

Observations to make and report for patients with drains are listed in Table 29-2.

TABLE 29-2 OBSERVATIONS RELATING TO DRAINS TO REPORT TO THE NURSE

- Drain is not intact or patent
- Drain appears blocked, dislodged, or kinked
- Surrounding skin appears abnormal (erosion, red, hot, swollen, macerated)
- Drainage is eroding surrounding healthy skin
- Drainage is purulent, cloudy, or foul smelling
- Drainage color changes or appears abnormal
- Amount of drainage decreases markedly or stops entirely
- Amount of drainage increases markedly
- Patient has fever, tachycardia, hypotension
- Urinary output decreases

Dressings and Bandages

Dressings are gauze, film, or other synthetic substances that cover a wound, ulcer, or injury. Some have an adhesive backing. Some are affixed with tape. **Bandages** are fabric, gauze, net, or elasticized materials that are wrapped around an extremity to hold a dressing securely in place. Gauze bandages may be used to cover dressings. Elastic bandages are used to reduce edema and support injured body parts. Monitor bandages to be sure they do not restrict circulation. Inform the nurse if wound drainage seeps through the bandage. Review the information in Unit 35 if you will be responsible for changing clean dressings and bandages.

Montgomery straps (Figure 29-9) are long strips of adhesive attached to the skin on either side of the wound to hold dressings in place. They are less traumatic than tape

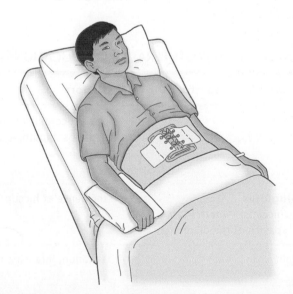

FIGURE 29-9 Montgomery straps hold dressings securely in place so they can be observed, changed, and reinforced without tape. This is much less traumatic for the patient. (© *Delmar/Cengage Learning*)

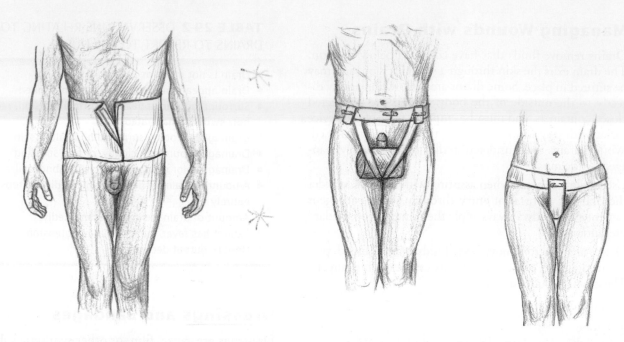

FIGURE 29-10 Various surgical binders support the body part and hold dressings in place. (© *Delmar/Cengage Learning*)

because the straps are not removed unless they are soiled. After the dressing is in place, the straps are tied to hold the dressing securely. **Binders** (Figure 29-10) may also be used to hold dressings in place.

PATIENT MONITORING AND OBSERVATIONS

The surgical patient must be carefully observed, especially during the first 24 hours, for possible complications.

Possible postoperative discomfort and complications and appropriate nursing assistant actions are summarized in Table 29-3.

DEEP BREATHING AND COUGHING

Deep breathing and coughing clear the air passages to prevent respiratory complications. However, they increase discomfort when the patient has a new incision

TABLE 29-3 POSTOPERATIVE COMPLICATIONS AND NURSING ASSISTANT ACTIONS

Possible Discomfort	Report	What You Can Do*
Thirst	Patient complaints of dryness of lips, mouth, and skin	Carefully check I&O. Give ice chips or increase fluid intake by mouth with permission. Monitor IV if ordered. Give mouth care. Check BP and pulse. Watch for signs of shock and hemorrhage.
Singultus (hiccups)—intermittent spasms of the diaphragm	Incidence of hiccups	Allow the patient to rest; hiccups can be tiring. Support the incisional area. Assist the patient to breathe into a paper bag.
Pain	Location, intensity, type	Change patient's position. Apply warmth if instructed. Monitor carefully for and report effects of medication given by nurse.
Distention (accumulation of gas in bowel)	Distention of abdomen, complaints of pain	Increase mobility. Insert a rectal tube if instructed and permitted.

TABLE 29-3 continued

Nausea, vomiting	Nausea, character of vomitus	Keep an emesis basin at the bedside. Monitor IV fluids, which are substituted for oral fluids. Give mouth care. Limit fluids by mouth. Encourage the patient to breathe deeply.
Urinary retention	Amount and time of first voiding. Distention, restlessness, imbalance between I&O	Monitor I&O carefully. Check for distention.
Hemorrhage (excessive blood loss)	Fall in blood pressure; cold, moist skin; weak, rapid pulse; restlessness; pallor/cyanosis; condition of dressing; thirst	Report immediately to nurse. Keep the patient quiet. Check vital signs.
Shock	Fall in blood pressure; weak, rapid pulse; cold, moist skin; pallor	Report immediately to nurse. Keep the patient quiet. Monitor ordered oxygen. Be prepared to follow additional instructions.
Hypoxia (lack of oxygen)	Restlessness, dyspnea, crowing sound to respirations, pounding pulse, perspiring	Report immediately to nurse. Monitor oxygen, if ordered.
Atelectasis (decreased or absent air in all or part of a lung, resulting in loss of lung volume and inability to expand lung fully)	Dyspnea; cyanosis/pallor	Report immediately to nurse.
Wound infection	Increased pain in incisional area; fever; chills, anorexia, increased drainage on dressing	Be observant. Report findings promptly to nurse. Check dressing.
Wound **disruption** (separation of wound edges)	Pinkish drainage. Complaints by patient that he "feels open," "broken," "given away"	Report immediately to nurse. Keep the patient quiet. Support incisional area.
Pulmonary emboli	Anxiety, difficulty breathing; feelings of "heaviness" in chest, cyanosis, chest pain	Keep the patient quiet. Report immediately to nurse. Elevate head of bed.

*In all cases, be prepared to follow the nurse's additional instructions.

and feels fatigued. (See Procedure 80.) You can best assist the patient by:

- Checking to see if pain medication is needed before the exercise. If so, wait for 45 minutes after the medication has been given before carrying out the exercise.
- Learning how many deep breaths and coughs should be attempted. The usual number is 5 to 10 breaths and 2 to 3 coughs.
- Using a pillow or binder to support the incision during the procedure.

Safety ALERT

If you work with postoperative patients, encouraging coughing and deep breathing will be automatic. There are a few exceptions you must be aware of. Avoid this procedure with patients who have had eye, nose, or neurologic surgery. Coughing and deep breathing will increase pressure, causing complications in these patients. Check with the nurse if you are unsure of what action to take. ■

PROCEDURE

80

ASSISTING THE PATIENT TO DEEP BREATHE AND COUGH

1. Carry out initial procedure actions.

2. Assemble equipment:
   - Disposable gloves
   - Pillowcase-covered pillow
   - Binder, if ordered
   - Tissues
   - Emesis basin

3. Elevate the head of the bed and assist the patient to assume a comfortable semi-Fowler's position.

4. Have the patient place his hands on either side of the rib cage or over the operative site (Figure 29-11).

5. Ask the patient to take as deep a breath as possible and hold it for 3 to 5 seconds; then exhale slowly through pursed lips.

6. Repeat this exercise about 5 times unless the patient seems too tired. If so, stop the procedure and report to the nurse.

7. Place the pillow across the incision line as a brace. Assist the patient to hold the sides or interlace his fingers across the incision (Figure 29-12).

8. Provide tissues and instruct the person to take a deep breath and cough forcefully twice with the mouth open, collecting any secretions in the tissues.

9. Put on disposable gloves to handle the tissues.

10. Dispose of tissues in an emesis basin.

11. When finished, assist the patient to assume a comfortable position.

12. Clean the emesis basin.

13. Remove and dispose of gloves according to facility policy.

14. Carry out ending procedure actions.

15. Report to the nurse on the number of times the patient performed each exercise, how the patient tolerated the exercise, and the type and amount of sputum coughed up.

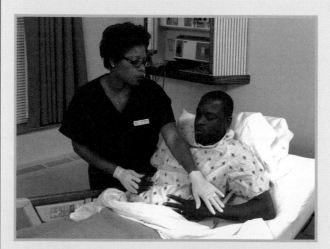

FIGURE 29-11 Remind, encourage, and assist the patient to perform deep breathing exercises. *(© Delmar/Cengage Learning)*

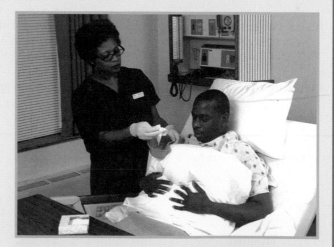

FIGURE 29-12 A pillow helps support the abdomen and splint the incision during coughing and deep breathing. *(© Delmar/Cengage Learning)*

LEG EXERCISES

Leg exercises improve blood flow, preventing blood clots, which are a serious postoperative complication. A blood clot or **deep vein thrombosis (DVT)** could develop in the venous system and block the essential blood flow. A small piece of thrombus broken off (**embolus**) could travel throughout the vascular system and block a vessel in the lungs.

A specific order must be written for leg exercises when a patient has had leg surgery. Otherwise, leg exercises are done routinely. If the patient is very weak, you may need to assist.

- Encourage leg exercises and be sure they have been performed.
- Remind the patient to do each exercise 3 to 5 times every 1 or 2 hours, or as specified on the care plan.
- Have the patient carry out leg exercises during position changes.
- Apply or reapply support hose, as ordered.

PROCEDURE

PERFORMING POSTOPERATIVE LEG EXERCISES

1. Carry out initial procedure actions.

2. Lower the side rail.

3. Cover the patient with a bath blanket and draw the top bedding to the foot of the bed.

4. Explain how the exercise is to be performed. Have the patient:
   a. Brace the incisional area with laced hands.
   b. Dorsiflex (bring the toes toward the knee) and plantar flex (point the toes and foot down) each ankle (Figure 29-13A).
   c. Rotate each ankle by drawing imaginary circles with the toes (Figure 29-13B).

   d. Flex and extend each knee (Figure 29-13C).
   e. Flex and extend each hip.
   f. Repeat each exercise 3 to 5 times. Assist as needed.

5. Supervise exercises or assist. Apply or reapply support hose as ordered.

6. Draw bedding up and remove the bath blanket.

7. Fold the bath blanket and place it in the bedside stand for reuse.

8. Carry out ending procedure actions. Report to the nurse on the number of exercises done and how the patient tolerated them.

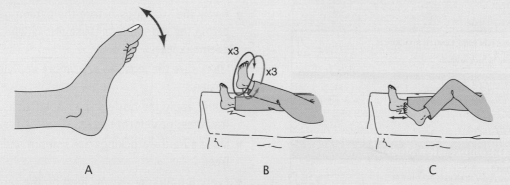

A   B   C

FIGURE 29-13 Help the patient perform leg exercises to encourage circulation. (© Delmar/ Cengage Learning)
A. Curl the toes down and up. Repeat 5 times.
B. Make circles with the feet clockwise 3 times and counterclockwise 3 times. Repeat 5 times.
C. Slide one leg up and down in bed. Do the same with the other leg. Repeat 5 times.

ELASTICIZED STOCKINGS

Elasticized stockings are called **TED hose**, **anti-embolism hose**, or *graduated compression stockings (GCS)*. This name refers to the pressure, which is tightest at the foot and ankle and becomes looser as the stockings extend up the leg. The hose are worn from the ankle or foot to calf or midthigh. They are often applied during the perioperative period to support the veins of the legs. This reduces the incidence of **thrombophlebitis**, an inflammation of the veins that can lead to blood clots. The stockings must be applied smoothly and evenly before the patient gets out of bed. Remove and reapply them every 8 hours, or as specified on the care plan.

Several different types of anti-embolism hose are used. Some have closed toes, but most have an opening near the toe end. The hole is positioned on the top or the bottom of the foot, just proximal to the toes. Use the heel of the stocking as a landmark so you can see where to position the hole.

Preventing Complications

A physician's order is needed to apply special hosiery. The ordering physician will specify if knee-high or thigh-high hose should be used. The size is based on each patient's leg measurements (Figure 29-14). Make sure you apply the correct hosiery and the correct size.

The risk of complications from anti-embolism hosiery is low. However, they are not totally risk-free. Ill-fitting hosiery is the most common cause of complications. The greatest risk is a reduction in blood flow from pressure, which increases the potential for blood clots. Other complications are pressure ulcers, gangrene, and arterial occlusion. These usually occur when the patient sits for a prolonged period without moving. In one reported case, the tourniquet effect created by bunched-up hosiery, combined with swelling of the leg, caused serious skin breakdown that led to amputation.

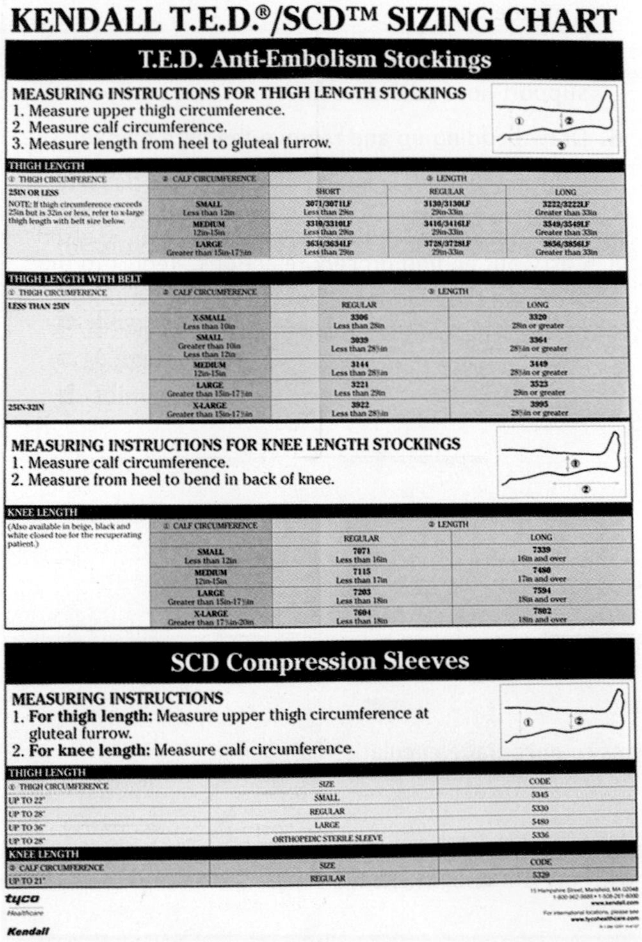
KENDALL T.E.D.®/SCD™ SIZING CHART

T.E.D. Anti-Embolism Stockings

MEASURING INSTRUCTIONS FOR THIGH LENGTH STOCKINGS
1. Measure upper thigh circumference.
2. Measure calf circumference.
3. Measure length from heel to gluteal furrow.

THIGH LENGTH

① THIGH CIRCUMFERENCE	② CALF CIRCUMFERENCE	③ LENGTH		
25IN OR LESS		SHORT	REGULAR	LONG
NOTE: If thigh circumference exceeds 25in but is 32in or less, refer to x-large thigh length with belt size below.	SMALL Less than 12in	3071/3071LF Less than 29in	3130/3130LF 29in-33in	3222/3222LF Greater than 33in
	MEDIUM 12in-15in	3310/3310LF Less than 29in	3416/3416LF 29in-33in	3349/3349LF Greater than 33in
	LARGE Greater than 15in-17½in	3634/3634LF Less than 29in	3728/3728LF 29in-33in	3856/3856LF Greater than 33in

THIGH LENGTH WITH BELT

① THIGH CIRCUMFERENCE	② CALF CIRCUMFERENCE	③ LENGTH	
LESS THAN 25IN		REGULAR	LONG
	X-SMALL Less than 10in	3306 Less than 28in	3320 28in or greater
	SMALL Greater than 10in Less than 12in	3039 Less than 28½in	3364 28½in or greater
	MEDIUM 12in-15in	3144 Less than 28½in	3449 28½in or greater
	LARGE Greater than 15in-17½in	3221 Less than 29in	3523 29in or greater
25IN-32IN	X-LARGE Greater than 15in-17½in	3922 Less than 28½in	3995 28½in or greater

MEASURING INSTRUCTIONS FOR KNEE LENGTH STOCKINGS
1. Measure calf circumference.
2. Measure from heel to bend in back of knee.

KNEE LENGTH

	① CALF CIRCUMFERENCE	② LENGTH	
(Also available in beige, black and white closed toe for the recuperating patient.)		REGULAR	LONG
	SMALL Less than 12in	7071 Less than 16in	7339 16in and over
	MEDIUM 12in-15in	7115 Less than 17in	7480 17in and over
	LARGE Greater than 15in-17½in	7203 Less than 18in	7594 18in and over
	X-LARGE Greater than 17½in-20in	7604 Less than 18in	7802 18in and over

SCD Compression Sleeves

MEASURING INSTRUCTIONS
1. **For thigh length:** Measure upper thigh circumference at gluteal furrow.
2. **For knee length:** Measure calf circumference.

THIGH LENGTH

① THIGH CIRCUMFERENCE	SIZE	CODE
UP TO 22"	SMALL	5345
UP TO 28"	REGULAR	5330
UP TO 36"	LARGE	5480
UP TO 28"	ORTHOPEDIC STERILE SLEEVE	5336

KNEE LENGTH

② CALF CIRCUMFERENCE	SIZE	CODE
UP TO 21"	REGULAR	5329

tyco Healthcare Kendall

FIGURE 29-14 Measure the patient's leg with the disposable paper tape measure, then compare the measurements to the manufacturer's chart to determine the correct size hosiery. Discard the tape measure. *(© Delmar/Cengage Learning)*

GUIDELINES *for* Applying Anti-Embolism Stockings

- The care plan will specify the wearing schedule for the stockings. For most patients, hosiery is removed at bedtime.
- If the patient has a latex sensitivity, be sure the hosiery used is latex free.
- Apply the stockings before the patient gets out of bed in the morning, because this is when the edema is least.
- Make sure the legs are dry before applying the hosiery.
- Never apply the hosiery over open areas, fractures, or deformities.
- Make sure the stockings are smooth and wrinkle free.
- Every 8 hours (or as specified on the care plan), monitor circulation in the toes and be sure the hosiery tops have not rolled down. Note color, sensation, swelling, temperature, and ability to move. *Document that you have done regular skin and circulation checks.*
- Avoid contact with lotions, ointments, or oils containing lanolin or petroleum products. These products deteriorate the elastic in the hosiery.

PROCEDURE

82

APPLYING ELASTICIZED STOCKINGS

1. Carry out initial procedure actions.

2. Assemble equipment:
   - Elasticized stockings of proper length and size

3. Apply stockings with the patient lying down. Expose one leg at a time.

4. Grasp the stocking with both hands at the top and roll it toward the toe end (Figure 29-15A).

5. Adjust the stocking, positioning the opening at the top or base of the toes (unless the toes are to be covered) (Figure 29-15B).

6. Continue rolling the stocking upward toward the body (Figure 29-15C).

7. Be sure the stocking is smooth, even, and wrinkle free (Figure 29-15D).

8. Repeat the procedure on the opposite leg.

9. Carry out ending procedure actions.

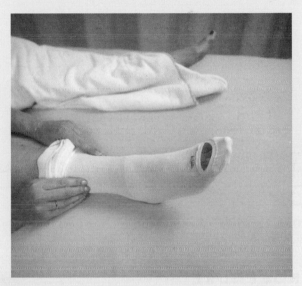

FIGURE 29-15C Draw the stocking smoothly up to the knee. (© Delmar/Cengage Learning)

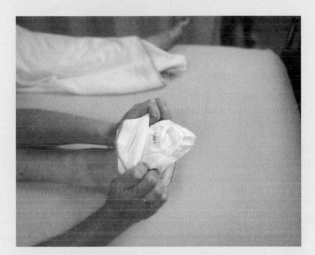

FIGURE 29-15A Gather the stocking and slip it over the patient's toes. (© Delmar/Cengage Learning)

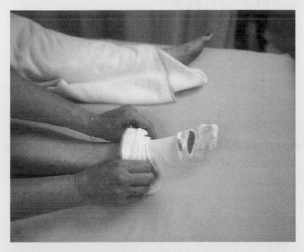

FIGURE 29-15B Position the opening on the top of the foot, at the base of the toes. (© Delmar/Cengage Learning)

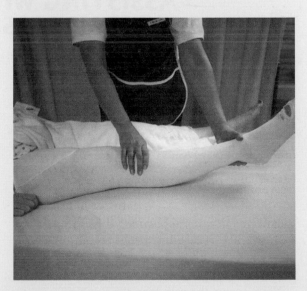

FIGURE 29-15D Check to make sure the stocking is free from wrinkles. (© Delmar/Cengage Learning)

SEQUENTIAL COMPRESSION THERAPY

Deep vein thrombosis and **pulmonary embolism** (blood clot in the lungs) are serious postoperative complications. Approximately 10% of all patients with DVT die from pulmonary embolism. Most have no symptoms until they develop the pulmonary embolus. The femoral vein, the large blood vessel in the groin, is particularly susceptible to clot formation. Because of the high risk, the physician may order sequential compression therapy. **Sequential compression therapy** (Figure 29-16) massages the legs and keeps blood flowing, making blood clots less likely. The device is applied over anti-embolism hosiery, if the patient is wearing them.

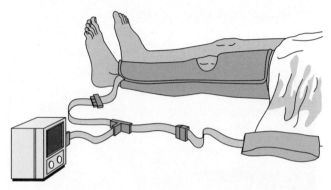

FIGURE 29-16 Pneumatic compression hosiery is used to prevent blood clots. *(© Delmar/Cengage Learning)*

INITIAL AMBULATION

Some time after surgery, a patient is permitted to sit up with the legs over the edge of the bed. This position is called **dangling**. Assist the patient to assume the position slowly.

The first **ambulation** (walk) is usually short. The patient usually dangles for a short time before ambulating. Dangling is an important part of postoperative care because it stimulates circulation. (Refer to Procedure 84.)

The patient may need assistance the first few times he stands to ambulate. Be familiar with the location of tubes and move them with the patient (Figure 29-17).

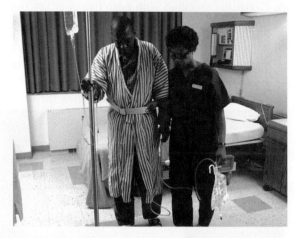

FIGURE 29-17 Drainage tubes and IV lines may be in place after surgery. Carefully move these with the patient. *(© Delmar/Cengage Learning)*

PROCEDURE

83

ASSISTING WITH SEQUENTIAL COMPRESSION HOSIERY

 Note: Be certain this is a nursing assistant procedure in your facility.

1. Carry out initial procedure actions.

2. Assemble equipment:
   - Hosiery of proper size
   - Compression controller

3. Open the hose, laying them flat on the bed with the markings opposite the knee and ankle.

4. Lift the patient's leg and slide the hose under it. Wrap the sleeve smoothly around the leg with the opening in front, over the knee.

5. Beginning at the ankle, fasten the Velcro securely. Next, secure the calf, then the thigh.

6. Check the fit by inserting two fingers between the sleeve and the patient's leg. The fit should feel snug and secure, but not tight.

7. Wrap the other leg in the same manner, beginning on the side opposite the plastic tubing. Check the fit.

8. Attach the plastic tubing on each leg by lining up the arrows on the tubing.

9. Plug the controller in and turn on the power.

10. Remain in the room for one complete cycle (usually 60 to 90 seconds) to ensure that the patient tolerates the procedure.

11. Carry out ending procedure actions.

PROCEDURE

84

ASSISTING THE PATIENT TO DANGLE

1. Carry out initial procedure actions.

2. Assemble equipment:
   - Bath blanket
   - Pillow

3. Lower the side rail nearest to you. Lock the bed at the lowest position.

4. Drape the patient with a bath blanket and fanfold the top bedcovers to the foot of the bed.

5. Gradually elevate the head of the bed.

6. Help the patient to put on a bathrobe.

7. Place one arm around the patient's shoulders and the other arm under the knees.

8. Gently and slowly turn the patient toward you. Allow the patient's legs to hang over the side of the bed.

9. After putting slippers on the patient, ask the patient to swing the legs.

10. Have the patient dangle as long as ordered. If he becomes dizzy or faint, help him lie down.

11. Rearrange the pillow at the head of the bed. Remove the patient's bathrobe and slippers.

12. Place one arm around the patient's shoulders and the other arm under the knees. Gently and slowly swing the patient's legs onto the bed.

13. Check the patient's pulse. Lower the head of the bed and raise the side rails, according to the care plan.

14. Carry out ending procedure actions.

Safety ALERT

Remain next to the patient during the first dangling and ambulation. Do not turn your back or leave the bedside. These precautions will probably not be necessary as the patient recovers and gains strength. Use common sense and follow the care plan and the nurse's instructions. ■

HEAT AND COLD APPLICATIONS

Heat and cold applications are used for many different purposes. A localized application is used to apply heat or cold to a specific area of the body. An example of this type of application is an ice bag applied to a swollen ankle. A **generalized** application is used to apply heat or cold to the patient's entire body.

Heat applications **dilate** or enlarge the blood vessels, bringing oxygen and nutrients to the area, relieving pain and

GUIDELINES *for*

Assisting the Patient in Initial Ambulation

- Check with the nurse to see if a transfer belt can be used.
- Assist the patient to sit on the edge of the bed with the bed in low position.
- Assist the patient to put on footwear appropriate to the floor surface. Never allow a patient to ambulate with bare feet or just socks.
- Take the patient's pulse before and after standing. If there is more than 10 points difference, return the patient to bed and inform the nurse.
- If the patient becomes dizzy or faint, return the patient to bed and inform the nurse.
- Walk with the patient as instructed in Unit 17.

speeding healing. They are commonly used when IV fluid has accidentally entered the tissue.

Local cold applications are used to control bleeding, relieve pain, and prevent or relieve edema, which is common after an injury. Cooling causes blood vessels to **constrict**, making them smaller. Generalized cooling is used to reduce temperature. Blankets may also be used for heating, but this is less common.

Dry or moist treatments may be ordered. Moist treatments (those in which water touches the skin) penetrate more deeply than dry. Some dry applications have water inside them, but the outer surface remains dry. Dry applications may be used to maintain the temperature of moist applications. Common types of heat and cold treatments are:

- Ice bags, ice collars, hot water bottles (Figure 29-18).
- Aquamatic K-Pads. K-Pads (Figure 29-19) come in many shapes and sizes. Distilled water circulates through the pad continuously. The temperature can be set by the user. They are commonly used to apply heat. With a special attachment, they can also be used for cooling.
- Prepackaged, single-use chemical packs (Figure 29-20) for the application of heat or cold. Squeezing or striking

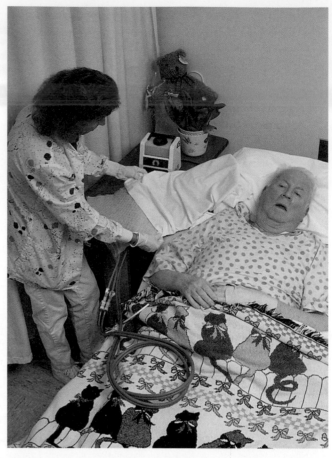

FIGURE 29-19 The Aquamatic K-Pad is usually used for heat treatments. (© *Delmar/Cengage Learning*)

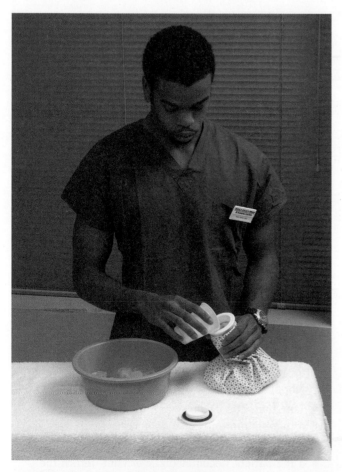

FIGURE 29-18 An ice bag. (© *Delmar/Cengage Learning*)

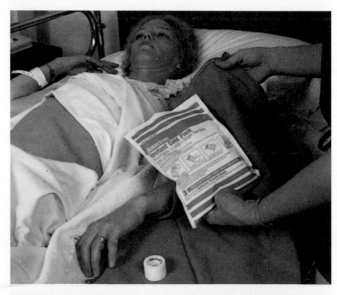

FIGURE 29-20 The chemical cold pack is activated by squeezing or striking away from your face. Cover the pack before using. (© *Delmar/Cengage Learning*)

the surface activates the contents, providing a controlled temperature.

- Reusable gel packs that can be cooled or heated as needed.
- The **hypothermia-hyperthermia blanket** (Figure 29-21), a generalized treatment that is usually used to cool the patient to reduce a high fever. The blanket may also be used to warm a patient in cases of hypothermia.
- Warm or cool compresses or soaks (less commonly used).

ELIMINATION

Some patients experience difficulty with elimination postoperatively. Abdominal distention may also occur. Monitor the patient's bladder and bowel elimination and inform the nurse when the patient voids for the first time after surgery. Inform the nurse if abdominal distention develops, as well as if the patient complains of constipation.

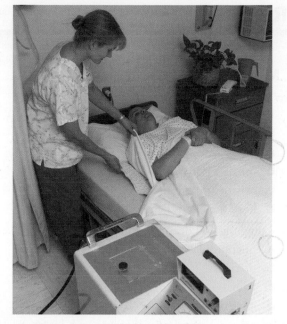

FIGURE 29-21 The hypothermia-hyperthermia blanket is usually used to reduce body temperature, but may also be used for warming. (© *Delmar/Cengage Learning*)

GUIDELINES *for*

Applying Heat and Cold

- Before using a heat or cold application, be sure you know the:
  - type of application
  - area to be treated
  - length of time for the treatment
  - proper temperature of the application
  - safety precautions
  - side effects
  - special precautions or monitoring
- Follow safety rules to prevent spills and falls.
- Apply the principles of standard precautions.
- Always check the temperature of the treatment with a thermometer.
- Cover the application with a protective cover. Covers may be flannel or foam. Towels and pillowcases are also used.
- Assist the patient into a comfortable position that he or she can maintain during the treatment.

- Cover the patient with a bath blanket.
- Expose only the part of the body that you will be treating.
- A metal cap conducts heat and cold. Face it away from the person.
- Remove or reposition metal zippers, buttons, jewelry, or other materials that may conduct heat or cold.
- Check the skin under the application every 10 minutes or more often.
  - If the skin under a heat application is very red, or if a dark area appears, stop the application and inform the nurse.
  - If the skin under a cold application is blue, pale, white, or bright red, or if the person is shivering, stop the application and notify the nurse.
- Treatments are usually applied for 20 minutes. Check the care plan or with the nurse to learn the length of time the application is to be applied.

REVIEW

A. Multiple Choice

Select the one best answer for each of the following.

1. When assisting a patient with coughing and deep breathing exercises, teach him or her to
   - **a.** inhale through the nose.
   - **b.** inhale through the mouth.
   - **c.** exhale through the nose.
   - **d.** keep the hands behind the neck.

2. Coughing and deep breathing exercises help prevent
   - **a.** pneumonia.
   - **b.** dizziness.
   - **c.** pain.
   - **d.** anxiety.

3. The main purpose of sequential compression hosiery is to prevent
   - **a.** edema.
   - **b.** pneumonia.
   - **c.** blood clots.
   - **d.** pain.

4. Sequential compression hosiery should not be used
   - **a.** on patients who have had abdominal surgery.
   - **b.** if the patient is using oxygen.
   - **c.** if a rash is present on the legs.
   - **d.** for patients wearing support hosiery.

5. Check the postoperative patient's vital signs every
   - **a.** 5 minutes for the first hour, then every 15 minutes for 4 hours.
   - **b.** 15 minutes for an hour, then every 30 minutes for an hour.
   - **c.** 30 minutes for 4 hours, then every 8 hours for 72 hours.
   - **d.** 60 minutes for 4 hours, then every 4 hours for 16 hours.

6. Heat affects the body by
   - **a.** causing constriction.
   - **b.** increasing blood supply.
   - **c.** reducing oxygen in tissues.
   - **d.** increasing white blood cells.

7. Heat and cold treatments are usually applied
   - **a.** continuously.
   - **b.** every 2 hours.
   - **c.** as desired.
   - **d.** for 20 minutes.

8. Cold affects the body by
   - **a.** reducing pain sensations.
   - **b.** stimulating life processes.
   - **c.** promoting inflammation.
   - **d.** increasing the oxygen supply.

9. An example of a moist cold application is
   - **a.** ice bags.
   - **b.** ice caps.
   - **c.** ice collars.
   - **d.** soaks.

10. When applying heat and cold treatments, the nursing assistant should
    - **a.** always remain in the room for the duration of the treatment.
    - **b.** check the temperature of the solution with an elbow.
    - **c.** monitor the skin under the application every 30 minutes.
    - **d.** remove jewelry, buttons, or zippers that may conduct heat or cold.

B. Nursing Assistant Challenge

Mr. Dovetski is a 47-year-old patient on the surgical unit. He has had abdominal surgery. When he is returned to his room from surgery, you note that he has a Foley catheter, an intravenous feeding running, dressings on an abdominal incision, and elastic stockings. Think about what procedures you will include in your care of Mr. Dovetski.

11. How often will you take his vital signs? Which procedures are included in vital signs? What are the "normal" ranges for each vital sign for a person of this age? If there are changes in the vital signs, these changes may be indications of what complications?

12. What observations will you make regarding the Foley catheter? Why do you think he has the catheter in place?

13. You know you will need to have Mr. Dovetski perform deep breathing exercises and deep coughing. Why is this important? How can you help him do the exercises with the least discomfort?

14. Why do you think he has elastic stockings on? How often should you take the stockings off and reapply them? What do you need to remember when putting the stockings back on?

15. How will you check for bleeding from the incision?

UNIT 30

Caring for the Emotionally Stressed Patient

OBJECTIVES

After completing this unit, you will be able to:

- Spell and define terms.
- Define mental health.
- Explain how physical and mental health are related.
- Identify common mental health problems.
- Describe nursing assistant actions and observations related to the care of patients with mental health needs.
- Describe ways of helping patients cope with stressful situations.
- Identify professional boundaries in relationships with patients and families.

VOCABULARY

Learn the meaning and the correct spelling of the following words and phrases:

adaptation	bulimia nervosa	maladaptive behavior	reality orientation
affective disorders	compulsion	mental illness	reminiscing
agitation	coping	obsession	schizoaffective disorder
alcoholism	defense mechanisms	obsessive-compulsive	seasonal affective
anorexia nervosa	delirium	disorder (OCD)	disorder (SAD)
anxiety	delirium tremens (DTs)	panic disorder	stressors
anxiety disorder	depression	phobia	substance abuse
bipolar affective disorder	disorientation	posttraumatic stress	suicide
borderline personality	eating disorders	disorder (PTSD)	suicide precautions
disorder (BPD)	enabling	professional boundaries	validation therapy

INTRODUCTION

There are varying degrees and differing aspects of health. A person who is in poor physical health may be mentally healthy. Because of good mental health, the person may be self-reliant, able to make decisions and to live an effective, productive life (Figure 30-1).

In contrast, a person with good physical health may not be able to cope with and adapt to changes. This inability limits the person's ability to participate successfully in society.

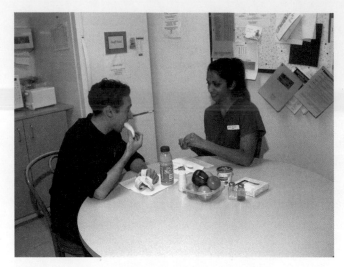

FIGURE 30-1 A mentally healthy person leads a productive life. (© *Delmar/Cengage Learning*)

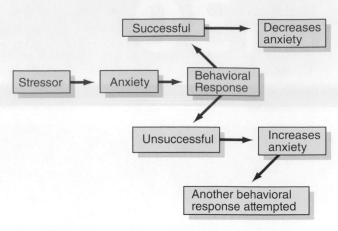

FIGURE 30-2 Each individual has ways of coping with stress. (© *Delmar/Cengage Learning*)

Culture ALERT

Patients from various cultures have different views about how disabling certain conditions are. In some cultures, mental illness is considered shameful, or a punishment from a higher power or supernatural force. They may not tell anyone outside the family. Some fear that the mental problem is contagious, or that others will develop a similar problem. ■

ANXIETY DISORDERS

Anxiety is fear, apprehension, or a sense of impending danger. It is often marked by vague physical symptoms, such as tension, restlessness, and rapid heart rate. An **anxiety disorder** is one of a group of recognized mental illnesses involving anxiety reactions in response to stress. These are listed in Table 30-1.

MENTAL HEALTH

Mental health means exhibiting behaviors that reflect a person's **adaptation** or adjustment to the multiple stresses of life. Stresses or **stressors** are situations, feelings, or conditions that cause a person to be anxious about his or her physical or emotional well-being. Good mental health leads to positive adaptations. Poor mental health is demonstrated by behaviors that harm the person or her adjustment.

Physical and mental health are interrelated. Physical illness is often preceded by stressful life situations. Ill health causes emotional stress. It is easy to understand that each of these factors contributes to the total health pattern of each person.

Ways of **coping** with (handling) stressful situations (Figure 30-2) are learned early in life. As people grow, they find the behaviors that work best for them. They learn to use those behaviors to reduce stress and protect self-esteem. These coping patterns become part of the individual's habitual responses, becoming more and more obvious as the person ages.

GUIDELINES *for*

Assisting a Patient Who Is Upset, Anxious, or Agitated

- Attempt to identify and eliminate stressors.
- Do not argue with or confront the patient.
- Make the environment safe.
- Keep a recent photo of the patient in case he or she wanders off.
- Monitor the patient's activities. Such a patient is at risk of injury.
- Notify the nurse promptly if the patient wanders away from the unit, facility, or home.
- Assign the patient brief tasks, or engage the patient in activities that enhance self-esteem.
- Use bean-bag seats and rocking chairs in the long-term care facility or the patient's home.
- Watch for injuries.
- Prevent the patient from becoming exhausted.

TABLE 30-1 ANXIETY DISORDERS

Generalized anxiety	The most common anxiety disorder; a common trigger of agitation.
Panic disorder	Condition in which a person has panic attacks, or bouts of overwhelming fear with no specific cause or basis.
Obsessive-compulsive disorder (OCD)	An anxiety disorder in which the patient has recurrent obsessions and/or compulsions. An **obsession** is a frequent idea, impulse, or thought that does not make sense. The person cannot suppress it. A **compulsion** is a purposeful, repetitive behavior that is done many times, such as washing the hands hundreds of times each day. This is called *repeated ritualistic activity*. The person cannot control this behavior.
Posttraumatic stress disorder (PTSD)	Common in survivors of major trauma—the person has nightmares or flashbacks, and may have trouble with normal emotional responses.
Phobias	A **phobia** is an unfounded, recurring fear that causes the person to feel panic. The fear can be mildly annoying to severely disabling.
Agitation	Inappropriate verbal, vocal, or motor activity due to causes other than disorientation or real need.

AFFECTIVE DISORDERS

Affective disorders are a group of mental disorders characterized by a disturbance in mood. They may also be called *mood disorders*, and are usually marked by a profound and persistent sadness. Common affective disorders are listed in Table 30-2.

Note: Figures 30-4 and 30-5 were a gift to the author from a severely depressed patient who chronicled her feelings through her art. Each caption reflects her feelings at the time the picture was drawn.

Nursing Care of a Patient with the Potential for Suicide

Never assume that a suicide attempt is a means of getting the attention of staff or family. At least 15% of people who try to commit suicide do it again. The suicide rate is higher in acute medical units than it is on psychiatric units. Most suicides occur while the person is being supervised by a health provider, who either misses or ignores the clues.

TABLE 30-2 AFFECTIVE DISORDERS

Bipolar affective disorder (may also be called *manic depression*)	A condition in which the person has marked mood swings, ranging from elation (also called *mania*) to severe depression (Figure 30-3).
Schizoaffective disorder	Believed to be a combination of schizophrenia and a mood disorder. It is a chronic, disabling mental illness that is often difficult to diagnose.
Seasonal affective disorder (SAD)	A depression that recurs at the same time each year. The cause is not known.
Borderline personality disorder (BPD)	A condition in which the person is very unstable. He or she is manipulative, impulsive, and prone to self-injury.
Depression	The most common functional disorder in older persons, but seen in all age groups (Figures 30-4 and 30-5). May be masked by symptoms of physical illness.

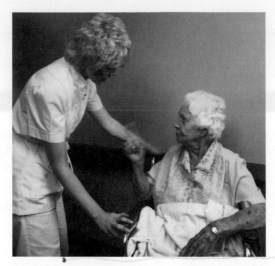

FIGURE 30-3 This patient is very frustrated because she feels as if she is powerless and lacks control over her life. *(© Delmar/Cengage Learning)*

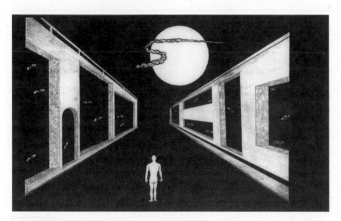

FIGURE 30-4 It is so lonely here. I struggle to communicate but there are no words for what I feel. I withdraw further and feel that I am being watched. I know that they laugh at my plight. *(Courtesy of Barbara Acello)*

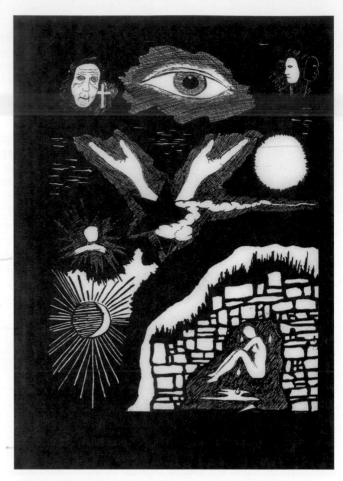

FIGURE 30-5 Depression's cave. It smothers me with thoughts of death, of futility. I feel so low and imagine that everyone thinks that it is all I deserve. Their looks are heavy and weigh me down. Which side of me do they judge or can they see all of me? Do they know how weak I am? Do they laugh at my inability to cope with life? I, also, have judged myself . . . it is the verdict which weighs me down. *(Courtesy of Barbara Acello)*

GUIDELINES *for*

Assisting the Patient Who Is Depressed

- Be honest, supportive, and caring.
- Be a good listener. Encourage the patient to express feelings. Avoid passing judgment or criticizing what the patient feels. Avoid interrupting or changing the subject.
- Give positive feedback on the patient's strengths and successes.
- Acknowledge the patient's feelings.
- Avoid comments like, "Cheer up. Things could be worse."

- Encourage physical activity to the extent possible. Exercise reduces stress.
- Encourage the patient to laugh regularly. Laughter is therapeutic and reduces stress. Turn on a funny television program or tell a joke.
- Monitor the patient's appetite and report overeating or undereating to the nurse.
- Reinforce the patient's self-concept by emphasizing the patient's value to society and helping the patient to use his or her support systems.

GUIDELINES *continued*

- Encourage and allow the patient to make decisions about daily routines and activities. Give him or her as much control as possible.
- Do not act sympathetic. This validates the patient's poor self-image and depressed feelings.
- Report complaints so that problems may be identified and corrected rather than being attributed to the depression.
- Provide the patient with activities within his or her limitations.
- Use simple language and speak slowly when giving instructions.
- Monitor elimination carefully; constipation is common.
- Provide fluids frequently; the patient may be too preoccupied to drink.
- Be alert to the potential for **suicide** (the taking of one's own life). Watch for and report:
  - Change in mood or behavior, such as deepening depression or suddenly seeming happy and calm

  - Withdrawal or secretiveness
  - Repeated, prolonged, or sporadic refusal of food, care, medications, or fluids
  - Hoarding of medications
  - Sudden decision to donate body parts to a medical school
  - Sudden interest or disinterest in religion
  - Purchase of a gun, razor blades, or other harmful items and hiding them
  - Statements such as: "I just want out," or "I want to end it all"
  - Increased use of alcohol and drugs
  - Deep preoccupation with something that cannot be explained

GUIDELINES *for*

Suicide Precautions

When a person is suicidal, the care plan will list certain **suicide precautions**. These are checks and practices a facility follows if a patient is a suicide risk. The precautions are continued until the patient is believed to be out of danger. When a patient is on suicide precautions, you should:

- Monitor for and report clues to suicide attempts; never ignore a patient's statements or threats about suicide.
- Be consistent in approaches and care.
- Emphasize positive aspects of the patient's life, and give the patient hope while being realistic (Figure 30-6).
- Work to restore the patient's self-esteem, self-worth, and self-respect.
- Make the patient feel accepted and valued as a unique individual.

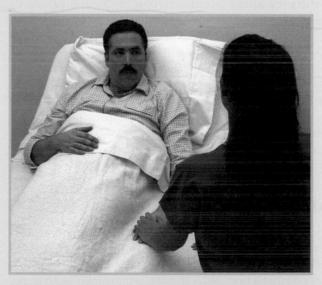

FIGURE 30-6 Be helpful but realistic with a depressed patient who is at risk of suicide. (© Delmar/Cengage Learning)

TABLE 30-3 COMMON EATING DISORDERS

Anorexia nervosa	Condition in which the person views his or her body as fat and limits food intake through diet, exercise, purging, and taking laxatives and diuretics.
Bulimia nervosa	Condition in which the person binge-eats huge amounts, then vomits (*purges*), or takes laxatives and diuretics to undo the binge.

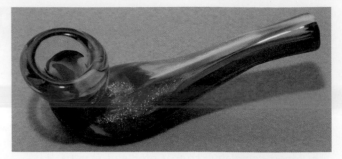

FIGURE 30-7 A pipe for smoking methamphetamine *(Courtesy of U.S. Drug Enforcement Administration)*

EATING DISORDERS

Eating disorders are a group of conditions in which the person has disturbances of appetite or food intake. The two most common are **anorexia nervosa** and **bulimia nervosa.** These conditions can occur in both males and females. They are summarized in Table 30-3.

Eating disorders are common in persons with borderline personality disorder. The conditions often overlap and are difficult to identify. People with eating disorders are usually very secretive, so family and close friends may not become aware of the condition until weight loss is profound. The electrolyte imbalance and starvation caused by these conditions can lead to death.

SUBSTANCE ABUSE

Substance abuse is characterized by the use of one or more substances (such as alcohol or drugs) to alter mood or behavior, resulting in impairment and poor judgment. Over time, the behavior strains finances, causes irresponsibility, and interferes with the person's ability to function normally. Drug abuse can be by use of illegal (street) drugs, such as marijuana, cocaine, or heroin; or misuse of prescription drugs, such as narcotic pain medications, without proper physician knowledge or oversight. Drugs may be swallowed, chewed, inhaled, injected, or smoked (Figure 30-7).

Alcoholism

Alcohol is a drug and **alcoholism** is a disease. Some people use alcohol as a means of coping with stress. It slows brain activity and alters alertness, judgment, coordination, and reaction time. It mixes unfavorably with many other drugs. Persons who are quitting the use of alcohol may have **delirium tremens (DTs)**. DTs are serious withdrawal symptoms seen in persons who stop drinking

suddenly following continuous and heavy consumption. These symptoms usually begin 48 to 96 hours after the person takes the last drink. They can become life-threatening and require immediate treatment. Common signs and symptoms of DTs are confusion, tremors, and hallucinations.

DEFENSE MECHANISMS

The inability to cope with stress threatens self-esteem, causing the person to act in protective ways. These actions are called **defense mechanisms**. The defense mechanisms temporarily reduce the stress, but do not resolve it.

Everyone uses defense mechanisms from time to time. Most people use a combination of defenses. People are usually unaware that they are behaving defensively. This behavior becomes harmful only when it is the major or sole means of coping with stress and the person avoids using problem-solving to respond to reality.

ASSISTING PATIENTS TO COPE

The nursing assistant can help patients become better able to cope and adapt by:

* Being a good listener.
* Trying to identify the source of stress so it can be removed.
* Being sensitive to body language that may give clues to the source of stress.
* Recognizing the patient as a unique individual and treating him or her with respect.
* Trying to understand the patient's point of view without passing judgment.
* Showing that you are dependable and respect the patient's privacy and feelings.
* Being supportive (Figure 30-8).

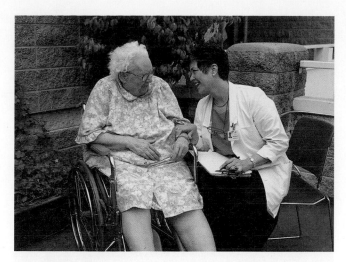

FIGURE 30-8 Be supportive while the patient works through her problem. (© Delmar/Cengage Learning)

THE DEMANDING PATIENT

In every nursing care situation, you will meet patients who are very demanding. This can be a difficult experience for everyone if it is not handled correctly.

Being demanding is a coping behavior that some patients use when they are frustrated. Persons who are very demanding are usually feeling as if they have lost control. To be successful in caring for these patients, the nursing assistant can use several tactics:

* Reassure the patient that you understand the complaint or problem and will report it to the appropriate person.
* If the complaints are about care given by others, remain neutral and do not criticize other workers. If complaints are about your care, listen, but do not argue or become defensive.
* Attempt to determine the cause of unjustified complaints and correct it, if possible.
* Try to identify the triggers of the demanding behavior.
* Show that you care, but control your emotions.

* Support the patient; be a good listener and be sensitive to the patient's body language.
* Provide opportunities for the patient to regain some control.
* Encourage and allow the patient to make decisions about things that affect him or her.
* Be consistent in the manner of care.
* Do not take the patient's demands personally.
* Stop and check on the patient without being asked.
* Keep your promises.
* Report observations to the nurse with suggestions for changes in the care plan.

MALADAPTIVE BEHAVIORS

Mental illness or **maladaptive behavior** occurs when behaviors and responses disrupt the person's ability to function smoothly within the family, environment, or community. Avoid labeling anyone as mentally ill. Even when an official diagnosis of mental illness has been made, avoid stereotyping the person. Note and report any unusual behavior or symptoms. Be objective and do not make judgments. Blaming and judging a patient is not helpful.

Evaluating the Patient's Behavior

An initial assessment of the patient's mental and emotional state will be made by licensed personnel. You contribute to the nursing process through careful and sensitive objective observations. Report:

* Physical responses related to eating, personal hygiene, sleeping, participation in activities, or any strange or unusual behaviors.
* Emotional responses related to interactions between the patient and yourself or between the patient and other patients. Also report emotional outbursts and inappropriate responses.
* Patient behavior as it relates to judgment and affects memory, orientation, and comprehension.

Difficult SITUATIONS

Patients with coping and behavior problems usually have a behavior management care plan that lists steps to follow when certain problems are exhibited. Implement the plan in the order listed as soon as the behavior starts, before it is out of control. Modify your behavior in response to the patient's behavior by monitoring how the patient responds to you, then adjusting your approach. ■

Difficult SITUATIONS

Reward patients for positive behavior. Behavior that is rewarded is usually repeated. The goal is to show the patient a healthy way of directing energy. Verbal praise, positive feedback, and other signs of approval are rewards. Nonverbal rewards such as a hug, smile, or pat on the back may also be used, when appropriate. Snacks and privileges are sometimes used as rewards. ■

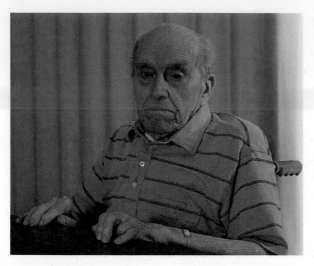

FIGURE 30-9 Disorientation is lack of awareness of time, place, or person. The patient may be oriented in one sphere, such as who he is, but not know the day, date, or where he is. (© *Delmar/Cengage Learning*)

Disorientation (Disordered Consciousness)

Disorientation is a condition in which a person shows a lack of reality awareness with regard to time, person, or place (Figure 30-9). It may be mild or severe, temporary or prolonged. The person has impaired judgment, memory, and understanding.

Delirium is an acute confusional state caused by reversible medical problems. It is often hard to tell whether a person is disoriented, has delirium, or both. Delirium is common in elderly persons as a result of medical problems such as infection and dehydration. Anesthesia, some medications, and uncorrected vision or hearing may cause the patient to misinterpret the environment. Delirium goes away when the physical and mental triggers of the problem are identified and eliminated. This can be confusing, because delirium often has multiple causes. All must be treated before the mental status returns to baseline.

Nursing Assistant Responsibilities

People with disorientation and delirium are not responsible for their actions, and cannot protect themselves. The patient's sensory problems (delusions or hallucinations) may put others at risk. *Protecting the patients is the most important nursing responsibility.*

Assist disoriented patients with reality orientation activities (Figure 30-10). **Reality orientation** (Unit 31) involves making the patient aware of person, place, and time by visual reminders, activities, and verbal cues. This approach reduces agitation in some patients, but increases agitation in others. Follow the care plan and the nurse's instructions.

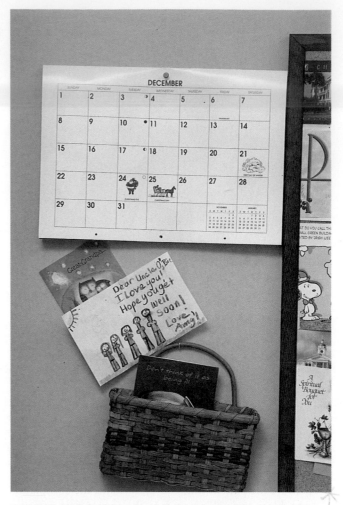

FIGURE 30-10 Calendars, clocks, and current magazines and newspapers may help maintain orientation in some patients. (© *Delmar/Cengage Learning*)

Reminiscing is an approach you may see listed on the care plans of some patients. **Reminiscing** (remembering past experiences) is a natural activity for people of all ages. We reminisce when we see old friends or get together with families.

Validation therapy is a technique that maintains dignity by acknowledging the patient's memories and feelings. It involves encouraging patients to express their feelings, and reassuring the patient that their feelings are worthwhile. When the patient describes an emotion, assure him or her that it is okay.

Your facility will teach you how to provide reality orientation, reminiscing, and validation therapy if you will be using these techniques in patient care. You may also wish to review the information on managing behavior problems, sleeping problems, dementia, aggression, yelling and calling out, sexual behavior problems, wandering, reality orientation, reminiscence, and validation therapy in the Online Companion to this book.

Table 30-4 lists observations to make of patient behaviors. Report your observations to the nurse.

TABLE 30-4 BEHAVIOR OBSERVATIONS
TO MAKE AND REPORT

- Always report abnormal behavior to the nurse, even if you believe that the behavior is "normal for the patient."
- Who? Does the behavior involve another person or specific types of people? How are these individuals alike?
- What? Describe the behavior. What were the circumstances in which the behavior occurred?
- Where? Did the behavior occur in one specific location?
- When? What is the time of day? Does the behavior occur at predictable times or in predictable situations, such as during bathing? When the patient is tired, when the patient awakens, etc.?
- What were the environmental conditions? Was it light, dark, hot, cold, noisy, quiet?
- How do others respond to the patient's behavior? Is there anyone who is never approached by the patient? If so, how does this person manage or prevent the behavior?
- Is there a pattern to the behavior? Can you identify clues or signals that the behavior is about to begin?

PROFESSIONAL BOUNDARIES

As a nursing assistant, you must stay within certain **professional boundaries** in the care of each patient. *Boundaries* are unspoken limits on your physical and emotional relationship with patients. It takes good judgment and experience to identify boundaries and keep from crossing them. Boundaries are like traveling from town to town on a one-way street. You cannot see a line marking when you leave one town and enter another. Once you have crossed the line, though, turning around on the one-way street is impossible. Learn how to identify boundaries and avoid crossing them.

Ethical Behavior with Patients and Families

As a nursing assistant, patients expect you to act in their best interests and treat them with dignity. You do this by not taking advantage of a patient's situation and by avoiding inappropriate involvement in the patient's personal and family relationships. Some relationships with patients and families are not healthy. It is not always easy to recognize unhealthy relationships until it is too late. Strive to keep your relationships professional. Actively work to find a balance in your relationships with patients and families. If any of the following occur, you are probably crossing professional boundaries and may be in a relationship danger zone:

- Discussing your personal problems with the patient or his or her family members

- Being flirtatious with a patient, including using sexual innuendoes, telling jokes that are sexual in nature, or using offensive language
- Discussing your feelings of sexual attraction with a patient
- Feeling that you may become involved in a sexual relationship with the patient
- Keeping secrets with a patient and becoming defensive when someone questions your relationship or involvement in the patient's personal life
- Thinking that you are immune from having an unhealthy relationship with a patient
- Believing that you are the only nursing assistant who can meet the patient's needs
- Spending an inappropriate amount of time with the patient, including off-duty visits or trading assignments with others to be with the patient
- Reporting only partial information about the patient to the nurse, because you fear disclosing unfavorable information or secrets the patient has told you
- Feeling that you must protect the patient from other workers and always siding with the patient's position

If you have trouble staying objective, or think you may cross a boundary, seek help from the nurse, your clergy-person, or another professional person whom you trust.

Consequences of Boundary Violations

Boundary violations lead to inappropriate relationships. These cloud your clinical judgment, and often carry over into your personal life. The improper relationship may cause you to do things that you would not ordinarily do (such as stealing from your employer). There are many serious personal, legal, and professional consequences to inappropriate relationships. For your own well-being, be aware that professional boundaries exist, and actively take steps to keep from crossing them.

Enabling *: Don't make promise you can't keep.*

Enabling behavior is a method of shielding a patient from the consequences of his or her behavior. Enabling differs from helping because it allows the patient to be irresponsible. By respecting professional boundaries, you will avoid helping others inappropriately. Enabling behavior causes dependency rather than moving the patient toward independence and good mental health. Strive to keep your behavior in the zone of helpfulness (Figure 30-11) to avoid crossing professional boundaries and enabling patients.

You will find additional information about communicating with patients who have mental health problems and other special needs in Units 7 and 31, as well as in the Online Companion to this book.

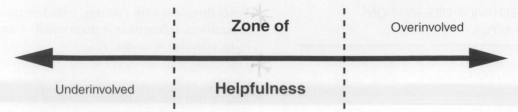

FIGURE 30-11 Keep your relationship with patients and families in the zone of helpfulness. (© *Delmar/Cengage Learning*)

GUIDELINES *for*

Assisting Patients Who Have Behavior Problems

- Follow the care plan.
- Control your own responses and reactions.
- Be a good communicator.
- Practice empathy.
- Avoid lying to the patient.
- Avoid making promises you cannot keep.
- Do not give a patient false hope.
- Avoid making a patient feel as if her problems, feelings, or hopes are unimportant.
- Avoid discussing facility or staff problems with the patient.
- Protect the safety of the patient and others.
- Follow the care plan when the target behavior starts.
- Attempt to learn the cause (trigger) of the behavior, and remove it if known.

- Inform others know if you discover an approach that works.
- Modify your own behavior in response to the patient's behavior.
- Watch the patient's response to your approaches. Adjust your approach, if necessary.
- Meet the patient's physical needs. Anticipate needs for patients who cannot communicate.
- Give patients as much control as possible. Offer choices in care and routines. Encourage patients to direct their own care.
- Be patient. Make sure your body language does not send the wrong message.
- Be happy. Smile. Positive behavior is contagious.

REVIEW

A. Multiple Choice

Select the one best answer for each of the following.

1. The patient is depressed. You can best help him by
   a. pitying him.
   b. keeping him from interacting with others.
   c. agreeing that he probably deserves the way he feels.
   d. stressing his continued value to society.

2. Professional boundaries
   a. apply only to licensed nursing personnel.
   b. involve assisting patients with activities of daily living.
   c. are set out in the job description.
   d. are unspoken limits on relationships with patients.

3. Enabling behavior
   a. is used when caring for patients who require total care.
   b. shields an individual from the consequences of his or her actions.
   c. involves orienting patients to person, place, and time.
   d. is used to help patients relieve stress.

4. Purging behavior is
   a. self-induced vomiting.
   b. refusing to eat.
   c. exercising vigorously.
   d. a form of substance abuse.

5. Substance abusers use alcohol or drugs to
   a. relieve chronic pain.
   b. alter their mood.
   c. get back at family members.
   d. treat medical problems under physician supervision.

6. An unfounded, recurring fear that causes the person to feel panic is a/an
   a. obsession.
   b. phobia.
   c. compulsion.
   d. delusion.

7. Patients with borderline personality disorder are often
   a. manipulative.
   b. depressed.
   c. compulsive.
   d. delusional.

8. The most common functional disorder in older people is
   a. agitation.
   b. delirium. — dehydration
   c. dementia.
   d. depression.

9. Which of the following patients is at high risk of suicide?
   a. A new mother who is feeling overwhelmed
   b. The 30-year-old who was just told that he has HIV
   c. The 53-year-old with chronic, unrelieved pain
   d. A 45-year-old female who has never married

10. DTs are a problem that is seen in
    a. obsessive-compulsive disorder.
    b. withdrawal from alcohol.
    c. depressed patients.
    d. drug overdose.

B. Nursing Assistant Challenge

You are assigned to care for Mr. Simonson, who was recently diagnosed with diabetes. He is a top executive in a large corporation and has a wife and three adult children. He is learning how to administer his insulin, how to plan his diet, and how to test his blood sugar. He has been very quiet and keeps his eyes closed most of the time, although he is not sleeping. One day, as you enter the room, he screams at you to get out and then picks up his water pitcher and throws it. Think of what you learned in this unit about human behavior as you consider these questions.

11. What examples of nonverbal communication is Mr. Simonson displaying? eyes are closed.

12. Do you think he is using defense mechanisms to cope with his diagnosis?

13. How can the nursing assistant show respect and concern for this patient?

Caring for Patients with Cognitive Impairment and Related Conditions

OBJECTIVES

After completing this unit, you will be able to:

- Spell and define terms.
- Describe the care of persons with mental retardation or developmental disability.
- List eight diseases that may cause dementia, and give an overview of each.

- List the stages of Alzheimer's disease and briefly describe each stage.
- Describe actions to use when working with persons who have dementia.
- Describe the management of patients who wander.

VOCABULARY

Learn the meaning and the correct spelling of the following words and phrases:

Alzheimer's disease
catastrophic reaction
cognitive impairment

dementia
developmental disability (DD)
eloping

mental retardation (MR)
sundowning

INTRODUCTION

The term **cognitive impairment** is used to describe changes in mental function caused by injury or disease. Some degree of cognitive impairment occurs in many different conditions. Persons who are cognitively impaired may have difficulty learning, processing, and remembering information. Their ability to plan and carry out activities of daily living is usually reduced. With some conditions, the person's short-term memory, intellectual capacity, and safety judgment are impaired.

PATIENTS WHO ARE MENTALLY RETARDED OR DEVELOPMENTALLY DISABLED

You will care for some patients who have been diagnosed with *mental retardation and developmental disability* (MRDD).

Patients with Mental Retardation

Mental retardation (MR) is a condition in which a person has lower-than-average intelligence. This condition causes the person to have limited ability to learn and social immaturity. Persons with this condition may be unable to care for themselves or live independently. Most can learn new things, but learning may take a long time.

Those who are severely retarded are usually cared for at home or a special facility for persons with similar problems. The current trend in health care is to place these individuals in homelike group settings, where four to six individuals live together with a caregiver. Over time, they learn skills that help them to function at their maximum potential. Although persons with mental retardation require lifelong care, many can feed, bathe, and dress themselves. Some are very high functioning and can go to work, use public transportation, and do many of the things that adults with normal mental functioning do each day.

Patients with Developmental Disability

Some patients have a **developmental disability (DD)**. This condition first occurs in the developmental period, which is before the age of 22. The person may have a physical impairment, mental impairment, or a combination of both. Some individuals are born with the condition, but others acquired their medical problems before the age of 22. For example, a child with a traumatic brain injury from an auto accident at age 7 may be considered developmentally disabled. Individuals with mental retardation or developmental disabilities may not be admitted to skilled nursing facilities unless their medical needs require skilled nursing care. If they do not require skilled care, they are usually admitted to special facilities that provide services to meet their highly individual needs and provide training in skills to make them as independent as possible.

Caring for Patients with Mental Retardation or Developmental Disability

Children and young adults with mental and physical problems often need the skills of an occupational therapist. Some need special teachers, but many go to regular schools. Those with highly specialized needs may have to go to a special school. Total independence is often not possible for some. Some will need help with activities of daily living throughout their lives. Care is designed to enhance self-esteem and provide the highest quality of life possible. Nursing assistant care for the patient with mental retardation or developmental disabilities includes:

- Ensuring a safe environment and teaching safety
- Providing information in a slow, simple manner
- Promoting self-esteem

- Being patient and repeating simple instructions as needed
- Assisting and supervising the patient with activities of daily living
- Using praise and rewards liberally
- Smiling and showing support and affection (as appropriate)

MENTAL CHANGES ASSOCIATED WITH AGING AND DISEASE

Mental decline is not a normal part of aging. However, the risk of mental deterioration increases with age. Mental decline may be the result of physical (organic) or emotional causes, or a combination of both. Periods of mental confusion are often temporary. They may be due to unusual stress, such as an infection; sudden injury, such as a fracture; or transfer to an unfamiliar environment. In some situations, the changes may signify a progressive deterioration of mental abilities. The term **dementia** refers to any disorder of the brain that causes deficits in thinking, memory, and judgment.

CARING FOR PATIENTS WHO HAVE DEMENTIA

You will care for many patients who have dementia (Figure 31-1). Dementia is not a disease in itself; rather, it is a group of symptoms caused by a number of different diseases. Recall that delirium is a temporary condition, usually caused by medical problems. Dementia is a permanent condition that is not related to acute physical

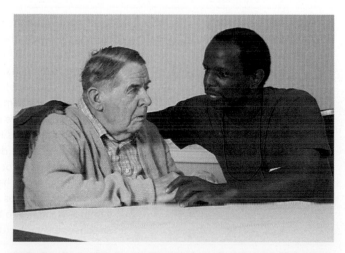

FIGURE 31-1 Persons with delirium develop confusion and decreased awareness of the environment. (© Delmar/Cengage Learning)

problems. Persons who have dementia may also develop delirium (Unit 30) when they become acutely ill. In such cases, their confusion worsens, but it returns to baseline when the problem is resolved. Unlike delirium, dementia progresses slowly, over a much longer period of time.

Alzheimer's disease is the most common form of dementia. Other types of dementia are listed in Table 31-1. The term *dementia* is used here when referring to symptoms, behavior, and nursing actions that are appropriate for people with any dementia. *Alzheimer's* is used when the information is specific to that dementia.

TABLE 31-1 DESCRIPTION OF MAJOR FORMS OF DEMENTIA

Disease	Features	Course
Alzheimer's disease (*Senile dementia* is an older term for this condition. Some professionals call this disorder "Senile Dementia, Alzheimer's Type [SDAT].")	The most common type of dementia. Lack of chemical in brain causes neurofibrillary tangles, neuritic plaques. The patient has progressive memory loss, behavioral changes, poor judgment, loss of abstract thinking ability. Eventually may cause loss of speech, loss of self-care ability, and apathy.	Onset age: 60–80 Slowly progressive and irreversible. Most people die within 4 to 6 years after diagnosis, but the illness can last from 3 to 20 years.
Vascular dementia (also called multi-infarct dementia)	Interference with blood circulation in brain cells due to arteriosclerosis or atherosclerosis. The most common form of dementia after Alzheimer's disease. Believed to be caused by a series of strokes. Each stroke involves a progressive mental decline. (For additional information, see Unit 37.)	Onset age: 55–70 Outcome depends on rate of damage to brain cells. People who have had a stroke have a 9 times greater risk of dementia compared with people who have not had a stroke. About 1 in 4 people who have had a stroke develop signs of dementia within 1 year.
Huntington's disease	Inherited from either parent who carries a gene for the disease. Causes progressive mental decline. (For additional information, see Unit 37.)	Onset age: 25–45 Average duration 15 years.
Lewy body dementia	Gets its name from the round nerve-cell deposits found in the brain after death. These are different from Alzheimer's deposits. Agitation, delusions, and problems with speech are early symptoms. Involves progressive mental decline, fluctuations in alertness and attention span, drowsiness, staring into space for long periods, and visual hallucinations. The person develops motor symptoms similar to those of Parkinson's disease (Unit 37).	Tends to develop later in life than other types of dementia, usually between the ages of 68 and 80.

TABLE 31-1 continued

Disease	Features	Course
Parkinson's disease	Deficiency of chemical in brain (dopamine). Causes progressive mental decline in some persons. Signs of dementia include memory loss, distractibility, slowed thinking, disorientation, confusion, moodiness, and lack of motivation. (For additional information, see Unit 37.)	Dementia affects approximately 20% of people who have Parkinson's, usually those who develop the condition after the age of 70. There is usually a delay of 10 to 15 years between the diagnosis and the onset of dementia. This condition is also caused by Lewy bodies, but they are in a different area of the brain than Lewy body dementia.
Tertiary syphilis	Untreated syphilis causes neurological problems as the spirochete (bacteria) causes brain damage. The internal organs are also affected. At this stage, the person cannot be cured.	Occurs 15–20 years after primary infection, but can occur as early as one year after infection in some people. Although the person is highly symptomatic, the condition is not contagious and only standard precautions are used.
Creutzfeldt-Jakob disease	A rare and incurable disorder that causes changes in the brain. Thought to be viral in origin for many years; now believed to be caused by prions (Unit 12). Harmless and infectious prions are nearly identical, but the infectious form has a folded appearance.	Onset age: 50–60 Rapidly progressive. About 90 percent of patients die within 1 year.
Prion diseases	The existence of prions was only recently discovered. *Prion* is an abbreviation for *proteinaceous infectious particle.* Prions may be ingested through infected food, such as meat. Much research is needed to identify factors that influence prion infectivity and determine how they cause brain damage. Researchers are also trying to identify risk factors for the condition and determine when in life the disease appears.	Usual onset age: 50–60 Rapidly progressive and incurable.

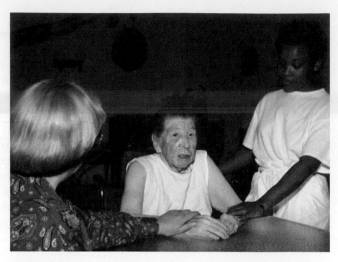

FIGURE 31-2 People with dementia exhibit indifference and loss of spontaneity. (© *Delmar/Cengage Learning*)

Alzheimer's Disease

Alzheimer's disease can begin during middle age, but is more common in older persons. It has been called a "slow death of the mind." The cause is not known. The disease affects people of all races, levels of intelligence, and education. It is progressive and cannot be cured. In the past, the term *senility* was used to describe these symptoms. We know now that this dementia is a disease of the brain cells and is not a normal part of aging.

Despite having a healthy appearance, persons with Alzheimer's have changes in the structure and function of the brain, which shrinks and becomes smaller. An autopsy performed after death reveals areas resembling spider webs, called *neuritic plaques* and *neurofibrillary tangles,* in the brain.

Alzheimer's disease generally has three main stages, with symptoms becoming progressively worse. These stages have been further divided into seven categories. However, there are many individual variables, and the course of the disease varies markedly from person to person. The symptoms progress in a general way, related to the underlying nerve cell degeneration that characterizes the condition. Damage begins with cells used for memory and learning and gradually spreads to brain cells that control behavior, thinking, and judgment. The best-learned skills tend to remain the longest. An English teacher, for example, may maintain verbal skills longer than usual. However, once a skill is lost, it is lost forever. As the disease progresses, the ability to speak deteriorates. The ability to walk is lost. In late stages, physical ability needed for daily life skills, coordination, and voluntary movement are also affected.

Stage I: Mild Dementia During the first stage, most people remain at home if they have a supportive family to provide assistance. They are usually physically capable and can attend to the activities of daily living with supervision. Characteristics of stage I include:

- Short-term memory loss
- Personality changes, with indifference and loss of spontaneity (Figure 31-2)

- Decreased ability to concentrate; shortened attention span
- Disorientation as to time and space
- Poor judgment
- Lack of safety awareness
- Carelessness in actions and appearance
- Anxiety, depression, and agitation
- Delusions of persecution—the person thinks that others are conspiring to do him harm
- Enough alertness to recognize that the person has a memory problem; may fabricate stories and make excuses to cover for memory loss

Stage II: Moderate Dementia Symptoms of this stage are:

- Increased short-term memory loss and deterioration of memory for remote events.
- Complete disorientation.
- Wandering and pacing.
- **Sundowning** (confusion and restlessness that occur during the late afternoon, evening, or night).
- Sensory/perceptual changes. The person becomes unable to recognize and use common objects, such as eating utensils, combs, and pencils. He or she cannot distinguish between right and left, up and down, hot and cold.
- Perseveration phenomena. *Perseveration* refers to repeating an action. Examples are repeating the same word or phrase, lip-licking, chewing, or finger-tapping.
- Problems with walking.
- Problems with speech, reading, writing.
- Incontinence of bowel and bladder.
- Catastrophic reactions, hallucinations, delusions. A **catastrophic reaction** is the response of a person with dementia to overwhelming stimuli (Figure 31-3).

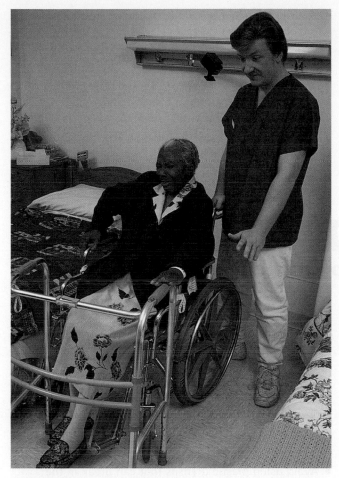

FIGURE 31-3 Catastrophic reactions can occur when the patient with dementia feels overwhelmed.
(© Delmar/Cengage Learning)

Most people with Alzheimer's are admitted to long-term care facilities during the second stage. Although they are healthy physically, they require constant care. Most families do not have the emotional resources and physical energy to cope. Wandering incontinence, and poor safety judgment are usually the problems that cause the family to seek outside care. Nevertheless, admission is often traumatic to families. Families are vital members of the interdisciplinary team. They can provide staff with insights about the patient and how to deal with the problems.

Stage III: Severe Dementia The person in Stage III:

- Is totally dependent
- Is verbally unresponsive
- May have seizures
- May refuse to eat and drink

In this stage, the ability to speak and swallow are lost, and the person is totally dependent. Caregivers must be compassionate, calm, and have a sense of humor. When you are caring for patients with dementia, remember to:

- Protect these patients from physical injury.
- Encourage independence for as long as possible.

- Support dignity and self-esteem.
- Maintain nutrition and hydration for as long as possible. Follow the care plan and the speech therapist's recommendations to prevent choking.

To meet these goals, the care must be consistent and structured with a flexible routine. Care should be given in an environment that is calm, quiet, and simple.

It is helpful to:

- Make eye contact.
- Be accepting of the patient without being judgmental or critical.
- Monitor your body language. Patients with dementia get clues from your body language. When this occurs, the patient's behavior tends to reflect the mood of the staff (Figure 31-4).
- Remember that when the ability to use speech is lost, communication occurs through nonverbal means.
- Biting, scratching, and kicking may be the only way the person can express displeasure.
- Use touch appropriately. However, avoid startling the patient. Make sure he or she knows you are approaching. Do not try to touch the patient if he or she is agitated. Surprising the patient with body contact can trigger a catastrophic reaction.

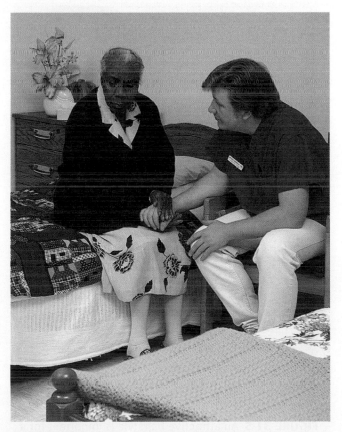

FIGURE 31-4 Patients who have dementia are in tune with the body language of the caregiver.
(© Delmar/Cengage Learning)

- Avoid using logic, reasoning, or lengthy explanations.
- Watch for facial expressions and body language for clues to the patient's feelings and moods.
- Learn what triggers agitation or anger. Work on preventing those situations.
- Use techniques of diversion and distraction. For example, calmly take the patient by the hand and walk together or direct the patient's attention to another activity. These techniques work well because of the shortened attention span.

- Realize that patients with dementia are not responsible for what they do or say.
  - Their behavior is not intentional, and they cannot change.
  - They lose the ability to control their impulses.
  - Avoid confrontations and always allow them to "save face"—that is, keep their dignity.
- No one really knows what is happening in the minds of people with dementia.

GUIDELINES *for*

Activities of Daily Living for Patients with Dementia

- Allow the patient to do as much as possible.
- Give only one short, simple direction at a time.
- Observe the patient's physical condition. People with dementia are usually unaware of signs of illness.
- Assist the patient to maintain a dignified, attractive appearance (Figure 31-5).
- Monitor food and fluid intake.

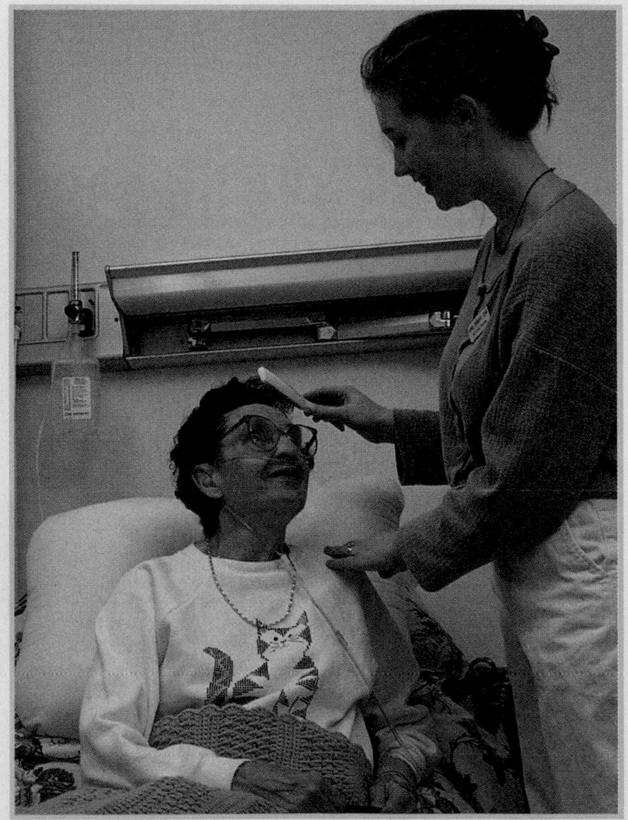

- Encourage and provide sufficient fluids to prevent dehydration.
- Offer the patient a drink each time you enter the room.
- Some patients do not like water, but will drink fruit juice, soda, or sugarless beverages. Provide fluids that the patient likes and will consume readily.
- Too many foods at once are confusing.
- Placing one food at a time in front of the patient may improve food acceptance.
- Avoid using plastic utensils that can break in the patient's mouth.
- Provide nutritious finger foods when the patient is unable to use utensils.
- Avoid pureed foods as long as possible.
- Check food temperatures (Figure 31-6). If the patient is a slow eater, you may have to reheat the food.
- Prepare foods for eating as needed by buttering bread, cutting meat, removing wrappers, and opening cartons.

FIGURE 31-5 An attractive hairstyle is important for a patient's self-esteem. (© *Delmar/Cengage Learning*)

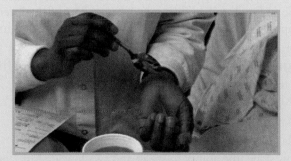

FIGURE 31-6 Serve foods promptly to maintain temperature. Check hot food temperature by dropping a small amount on your wrist. (© *Delmar/Cengage Learning*)

GUIDELINES *continued*

- Check the patient's mouth after eating. "Squirreling" food (hoarding food in the cheeks) can cause aspiration.
- Weigh patients regularly to identify patterns of weight gain or loss.
- Keep the dining area quiet and calm.
- Patients with dementia eventually lose bowel and bladder continence. Taking them to the bathroom regularly helps them remain dry and maintains dignity.
- Patients with dementia need activities geared to their abilities.
- Avoid large groups or competitive activities.
- In later stages, use sensory stimulation with quiet music, soft touching, and calm talk.
- Holding puppies or kittens (pet therapy) often brings pleasure to severely impaired patients.
- Provide daily exercise according to the care plan and the patients' habits and abilities (Figure 31-7).

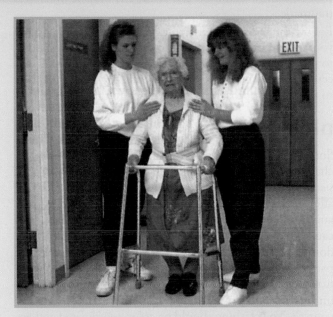

FIGURE 31-7 Daily exercise is important to maintain physical health and well-being. (*© Delmar/Cengage Learning*)

SPECIAL PROBLEMS

Patients who have dementia often present problems different from those of other patients. Procedures and activities that are normal for and acceptable to other patients may frighten or upset a patient with dementia.

Problems with Bathing

Resistance to bathing is common in patients with dementia. The patient may have forgotten the purpose of bathing, or may resist removing clothing. They may misinterpret your assistance as a sexual assault. Staff may label this behavior "uncooperative," "combative," or "aggressive" when in fact the patient is just using normal defense mechanisms. The behavior may worsen if the patient's requests to stop are ignored. Try to view the procedure from the patient's perspective. Observe and listen to the patient's verbal and nonverbal behavior.

If a patient steadfastly refuses a bath, consider whether it is really necessary to bathe the patient in this way at this time. Return and try again later, or consult the nurse. Try to avoid agitating the patient further. Consider a different method of bathing, such as using a towel bath or bag bath (Unit 24). Modify the environment so it is comfortable and pleasurable, and be flexible in your approach to and communication with the patient.

Prepare the tub room before attempting to bathe a patient with dementia. Your best approach is to be sure the room is warm, quiet, and private. Monitor for equipment noises, such as from the whirlpool, heater, or running water. Sound tends to echo in shower and tub rooms, and this may frighten or agitate the patient. Some are afraid of water. Encouraging the patient to sing an old song with you or playing pleasant music may help. (You may also use a special battery-operated shower radio, or a regular radio if you keep the plug away from sources of water.)

Patients in the early stages of Alzheimer's disease may also be sensitive with an unfamiliar nursing assistant. Wrapping a towel or bath blanket around the shoulders and pinning it securely may help with modesty problems. Leave it in place during the bath. Dementia causes problems with sensation, so bathing may be uncomfortable. A person with Alzheimer's may not be able to identify the warm, comfortable sensation. Say something like, "This feels good." Bathing is a complex task involving many steps. Explain what you are going to do and what you want the patient to do, one step at a time. Avoid giving too many directions at once, which may overwhelm the patient and trigger a catastrophic reaction. Giving the patient a washcloth or sponge to occupy the hands may be helpful. Taking a bath may simply be too overwhelming for an Alzheimer's patient. You may have to use creative alternatives (Unit 24).

Washing the hair may also be frightening. Use the patient's responses to guide your actions. Washing the hair in the sink or using a shampoo cap (Unit 24) may be much less traumatic.

Follow the bathing instructions on the care plan. Modify your behavior and care according to the patient's responses to the procedure. Be slow, calm, and reassuring. Share successful approaches with the nurse and other team members so that these approaches can be added to the care plan.

Dressing Problems

Some patients with dementia are resistant to dressing or changing clothes. As with bathing, they may view your assistance as a form of assault. Others remove their clothing after they are dressed. Keep the morning routine consistent and familiar. Once you start, avoid interruptions, which cause the patient to forget what she is supposed to be doing. Make sure the room is warm and private. Ask the patient to select clothing by giving her a choice between two outfits. More than this may be overwhelming. If making decisions overwhelms the patient, select the clothes yourself. The clothing should be color-coordinated and appropriate for the patient's age and the season. Lay out clothing in the order in which it will be put on. Break the task down into simple, manageable steps and give the patient easy instructions, one step at a time. Assist with dressing, if needed. Allow the patient to do as much for herself as possible, but intervene promptly if she starts to become frustrated.

Understand the patient's need for privacy and unwillingness to disrobe in front of you. Be sensitive to grooming issues and encourage the patient to comb hair, shave, or wear cosmetics and jewelry. Praise the patient and compliment her appearance.

Sexual Behavior

Sexuality is a basic human need. It does not diminish with age. Sexual expression may be physical or psychological. Maintaining an attractive appearance is one way of expressing one's sexuality. Some people may touch certain areas of their bodies because doing so results in pleasurable sensations. Many health care workers feel that masturbation is inappropriate behavior. However, masturbation is satisfying to the patient and is not harmful. It is an acceptable behavior as long as it is done in a private area. Always knock before entering a patient's room and wait for a response before entering. If you enter a patient's room and find the patient masturbating, provide privacy and leave the room.

If you enter a room and find two consenting adults engaged in a sexual act, provide privacy and leave. Adults have a legal right to do whatever is pleasing to them, as long as it is not medically contraindicated and both partners are mentally capable of consent. Do not pass judgment on the patient's choice of partner or methods of sexual expression.

Facility staff is responsible for protecting patients who are physically or mentally vulnerable to unwanted sexual contact. Sexual contact with unwilling, alert persons who are physically unable to defend themselves, or with confused patients who cannot give full informed consent, is sexual abuse. Sexual abuse is a violation of the patient's rights and is illegal. No health care worker, resident, visitor, or other person may sexually abuse others. If sexual abuse occurs, the police are notified. Anyone who sexually harasses or abuses a patient or care provider should be reported to the nurse, manager, or other appropriate person.

Sometimes patients make unwanted sexual advances toward the nursing assistant. The patient's desire for sexuality is normal, but the choice of partner is not. Evaluate the situation to determine whether the patient is misinterpreting your use of touch. If a patient makes sexual advances, do not ridicule or belittle him or her. Be calm, understanding, and matter-of-fact. Tactfully inform the patient that the behavior is not acceptable. Follow your facility policy for reporting sexual advances.

Disrobing

Sometimes mentally confused patients disrobe in public areas. When in bed, they may remove the covers many times each day, exposing themselves to anyone who looks in the door. This sight is offensive to adults, and can be traumatic to a young child who is visiting. It is your responsibility to keep the patients covered. This may be a difficult task. As with all other behavior problems, look for a cause. Common causes of disrobing are boredom, need to use the bathroom, being tired and ready for bed, uncomfortable clothing, and very warm room temperature. Evaluate the situation and common triggers. Sometimes there is no apparent cause, but rule out all logical triggers before arriving at this conclusion.

You cannot put a patient's clothing on backward to keep him or her from disrobing. Consult the care plan and nurse about approaches to use. Find out whether tying the sheet to the side rails of the bed constitutes a restraint. Tying a sheet to the bed or chair is usually considered a restraint, but wrapping it around the patient's body only, then tying it in back, may be effective. If the sheet does not limit the patient's movement or access to his own body, it is not a restraint. Monitor the patient who disrobes frequently and do your best to keep him or her covered.

Wandering and Pacing

Patients with Alzheimer's may wander or pace for hours at a time (Figure 31-8). The patient may repeatedly try to leave the facility. No one knows why this occurs. The patient may not know where he is, but knows he does not want to be there. He is seeking a state of mind, not a physical location. Ask the patient the intended destination. A man may tell you he is going to work. A woman may

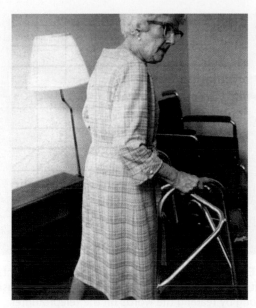

FIGURE 31-8 Some patients with Alzheimer's disease wander continually. They must be reminded to rest, to eat, and to drink. (© Delmar/Cengage Learning)

say she is going home to cook dinner for the children. Avoid arguing or providing reality orientation, which will agitate the patient. Instead, talk about the patient's activities, work, meal preparation, or cooking. Make comments such as, "That must be very interesting work," or "You must be a very good cook." Ask the patient about his former work routines. Ask what the patient likes to cook, what foods are family favorites, and other related questions. This restores the state of mind the patient seeks, reducing stress and the risk of **eloping** (wandering away from the facility).

Triggers of Wandering Many different things trigger wandering behavior. The facility may keep a log to help identify the patient's wandering triggers. You will record information such as the patient's behavior, staff on duty, and temperature and noise in the environment on the log. The nurse will use this important information to develop a plan of care. Several studies have shown that a noisy environment increases wandering. Health care facilities can be very noisy at times (Unit 10). Loud talking, using the intercom, loud televisions, and persons yelling or calling out for help can be very upsetting to wanderers. Hot or cold environmental temperature may also be a problem. If patients are uncomfortable, they may wander to escape.

Nursing Assistant Approaches Seeing items associated with going outdoors may also trigger wandering. Remove purses, hats, coats, shoes, or other outerwear from sight. Allow the patient to wander. Using restraints increases anxiety and frustration, worsening the problem. Walk with the patient and subtly guide her to circle back. Adapt the environment so it is safe and secure. Keeping the patient's stress as low as possible is important because if he feels overwhelmed, he may wander to elope.

Thinking is a very complex process. If someone tells you *not to think* of a purple dog, you will think of it, then have to unthink it. "Unthinking" is much more complex, especially for a patient who is cognitively impaired. Avoid saying, "Don't go outside," or "Don't go in that room," because that will cause the patient to think about doing exactly what you told him not to. A better approach is to say, "Stay inside," or "Stay here." Communication is best if it is concrete and does not require abstract thinking.

Avoid forcing your own agenda on the patient, which will cause agitation and worsen the behavior. Instead, use gentle persuasion (Figure 31-9). Avoid making too many demands during direct care and assistance with activities of daily living (ADLs). Keep instructions simple and brief. As the patient completes one task, give her another. Be patient, calm, and reassuring. Tell the patient that she is in the right place, safe, and you will help her. Compliment her on her successes, even if they are small. The patient will probably not remember the compliment, but will feel good about herself. She will be more cooperative and less likely to act out or wander.

There is no single effective approach for all wandering behavior. Use the strategies listed here and see if they work. If you discover an effective approach, inform the nurse so he or she can add it to the care plan. Try the approaches you learned in Unit 30. Remember that identifying and modifying the patient's agenda, feelings, and unmet needs will usually modify or stop the behavior.

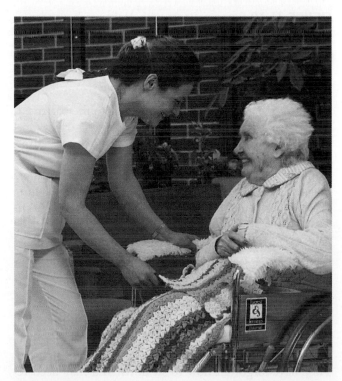

FIGURE 31-9 A friendly smile and a gentle touch are very persuasive, and many patients with dementia will respond to the smile. (© Delmar/Cengage Learning)

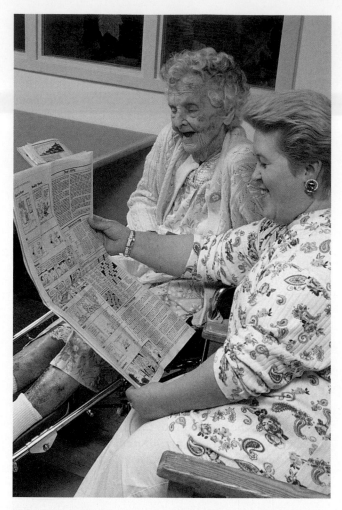

FIGURE 31-10 Some patients with Alzheimer's wander in their wheelchairs. Distracting such a patient with a newspaper will provide an opportunity to rest. (© Delmar/Cengage Learning)

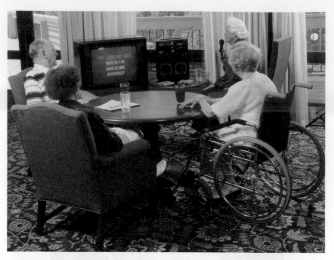

FIGURE 31-11 Singing is an activity that most patients with dementia thoroughly enjoy. They can listen to the music or sing along by reading the words on the teleprompter. (Courtesy of Briggs Corporation, Des Moines, IA; (800) 247–2343)

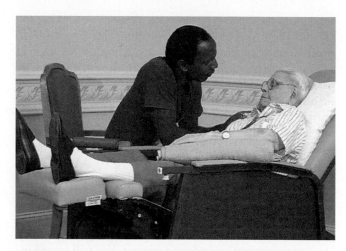

FIGURE 31-12 Some patients wander until they are physically exhausted. Seating the patient in a recliner enables him to rest. (© Delmar/Cengage Learning)

Effective management is individualized to the patient. It is often the result of trial and error. As a rule, try to meet the patient's needs relating to hunger, thirst, and elimination first. Consider whether he is having pain, and inform the nurse. Try distraction, such as by providing a magazine, newspaper, book, or picture album (Figure 31-10). Take the patient to activities that he or she enjoys (Figure 31-11). If you meet the need, the wandering will cease.

Remember that patients who wander will burn extra calories and are at risk for weight loss. Some are so busy wandering that they will not sit long enough to eat a meal. Give them finger foods and walk with them, if necessary. Follow the care plan to ensure that the patient takes in enough nutrients.

Patients who wander may become physically exhausted. They have forgotten how to sit down and may need reminders. Special reclining chairs (Figure 31-12) and bean-bag-type chairs may be used to allow patients to rest. Again, the care plan will specify the method to use.

Agitation, Anxiety, and Catastrophic Reactions

Agitation and anxiety are shown by an increase in physical activity, such as pacing, or the perseveration behaviors described for Stage II. If appropriate interventions are not implemented in time, a catastrophic reaction will likely occur. When agitation or catastrophic reactions occur:

- Do not use physical restraints or force to subdue the patient. This increases agitation and can result in injury to the patient or staff.
- Avoid having several staff persons approach the patient at the same time. This is frightening. The patient may react violently.

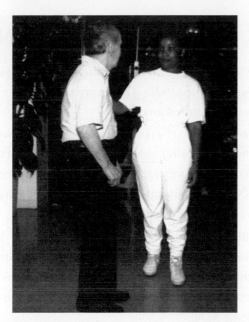

FIGURE 31-13 Your demeanor has a powerful effect on patients with dementia. Approach the patient slowly, calmly, and in a nonthreatening manner. *(© Delmar/Cengage Learning)*

- Use a soft, calm voice. Do not try to reason with the patient. Using touch may or may not be appropriate (Figure 31-13). Some patients respond to smooth stroking of the arms or back with lotion. Others may strike out if they are already agitated when they are touched.

Sundowning

Sundowning is increased confusion, restlessness, and wandering during the late afternoon, evening, or night. It is sometimes prevented by avoiding too much activity before bedtime and by establishing a consistent bedtime routine. Provide a light bedtime snack that is easily chewed and digested (Figure 31-14). Take patients to the bathroom before putting them in bed for the night. Check the lighting. Shadows and reflections are disturbing. If the patient awakens during the night, repeat the bedtime routine. If this is ineffective and the patient does not remain in bed, try a recliner or Alzheimer's chair.

Pillaging and Hoarding

Pillaging (taking possession of items) and hoarding (saving or stockpiling multiple items) do not present a major problem unless patients collect items from other patients' rooms or hide things that are difficult to find. This patient usually believes that he is in his own home, and he can explore and take whatever he wants because everything in the "house" belongs to him. The patient has very poor safety awareness and is at high risk of injury from entering housekeeping closets and service areas

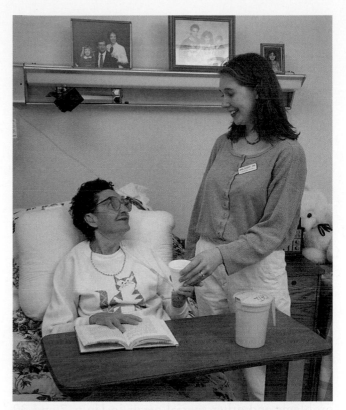

FIGURE 31-14 Provide light foods, such as graham crackers or plain vanilla wafers and juice if the patient wants a bedtime snack. *(© Delmar/Cengage Learning)*

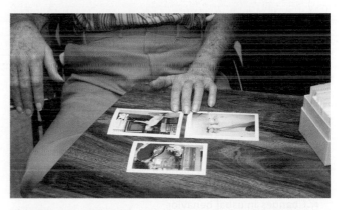

FIGURE 31-15 Patients with dementia retain long-term memory even though short-term memory is lost. Looking at family pictures is an excellent way to reminisce. *(© Delmar/Cengage Learning)*

and ingesting chemicals or becoming injured by sharp objects. Others may harm this patient, such as by hitting him, because they believe that he is stealing their belongings. Check the room daily for stale food and items belonging to others. Keep the patient's hands busy. Activities like folding washcloths, "fiddling" with keys on a ring, clipping coupons, or sorting junk mail may help. Provide a dresser, nightstand, suitcase, or box in the hallway with items that he can safely rummage through. Try distracting the patient with pictures (Figure 31-15).

Clinical Information ALERT

You may also wish to review the information on managing behavior problems, problems sleeping, dementia, aggression, yelling and calling out, sexual behavior problems, wandering, reality orientation, reminiscence, and validation therapy in the Online Companion to this book. ■

OBSERVATIONS

Your observations are critically important in the care of patients who have cognitive impairment, both for improved care and sharing with the rest of the health care team. Table 31-2 lists some that should always be reported to the nurse.

You will find additional information about communicating with patients who have mental health problems and other special needs in Units 7 and 30 of this book, as well as in the Online Companion to this book.

TABLE 31-2 OBSERVATIONS TO MAKE AND REPORT ABOUT PATIENTS WITH COGNITIVE IMPAIRMENT

- Change in consciousness, awareness, or alertness
- Changes in mood, behavior, or emotional status
- Changes in orientation to person, place, time, season
- Change in communication
- Changes in ability to respond verbally or nonverbally
- Changes in memory
- Changes in usual behavior
- Increasing agitation
- Excessive drowsiness; sleepiness for no apparent reason
- Sudden onset of wandering, worsening of wandering, or trying to leave facility
- Refusal of food or fluids
- New onset of incontinence or change in usual pattern of incontinence
- Loss of ability to recognize familiar persons
- Sudden onset of mental confusion (or worsening confusion)
- Abnormal vital signs
- Signs or symptoms of illness or infection

Difficult SITUATIONS

The Velveteen Rabbit is a children's story that was copyrighted in 1922. This is a conversation between two stuffed animals:

"What is REAL?" asked the Rabbit one day, when they were lying side by side near the nursery fender, before Nana came to tidy the room. "Does it mean having things that buzz inside you and a stick-out handle?"

"REAL isn't how you are made," said the Skin Horse. "It's a thing that happens to you. When a child loves you for a long, long time, not just to play with, but REALLY loves you, then you become REAL."

"Does it hurt?" asked the Rabbit.

"Sometimes," said the Skin Horse, for he was always truthful. "When you are REAL you don't mind being hurt."

"Does it happen all at once, like being wound up," he asked, "or bit by bit?"

"It doesn't happen all at once, like being wound up," said the Skin Horse. "You become. It takes a long time. . . . Generally, by the time you are REAL, most of your hair has been loved off, and your eyes drop out and you get loose in the joints and very shabby. But these things don't matter at all, because once you are REAL you can't be ugly, except to people who don't understand."

There is a lesson for all health care workers in this old children's story. The patients entrusted to your care may be loose in the joints and shabby in appearance, but they have shaped the communities and the world in which we live. They have families and others who love and value them just as they are: shabby, balding, hard of hearing, slow, confused, even combative. They are worth your investment, even if they do not always appreciate it. They are REAL. ■

Bianco, Margery Williams. (1880–1944). The Velveteen Rabbit. Not copyrighted in the United States. Electronic copy courtesy of Project Gutenberg Literary Archive Foundation. http://www.gutenberg.org/etext/23980.

REVIEW

A. Multiple Choice

Select the one best answer for each of the following.

1. Which statement is true of catastrophic reactions?
   a. They are unavoidable in patients with dementia.
   b. They may be precipitated by too much sensory stimulation.
   c. Providing activity will subdue the catastrophic reaction.
   d. They are always expressions of violence.

2. An 89-year-old patient tells you that her grandmother visited today. Your best response is to
   a. tell her the grandmother died years ago.
   b. change the subject as quickly as possible.
   c. tell her the visitor was a staff person.
   d. ask if she is thinking about her grandmother.

3. A patient tells you she is going home to prepare dinner for her children, then proceeds to go toward the front door. Your best response is to walk with her and say
   a. "Don't go outside."
   b. "Your children live in another state."
   c. "Stay inside. What do you like to cook?"
   d. "Your children are spending the night at a friend's house."

4. Dementia is
   a. a symptom, not a disease.
   b. the result of mental illness.
   c. a temporary condition.
   d. the result of physical illness.

5. Alzheimer's disease is
   a. never seen in middle-aged adults.
   b. a progressive condition.
   c. a genetic disorder.
   d. most common in men.

6. A person in the first stage of Alzheimer's disease
   a. will not recognize her relatives.
   b. will have seizures and weight loss.
   c. displays perseveration phenomena.
   d. may try to cover the memory loss.

7. A whirlpool bath
   a. is soothing and refreshing to a patient with Alzheimer's disease.
   b. is the preferred method of bathing for patients with dementia.

   c. may frighten some individuals who have Alzheimer's disease.
   d. will increase confusion because of the high water temperature.

8. When assisting a patient who has Alzheimer's with dressing,
   a. take the patient to the closet and have her select the clothes.
   b. lay out clothing in the order in which it will be used.
   c. give the patient a series of instructions before beginning.
   d. put the shoes on first to reduce the risk of agitation.

9. When caring for a patient who disrobes frequently,
   a. put the clothes on backwards, making them hard to remove.
   b. turn the air conditioner up so the patient is too cold to disrobe.
   c. evaluate the environmental temperature to see if it is too warm.
   d. tie a sheet to the rails to keep the patient in bed and prevent exposure.

10. A patient with Alzheimer's disease who wanders is probably
   a. looking for a state of mind.
   b. trying to find her family.
   c. looking for her clothing.
   d. trying to go home.

B. Nursing Assistant Challenge

Mr. Wardlaw is one of your assigned patients. He is in the second stage of Alzheimer's disease, and keeps setting off the door alarm. He says he must go rewire his house so it does not burn down. Your unit is very busy. To make matters worse, you are short one nursing assistant, and you fear Mr. Wardlaw will elope.

11. What is your best immediate response to keep Mr. Wardlaw in the building?

12. Should restraints be used to keep this patient safe?

13. How will you reduce Mr. Wardlaw's agitation?

14. What will you do to ensure that someone monitors Mr. Wardlaw while you are giving a complete bath to another patient?

UNIT 32

Caring for the Bariatric Patient

OBJECTIVES

After completing this unit, you will be able to:

- Spell and define terms.
- Define the terms *overweight, obesity,* and *morbid obesity,* and explain how these conditions differ from each other.
- Explain why weight affects life span (longevity) and health.
- Define comorbidities and explain how they affect a person's health.

- Describe nursing assistant actions and observations related to the care of patients of size.
- Explain why environmental modifications are needed for bariatric patient care.
- Describe observations to make and methods of meeting bariatric patients' ADL needs.
- List precautions to take when moving and positioning bariatric patients.

VOCABULARY

Learn the meaning and the correct spelling of the following words and phrases:

advocate	comorbidities	obesity	pannus
bariatrics	ideal body weight (IBW)	overweight	
body mass index (BMI)	morbid obesity	panniculus	

INTRODUCTION

Being **overweight** (Figure 32-1) is a condition in which a person weighs more than he or she should, according to standards based on height and bone (frame) size. When a person is overweight, he or she weighs more than is considered desirable or medically advisable.

Obesity is a very misunderstood disease. Definitions vary, but most experts consider **obesity** being overweight by 20% to 30% of the ideal body weight. It is a complex condition with many causes. Heredity may account for up to 70% of all weight problems. Some experts believe that the

hormones used in production of our meat supply are also affecting the humans who consume the meat.

Environmental factors are also very important. Obesity negatively affects every system of the body and increases the risk for many other serious medical conditions and diseases. Untreated, it results in a shorter life span.

In addition to health risks, obese persons often experience emotional problems, including depression; low self-esteem; social isolation; and affective, anxiety, substance abuse, and eating disorders (see Unit 30). Experts believe that society's treatment of and response to obese persons increases their risk for emotional problems. Overweight people often feel

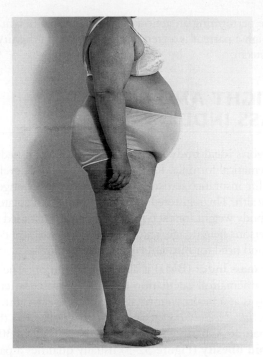

FIGURE 32-1 Obesity is a very misunderstood condition, in which the person is 20 to 30% above ideal body weight. Heredity may account for up to 70% of all weight problems. *(Courtesy of the Armed Forces Institute of Pathology)*

TABLE 32-1 GENERAL NURSING ASSISTANT OBSERVATIONS TO MAKE AND REPORT RELATED TO THE CARE OF BARIATRIC PATIENTS

- Skin problems, rashes, red areas in skin folds
- Open areas
- Weeping skin
- Wounds that do not heal
- Pain
- Apathy or signs of depression
- Binging, purging, and other behaviors for dietary regulation
- Excessive thirst
- Unexplained weakness
- Increased urination
- Hypoventilation (shallow breathing)
- Respiratory distress
- Unexplained hypoxia (pulse oximeter values below 90; see Unit 36)
- Rapid respirations
- Complaint of chest pain or discomfort
- Dyspnea
- Sleep apnea
- Complaints of heartburn or esophageal reflux
- Change in leg color, sensation, swelling, and temperature
- Change in patient's ability to move legs
- Signs of fatigue, becoming quieter, lethargy, progressive sleepiness

Age-Appropriate Care ALERT

Expressions such as "A fat baby is a healthy baby" are myths, with no basis in fact. The opposite is true. Obese children are also at risk for the medical problems that obese adults experience. ■

deep emotional pain caused by the insensitivity of others. Discrimination is a great obstacle for them.

Persons with obesity experience discrimination and prejudice in social and employment situations. Activities of daily living are difficult. Obese individuals have limited access to public facilities. They often have difficulty forming and maintaining personal relationships. Many are victims of physical and psychological abuse. When they are hospitalized, they know that their size makes it hard for staff to care for them, and when admitted to your unit they may bring with them feelings of shame, embarrassment, and fear.

You will be caring for bariatric patients who have medical and surgical problems. General nursing assistant observations related to the care of bariatric patients are listed in Table 32-1. Refer also to the chapters describing care of patients with specific conditions (such as problems related to the cardiovascular system or care of the perioperative patient), as appropriate.

Bariatrics is a relatively new field of medicine that focuses on the treatment and control of obesity and medical conditions and diseases associated with obesity. Treatment may be medical, surgical, or both. Some facilities have special bariatric treatment units. Regardless of the setting, as a nursing assistant you are likely to encounter bariatric patients, and must know how to care for them correctly.

Providing quality care for the bariatric patient presents many challenges and risks, both physical and emotional.

Care that is routine for normal-size patients often cannot be done the same way for the bariatric population. Simple activities such as standing up, sitting down, and walking to the bathroom can be strenuous (Figure 32-2A) or painful (Figure 32-2B) for the bariatric patient. These patients share the challenges and frustrations of care with you. Certain aspects of care can be frustrating or humiliating for them. For example, many hospitals do not have scales to weigh patients who are more than 350 pounds. Some patients have been taken to the laundry, loading dock, or maintenance department, where a freight scale was used to weigh them. Think carefully about the patients' feelings

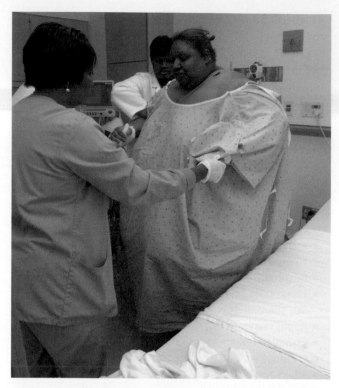

FIGURE 32-2A Many activities of daily living are difficult or painful for the patient. *(© Delmar/Cengage Learning)*

before performing an action like this. Using a freight scale to weigh a patient is a tremendous assault on dignity and self-esteem.

WEIGHT AND BODY MASS INDEX

A person's **ideal body weight (IBW)** is determined by a mathematical formula. Ideal weight is a concept developed from life insurance statistics related to life span (longevity) and health. The registered dietitian routinely calculates the ideal body weight for each patient. The formula used takes the person's height, age, sex, build, activity, medical condition, and need for nutrients into consideration.

Body mass index (BMI) is also a consideration. The BMI is a mathematical calculation used to determine whether a person is at a healthy, normal weight; is overweight; or is obese. *Ideal weight* is considered as having a BMI that is less than 26. Obesity is often defined as a BMI of 30–39. **Morbid obesity** (Figure 32-3) usually qualifies a patient for surgical treatment. Patients who are morbidly obese have a BMI of 40 or higher and are 100 pounds or more over their ideal body weight. Refer to the Online Companion for BMI information.

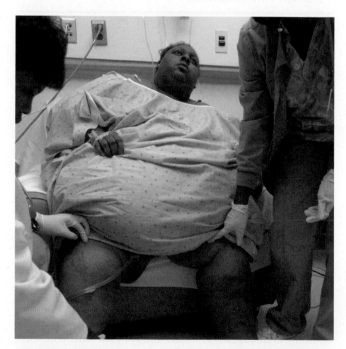

FIGURE 32-2B The patient's large body is surrounding a normal-size frame. This causes wear on the musculoskeletal system and pain in the joints. Researchers theorize that each extra pound applies 4 to 5 pounds of pressure on the spine, making complaints of back pain common. Activities such as sitting in a chair can also be difficult and painful. *(© Delmar/Cengage Learning)*

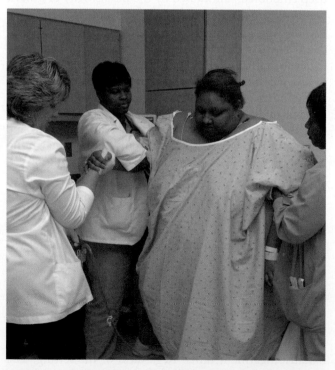

FIGURE 32-3 Patients who are morbidly obese qualify for bariatric surgery, but their medical problems must be stabilized first. Most have a BMI of 40 or higher and are 100 pounds or more over their ideal body weight. *(© Delmar/Cengage Learning)*

COMORBIDITIES

Being overweight or obese increases the risk for many health conditions. These conditions are called comorbidities. **Comorbidities** are diseases and medical conditions that are either caused by or contributed to by morbid obesity, such as diabetes, sleep apnea, and heart disease. The comorbidities associated with obesity are very serious. Weight loss often improves or eliminates many comorbid conditions.

Some bariatric patients will be admitted for weight-loss surgery. They may also be admitted to your facility for management of medical problems and complications of comorbidities. Because getting out of the house and to the hospital is very difficult, they tend to wait a long time before seeking treatment. Because of this, they are often very ill and unstable upon admission.

PATIENT CARE

The expertise of many professionals and support workers is needed to successfully care for bariatric patients. In addition, environmental adaptations must be made. Some facilities have specialists called *advocates* who work only with bariatric patients. An **advocate** is a person who speaks on behalf of the patient. He or she will have special knowledge and skill in this area of health care.

Many hospitals admit bariatric patients to private rooms that have been modified and equipped to meet their needs. The furnishings and equipment are designed for safe use with persons of size. The room is designed for patient safety and to prevent injury to caregivers. The private room upholds the patient's dignity, and prevents potential infringement on the rights of other patients.

Specialized Equipment and Supplies

The obese patient may be unable to fit into regular hospital furniture without getting stuck. This is not a laughing matter. Regular furnishings may be unsafe and break under the patient's weight. Items that are marked "large size" may still be unsafe for a bariatric patient. Specially manufactured equipment is usually necessary. Bariatric furnishings reduce the risk of injury to patients and workers, and increase patient comfort.

The Bed The bed is the most important piece of equipment in the hospital room. It is literally the center of the hospital patient's universe. You know that most daily activities are modified so they can be done when the patient is in bed. Because of concern for patient comfort and the risk of staff injury, special bariatric beds (Figure 32-4) have been developed that will safely support patients who are morbidly obese, and allow enough space for turning.

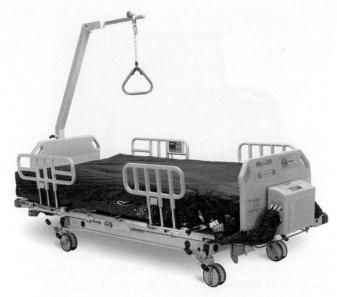

FIGURE 32-4 The Excel Care bed is manufactured for the care of bariatric patients. The trapeze is an accessory for the bed. *(The Excel Care™ bed is a registered trademark of Hill-Rom Services, Inc. ©2007 Hill-Rom Services, Inc. Reprinted with permission. All rights reserved.)*

Become familiar with the beds your facility uses. Special bariatric beds enable staff to move the bed from the flat position into the sitting position. After the patient is seated, the footboard to the bed can be removed so the patient can take a step and walk out of the bottom of the bed. Bariatric wheelchairs (Figure 32-5) and walkers can be used when the patient is up, if needed.

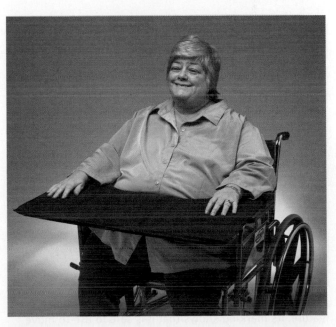

FIGURE 32-5 A wide wheelchair is needed for bariatric patients. This chair also has a self-releasing tray that the patient leans on for upper body support. *(Courtesy of Skil-Care Corporation, Yonkers, NY; (800) 432–2972)*

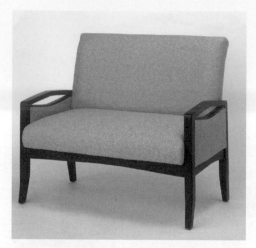

FIGURE 32-6 The furniture in the patient's room is usually oversized to accommodate large-size family and friends. *(Courtesy of Medline Industries, Inc.; (800) MEDLINE)*

Bedside Chairs The room should be equipped with a chair that the patient can sit in. Many of the bariatric patient's visitors will also be large. Chairs in the patient's room should have expanded capacity for the patient and visitors. Chairs the size of loveseats (Figure 32-6) and chairs without arms give the best fit, although the lack of arms will make standing difficult for some people.

Mechanical Lift The mechanical lift you normally use may not support the bariatric patient's weight. The hydraulic mechanical lift is normally safe for about 350 pounds. A special high-capacity lift (Figure 32-7A) is necessary to safely transfer bariatric patients. Some

facilities mount a ceiling lift (Figure 32-7B) in each dedicated bariatric room.

Gowns Regular hospital gowns do not fit bariatric patients. Extra-large gowns (Figure 32-8) are needed, and are

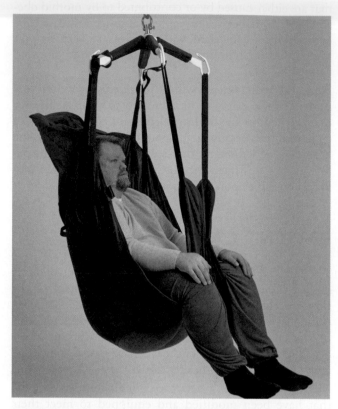

FIGURE 32-7B This sling is suspended from a ceiling-mounted hoist that slides on a track to move from one location to another. A switch in the hoist releases a cord to lower the sling to seat the patient in the bed or chair. *(Photo courtesy of Alpha Modalities)*

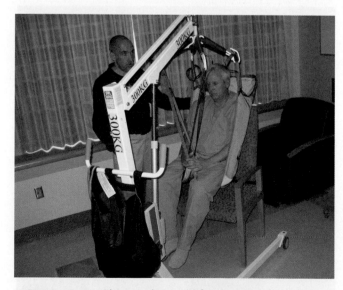

FIGURE 32-7A This mechanical lift also has a digital scale feature. Its marking shows that it is safe to use to move patients weighing as much as 300 kilograms, or 660 pounds. It may also be used for normal-size adults, but the sling size is larger and may be more cumbersome for both staff and patient. *(Photo courtesy of Alpha Modalities)*

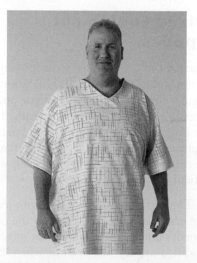

FIGURE 32-8 Oversize gowns are available for bariatric patients. These are much more comfortable than having to wear two regular-size gowns. *(Courtesy of Medline Industries, Inc.; (800) MEDLINE)*

stocked by most hospitals. If no large-size gown is available, use two regular gowns, with one on backward. However, this is an assault on the patient's dignity that should be avoided if at all possible.

Ventilation Bariatric patients often sweat profusely and may feel as if they are chronically short of breath. The discomfort is often relieved by using an electric fan. However, few hospitals provide fans, for a variety of reasons. Some hospitals have ceiling fans. Many patients prefer portable, oscillating fans that they can position to blow directly on the face or upper body. Some facilities provide small plastic fans that fasten to the overbed table or side rail with a large clip. The patient takes the fan home at discharge. Whatever fan is being used, the patient should be able to control fan position and speed.

Toileting and Bathing Double-size bedside commodes (Figure 32-9), shower chairs or benches, wheelchairs, and stretchers are also necessary. These devices normally cannot support more than 300 pounds. Many will not support even that much. A wall-mounted toilet is dangerous for a bariatric patient, as the extra weight may tear it off the wall.

Scales A number of scale options have become available for weighing bariatric patients without offending their dignity. Some bariatric beds and mechanical lifts have built-in scales. These are the best options for weighing the patient of size.

Anticipating Patient Care Needs

When you are assigned to care for a bariatric patient, try to anticipate your needs in advance. You may have to request equipment from central supply. Inform the nurse if you

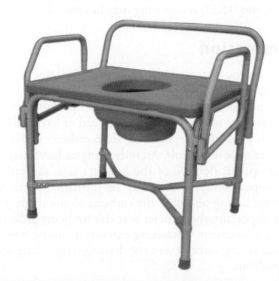

FIGURE 32-9 Oversize commodes often have drop arms so sliding transfers can be done. If the patient does sliding transfers, no lid is used. (The lid would be dislodged during sliding.) *(Courtesy of Medline Industries, Inc.; (800) MEDLINE)*

Clinical Information ALERT

The care of medical and surgical bariatric patients differs in many ways from the care of adults with no weight problems. Avoid assuming that bariatric patients are just larger versions of the normal adult. Bariatric patients have many problems and risk factors not seen in adults of normal weight. They have a higher risk of blood clots and skin-related problems. The weight of the chest may make it difficult to breathe, and the patient may need to use oxygen regularly (Figure 32-10). ∎

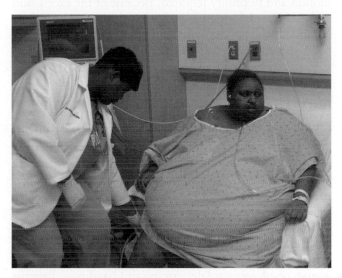

FIGURE 32-10 The weight of the chest makes breathing difficult, so supplemental oxygen is often necessary. *(© Delmar/Cengage Learning)*

will need additional items that are not routinely stocked on the unit. Expect care of bariatric patients to take more time than care of the average medical or surgical patient.

Patient Transport

When you must transport a patient to another area of the facility, evaluate the route you will take to make sure that doors, elevators, and other areas are wide enough for the patient and extra equipment. If you will encounter ramps or inclines, have another assistant help you. Alert the receiving department so they can accommodate the patient's special needs.

Taking Blood Pressure

Regular blood pressure cuffs are too small for bariatric patients, and will give inaccurate readings. A large, extra-large, or thigh-size cuff may be necessary. Occasionally, even these will not solve the problem. The upper arm is triangular in shape. Because the narrow part is near the elbow, the cuffs may slip off. In this case, the care plan will identify how the blood pressure should be taken. Some facilities use a regular-size manual or electronic cuff on the forearm. Occasionally, the lower leg is used. Review the guidelines for blood pressure monitoring in Unit 20.

Assisting with ADLs

Protect the patient's dignity at all costs. Some patients may refuse an offer of help with personal care because they are embarrassed by their inabilities or ashamed of their bodies. However, some patients are so large that they cannot complete their own personal hygiene. They may be unable to reach everywhere that needs washing, or lack the range of motion and flexibility required. Because of the excess skin and moisture, it is essential to keep patients' skin very clean and dry. If the patient is perspiring heavily, he or she may need special skin care several times during your shift. Check the care plan for instructions.

Nutrition and Hydration

Obese patients often have nutritional problems. Surprisingly, many are malnourished, with a protein deficiency. For many, carbohydrates are dietary staples. This may be a financial issue. High-carbohydrate items stop hunger pangs and often cost less than foods with higher nutrient value. The dietitian will evaluate the patient and the physician will write a diet order. A patient may have signs or symptoms of an eating disorder, such as binging and purging. Bariatric patients are at risk for type 2 diabetes. Many young, obese teens are developing this condition. Patients who are bedfast may have difficulty feeding themselves because of their size or position, or because they cannot

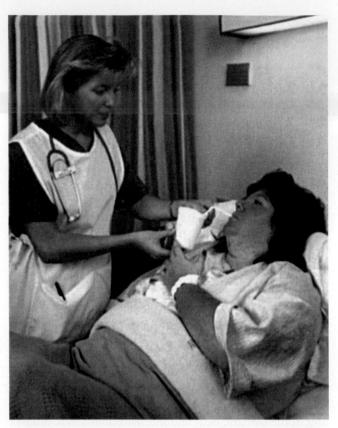

FIGURE 32-11 Assist the patient if her position prevents her from reaching the cup. (© Delmar/Cengage Learning)

use the overbed table. Assist the patient as necessary (Figure 32-11).

Many bariatric patients perspire excessively and eliminate a large amount of fluid through the skin. These patients need a large amount of fluid to support body needs. Intake and output (I&O) monitoring may be ordered.

Elimination

The bariatric patient may be catheterized for accurate monitoring of kidney function and fluid balance. Because of the patient's size, it may be easier to perform perineal care using the side-lying position instead of having the patient on the back. Keeping a condom catheter in place on an obese male is difficult. An indwelling catheter may be a better option. Because of the patient's size, the catheter may appear short, and it may be difficult to attach to drainage tubing or secure the catheter to the thigh. Even more important, the catheter is at risk for being pulled out during movement. Attaching extension tubing between the indwelling catheter and the drainage bag tubing solves the problem.

Skin Care

The skin is the largest organ of the body, and the bariatric patient has much extra skin. Usually, it has been stretched,

Difficult SITUATIONS

Keeping the skin clean is essential. However, if the skin is very sensitive, a washcloth and towel will be irritating. Using a soft disposable washcloth and gently patting skin dry with a flannel bath blanket may be easier on the skin. You can put a sock over your hand to wash and rinse the skin, then use a second sock for drying. You may also use a dry sock for padding to absorb moisture in skin folds. As you gain experience working with bariatric patients, improvising in this manner will become second nature to you. ■

is in poor condition, and is easily injured. You know that the skin is very sensitive to the effects of moisture, pressure, friction, and shearing force. The buttocks are at high risk of breakdown because patients tend to sit for long periods without moving or shifting their weight. A pressure-relieving cushion (Figure 32-12A) is much more comfortable to sit on and helps protect the skin (Figure 32-12B). The hips are also a high-risk area because of pressure from sitting for long periods in a chair or wheelchair that is too small or narrow. Bariatric patients have many skin folds (Figure 32-13). The patient's skin must be kept very clean and dry to reduce the risk of complications.

Each time you turn the patient to the side, check the skin folds to make sure they are not red or "weeping" (overly moist). The warm, moist, dark environment of a skin fold creates a great risk of a painful yeast infection (Figure 32-14). Keep the areas dry. If necessary, cut a flannel bath blanket

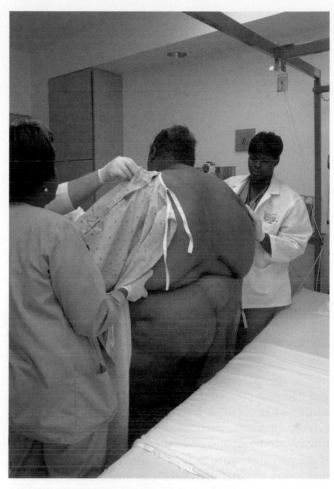

FIGURE 32-13 Bariatric patients have many skin folds. *(© Delmar/Cengage Learning)*

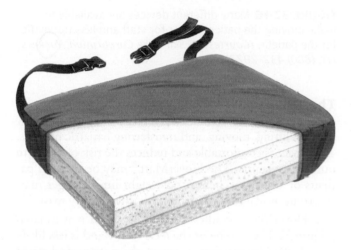

FIGURE 32-12A The bariatric cushion comes with an internal leveling pad for sling-seat chairs or a contoured base for chairs with flat seats. The foam layer is comfortable to sit on. *(Courtesy of Skil-Care Corporation, Yonkers, NY; (800) 432–2972)*

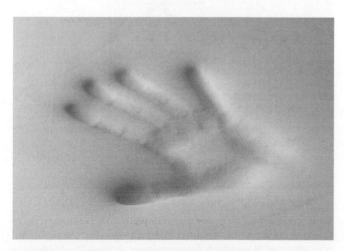

FIGURE 32-12B The internal layer of visco foam provides excellent pressure relief. *(Courtesy of Skil-Care Corporation, Yonkers, NY; (800) 432–2972)*

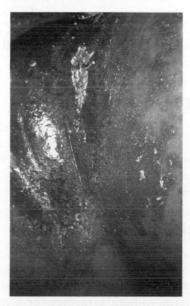

FIGURE 32-14 This painful condition is called *candidiasis* or *intertrigo.* It commonly develops in warm, moist skin folds, such as under the arms, breasts, abdominal apron, and groin. *(Courtesy of Centers for Disease Control and Prevention)*

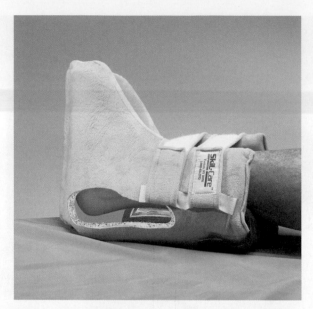

FIGURE 32-15 The bariatric heel float eliminates all pressure from the heels. *(Courtesy of Skil-Care Corporation, Yonkers, NY; (800) 432–2972)*

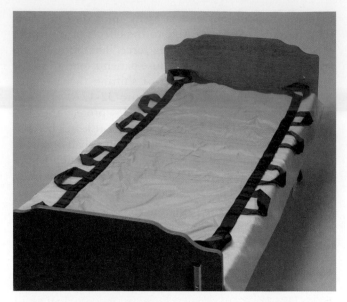

FIGURE 32-16 Many different devices are available to make moving the patient easier for staff and less traumatic for the patient. *(Courtesy of Skil-Care Corporation, Yonkers, NY; (800) 432–2972)*

and fold it to place in the skin folds. A better alternative to cutting a bath blanket is to obtain a supply of flannel receiving blankets, such as those used in the newborn nursery, and fold and place them between the skin folds. If the patient is unconscious or using ventilator support, make sure to carefully check the skin folds behind the neck. These tend to become wet from sputum and saliva, and the position causes constant pressure, increasing the risk of both yeast infection and pressure ulcers. Elevate the heels off the surface of the bed, or use a pressure-free bariatric heel elevator (Figure 32-15). The heels are a very high-pressure, high-risk area. Remember, fleece and sock-type heel protectors prevent friction and shearing, but do not relieve pressure.

Dressing the Patient

Because some bariatric patients feel warm and perspire, they may want to remain in a hospital gown or light pajamas all day. Some prefer to wear nothing and be covered only with a sheet. Make sure the patient is fully covered if he or she has visitors or must leave the room.

Moving the Bariatric Patient

Bariatric patients have many individual needs and many types of equipment are used in patient care. One staff person should never lift or move more than 35 pounds of patient body weight without extra help or a mechanical device. A variety of devices have been developed to make procedures as easy as possible for the patient and the nursing assistant (Figure 32-16).

The HoverMatt® The HoverMatt® Lateral Transfer and Repositioning System (Figure 32-17A) is commonly used for lifting, moving, and transferring bariatric patients. The device is comfortable and reduces the risk of injury to nursing assistants. The HoverMatt® may be used on patients of any size. There is no weight limit. Larger mattresses are available for patients with greater body mass.

The HoverMatt® cradles the patient when it is inflated (Figure 32-17B), so he or she feels secure and is less likely to roll off. Nevertheless, reassure the patient and never

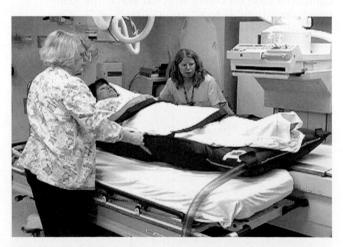

FIGURE 32-17A The HoverMatt® Lateral Transfer and Repositioning System reduces friction, so it seems as if you are moving only about 10% of the patient's weight. *(Courtesy of HoverTech International; 800–471–2776; http://www.hovermatt.com)*

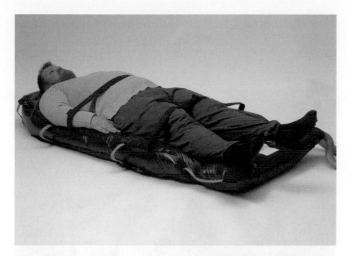

FIGURE 32-17B The edges of the HoverMatt curve up and in, making the patient feel secure and less likely to roll off. Nevertheless, patients should not be left alone when the mat is inflated. *(Courtesy of HoverTech International; 800–471–2776; http://www.hovermatt.com)*

Infection Control ALERT

The HoverMatt® is a safe, effective device. Like many other useful products, it is also very costly. *It is not disposable.* After a patient is discharged, the HoverMatt® is disinfected and reused. Never discard it or send it home with a patient! Consult the nurse or central supply clerk about how to care for the device after the patient is discharged. ▪

leave him or her alone when the mattress is inflated. Many facilities apply this mattress to the bed at the time of admission, so it is quickly available when the patient needs lifting and moving assistance. If the patient slides down in bed, the HoverMatt® slides as well. Inflating the mattress and using the handles on the sides is all that is necessary to move the patient up in bed.

Moving the Patient: Bed Mobility Review the guidelines for moving patients in Units 15 through 17 of this book. Apply the principles of good body mechanics for yourself and the patient. Moving procedures present a high risk of injury to the patient and the nursing assistant. Bedfast patients must be turned every 2 hours or more often, even if a special bed or mattress is used. If the patient turns herself, check to ensure that she is turning often enough, and that pressure is relieved from all high-risk areas.

Make sure that all tubes are firmly secured, and monitor them for proper placement each time you are in the room. Because the patient uses the arms for bed mobility, try to

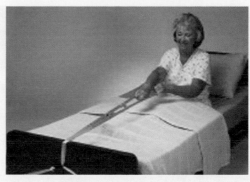

FIGURE 32-18 The bed ladder fastens to the frame and enables the person to sit up in the bed. *(Courtesy of Skil-Care Corporation, Yonkers, NY; (800) 432–2972)*

avoid devices that limit movement of the hands and arms. For example, having an IV in the left arm and an electronic blood pressure monitor on the right arm acts as a method of restraint and will restrict the patient's ability to move about in bed. Accessories such as the bed ladder (Figure 32-18) will help facilitate movement.

Manual Patient-Handling Devices Many bariatric patients prefer to keep the bed positioned in the high Fowler's position (Figure 32-19), which relieves pressure on the chest and eases breathing. However, this position promotes slipping down in bed. Elevating the knee of the bed slightly will reduce strain and help prevent downward sliding. If the patient complains of back pain when the head is

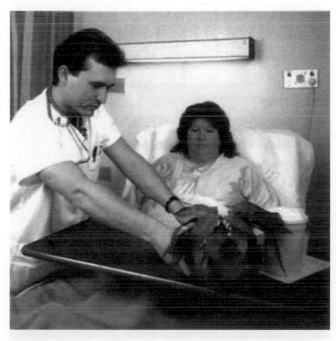

FIGURE 32-19 Positioning the bed in the high Fowler's position makes breathing easier. *(© Delmar/Cengage Learning)*

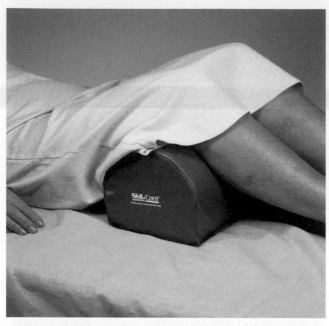

FIGURE 32-20 A knee elevator relieves pressure and pain on the back. *(Courtesy of Skil-Care Corporation, Yonkers, NY; (800) 432–2972)*

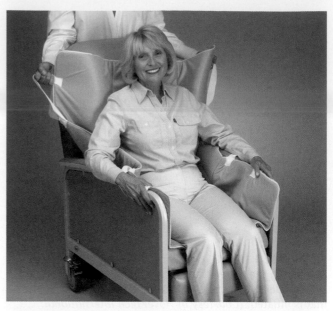

FIGURE 32-21B A regular-size patient can be moved by a single caregiver. Two to four workers may be necessary to move the bariatric patient up in a bed or chair. *(Courtesy of Skil-Care Corporation, Yonkers, NY; (800) 432–2972)*

elevated, elevating the knee of the bed will not provide sufficient relief. A commercial knee elevator (Figure 32-20) will relieve pressure on the back.

The TLC Pad (Figure 32-21A) and other similar patient-handling devices can be used for moving patients up in the bed or chair, and from side to side in bed. A regular-size patient can often be moved by a single caregiver (Figure 32-21B). Two to four workers may be necessary to move a bariatric patient up in bed or chair using this

type of device. The handles make the job easier, and using a sturdy lifting device reduces the risk of injury.

Some bariatric beds have an adjustable length feature at the foot end, which makes slipping down in bed less of a problem than it is in a regular bed. If slipping down in bed is a problem, consider using the modified Trendelenburg position (Unit 15) before moving the person. However, remember that this position places greater pressure on the lungs, so use it only under the direction and supervision of the nurse.

Moving the patient by tugging on his or her body increases the risk of injury to patient and staff. Use a lifting device for moving the patient in bed. Supporting the patient's body reduces the effects of gravity, making the move easier for both patient and staff. Four to six people may be needed to reposition a total-care patient safely. One person lifts the head. A second and third are positioned on each side, and a lift sheet or other device is also used. Another assistant positioned at the foot of the bed lifts the heels to eliminate friction and shearing.

When the patient is on the side, support the upper leg on pillows. The extra support reduces the risk of skin problems caused by the legs rubbing together, as well as preventing pressure on the bony prominence at the knee. Supporting the upper leg helps relieve pain in the hip joint and lumbar area of the spine. Unsupported, the weight of the leg exerts a downward pull on both the hip and the spine, which can be very painful.

The patient's skin and extremities are heavy and will not move on their own. You must move his or her body parts manually. Some hospitals have an arrangement of slings

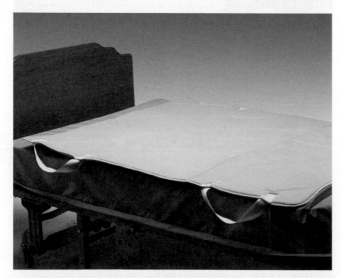

FIGURE 32-21A The TLC Pad is used for moving patients up in the bed or chair, and from side to side in bed. *(Courtesy of Skil-Care Corporation, Yonkers, NY; (800) 432–2972)*

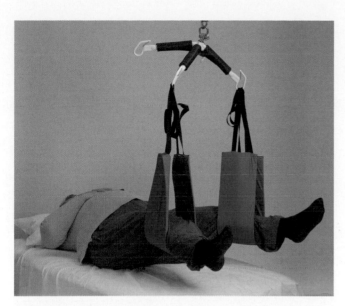

FIGURE 32-22 Various lifts, slings, and pulleys may be used to move the patient's extremities. This patient's legs are being elevated to relieve edema and pressure from the heels by using a ceiling-mounted hoist to hold them in place. *(Photo courtesy of Alpha Modalities)*

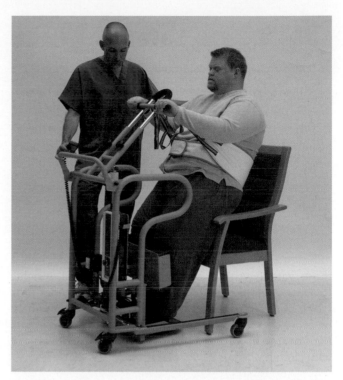

FIGURE 32-23 Devices are available to assist patients in rising to their feet or to perform a standing transfer, such as for pivoting the patient to sit on a chair. *(Photo courtesy of Alpha Modalities)*

and pulleys for moving the arms and legs (Figure 32-22). The patient is encouraged to assist by pulling on the rope to which the sling is attached.

Explaining positioning and moving techniques beyond the general principles of bariatric patient care is impossible; an entire book is necessary for this subject. Your facility will teach you how to use its special equipment. Even when a device is used, two or more nursing assistants are often needed for procedures that involve moving the patient, as well as for personal hygiene.

Moving the Patient: Transfers and Ambulation Some bariatric patients can walk for short distances. Some will use a walker for support. Others use mobility scooters. Some will need help or use a mechanical device to come to a standing position (Figure 32-23), and others will require assistance with transfers. The care plan will list instructions for mobilizing each patient. Some patients will be able to ambulate in their rooms with minimal assistance and support.

A gait/transfer belt may be used for transfers and ambulation if you have a long belt (Figure 32-24). A 72-inch belt will probably be necessary, in addition to two or three assistants to help. Avoid doubling a gait belt, if possible. If a long belt is not available and you must join two regular belts, make sure to lock the buckles down securely. Position both buckles close to your hands so you can see their position. If they begin to slip, even slowly, stop the procedure.

The nurse may instruct you to apply an abdominal binder before moving the patient so that the abdomen does not interfere with safe patient handling and movement. The

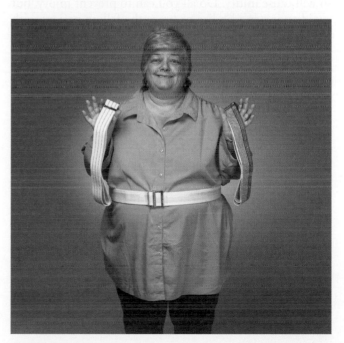

FIGURE 32-24 A long belt may necessary for transferring and ambulating bariatric patients. A cloth belt holds more securely than a plastic belt. *(Courtesy of Skil-Care Corporation, Yonkers, NY; (800) 432–2972)*

fatty apron of abdominal skin is called the **panniculus** or pannus. A **pannus** is a hanging flap of skin anywhere on the body. It is usually seen in overweight individuals and

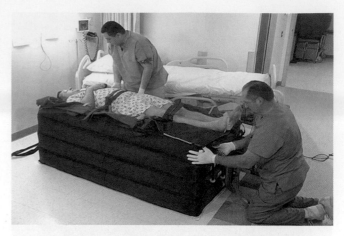

FIGURE 32-25 The HoverJack® is used to lift a patient from the floor to bed or stretcher. *(Courtesy of HoverTech International; 800–471–2776)*

those who have lost a significant amount of weight. Patients often like the feeling of support the binder provides. In this case, a cloth (cotton or flannel) binder may be more effective than a binder made of elastic. Binders tend to ride up on persons of size. There is less slippage with cloth binders.

Falls

If a standing patient starts to fall to the floor, you may instinctively try to hold him up or break the fall. Trying to do so will cause injury. Do all you can to prevent injury, but avoid trying to stabilize or brace the falling patient with your body. For example, quickly push items out of the way. Try to protect the patient's head. If you can ease the patient down your leg, do so. However, this may not be possible with a patient who is much larger than you are. When standing or ambulating the patient for the first time, have plenty of help. Monitor the patient for dizziness or weakness. If he experiences these problems, return the patient to bed.

If the patient falls to the floor, a team will be required to get him up. Several methods are used, depending on how much assistance the patient can provide. The HoverJack® (Figure 32-25) operates in a manner similar to the HoverMatt®. The HoverJack® is used to lift a patient from the floor to bed or stretcher. By placing the HoverMatt® on top, the patient is easily lifted from the floor and transferred back to bed.

A dependent patient may be rolled onto a bariatric sling (Figure 32-26) or a heavy blanket. The patient is lifted only

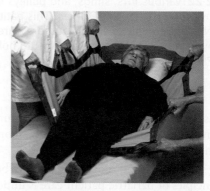

FIGURE 32-26 A dependent patient may be moved by rolling her onto a bariatric sling made of nylon or canvas. *(Courtesy of Skil-Care Corporation, Yonkers, NY; (800) 432–2972)*

enough to slide a backboard underneath. The backboard is used for moving the patient. If the patient can assist, a strong chair may be positioned against her back, then turned upright, or a team can lift the patient's arms and legs while another person slides a chair under her. Another option is to lift the patient to a sitting position with a manual lifting sling and four caregivers. Slide the chair underneath. These are potentially dangerous maneuvers for caregivers. Do not move an obese, dependent patient until you have proper instruction, supervision, adaptive mobility devices, and enough staff to accomplish the task.

REVIEW

A. Multiple Choice

Select the one best answer for each of the following.

1. The bariatric patient is at risk for
   a. fever and low blood pressure.
   b. bradycardia and increased urination.
   c. malnutrition and dehydration.
   d. diarrhea and constipation.

2. Bariatric patients who complain of feeling hot may obtain relief from
   a. removing the patient's clothes and top sheet, then closing the door.
   b. an electric fan that the patient can position and control.
   c. folding a newspaper to create a handheld fan.
   d. bathing the patient in ice water.

3. One staff person should never lift or move more than
   a. 5 pounds of body weight without extra help or a mechanical device.
   b. 35 pounds of body weight without extra help or a mechanical device.
   c. 65 pounds of body weight without extra help or a mechanical device.
   d. 90 pounds of body weight without extra help or a mechanical device.

4. When moving the bariatric patient up in bed, it may be helpful to position the bed in the
   a. modified Trendelenburg position.
   b. semi-Fowler's position.
   c. lithotomy position.
   d. Sims' position.

5. If a standing bariatric patient starts to fall to the floor, you should
   a. protect the patient's head, if possible.
   b. grab the patient under the arms.
   c. hold the patient up however you can.
   d. run for extra help.

6. When toileting a bariatric patient, never use a/an
   a. fracture bedpan.
   b. oversize commode.
   c. indwelling catheter.
   d. wall-mounted toilet.

7. Bariatric patients must be repositioned in bed every
   a. 4 hours.
   b. 3 hours.
   c. 2 hours.
   d. 1 hour.

8. When the patient is positioned on her side in bed, you should
   a. pad the underarm area.
   b. support the upper leg.
   c. apply heel protectors.
   d. keep the rails down.

9. The fatty apron of loose abdominal skin is the
   a. comorbidity.
   b. candidiasis.
   c. panniculus.
   d. intertrigo.

B. Nursing Assistant Challenge

You are assigned to care for Mrs. Esmerelda Gonsalves, a 32-year-old female who has been admitted to room 306 on your unit. She is scheduled for bariatric surgery tomorrow. Mrs. Gonsalves tells you that she has gradually gained weight since she was a child. She tells you she has tried every diet she could find and nothing worked for her. She gets teary-eyed and tells you that surgery is her last hope for a normal life. Her height on admission was 68 inches and her weight was 423 pounds. This calculates to a body mass index of 64.5. Her comorbidities include type 2 diabetes, sleep apnea, osteoarthritis of the lumbar spine and knees, and symptoms of depression.

10. The regular blood pressure cuff slips down every time you apply it, so you have not finished taking Mrs. Gonsalves's admission vital signs. No other vital signs monitoring equipment is available on the unit. What action will you take?

11. You finally obtain the patient's blood pressure. Your reading is 266/178. The patient has no history of hypertension. What action will you take?

12. After putting Mrs. Gonsalves to bed, you note that she has a large abdominal pannus. Under the pannus, the skin is bright red, with weeping and irritation. The patient tells you this is a chronic problem, which is painful for her. Is it necessary to notify the nurse? What else should you do to help this patient?

UNIT 33

Caring for the Patient Who Is Dying

OBJECTIVES

After completing this unit, you will be able to:
- Spell and define terms.
- Describe the grieving process and list the steps.
- Describe the nursing assistant's responsibilities for providing supportive care.

- Describe the hospice philosophy and method of care.
- List the signs of approaching death.
- Demonstrate the following procedure:
  - Procedure 85 Giving Postmortem Care

VOCABULARY

Learn the meaning and the correct spelling of the following words and phrases:

acceptance	critical list	life-sustaining treatment	Sacrament of the Sick
advance directive	denial	living will	supportive care
anger	depression	moribund	terminal
bargaining	DNR (do not resuscitate)	no-code order	
cardiac arrest	durable power of	postmortem	
cardiopulmonary	attorney for health care	postmortem care	
resuscitation (CPR)	hospice care	rigor mortis	

INTRODUCTION

Death is the final stage of life. It may come suddenly, without warning, or it may follow a long period of illness. It sometimes strikes the young but it always awaits the old. Death represents the final journey in the continuum of life. As a nursing assistant, you will be providing care throughout the period of dying and into the after-death (**postmortem**) period. Accepting the idea that death is the natural result of the life process may help you respond to your patients' needs more generously.

The concept of death and dying is handled differently by different people (Figure 33-1). There are many reactions to the diagnosis of a **terminal** (life-ending) illness.

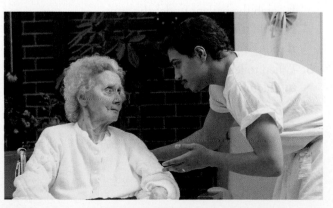

FIGURE 33-1 Each person handles death differently. (© *Delmar/Cengage Learning*)

Communication HIGHLIGHT

Health care workers may feel helpless when caring for a dying patient. Remember that active listening is a means of therapeutic communication. Listening shows honest and caring regard for the patient. Using touch also communicates caring and acceptance. When you are at a loss for words, consider these means of showing that you care. ■

FIVE STAGES OF GRIEF

Dr. Elisabeth Kübler-Ross (1926–2004) identified five stages of grief that can occur in a dying person. Family members, friends, and caregivers also experience the grieving process. The grief stages are denial, anger, bargaining, depression, and acceptance (Table 33-1). If there is adequate time and support, some patients may be able to move through each stage to a point of acceptance of their illness and death.

- **Denial** begins when the person is made aware that he is going to die. He may deny that the information is true. Making long-range plans suggests that the patient is in the denial stage. This stage is necessary and therapeutic.

Clinical Information ALERT

The grieving process begins immediately when someone is diagnosed with a life-threatening or terminal illness. Mourning before someone dies is called *anticipatory grief*. Patients and families grieve for their former way of life, recognizing that returning to it will be impossible. Roles and responsibilities within the family change. Illness may change body image. Friends and family may begin to separate themselves from the dying person. This is one way they deal with loss, but it makes the patient feel isolated. Losses are many. Some are very private and personal. Each loss triggers the grieving process, causing feelings of isolation, abandonment, anger, and depression. ■

- **Anger** (Figure 33-2) occurs when the patient can no longer deny the fact that she is going to die. The patient may blame others for her illness. She is angry about her diagnosis, not with you personally. Remain calm and avoid saying anything that may make her angrier.

TABLE 33-1 EMOTIONAL RESPONSES TO DYING

Stage of Grief	Response of the Nursing Assistant
Denial	Reflect patient's statements, but try not to confirm or deny the fact that the patient is dying. **Example:** *"The lab tests can't be right—I don't have cancer." "It must have been difficult for you to learn the results of your tests."*
Anger	Understand the source of the patient's anger. Provide understanding and support. Listen. Try to meet reasonable needs and demands quickly. **Example:** *"This food is terrible—not fit to eat." "Let me see if I can find something that would appeal to you more."*
Bargaining	If it is possible to meet the patient's requests, do so. Listen attentively. **Example:** *"If only God will spare me this, I'll go to church every week." "Would you like a visit from your clergyperson?"*
Depression	Avoid clichés that dismiss the patient's depression ("It could be worse—you could be in more pain"). Be caring and supportive. Let the patient know that it is all right to be depressed. **Example:** *"There just isn't any sense in going on." "I understand you are feeling very depressed."*
Acceptance	Do not assume that, because the patient has accepted death, she or he is unafraid, or that she or he does not need emotional support. Listen attentively and be supportive and caring. **Example:** *"I feel so alone." "I am here with you. Would you like to talk?"*

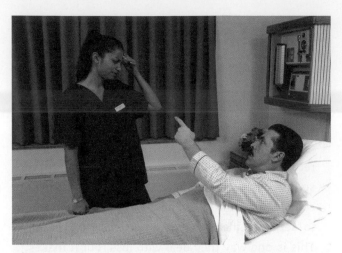

FIGURE 33-2 Patients may demonstrate feelings of frustration and anger. (© Delmar/Cengage Learning)

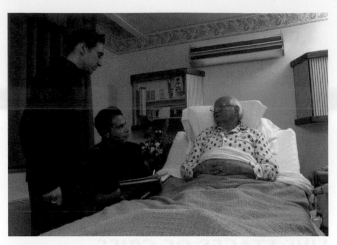

FIGURE 33-4 The patient may strive to complete unfinished business during the acceptance phase of the grieving process. (© Delmar/Cengage Learning)

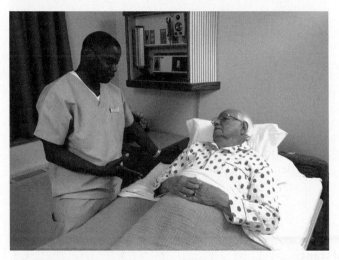

FIGURE 33-3 Depression is a normal part of the grieving process. (© Delmar/Cengage Learning)

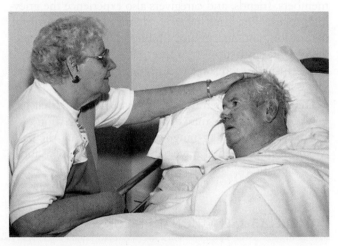

FIGURE 33-5 The support of family and friends is very important to the dying patient. (© Delmar/Cengage Learning)

- **Bargaining** is the stage in which the patient attempts to bargain for more time to live. Trying to make private "deals" with God or a higher power is also common. For example, "If you will let me live another two months, I promise I will try to be a better person." Bargaining frequently involves an important event, such as the birth of a grandchild. The patient is basically saying, "I know I'm going to die and I'm ready to die, but not just yet." This may be done in private and not stated verbally.

- **Depression** is the fourth stage of the grieving process. The patient comes to the realization that he will die soon (Figure 33-3). He is saddened by the thought of separation from family and friends, and that he could not do everything he wanted to do.

- **Acceptance** is the stage during which the patient understands and accepts the fact that he is going to die

(Figure 33-4). He may try to complete unfinished business. Having accepted his eventual death, he may also try to help those around him to deal with it.

Not all patients progress through these stages in sequential order. Movement from one level to the next does not mean that the previous level will be completely left behind. Patients sometimes move back and forth between stages several times before completely resolving one stage and moving ahead.

When all five stages have been passed, it is believed that the patient is better able to accept the termination of life. If there is adequate time and support (Figure 33-5), many patients can be helped to reach a more accepting frame of mind.

The family and staff also go through the grieving process. Seeing the patient in one stage and the family in another stage is difficult.

Common Fears

Dying can be a lonely business. We experience various losses throughout life, but when a person is dying, he or she is losing everything—family, friends, pets, and belongings. It is natural to be afraid of the unknown, regardless of religious and spiritual beliefs. Some people do not feel good about how they lived their lives or things they have done. This causes feelings of guilt, grief, and remorse. Common fears associated with dying are:

- Fear of dying alone
- Fear of severe, unrelieved pain
- Fear of inability to finish personal business or manage affairs

Some people feel incomplete because they have failed to achieve all they wanted to do. They may also have a strong desire to do something that is no longer possible in light of their imminent death.

THE PATIENT SELF-DETERMINATION ACT

The Patient Self-Determination Act of 1990 requires health care providers to supply written information about advance directives. An **advance directive** is a document that is put into effect if and when the person becomes unable to make decisions. The patient may or may not choose to execute an advance directive.

Decisions often must be made when a patient is terminally or critically ill. These decisions involve provision of supportive care or life-sustaining treatment. The Patient Self-Determination Act was passed to assure patients and their families that their wishes will be followed. With **supportive care**, the patient's life will not be artificially prolonged, but the patient will be kept comfortable physically, mentally, and emotionally.

All patients deserve supportive care, but for terminally ill patients, supportive care means the absence of life-sustaining treatment. **Life-sustaining treatment** involves giving medications and treatments for the purpose of maintaining life, such as using a ventilator to maintain breathing, or receiving **cardiopulmonary resuscitation (CPR)** if **cardiac arrest** occurs (the heart and lungs stop functioning).

There are two basic types of advance directives: the living will and the durable power of attorney for health care. The **living will** is a request that death not be artificially postponed if the person has an incurable, irreversible illness that the physician judges to be terminal. The **durable power of attorney for health care** assigns someone else the responsibility for making medical decisions for the patient if the patient becomes unable to do so. The person designated may be called the *agent*, *proxy*, or *health care proxy*. This person should make decisions in keeping with the patient's known wishes.

As a nursing assistant, you must be aware of the patient's status for supportive care or life-sustaining treatment. The person on supportive care will have a **no-code order** or **DNR (do not resuscitate)** order. This means that no extraordinary means, such as CPR, will be used to prevent death. If the patient (or proxy) changes his or her mind, the order in the chart is changed accordingly.

Witnessing Advance Directives

Become familiar with facility policies and state laws for witnessing advance directives. In many states, caregivers cannot witness advance directives. In most states, caregivers cannot legally be appointed to be the agent (medical decision maker or proxy) for a patient unless they are related by blood or marriage.

Legal ALERT

Health care workers sometimes become confused about the meaning of a living will in which the patient specifies that no heroic procedures are to be undertaken if the person is in terminal, irreversible condition. If the patient is not known to be in terminal condition, resuscitation will be done (unless otherwise ordered). For example, a 33-year-old patient in good health enters the hospital for a diagnostic procedure that involves the injection of contrast material into the veins. The patient has an allergic reaction to the contrast material and suffers a cardiac arrest. In this case, *CPR would be done*, because the person is not in terminal condition.

In another instance, an elderly patient enters the hospital for insertion of a central intravenous catheter to be used for pain management as part of terminal care. The patient is known to have inoperable cancer, as documented by two or more physicians. The patient experiences a complication during the procedure and has a cardiac arrest. In this case, the provisions of the living will would be observed, and *CPR would not be done*. ■

Legal ALERT

Your facility may have designations for different levels of emergency care, ranging from comfort care to full advanced life support. Become familiar with the criteria for these levels. ■

THE ROLE OF THE NURSING ASSISTANT

As a nursing assistant, you spend much time with the patient. You have a unique opportunity to be a source of strength and comfort. You must behave in a way that instills confidence in both the patient and the patient's family. Developing the proper attitude and approach for this type of situation is not easy. It will come with experience. There are some things to keep in mind:

- Your response should be consistent. It should be guided by the patient's attitude and the care plan.
- You must be open and receptive, because the terminal patient's attitude, feelings, and wishes may change from day to day.
- Your own feelings about death and dying influence your ability to care for dying patients. Your acceptance of death as a natural occurrence will enable you to meet patient needs in a realistic manner.
- Give your best and most careful nursing care, with special attention to comfort measures such as mouth care and fluid intake.
- Be quietly empathetic and carry out your duties in a calm, efficient way.

When a patient's condition is critical, the physician will place the patient's name officially on the **critical list**. The family and the chaplain will be notified.

PROVIDING FOR SPIRITUAL NEEDS

Many people find spiritual faith to be a source of great comfort during difficult times. Some religions have specific rituals that are carried out when a person is very ill or dying. (These are listed in the Online Companion to this book.) Your role is to cooperate so that these activities may be performed in a dignified, caring manner. Respect the beliefs or nonbeliefs of every patient. Treat religious items with respect.

When a Catholic patient is ill, a priest may be called for the **Sacrament of the Sick** (Figure 33-6). It is preferable that the family be present and leave the room while the confession is heard. Many patients recover completely, but this hope should not prevent reception of this sacrament if the patient so desires.

Dying is a lonely business, a journey each person must finish alone. Until the final moment comes, privacy, but not total solitude, should be the guiding rule (Figure 33-7). Remember the family when a patient is dying. Assist in the following actions:

- Allow family members to be with the patient as they desire.
- Allow the family to assist with some of the care, if they wish to do so and the patient does not object.

Culture ALERT

The medical system and views about death and dying in the United States are based on Western values, which often differ greatly from those of other cultures. Cultural beliefs and values run deep and usually cannot be changed. People from other cultures have many views about care of the dying person. Within each culture, there are often gender-specific differences. One commonality in people of all cultures is that they want their loved ones nearby as they live out their last days. Many believe that the family should care for the patient. Some cultures maintain that the patient should die at home, believing the spirit remains at the place of death and is comforted by the grieving of loved ones. People from some cultures open the window so the spirit can escape. ■

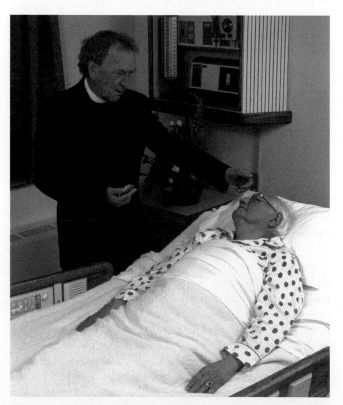

FIGURE 33-6 The Sacrament of the Sick may be administered to Roman Catholics who are gravely ill. (© *Delmar/Cengage Learning*)

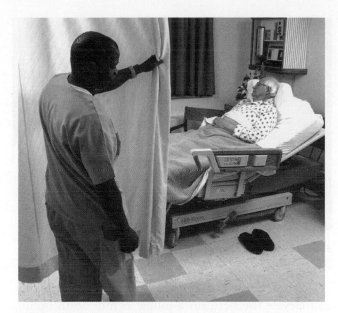

FIGURE 33-7 The dying patient needs privacy, but not total solitude. (© Delmar/Cengage Learning)

- Inform the family where they can get a cup of coffee or a meal.
- If a family member stays during the night, offer a pillow and blanket. Some facilities provide recliners or cots for family members.
- Avoid judging family members. Remember that each person grieves in his or her own way. The emotions that others see are not necessarily an accurate picture of what an individual is feeling.

HOSPICE CARE

Hospice care has evolved around the philosophy that death is a natural process that should neither be hastened nor delayed and that the dying person should be kept comfortable. **Hospice care** is:

- A program designed to meet many needs of the dying person and his or her family, in which an entire team of professionals provides services
- Provided to terminally ill people with a life expectancy of six months or less
- Involved with direct physical care when needed
- Supportive of both the family and the patient
- Provided in special hospice facilities, in other care facilities, and at home
- Largely carried out by a home health assistant or a nursing assistant under the direction of professional health care providers
- Available 24 hours a day, if needed
- A program that provides bereavement counseling to help survivors accept the death of a loved one

- A program in which volunteers play an important role, making regular personal visits to the patient and family

The goals of hospice care include:

- Control of pain
- Coordination of psychological, spiritual, and social support services for the patient and the family
- Making legal and financial counseling available to the patient and family

Because hospice care is a philosophy, it becomes part of the guide for your actions when caring for patients who are terminally ill. Give these patients the same care you would provide if a terminal diagnosis had not been made. Carry out all activities with dignity and respect.

Hospice care may seem to go against everything you have been taught. For example, a patient has bone cancer that is very painful, and is expected to die within a few days. Despite high doses of drugs, she remains in severe pain. Moving the patient worsens the pain, so the care plan instructs you to leave the patient on her back, rather than turning her every 2 hours. You know the patient has skin breakdown that will worsen if she is not turned. However, you must follow the care plan and *not turn* the patient. This shows respect for the patient's needs and supports the quality of her final hours of life.

PHYSICAL CHANGES AS DEATH APPROACHES

As death approaches, there are notable physical changes. Report the changes in Table 33-2 to the nurse promptly.

Hearing is the last sense to be lost. Do not assume that because death is approaching, the patient can no longer hear. Choose your words carefully. Do not say anything that you would not say to the patient. Continue to speak with the

TABLE 33-2 OBSERVATIONS OF IMPENDING DEATH TO MAKE AND REPORT

- The patient becomes less responsive (Figure 33-8).
- Body functions slow down.
- The patient loses muscle control.
- The patient involuntarily voids or defecates.
- The jaw tends to drop.
- Breathing becomes irregular and shallow.
- You cannot get a pulse or blood pressure, but the patient is still breathing.
- Circulation slows and the extremities become cold. The pulse becomes rapid and progressively weaker.
- Skin pales, or appears gray, mottled, or cyanotic.
- The eyes stare and do not respond to light.

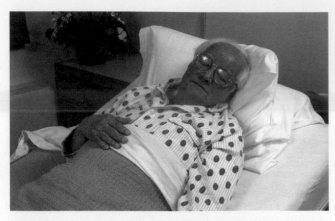

FIGURE 33-8 The patient becomes less responsive and body functions slow down as death approaches. *(© Delmar/Cengage Learning)*

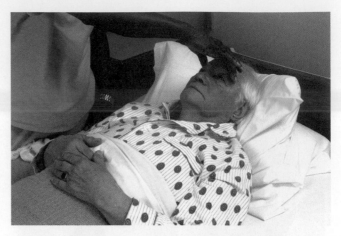

FIGURE 33-9 Postmortem care is given after death occurs. *(© Delmar/Cengage Learning)*

patient when you are in the room and inform her when you will be giving care.

As it becomes clear that death will occur very soon, you should call the nurse, who will supervise the care during the final moments of life.

Signs of Death

After death, changes continue to take place in the body. These changes are called **moribund** (dying) changes:

- Pupils become permanently dilated.
- There is no pulse or respiration.
- Heat is gradually lost from the body.
- The patient may urinate, defecate, or release flatus.
- Within 2 to 4 hours, body rigidity, called **rigor mortis**, develops.
- Unless the body is embalmed within 24 hours, there is progressive protein breakdown.
- When circulation stops, blood moves into the lowest areas of the body. This process can begin within 20 minutes of death. Over time, this will result in a stained appearance on the back of the body if the patient is in the supine position. To reduce the risk of staining about the head and neck, elevate the head of the bed 30°. Keep the head upright and not turned to the side. Some facilities do not use ties in the morgue pack to position the body. If used, tie them loosely.

POSTMORTEM CARE

Care of the body after death is called **postmortem care** (Figure 33-9). This is usually a nursing assistant responsibility. Treat the body with respect. Straighten the limbs

and elevate the head on a pillow before death occurs. Wash the body gently with warm water. If you are uncomfortable, you may find it easier if you ask a coworker to assist.

- Check the procedure manual before giving with postmortem care.
- Apply the principles of standard precautions when giving postmortem care. The body continues to be infectious following death.
- Treat the body with the same dignity you would a living person.
- Some facilities prefer to have the patient left alone until mortuary staff arrive. Your responsibility will be only to prepare the body for viewing by the family.
- One procedure for postmortem care is described in Procedure 85.

ORGAN DONATIONS

Some people desire to share their organs with others after death. They use an organ donor card and may have a notation on the driver's license. The card specifies if particular organs or the whole body is to be donated. In some facilities, the patient's family is asked to donate certain body organs. Such a request is made by the physician, nurse, or other licensed professional. If the patient or family make their wishes about organ donation known to you, inform the nurse promptly. He or she may have to make preparations before death.

PROCEDURE

85

GIVING POSTMORTEM CARE

1. Carry out initial procedure actions.

2. Assemble equipment:
   - Shroud, morgue pack, or clean sheet
   - Basin with warm water
   - Washcloth
   - Towels
   - Disposable gloves
   - Identification tags
   - Cotton
   - Bandages
   - Pads as needed

3. Put on disposable gloves.

4. Remove all appliances, tubing, and used articles, if permitted.

5. Work quickly and quietly; maintain an attitude of respect.

6. Position the body on the back, with head and shoulders elevated on a pillow. Straighten the arms and legs and place the arms at the sides.
   a. Close the eyes by grasping the eyelashes, gently pulling the eyelids down, and holding shut for a few seconds.
   b. Replace dentures in the patient's mouth, if used, or clean the dentures and place them in a denture cup. Make sure they are sent to the funeral home with the body. Send other artificial body parts to the funeral home, if used.
   c. Close the mouth. If the jaw will not stay closed, ask the nurse for instructions.

7. Bathe as necessary. Remove any soiled dressings and replace with clean ones. Groom hair.

8. Place a disposable pad underneath the buttocks. If the family is to view the body:
   a. Put a clean hospital gown on the patient.
   b. Cover the body to the shoulders with a sheet.
   c. Remove disposable gloves and wash your hands.

d. Make sure the room is neat.

e. Adjust the lights to a subdued level.

f. Provide chairs for the family.

g. Allow the family to visit in private.

9. Return to the patient's room after the family leaves. Wash your hands and put on disposable gloves.

10. Collect all belongings and make a list. Wrap properly and label. Valuables remain in the hospital safe until they are signed for by a relative.

11. Fill out the identification cards or tags in the morgue kit and attach them as follows:
    a. Place one card on the right ankle or right great toe.
    b. Attach one card to the bag with the patient's valuables.

12. Put the shroud on the patient and attach an identification card or tag to the outside.

13. Transport the body to the morgue, or leave in the room with the privacy curtain and door closed until the funeral home arrives. When it is time to move the body:
    a. Call an elevator to the floor, lock it off, and keep it empty.
    b. Close doors to other patients' rooms.
    c. Empty the corridor.
    d. With an assistant, transfer the body to a gurney or the mortuary cart.
    e. Keep the patient supine, with the head elevated.
    f. Cover the body with a sheet.
    g. Remove disposable gloves and discard according to facility policy. Wash your hands.
    h. Take the body to the morgue or assist the funeral home as directed.

REVIEW

A. Multiple Choice

Select the one best answer for each of the following.

1. Organs from a dead person may be
   a. harvested without permission.
   b. obtained on an as-needed basis.
   c. donated with permission at the time of death.
   d. donated only if listed in the person's will.

2. As death approaches, changes include
   a. constriction of the pupils.
   b. muscle spasm.
   c. slowing of circulation.
   d. skin developing a yellow hue.

3. Moribund changes include
   a. permanent pupil constriction.
   b. increased body heat.
   c. increase in pulse and respiration.
   d. blood pooling in the lower body.

4. A no-code order on a patient's chart means
   a. to start CPR immediately.
   b. do not resuscitate.
   c. to begin postmortem care at once.
   d. to call the family if the patient seems in danger of dying.

5. The person in the anger stage of the grieving process
   a. bargains with the higher power for more time.
   b. is trying to complete unfinished business.
   c. insists that the diagnosis is incorrect.
   d. may blame others for the terminal diagnosis.

6. A living will
   a. specifies a person's wishes if death is imminent.
   b. names a person to make medical decisions.
   c. may be used only if the person wants CPR.
   d. lists the doctor's wishes for the dying person.

7. A person who is designated as the agent in a durable power of attorney for health care
   a. takes care of the patient's legal, financial, and medical matters.
   b. makes all medical decisions for the remainder of the patient's life.
   c. makes medical decisions if the patient can no longer make them.
   d. must complete a living will on the patient's behalf.

8. Hospice
   a. is a philosophy of care.
   b. is available only at home.
   c. cannot care for children.
   d. is not available everywhere.

9. Rigidity of the body that occurs after death is
   a. moribund changes.
   b. rigor mortis.
   c. cyanotic mottling.
   d. muscular lividity.

10. The person who is actively dying probably
    a. cannot see.
    b. is not in pain.
    c. wants to be alone.
    d. can hear.

B. Nursing Assistant Challenge

Mrs. Goldstein is a patient in the hospital where you work. She was diagnosed with cancer of the ovaries two years ago. She has been at home but is admitted periodically for chemotherapy. You have taken care of her each time she has been in the hospital. The first time was right after Mrs. Goldstein was diagnosed. She seemed happy and made frequent comments like, "I'm glad I don't have cancer." The last time she was a patient, she refused to follow the suggestions of the nursing staff, but did allow her chemotherapy to be administered. When her family visited, she was irritated and hostile toward them. This time, she is agreeable with the staff on all matters and seems genuinely happy to see her family. She has told you that if she can live to see her granddaughter get married in two months, she will become a volunteer at the hospital so she can help other patients. She is not receiving chemotherapy anymore because the cancer is in an advanced stage. She is hospitalized for pain management now but plans to go home for hospice care. Consider these questions about Mrs. Goldstein:

11. Do you think she is preparing for her death?

12. How would you describe the stages of dying she has been experiencing?

13. What response is appropriate to her comments about the wedding?

14. Do you think hospice care will benefit Mrs. Goldstein? Give reasons for your answer.

Other Health Care Settings

UNIT 34
The Nursing Assistant in
Home Care

The Nursing Assistant in Home Care

OBJECTIVES

After completing this unit, you will be able to:

- Spell and define terms.
- Describe the characteristics that are important in the nursing assistant who provides home care.
- List at least 10 methods of protecting your personal safety when working as a home care assistant in the community.

- Describe the duties of the nursing assistant who works in the home setting.
- Describe the duties of the homemaker assistant.
- Carry out home care activities needed to maintain a safe and clean environment.

VOCABULARY

Learn the meaning and the correct spelling of the following words and phrases:

home health assistant   homemaker aide   homemaker assistant

INTRODUCTION

The health care of persons (clients) in their own homes is an age-old tradition. The permissive laws of the early 1900s placed few legal restrictions on people who provided care in private homes. In the 20th century, laws were passed that prohibited practicing nursing without a license. It was not until the middle of the 20th century that there was a massive trend toward moving patient care out of the home and into the community health care facility. Today, we have come full circle: home health care is provided by qualified caregivers and is a popular alternative to facility care.

THE HOME HEALTH CAREGIVER

The nursing assistant is an important part of the health team that provides home care. Nursing assistants who work in private homes are supervised by licensed nurses. This is called *remote supervision*, because the nurse is not on the premises. The nursing assistant may be called:

- **Home health assistant** or home health aide, when the primary role is to provide assistance with nursing care.
- **Homemaker assistant** or **homemaker aide**, when the primary role is to do housekeeping chores.

The nursing assistant who provides health care services may be asked to carry out homemaker assistant duties in some cases. As you learned from Unit 1, the recipient of care in the home is called the *client*.

THE HOME HEALTH ASSISTANT AND THE NURSING PROCESS

You continue to be part of the nursing process when working in a client's home. During:

- *Assessment*, your observations and careful reporting can make a valuable contribution to the data on which the analysis of the client's needs is based.
- *Planning*, you contribute as you actively share information with your supervisor and in meetings and care conferences (Figure 34-1).
- *Implementation*, you spend the most time with the client. You are therefore responsible for seeing that the plan is carried out.
- *Evaluation*, you also contribute to the nursing process when you share your observations about the success or lack of success of the care.

CHARACTERISTICS OF THE HOME CARE NURSING ASSISTANT AND HOMEMAKER ASSISTANT

As a home care nursing assistant or homemaker assistant, you must demonstrate:

- Honesty in managing the client's possessions and shopping money, and in reporting time.

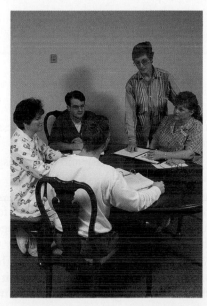

FIGURE 34-1 The home health assistant contributes to the client's care plan. (© *Delmar/Cengage Learning*)

- Self-starter ability in carrying out your assignment promptly and efficiently without reminders.
- Self-discipline in managing your time and doing the right thing.
- Accuracy and attention to details, so that each task is performed correctly.
- Organization, so that you plan your activities around the client's schedule, not your own, and make the best use of your time.
- Maturity, so that assessments can be made properly and you use good judgment.
- Insight that gives the ability to see the client as a whole person.
- Observational skills and the ability to recognize and report changes and abnormal signs and symptoms.
- Adaptability in modifying nursing assistant skills to the home situation.
- Acceptance of clients and their home environments.
- Ability to perform independently, making decisions within the limits of your responsibilities and the scope of the assignment.

THE NURSING BAG

Most home health care workers carry a nursing bag stocked with the supplies they use routinely in client care. Your bag should be stocked with enough supplies to carry you through the day without having to replenish it. Use a washable tote bag, backpack, or other carrying case that keeps supplies organized and easy to find. Clean and re-stock your bag daily. Never leave it in the car. Leaving it in the car invites theft, and heat and cold extremes may damage some of your supplies. Make it clear that you do not carry medications or syringes. When leaving your car for a short period of time, store the bag out of sight and lock the doors.

Surprisingly, some homes do not have running water. Alcohol-based hand cleaner is effective, but the CDC recommends washing hands with soap and water if the hands

GUIDELINES *for*

Nursing Bag Supplies

Your agency may have a basic supply list. If not, pack some basic supplies to get started.

- Cell phone
- Phone numbers
- Street map
- Pens
- Paper or memo book
- Extra forms for documentation
- Waterless (alcohol-based) hand cleaner
- Small bottle of liquid hand soap (antibacterial or antimicrobial type)
- Stethoscope
- Blood pressure cuff
- Thermometer and thermometer sheaths
- Pen light
- Tongue depressors, applicators, plastic bandage strips, adhesive tape, cotton balls, paper tape, 2 × 2 and 4 × 4 dressings (if you are responsible for applying simple dressings)
- Alcohol and povidone-iodine swabs
- Safety pins
- Newspapers
- Paper bag
- Plastic trash bags
- Small plastic bags

- Lubricant jelly or Vaseline
- Bandage scissors
- Rubber bands
- Disposable exam gloves
- Utility gloves, if you are responsible for dishwashing or cleaning
- Resuscitation mask
- N95 mask
- Goggles or face shield
- Disposable plastic aprons
- Disposable water-resistant gown
- Fingernail and toenail clippers in sheath
- Orangewood sticks
- Emery boards
- Household disinfectant
- Perineal cleanser ("peri-wash")
- Baby wipes
- Paper towels (carry a few folded dispenser towels, not an entire roll)

Some home health nursing assistants carry personal care items, such as aromatherapy soap, lotion, and shampoo. Grooming and hygiene products of this nature are not required, but they are certainly a bonus for the client's self-esteem.

---

are visibly soiled. Some workers carry a gallon jug of water in the car for this purpose.

When you bring your nursing bag into a home, you must place the bag and supplies on a barrier. You can use a piece of newspaper, a sheet of waxed paper, a disposable underpad ("blue pad"), or a plastic bag. Discard the barrier and a tied plastic bag of trash from supplies used during your visit when you leave the client's home.

Before using items from your bag:

1. Place your bag on the barrier, out of the reach of children.
2. Wash your hands or use an alcohol-based hand cleaner.

3. Put on a plastic apron and remove the necessary items from your bag.
4. When you are finished, wash and clean reusable equipment.
5. Wash your hands and replace equipment in your bag. Store contaminated supplies in a plastic bag for later cleaning and disinfection. If you used bandage scissors, wash them well with soap and water and dry them.
6. Discard contaminated disposable items. If the wastebasket is not lined with a plastic bag, it must be washed and thoroughly sanitized each time it is emptied.

PERSONAL SAFETY

Thousands of nursing personnel make daily home care visits, and incidents of violence are few. Still, personal safety is always a concern for home care workers. Be alert to conditions and people around you. Trust your instincts. If something does not feel right, it probably is not. There are several basic ways to protect your own safety:

- Map out the route in advance so you know where you are going.
- Inform the client what time you will be arriving.
- Lock your purse in the trunk of your car at the beginning of your day. Use pockets or a belt-type (fanny) pack for essentials such as driver's license and pens.
- Wear scrubs or clothing that identifies you as a nursing caregiver. Wear your name badge.
- In potentially dangerous areas, ask your agency if you can make joint visits with a coworker or use an escort.
- If neighbors, relatives, or others become a safety problem, make visits when they are away from the home.
- If a client suggests that a family member escort you, accept the offer, but never get into someone else's car.
- Keep your car's gas tank full.
- Avoid parking on deserted streets or in dark areas.
- Keep your car windows up and doors locked at all times.
- Attend classes on personal safety and self-defense.
- Always carry a cellular telephone, and keep the battery charged.

HOME HEALTH CARE DUTIES

The duties of the home health care assistant are planned around the client's and family's routine. These duties may include:

- Helping with the activities of daily living
- Giving special treatments
- Providing hygiene and comfort care
- Maintaining a safe environment
- Changing linen

Homemaker duties may include:

- Light housekeeping
- Shopping and preparing meals (Figure 34-2)

You may also have to transport the client to clinic or therapy visits (Figure 34-3). You must have permission from your agency to perform activities outside of the home. The homemaker duties *do not* include:

- Doing heavy housework, such as washing windows or moving heavy furniture
- Making decisions about food purchases, unless the client is unable to do so
- Becoming involved in family disputes

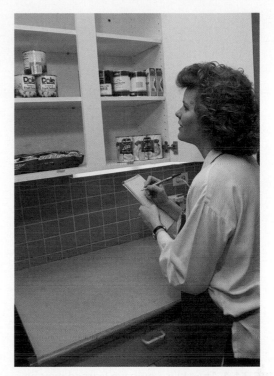

FIGURE 34-2 Homemaker duties may include grocery shopping. Prepare a shopping list before going to the store, to make sure you get everything. (© Delmar/ Cengage Learning)

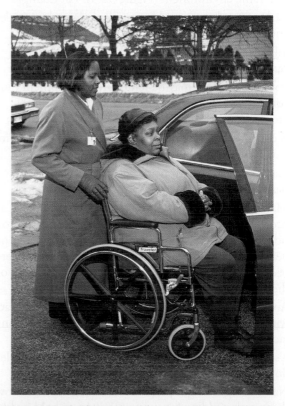

FIGURE 34-3 The home health assistant may have to transport clients to clinics for additional care and therapy. (© Delmar/Cengage Learning)

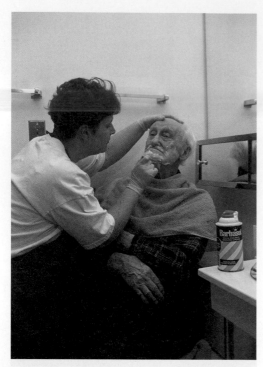

FIGURE 34-4 The skills you have learned may be adapted for care in the home. *(© Delmar/Cengage Learning)*

The skills you learned in the clinical setting can be adapted to the home environment (Figure 34-4). For example:

- Ice bags can be replaced by ice-filled plastic bags sealed and wrapped in a towel.
- Pillows can be used for support if the bed position cannot be changed.
- Some equipment may be rented from equipment rental companies (Figure 34-5) or borrowed from church groups or other organizations.
- A cotton blanket or lightweight spread can be used for a bath blanket.
- Plastic covered with a twin-size sheet can be used in place of a drawsheet.
- Making an occupied bed may be easier if you make a bedroll first. Lay the linen on the table. Roll it up from side to side, then top to bottom. Position the client on her side and unroll the linen halfway behind the client's back. Turn her on her other side and unroll the rest of the bedroll.
- Apply the principles of standard precautions if contact with blood, body fluids, mucous membranes, or nonintact skin is likely.
- Use a cardboard box or a straight chair turned upside down as a backrest (Figure 34-6A).
- Nail two lightweight pieces of wood together and cover them with padding for use as a footrest or hold bedding off the toes (Figure 34-6B).
- A bed tray can replace an overbed table for eating and activities.

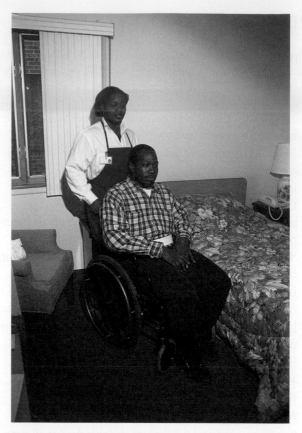

FIGURE 34-5 Equipment may be rented or borrowed from other organizations or agencies. *(© Delmar/Cengage Learning)*

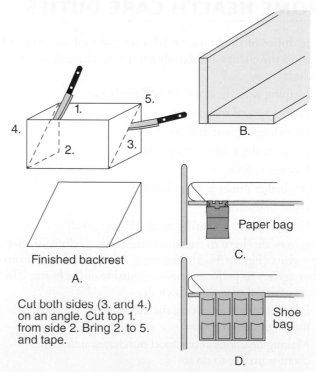

Cut both sides (3. and 4.) on an angle. Cut top 1. from side 2. Bring 2. to 5. and tape.

Finished backrest
A.

Paper bag
C.

Shoe bag
D.

FIGURE 34-6 Make equipment using readily available materials. *(© Delmar/Cengage Learning)*

- A paper bag can be taped to the table or bed to dispose of soiled tissues (Figure 34-6C).
- A shoe bag tucked under the mattress or hanging by the bedside (Figure 34-6D) can provide compartments for storage of and easy access to small personal articles.
- A pillowcase or plastic bag hung on the back of a chair can serve as a laundry bag.
- If you are assigned to do dressing changes on minor skin wounds, use a plastic bag. Place your hand inside the bag and gently remove the old dressing. Then turn the bag inside out, with the dressing on the inside. Tie or seal the bag and throw it away. This method may also be used for handling biohazardous or soiled material.
- Wind two rubber bands tightly around a slippery drinking glass to make it easier for a client to grasp. Place the rubber bands about an inch apart.
- Some clients cannot suck forcefully enough to draw liquids up through a straw. Wash and dry your bandage scissors, then cut the straw a few inches shorter. Place the cut end in the bottom of the glass and have the client suck from the smooth end. Removing a few inches is usually enough to enable them to drink successfully.
- Attach an inexpensive cloth tote bag or plastic grocery bag to the client's walker or wheelchair for carrying personal items.
- Cut a small foam hair curler lengthwise, then wrap the foam around oxygen tubing that rests on the ears, to reduce discomfort. Wrapping tubing with a corn or bunion pad will also relieve pressure.
- Place a large piece of plastic on the car seat (you can cut a large trash bag, if necessary) to enable the client to slide easily onto or off the seat.
- Use a wire coat hanger to hang a catheter bag on the bed.
- Use denture cleaner or dishwasher soap to remove sediment and stains on bedpans and urinals.
- Use a turkey baster (that is reserved for this purpose) and warm water to rinse reusable ostomy pouches and other items.

Difficult SITUATIONS

Dry, sore, burning, itchy eyes are a common problem in the elderly. The eyelids fill with matter, which worsens the problem. Washing the eyelids with tearless baby shampoo clears this condition quickly. ■

Difficult SITUATIONS

If the client or a family member informs you of new problems with eating, getting into or out of bed, incontinence, bathing, or dressing, notify the nurse. Clients with new problems related to these activities require further nursing assessment. ■

THE HOME ENVIRONMENT

You are responsible for maintaining a safe and comfortable environment for the client. This means that you must:

- Be alert to unsafe situations
- Control the spread of infection
- Care for and maintain the client's furnishings, supplies, and appliances
- Learn the locations of items that may be needed in an emergency (such as a flashlight or fire extinguisher)

Safety in the Home

Your first visit to the client's home gives you an opportunity to check safety factors. Tell a family member or supervising nurse about safety problems. Your job is to ensure a safe environment, not to reorganize the client's home. Discuss unsafe conditions and the need for additional equipment with the nurse. Offer suggestions for modifications that you believe may be useful.

Keep a list of emergency numbers close to the telephone. The list should include the:

- Agency
- Supervising nurse
- Physician
- Family member
- Emergency number 9-1-1 (in areas where this number is in use)

Safety ALERT

The most common locations of injury in the home are stairs and steps, bathroom(s), kitchens, and basements. If you feel there are hazards or other safety or security risks, inform your supervisor promptly. Do not attempt to make mechanical or environmental modifications yourself. ■

If the 911 number is not used in your area, you will need numbers for the:

- Ambulance
- Hospital
- Police department
- Fire department

Find out if the client:

- Uses a medical alert bracelet or necklace.
- Has out-of-hospital code papers, advance directives, or a living will.
- Has a special storage place in the house for important medical information that would be needed in an emergency. Some people keep these in the refrigerator so that they can be located easily.

ASSISTING WITH MEDICATIONS

The physician may prescribe medications for clients who receive home health care. You are not legally responsible for giving medications. However, you may have to supervise the client as she self-administers medications.

ELDER ABUSE

As a home health assistant, you may observe clients with signs and symptoms suggesting abuse. Unit 4 describes the various types of abuse that may be inflicted by staff members, family members, or others. Nursing assistants are not responsible for determining if abuse has occurred. Your responsibility is to report signs or symptoms to the nurse for further evaluation.

INFECTION CONTROL

Some of the methods used in daily cleaning help to control the spread of infection. Other requirements are:

- Washing your hands (Figure 34-7) or using an alcohol-based hand cleaner
- Keeping the kitchen and bathroom clean
- Caring for food properly
- Disposing of tissues and other wastes properly

Difficult SITUATIONS

Sometimes a client swallows a pill and complains that it "didn't go down all the way." A piece of banana works well for moving pills down the esophagus. ■

GUIDELINES *for*

Supervising Self-Administration of Medications

- Medications must be taken at the correct time. Note whether it should be taken before meals, with food, or after meals.
- Check the expiration date to be sure the medicine is not outdated.
- Note whether the client is also taking over-the-counter (nonprescription) medications and check with your supervisor to find out whether these medications will interact with the prescription drugs.
- Perform any monitoring activities required, such as checking the pulse, the blood pressure, or the blood sugar, *before* the drug is taken.
- Note how much medication is left in the container. Follow your instructions for getting the prescription refilled so that the client does not run out.

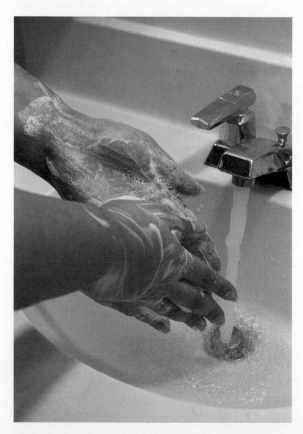

FIGURE 34-7 Handwashing is the most important infection control technique in health care. All handwashing rules and guidelines used in facilities also apply to home care. (© *Delmar/Cengage Learning*)

- Washing dirty dishes
- Dusting daily
- Not allowing clutter to accumulate
- Wearing a plastic apron
- Wearing latex gloves for client care if contact with blood, body fluids, mucous membranes, or nonintact skin is likely
- Wearing utility gloves when cleaning environmental surfaces or doing laundry contaminated with blood, body fluids, secretions, or excretions

DISCARDING MEDICAL WASTE

Your agency will have policies and procedures on discarding disposable, contaminated items, and on cleaning permanent items for reuse. Apply the principles of standard precautions and use personal protective equipment appropriate to the task. Follow your local regulations for disposal of all infectious medical waste.

HOUSEKEEPING TASKS

In some cases, the homemaker assistant (aide) will perform housekeeping tasks. In other cases, the home health care nursing assistant may be assigned some or all of these duties.

Cleaning the Client's Room

Keeping the client's room clean is a way to prevent infection. It also helps raise the client's morale. Do not rearrange the client's things without permission.

- Pick things up so clutter will not accumulate.
- Keep cleaning equipment in one place so that you do not waste time gathering it for each job as you move from room to room (Figure 34-8). A caddy or bucket is very helpful.
- Clean and put equipment away as soon as you have finished with it.
- Dust the room daily.
- Damp-dust noncarpeted floors weekly or vacuum carpeted floors.
- Remove used dishes and glasses when finished and rinse them right away.
- Put clean clothes away after laundering. Hang up robes when not in use.
- Line each wastepaper basket with a plastic bag and empty the baskets regularly.

Cleaning the Bathroom

The bathroom can be a source of infection, so you must be careful and thorough in your daily cleaning (Figure 34-9). Use a disinfectant solution (family's choice) for cleaning.

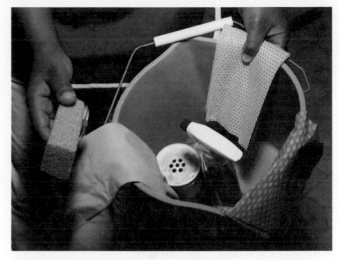

FIGURE 34-8 Keep cleaning equipment together for good organization and efficient time management. (© *Delmar/ Cengage Learning*)

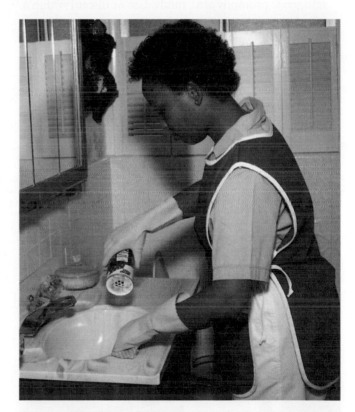

FIGURE 34-9 Clean the bathroom daily. (© *Delmar/ Cengage Learning*)

Place used towels in the laundry immediately after use. Replace them with clean towels and washcloths. Use a deodorizer to keep the bathroom smelling fresh and clean.

Cleaning the Kitchen

An unclean kitchen can be a source of infection.

- Clean up after each meal.

- Wash or rinse used dishes immediately. Do not allow them to accumulate in the sink.
  - After rinsing, wash by hand in detergent and hot water or in a dishwasher, if available. If using a dishwasher, rinse the dishes, load the dishwasher, and close the door. Run the dishwasher when it is full.
  - Wash glasses first, then silverware, then dishes, then cooking utensils such as pots and pans. Change the water as needed.
  - Rinse items with hot water and allow them to dry in a dish drainer.
  - Put away when dry.
- Wash pots and pans and utensils with wooden handles by hand; most are not dishwasher-safe.
- Clean sink, countertops, and stove.
- Dispose of garbage properly.
- Sweep the floor after each meal.
- Place leftover foods in small covered containers and refrigerate promptly after meals. Use or discard within a few days.
- Keep the refrigerator clean and keep food covered. Clean up spills in the refrigerator immediately (Figure 34-10).
- Keep the microwave oven clean (Figure 34-11). Use a damp cloth to wipe up spills immediately and to clean the microwave after each use. Heat food in microwave-safe dishes only. Do not use metal of any kind in a microwave oven. For example, never use dishes with metallic trim in a microwave.
- Wash the kitchen floor weekly, or more often if necessary.

Other Duties

Food management and laundry may be your responsibility in the home situation.

Food management Plan food purchases with the client or a family member. If consultation is not possible, keep these guidelines in mind:

- Plan menus a week in advance. Base them on good nutrition.

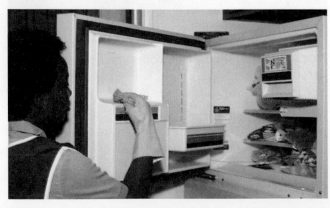

FIGURE 34-10 Wipe spills immediately. (© Delmar/ Cengage Learning)

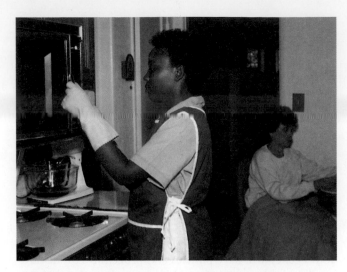

FIGURE 34-11 Wipe the microwave after each use. (© Delmar/Cengage Learning)

- Consider the client's ordered diet, digestive problems, and preferences. Take the client's cultural background and religious prohibitions into consideration.
- Spend only what the client's budget allows.
- Buy only what you need and what can be used.
- Look for quality bargains.
- Keep track of all money spent and a list of items purchased; keep receipts.

Using the weekly menu, prepare foods in such a way that the client's dietary needs are met. Also:

- Wash fresh fruits and vegetables that are to be used soon and store them in the refrigerator; store them unwashed if they will not be used right away. Remember to wash them before use.
- Keep dairy products and meats refrigerated until use.
- Allow frozen meats to thaw in the refrigerator before use.
- Keep dried and canned foods in cabinets.

Laundry Carefully launder the client's clothes. They represent a sizable investment. You may have to do laundry daily. Always:

- Read labels before laundering. Some clothes must be dry-cleaned or washed at special temperatures.
- Use the client's choice of detergent and read the label for instructions on the amount to use.
- Wear gloves when sorting clothing and loading the washing machine if contact with blood, body fluids, secretions, or excretions is likely.
- Separate and wash light and dark fabrics separately.
- Wash drip-dry fabrics separately so they can be hung and dried or folded.
- Be sure clothes can be dried in a dryer, and use the proper setting.
- Hang clothes after wiping off the clothesline, if a dryer is not available.

- After laundering, fold, iron, or hang clothes.
- Check for needed repairs and do mending before storing clothes.

- Ask the client or a responsible family member for operating instructions before using the client's washer or dryer.

REVIEW

A. Multiple Choice

Select the one best answer for each of the following.

1. Essential characteristics of the home health care nursing assistant include
   a. dependability and honesty.
   b. being a follower.
   c. being a fast worker.
   d. being able to take shortcuts.

2. The home health care nursing assistant *would not* be required to:
   a. shop for food.
   b. move heavy furniture.
   c. bathe and dress the client.
   d. prepare food for the client.

3. Home health assistant responsibilities include all of the following except:
   a. washing windows.
   b. cleaning the bathroom daily.
   c. documenting the care given.
   d. shopping for the client.

4. The home health assistant should carry a kit that contains
   a. a change of clothes and comfortable shoes.
   b. thermometers, stethoscope, blood pressure kit.
   c. gardening gloves.
   d. a policy and procedure manual.

5. Daily tasks may include
   a. sweeping the floor after each meal.
   b. watering the lawn and shrubs.
   c. shampooing the carpets.
   d. washing windows.

6. The home health nursing assistant's supervisor is the
   a. physician.
   b. licensed nurse.
   c. client's family.
   d. case worker.

7. Practicing nursing without a license
   a. applies only if medications are given.
   b. is acceptable in home care.
   c. is permitted in some states.
   d. is illegal.

8. The person receiving home health care is called the
   a. patient.
   b. resident.
   c. client.
   d. recipient.

9. Time management is important because
   a. you can get home earlier.
   b. you may have more than one client to care for during your shift.
   c. the client may have other business to tend to.
   d. the agency will make more money if you work faster.

10. Home care assistants must be able to
    a. know how to care for family pets.
    b. make accurate observations.
    c. manage the household bills.
    d. drive the client's car.

B. Nursing Assistant Challenge

You are working for a home health agency and Mrs. Fernandez is one of your clients. She has had a stroke and needs assistance with all activities of daily living. Your assignment includes: a bath, personal care, dressing, making the bed, making her breakfast, making her lunch so she can have it after you are gone, cleaning the bathroom, and general "picking up" around her apartment. She asks if you will go to the drugstore before you leave to get her prescriptions refilled.

11. Make a work plan that includes all of these tasks, as well as any other routine tasks you need to complete.

Body Systems, Common Disorders, and Related Care Procedures

Caring for Patients with Disorders of the Integumentary System

OBJECTIVES

After completing this unit, you will be able to:
- Spell and define terms.
- Review the location and function of the skin.
- Identify aging changes of the integumentary system.
- List common problems related to the integumentary system.
- Identify observations of signs and symptoms that the nursing assistant should make and report.

- Identify patients at risk for the formation of pressure ulcers.
- Describe the stages of pressure ulcer formation.
- Describe measures and identify appropriate nursing assistant actions to prevent pressure ulcers.
- Describe electrical, thermal, and chemical burns.
- Demonstrate the following procedure:
  - Procedure 86 Changing a Clean Dressing

VOCABULARY

Learn the meaning and the correct spelling of the following words and phrases:

abrasion	eschar	lesions	shearing
burns	excoriation	necrosis	skin tear
chemical burn	friction	pressure ulcer	thermal burn
contusion	hematoma	rash	
electrical burn	laceration	senile purpura	

INTRODUCTION

The integumentary system, or skin system, covers the body. It consists of the skin, hair, and nails. The skin protects against infection, maintains fluid balance in the body, excretes waste products, maintains temperature, and provides sensation for the body.

AGING CHANGES

The integumentary system changes with aging:
- The skin thins and becomes less elastic; wrinkles appear; skin becomes irritated and breaks more easily. The skin may appear translucent or pale.

The skin is the largest organ of the human body. In an average-size adult, the skin weighs approximately 4 kilograms (8.8 pounds). It covers an area of approximately 2 meters (78.4 inches). The average person's skin renews itself every 28 days. Human skin has about 100,000 bacteria per square centimeter; 10% of human dry weight is attributed to bacteria. The normal flora that live on the skin help to protect you from harmful bacteria. ∎

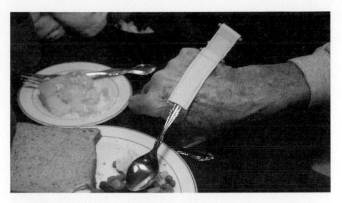

FIGURE 35-2 This is an elderly nursing home resident. The skin appears fragile, thin, and translucent. You can see the pronounced wrinkling and brown age spots. (© Delmar/Cengage Learning)

- Facial skin begins to sag from loss of elasticity. Jowls develop or worsen. *Jowl* is the word used to describe the jaw or cheek. When used in this context, *jowls* refers to loose, sagging skin about the lower cheek and jawline below the chin. Deep creases form on both sides of the mouth (Figure 35-1).
- Blood vessels that nourish the skin become more fragile and break more easily, resulting in bruising, senile purpura, and skin tears. **Skin tears** are irregular-shaped injuries in which the top layer of the skin peels back.
- Age spots (also called liver spots) (Figure 35-2) appear. These are brown areas that look like large freckles. They have little to do with aging. Age spots occur as a result of sun exposure earlier in life. People who have had significant sun exposure may develop these spots in their 20s or 30s, but they are commonly associated with aging skin.

Aging changes cause the skin to become very dry and fragile. The skin of elderly persons often tears, breaks, and bruises readily. Handle older patients very gently. ∎

- Blood flow in vessels that nourish the skin is reduced, resulting in slower healing.
- Oil glands that supply the skin secrete less, causing drying of the skin and itching.
- Perspiration decreases; the body's ability to regulate temperature is impaired.
- Subcutaneous fat diminishes.
- Blood supply to the feet and legs is reduced.
- Finger and toenail growth slows; nails thicken and become brittle.
- Hair thins and turns gray.

SKIN LESIONS

Injury or disease can cause changes in skin structures. These changes are called **lesions**. The lesions may be caused by disease, trauma, wear, or the aging process. Some lesions that occur as a result of injury are listed in Table 35-1.

Observation of the skin and accurate descriptions of what you see must be carefully charted. Abnormalities that should be reported to the nurse are listed in Table 35-2.

Use standard precautions when caring for patients who have skin lesions.

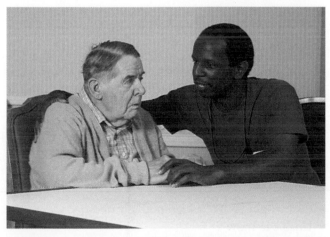

FIGURE 35-1 Aging changes to the skin are evidenced by deep creases on the sides of the mouth, sagging cheeks, and loose skin of the lower jaw and neck. (© Delmar/Cengage Learning)

TABLE 35-1 SKIN LESIONS

Abrasion	Injury that results from scraping the skin.
Contusion	Mechanical injury resulting in hemorrhage beneath unbroken skin.
Ecchymosis	A bruise.
Excoriation	A superficial mechanical injury caused by scraping or rubbing the skin surface. Excoriation may also occur as a result of skin exposure to irritating substances, such as urine or chemicals, or from burns.
Hematoma	Localized mass of blood that is confined to one area.
Laceration	Accidental break in the skin.
Rash	A change in the skin affecting color, appearance, or texture. The rash may cause pain and swelling. Rashes have many causes, such as allergies, infections (Unit 12), and parasites (Unit 12). A typical rash is red. The rash may be localized to one area of the body, or generalized, affecting the entire body. Rashes may itch, burn, feel hot to the touch, or appear bumpy, dry, cracked, or blistered.
Senile purpura	Dark purple bruises on forearms and backs of hands; common in older persons.
Skin tear	Shallow, irregular-shaped injury in which the epidermis is torn; common in older individuals.
Pressure ulcers (older names are *bedsore* and *decubitus ulcer*)	Open areas that develop over bony prominences as the result of pressure; can develop whether the patient is in bed or a chair.
Shearing	Injury that occurs when the skin moves in one direction while underlying structures move in the opposite direction, such as when being moved up in bed or sliding down in bed or in a wheelchair.
Friction	Rubbing the skin against another surface, such as bed linen.

TABLE 35-2 SIGNS AND SYMPTOMS OF SKIN CONDITIONS THAT SHOULD BE REPORTED TO THE NURSE IMMEDIATELY

- Rash
- Redness
- Redness in the skin that does not go away within 30 minutes after pressure is relieved from a bony prominence or pressure area
- In dark- or yellow-skinned patients, spots or areas that are darker in appearance than normal skin tone
- Pressure ulcers, blisters
- Abrasions, skin tears, lacerations
- Irritation
- Bruises
- Skin discoloration
- Swelling
- Lumps
- Abnormal skin growths
- Change in color of a wart or mole
- Abnormal sweating
- Excessive heat or coolness to touch
- Open areas/skin breakdown
- Drainage
- Foul odor
- Complaints such as numbness, burning, tingling, itching
- Signs of infection
- Unusual skin color, such as blue or gray color of the skin, lips, nail beds, roof of mouth, or mucous membranes
- Skin growths
- Poor skin turgor/tenting of skin on forehead or over sternum
- Sunken, dark eyes

PRESSURE ULCERS

Pressure ulcers occur most frequently over areas where bones come close to the surface. They are a serious problem for health care facilities. Although they are caused primarily by pressure on the skin, friction and shearing also contribute greatly to the problem. If the pressure on the skin is not promptly relieved, the ulcer can become very large and deep. Patients are at highest risk of pressure ulcers if they are:

- Elderly
- Very thin
- Overweight (also obese or morbidly obese)
- Unable to move
- Incontinent
- Debilitated
- Poorly nourished (eat less than half of meals and snacks)
- Confined to bed or wheelchair
- Disoriented

- Dehydrated
- In prolonged contact with moisture
- Circulation-impaired
- Subjected to friction and shearing

Patients who already have skin problems, such as discolored, torn, or swollen skin, are also at great risk of developing pressure ulcers.

Shearing (Figure 35-3) occurs when the skin moves in one direction while the structures under the skin, such as the bones, remain fixed or move in the opposite direction. This can happen when a patient is dragged rather than lifted up in bed, when a patient's positions is changed, or when the patient slides down in bed or in a wheelchair (Figure 35-4). Blood vessels become twisted and stretched, causing the tissues being served to lose essential oxygen and nutrients, leading to breakdown. In addition, shearing may cause painful tears in fragile skin. Skin tears are a portal of entry for infection, and commonly lead to further breakdown. **Friction** (rubbing the skin against

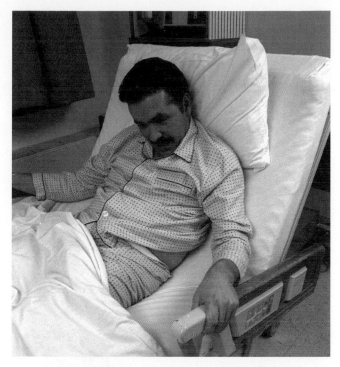

FIGURE 35-4 Shearing occurs when a patient slides down or is improperly pulled up in bed. *(© Delmar/Cengage Learning)*

another surface, such as bed linen) also contributes to pressure ulcer formation. It usually occurs when the patient is being moved.

Pressure ulcers occur most frequently over areas where bones come close to the surface. The most common sites (Figures 35-5A and 35-5B) are the:

- Elbows
- Heels
- Shoulders
- Sacrum, coccyx
- Hips
- Buttocks
- Ankles
- Ears
- Knees (inner and outer parts)
- Toes

Patients also tend to develop pressure ulcers where body parts rub and cause friction. Common sites are:

- Between the folds of the buttocks
- Legs
- Under the breasts
- Between abdominal folds
- Ankles
- Knees

The rubbing of tubing and other equipment used in long-term care of patients can also cause pressure sores (Figure 35-6).

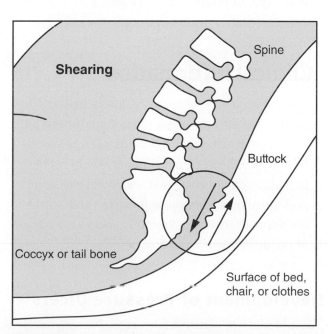

FIGURE 35-3 Shearing occurs when the skin is stretched in one direction and the underlying structures move in the opposite direction. *(© Delmar/Cengage Learning)*

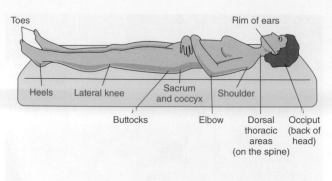

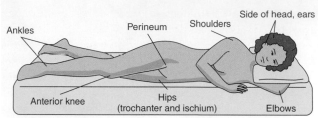

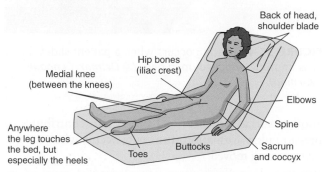

FIGURE 35-5A Potential areas of pressure when a patient is in bed. (© *Delmar/Cengage Learning*)

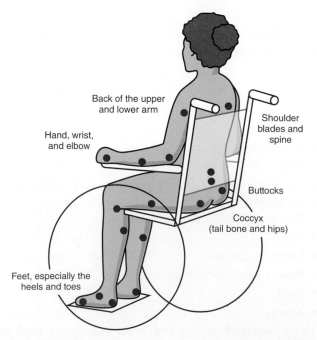

FIGURE 35-5B Potential areas of pressure when a patient is in a chair or wheelchair. (© *Delmar/Cengage Learning*)

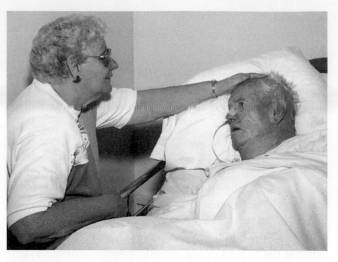

FIGURE 35-6 Rubbing and pressure from tubes can cause irritation and skin breakdown. (© *Delmar/Cengage Learning*)

Clinical Information ALERT

In 2006, government payers were billed for nearly 90% of hospitalizations during which pressure ulcers were noted. The average cost of stays for pressure ulcer care was $43,180, but charges varied by payer. The total cost of pressure ulcer care in the US was $11 billion. Pressure ulcers are preventable injuries. The government has announced that it will no longer pay for care of pressure ulcers that developed in the facility. ∎

Clinical Information ALERT

The red area on the patient's skin is believed to be the "tip of the iceberg" in a stage I pressure ulcer. The damage that cannot be seen below the skin may actually be much larger. Avoid rubbing or massaging red areas that are potentially stage I pressure ulcers. Rubbing will worsen and accelerate tissue destruction. Promptly inform the nurse of the presence of a red area. ∎

Development of Pressure Ulcers

Tissue breakdown occurs in four stages. Nursing intervention at each stage can limit the process and prevent further damage. Remember to continue all preventive measures throughout care.

Pressure Ulcer Stages

Stage I In stage I, the skin becomes red (Figures 35-7A and 35-7B) or blue-gray over the pressure area (usually a bony prominence). In dark-skinned people, the area may dry, and dark blue or black. The skin is intact, but the discoloration does not go away within 30 minutes after pressure has been relieved. The area may be hard, soft, warmer or cooler than adjacent tissue. It may be painful. At this stage, an ulcer is usually reversible if the area is identified promptly and pressure is relieved.

Stage II In stage II, the skin is reddened and there are abrasions, blisters, or a shallow crater at the site (Figures 35-8A and 35-8B). The surrounding area may be reddened. The skin may or may not be broken. (A serum-filled blister is an example of a stage II ulcer in which tissue is damaged but intact.) The epidermis alone or both the epidermis and the dermis may be involved. If the pressure ulcer is neglected at this stage, further and deeper damage occurs. Bruising of a stage II area suggests that deeper tissue damage may have occurred.

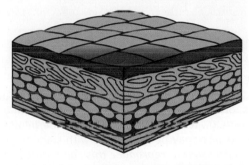

FIGURE 35-7A Cross-section of skin showing damage from stage I pressure ulcer. (© *Delmar/Cengage Learning*)

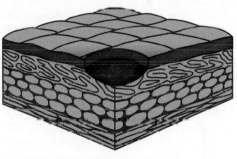

FIGURE 35-8A Cross-section of skin showing damage from stage II pressure ulcer. (© *Delmar/Cengage Learning*)

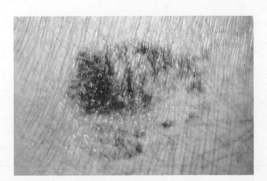

FIGURE 35-7B A stage I pressure ulcer has nonblanchable erythema of intact skin, the heralding lesion of skin ulceration. In individuals with darker skin, discoloration of the skin, warmth, edema, induration, or hardness may also be indicators. The lesion is not always round. Some pressure ulcers are irregular in shape. (*Permission to reproduce this copyrighted material has been given by the owner, Hollister, Inc.*)

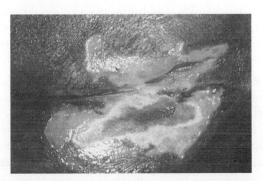

FIGURE 35-8B A stage II pressure ulcer has partial-thickness skin loss involving the epidermis, dermis, or both. The ulcer is superficial and presents clinically as an abrasion, blister, or shallow crater. The skin surrounding this ulcer is tender and inflamed and at very high risk of further breakdown. (*Permission to reproduce this copyrighted material has been given by the owner, Hollister, Inc.*)

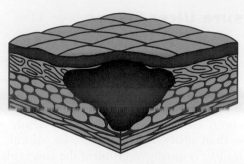

FIGURE 35-9A Cross-section of skin showing damage from stage III pressure ulcer. (© Delmar/Cengage Learning)

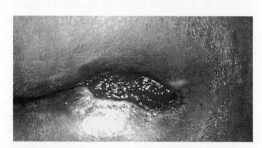

FIGURE 35-9B A stage III pressure ulcer has full-thickness skin loss involving damage to or necrosis of subcutaneous tissue that may extend down to, but not through, underlying fascia. The ulcer presents clinically as a deep crater with or without undermining of adjacent tissue. Although the diameter of this pressure ulcer is not large, the patient has experienced full-thickness skin loss. *(Permission to reproduce this copyrighted material has been given by the owner, Hollister, Inc.)*

Stage III In stage III, all the layers of the skin are destroyed and a deep crater forms (Figures 35-9A and 35-9B). Subcutaneous fat is visible, but other structures are not. Bone and tendon are not visible. An ulcer at stage III may include undermining (loose skin around the edge of the wound bed) or tunneling (tunnels running parallel into other tissue). The depth of this ulcer varies with the anatomical location. The ear, head, ankle, and bridge of the nose, do not have subcutaneous tissue, so stage III ulcers these areas can be shallow. However, areas with significant subcutaneous fat may develop very deep stage III pressure ulcers.

Stage IV In stage IV, the ulcer extends through the skin and subcutaneous tissues, and may involve bone, muscle, and other structures (Figures 35-10A and 35-10B). At this stage, the patient will experience fluid loss and is at great risk for infection. Tunneling and undermining may be present. The depth of this ulcer varies with the anatomical location. Because the ear, head, ankle, and bridge of the nose do not have subcutaneous tissue, so stage IV ulcers these areas can be shallow. However, areas with significant subcutaneous fat may develop very deep stage IV pressure ulcers. Bone and/or tendon may be visible or palpable.

Unstageable An unstageable pressure ulcer may cause full-thickness tissue loss in which the base of the ulcer is covered by slough (yellow, tan, gray, green, or brown)

and/or eschar (tan, brown, or black) in the wound bed. **Eschar** (Figure 35-11) is a thick crust or slough caused by the death of cells. The word **necrosis** may also be used to describe this condition. Both words are translated from Greek and mean "tissue death" or "scab." Once this condition has developed, it is irreversible. The wound-covering

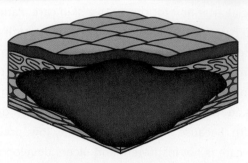

FIGURE 35-10A Cross-section of skin showing damage from stage IV pressure ulcer. (© Delmar/Cengage Learning)

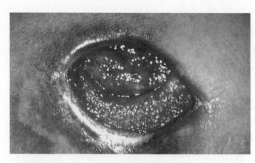

FIGURE 35-10B A stage IV pressure ulcer has full-thickness skin loss with extensive destruction, tissue necrosis, or damage to muscle, bone, or supporting structures (e.g., tendon, joint capsule). Undermining and sinus tracts also may be associated with stage IV pressure ulcers. *(Permission to reproduce this copyrighted material has been given by the owner, Hollister, Inc.)*

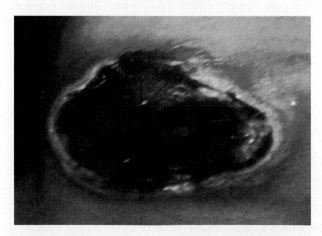

FIGURE 35-11 Necrotic tissue (eschar) is dead, devitalized tissue. It is usually hard, thick, and leathery. The wound covering is usually black or brown in color, but is occasionally red. A pressure ulcer cannot be accurately staged and healing will not occur until necrosis is surgically, chemically, or mechanically removed. *(Courtesy of Emory University Hospital, Atlanta, GA)*

Clinical Information ALERT

Pressure ulcers are very painful. A common health care myth is that stage IV ulcers do not hurt because they are below the nerve endings. This is not true. Although the base of the ulcer is stage IV, the nerve endings are exposed around the edges, which are usually the depth of a stage II or III ulcer. The ulcer has passed through stages I, II, and III before becoming a stage IV. In each of these stages, nerve endings were exposed and painful. Depending on the area of the ulcer on the body, even a minor stage I pressure ulcer can be very painful. ■

scab is commonly black, but may be other colors. It is often thick and leathery, and must be removed before a pressure ulcer can be staged or healing can occur. Eschar may also develop on burns and other nonpressure-related wounds.

Suspected Deep Tissue Injury

With a deep tissue injury, the skin remains intact, but a localized area usually turns purple or maroon in color, or looks like a blood-filled blister. Prior to these skin changes, the patient may complain of pain. The tissue may appear firm, mushy, boggy, or warmer or cooler compared with adjacent tissue. A deep tissue injury may be difficult to identify in persons with dark skin. The wound may worsen quickly, involving and exposing additional layers of tissue and underlying structures.

Preventing Pressure Ulcers

Because pressure ulcers are far easier to prevent than to cure, everyone caring for the patient is responsible for preventing skin breakdown.

When a patient is admitted, the nurse will assess the patient's potential for skin breakdown. This assessment gives a baseline against which all future assessments may be measured. The assessment may be described on the patient's chart in words, pictures, diagrams, or as a score. If a nursing diagnosis of "impaired skin integrity" or "risk for impaired skin integrity" is made, every staff member must make extra efforts to prevent skin breakdown, limit any breakdown that has already occurred, and promote healing. The care plan will list approaches to use and the person's skin condition will be evaluated daily. Report changes and abnormalities promptly.

GUIDELINES *for*
Preventing Pressure Ulcers

Nursing assistants are vital in preventing skin breakdown. Care should include:

- Changing the patient's position at least every 2 hours or more often. When moving a patient, avoid friction and shearing, such as sliding the patient over the sheets. Avoid dragging the heels when moving the person up in bed. Use lifting devices to avoid dragging. Follow the care plan.

- Encourage patients sitting in chairs or wheelchairs to raise themselves every 15 minutes to relieve pressure, or assist patients to do so.

- Encourage proper nutrition and adequate intake of fluids. Breakdown occurs more readily and healing is delayed when the patient is poorly nourished or fluid intake is inadequate.

- Cleanse the skin promptly if urinary or fecal incontinence occurs. These waste products are very irritating to the skin.

- Carefully check the skin daily and when giving personal care. Report abnormalities.

- Keep the skin and bedding clean and dry. The bed should be free from wrinkles and hard objects such as crumbs and hairpins.

- Keep the skin well lubricated with lotion. Do not massage an ulcer site, and avoid alcohol. Apply moisturizers by patting. Do not rub vigorously. Do not use lotion on broken skin.

- Separate body areas that are likely to rub together, especially over bony prominences, by using pillows, foam wedges, or folded bath blankets, according to the care plan.

- Use mechanical aids, pillows, and props to maintain position and relieve pressure, friction, and shearing.

- Protect areas at risk, such as heels and elbows.

continues

GUIDELINES *continued*

- Use a turning sheet or special moving device (Units 15 and 32) to move dependent patients in bed.

- Elevate the head of the bed no higher than 30°, to prevent a shearing effect on the tissues. If the patient must have the head elevated, relieve pressure from the buttocks, hips, and torso regularly. Monitor the skin condition closely.

- Carry out range-of-motion exercises at least twice daily to encourage circulation.

- Check all tubes that enter the body, to be sure they are not a source of pressure and irritation.

- Use pressure-reducing cushions between patients and bottom linen and wheelchair seats where excess pressure may be expected.

- Make sure bed linen is not too tight on the feet. Use a bed cradle, if needed to keep the bedding away from the skin.

- For patients in bed, relieve pressure on heels by supporting feet off the bed or using heel floats (Unit 32) and other devices to eliminate pressure on the sensitive, thin skin of the feet.

- For patients in chairs, avoid pressure from buttons and zippers, bulky seams, objects pockets, catheters, and clamps.

ACTIONS TO TAKE WHEN BREAKDOWN OCCURS

Nursing assistant actions when skin breakdown occurs include:

- Performing the actions listed in the guidelines to prevent further breakdown
- Following the care plan exactly
- Reporting fever, odor, drainage, bleeding, and changes in size or appearance of the breakdown area
- Keeping the area around the breakdown clean and dry

Positioning

Five basic in-bed positions are used to relieve pressure as the patient's condition permits. Each position must be supported for comfort. Review the positions in Unit 15 and follow each patient's care plan.

Note: The prone position is a sixth position, but it is not used by many facilities because it has the potential to cause respiratory distress. Follow your facility policies for use of the prone position.

Protecting the Feet

Bedfast patients are at very high risk for developing pressure ulcers on the feet and ankles. Although the heels and ankles are at greatest risk, ulcers may develop on the toes and the sides of the feet. Patients with hip fractures are at great risk. The skin on the feet and lower legs is thin, and there is little fatty padding. A shallow injury or pressure ulcer can become a deep stage IV ulceration very quickly. Foot ulcers are easy to prevent by propping the calves on pillows positioned lengthwise. This suspends the heels over the surface of the bed, relieving all pressure.

Mechanical Aids

Various props and mechanical aids are used to relieve pressure and protect the skin.

Heel and elbow protectors Heel (Figure 35-12A) and elbow (Figure 35-12B) protectors prevent friction and shearing, but do not relieve pressure.

Sheepskin pads Sheepskin (Figure 35-12C), or artificial sheepskin, absorbs moisture and reduces friction and shearing. It does not relieve pressure. Sheepskin also works well to prevent skin tears and bruises when the patient is up in a wheelchair (Figure 35-12D).

Foam pads, pillows, and overlays Foam pads and pillows are used to bridge areas to reduce pressure. Foam overlays (Figure 35-12E) are large foam pads that are placed on top of the mattress to provide a pressure-reducing surface. Some of these are cooler than other pads, which is important because trapped heat contributes to skin breakdown. Many foam overlays and pads lose their fire-retardant properties when washed, and must be replaced if they become soiled. Protect the surface of the overlay with incontinent pads to prevent accidental soiling.

Bed (foot) cradles Cradles lift the weight of bedding from the lower legs and feet. The reduction of pressure assists in preventing pressure ulcers.

Low air loss therapy beds and mattress overlays A low air loss bed (Figure 35-12F) provides pressure relief for patients who have special skin problems and risk factors. Low air loss beds relieve pressure and keep the patient cooler and drier than other types of beds. Most have special features, such as an instant deflate switch in the event that CPR is necessary. Some are equipped with bed scales. A low air loss mattress overlay (Figure 35-12G) is also available. The overlay replaces the mattress on a regular hospital

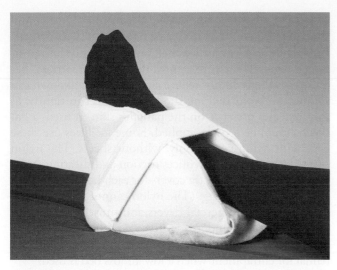

FIGURE 35-12A Heel protector. *(Courtesy of Skil-Care Corporation, Yonkers, NY; (800) 431–2972)*

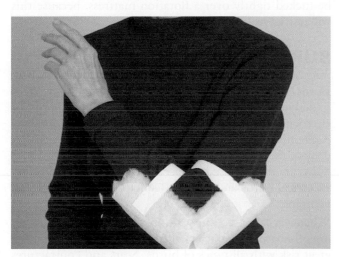

FIGURE 35-12B Elbow protector. *(Courtesy of Skil-Care Corporation, Yonkers, NY; (800) 431–2972)*

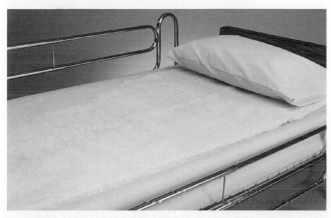

FIGURE 35-12C A synthetic sheepskin pad prevents friction. It does not relieve pressure. *(Courtesy of Skil-Care Corporation, Yonkers, NY; (800) 431–2972)*

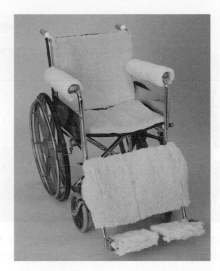

FIGURE 35-12D Padding the wheelchair with sheepskin protects the skin of patients who are at high risk of conditions such as skin tears. *(Courtesy of Skil-Care Corporation, Yonkers, NY; (800) 431–2972)*

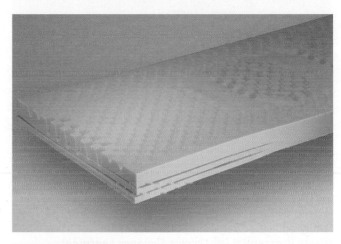

FIGURE 35-12E A foam mattress overlay has pressure-relieving properties and is comfortable for the patient. *(Courtesy of Medline Industries, Inc.; (800) MEDLINE)*

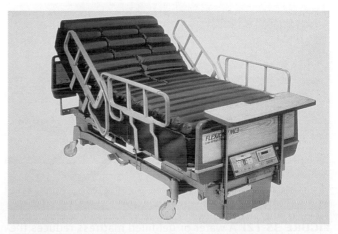

FIGURE 35-12F The low air loss bed. *(Courtesy of Hill-Rom, Charleston, SC)*

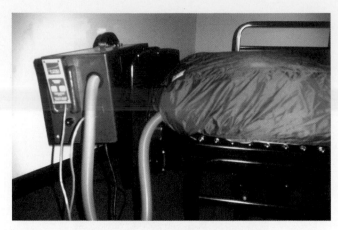

FIGURE 35-12G A low air loss mattress overlay can be used in place of a regular mattress. (© Delmar/Cengage Learning)

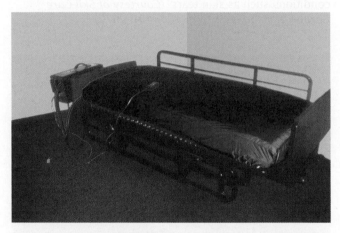

FIGURE 35-12H The nylon cover for the low air loss bed is used without sheets in some facilities. Patient and family education regarding the reasons for not using sheets is essential. (© Delmar/Cengage Learning)

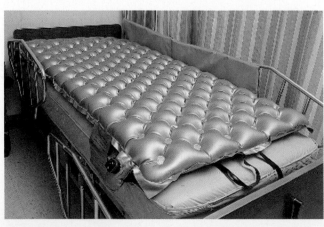

FIGURE 35-12I A water or gel-filled mattress reduces the risk of trapped heat and reduces pressure on bony prominences. (© Delmar/Cengage Learning)

bed. Low air loss beds reduce pressure, friction, and shearing, which are primary causes of skin breakdown. Patients using a low air loss bed must be turned and positioned regularly, despite using a therapeutic mattress. Because these beds do not relieve all pressure, breakdown can still occur. Avoid tucking the bottom sheet in tightly, as this increases pressure on the patient's skin. If used, a flat sheet should be loosely applied. Some facilities use these beds with nylon covers only, without sheets. The nylon cover (Figure 35-12H) reduces friction and shearing. Most facilities have several extra covers for each bed, to allow for washing and air-drying. (The nylon cannot withstand the heat of some commercial dryers and must be air-dried.) Special disposable underpads are used with the low air loss bed. Review the information in Unit 15 related to the potential for entrapment when a low air loss bed is used.

Flotation mattress A flotation mattress is a water bed with controlled temperature (Figure 35-12I). The weight of the patient's body displaces water so that pressure is consistently equalized against the skin. Sheets should not be tucked tightly over a flotation mattress, because this will restrict its function.

BURNS

Burns (Figure 35-13) are traumatic injuries to the skin and underlying tissues. They are caused by heat, chemicals, or electricity. A **thermal burn** is caused by heat, fire, or flame. A **chemical burn** is caused by exposure to chemicals that damage the skin and mucous membranes. The most severe burns are those caused by electricity, including lightning. **Electrical burns** are caused by contact with electricity and lightning.

Whenever large sections of skin are destroyed, the body loses fluids and chemicals called electrolytes. Infection is a great risk with all types of burns. Scars and contractures

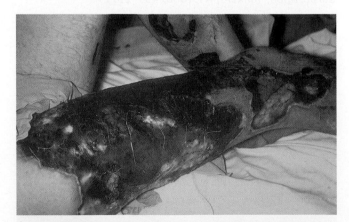

FIGURE 35-13 Burns are at high risk for infection and many other complications. They are usually very painful and take a long time to heal. Surgery and many other procedures are often necessary to treat the patient. (Courtesy of Emory University Hospital, Atlanta, GA)

are common complications. Burns to the face can cause disfigurement and emotional trauma. Extensive treatment is often required. Special nursing assistant care for burn patients emphasizes:

- Reporting pain so that appropriate analgesics may be prescribed and given
- Maintaining proper alignment
- Gentle positioning, as ordered, to prevent contractures
- Encouraging a high-protein diet
- Carefully measuring intake and output
- Giving emotional support and encouragement
- Carrying out procedures that prevent infection
- Applying the principles of standard precautions and wearing the correct protective apparel if contact with burned skin areas is likely

Note: A burn patient may be on a CircOlectric bed, Stryker frame, or Clinitron bed to permit frequent rotation to relieve pressure.

APPLYING A CLEAN DRESSING

Clean dressings are used on minor, uninfected wounds. Handle only the corners of the dressings. Avoid touching the center, which contacts the wound. Be sure to wash your bandage scissors and dry them well before and after using them for a dressing change.

Infection Control ALERT

Your bandage scissors, stethoscope, and other personal items may transfer pathogens from one patient to the next. If personal equipment items will be used during a procedure, wash them with an alcohol product or soap and water before and after each use. ∎

PROCEDURE

86

CHANGING A CLEAN DRESSING

1. Carry out initial procedure actions.
2. Assemble equipment:
   - 2 pair clean, disposable exam gloves
   - Cleansing solution
   - Plastic bag for used supplies
   - Clean or sterile gauze pads or other dressing, as ordered, and according to facility policy
   - Tape or bandage material
3. Holding gentle traction on the skin, loosen the tape by pulling the ends toward the wound, and remove the dressing. Discard in the plastic bag.
4. Cleanse and rinse the wound as ordered. If the wound appears abnormal or infected, notify your supervisor.
5. Remove your gloves and discard them in the plastic bag.
6. Wash your hands.
7. Set up your dressing supplies, and open packages.
8. Apply clean exam gloves.

9. Pick up the gauze dressing, holding it only by the corners.
10. Center the dressing over the wound.
11. Tape the dressing securely in place, or cover it with a bandage, as instructed.
12. Perform your procedure completion actions.

Applying a Bandage

After applying the dressing, apply the bandage. Most bandaging materials are conforming, self adhering gauze. Brand name products, such as Kling® and Kerlix®, or generic products, such as conforming gauze, are commonly used in health care facilities. The bandage must cover the dressing completely.

13. Begin by holding the bandage in your dominant hand. Hold the bandage against the skin with your nondominant thumb, approximately 1 inch below the dressing.
14. Wrap the bandage around the extremity two or three times to hold it securely in place. Wrap the bandage from distal to proximal, in overlapping spiral turns

continues

PROCEDURE 86 CONTINUED

(Figure 35-14). Each turn should overlap ½ to ¾ of the previous turn. The bandage should be snug enough that it does not fall off. However, it must not be so tight that it restricts blood flow.

15. Wrap the bandage at least 1 inch above the top of the dressing. Wrap it completely around the

extremity twice, then cut the end. Tape the end to the bandage, not the skin.

16. Check the circulation distal to the bandage to ensure that the circulation is adequate.

17. Perform your procedure completion actions.

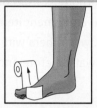

Foot and ankle: Use 3-inch width. Hold foot at right angle to leg. Start bandage on ridge of foot just back of the toes.

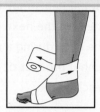

Pass bandage around foot from inside to outside. After two or three complete turns around foot, ascending toward the ankle on each turn, make a figure eight turn by bringing bandage up

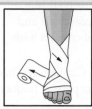

over the arch–to the inside of the ankle–around the ankle–down over the arch–and under the foot.

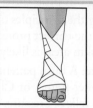

Repeat the figure eight wrapping two to three times. Fasten end by pressing the last 4 to 6 inches of unstretched bandage to the preceding layer.

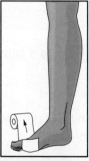

Lower leg: Use 3-4 inch width depending on the size of the leg. A leg wrap requires two rolls of bandage. Hold foot at right angle to leg. Start bandage on ridge of foot just back of the toes.

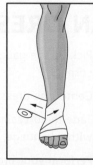

Pass bandage around foot from inside to outside. After two complete turns around foot, make a figure eight turn by bringing bandage up over the arch–to the inside of the ankle– around the ankle–

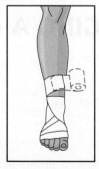

down over the arch–and under the foot. Start circular bandaging, making the first turn around the ankle. To begin the second roll of bandage, simply overlap the unstretched ends by 4 to 6 inches, press firmly, and continue wrapping.

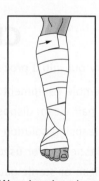

Wrap bandage in spiral turns to just below the kneecap. Fasten end by pressing the last 4 to 6 inches of unstretched bandage to the preceding layer.

FIGURE 35-14 Bandage-wrapping techniques. Always wrap from distal to proximal using spiral, circular, and figure-eight turns. *(Courtesy Becton Dickinson, and Co., Rutherford, NJ)*

PROCEDURE 86 CONTINUED

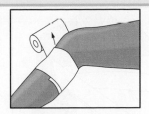

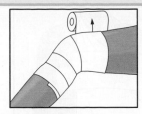

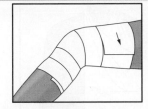

Knee: Use 4 inch width. Bend knee slightly. Start with one complete circular turn around the leg just below the knee.

Start circular bandaging, applying only comfortable tension. Cover kneecap completely.

Continue wrapping to thigh just above the knee. Fasten end by pressing the last 4 to 6 inches of unstretched bandage to the preceding layer.

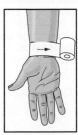

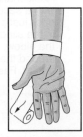

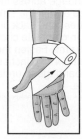

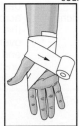

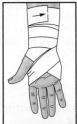

Wrist: Use 2- or 3-inch width. Anchor bandage loosely at the wrist with one complete circular turn.

Carry the bandage across the back of the hand, through the web space between the thumb and index finger

and across palm to the wrist. Make a circular turn around

the wrist and once more carry the bandage through the web space and back to the wrist.

Start circular bandaging, ascending to the wrist. Fasten the end by pressing the last 4 to 6 inches of unstretched bandage to the preceding layer.

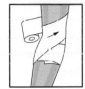

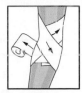

Elbow: Use 3- or 4-inch width, depending on the size of the arm. Two rolls of bandage are required to complete the wrap. Start with a complete circular turn just below the elbow.

Wrap bandage in loose figure eights

to form a protective bridge across the front of the elbow joint.

Fasten end by pressing 4 to 6 inches of unstretched bandage to preceding layer. Start second bandage with a circular turn below the elbow

over the first wrap. Continue spiral bandaging over the elbow, ascending to the lower portion of the upper arm. Fasten end with circular turn.

FIGURE 35-14 continued

PROCEDURE 86 CONTINUED

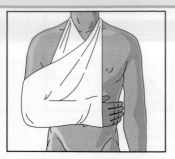

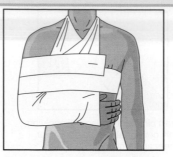

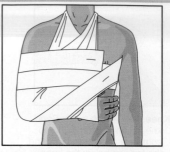

Shoulder: A shoulder wrap is used to provide additional support for an arm in a sling. Use 4- or 6-inch width. One or two rolls of bandage may be used. Start under the free arm.

Carry the bandage across the back, over the arm in the sling, across the chest and back under the free arm in complete circular, overlapping turns. Fasten the end by pressing 4 to 6 inches of unstretched bandage to under-lying bandage.

Additional support can be obtained with a second bandage. Start at the back just behind the flexed elbow in the sling. Carry the bandage under the elbow, up over the forearm, around the chest and back, and repeat. Fasten end.

FIGURE 35-14 continued

REVIEW

A. Multiple Choice

Select the one best answer for each of the following.

1. To help ensure adequate circulation to prevent skin breakdown, you could
   a. change the patient's position frequently.
   b. position the patient on bony prominences.
   c. rub red areas well.
   d. apply rubbing alcohol to the skin after bathing.

2. In a dark-skinned person, a stage I pressure ulcer may appear
   a. red or pink.
   b. gray or green.
   c. blue or black.
   d. shiny and oily.

3. Patients using low air loss beds
   a. do not require repositioning, as the bed relieves pressure.
   b. should be turned and positioned at least every 2 hours.
   c. should be turned and positioned twice each shift.
   d. should be turned and positioned every 30 to 45 minutes.

4. Shallow, irregular-shaped injuries in which the skin is torn that are common in older persons are
   a. lacerations.
   b. skin tears.
   c. pressure ulcers.
   d. senile purpura.

5. An injury that occurs when the skin is moved in one direction and underlying structures move in the opposite direction is
   a. shearing.
   b. excoriation.
   c. friction.
   d. eschar.

6. Dark purple bruises seen on the backs of the forearms and hands of older persons are
   a. skin tears.
   b. abrasions.
   c. senile hematomas.
   d senile purpura.

7. When a person has a stage I pressure ulcer, the skin is
   a. barely scratched.
   b. usually blistered.
   c. not broken.
   d. draining slightly.

8. A patient has a pressure ulcer on the hip in which bone is visible. You know this ulcer is a stage
   a. IV.
   b. III.
   c. II.
   d. I.

9. An intact blister on a bony prominence suggests that the bedfast person has a
   a. skin tear.
   b. stage I pressure ulcer.
   c. stage II pressure ulcer.
   d. contusion.

10. An ulcer that extends to the subcutaneous fat is a
   a. stage III pressure ulcer.
   b. stage II pressure ulcer.
   c. stage IV pressure ulcer.
   d. stage I pressure ulcer.

B. Nursing Assistant Challenge

Agnes Finlay has been transferred to your hospital unit from a long-term care facility. She uses a wheelchair but fell and fractured her arm. You notice a reddened area around the base of her spine. Answer the following by selecting the correct word.

11. People sitting in wheelchairs should raise themselves every _____ minutes.

   (60)   (15)

12. While she is in bed, Ms. Finlay's position should be changed at least every _____ hours.

   (3)   (2)

UNIT 36

Caring for Patients with Cardiopulmonary Disorders

OBJECTIVES

After completing this unit, you will be able to:

- Spell and define terms.
- Identify aging changes of the circulatory and respiratory systems.
- Describe some common disorders of the circulatory and respiratory systems.
- Describe nursing assistant observations and actions related to care of patients with disorders of the circulatory and respiratory systems.

- Identify patients who are at high risk of poor oxygenation.
- Describe nursing assistant care of a patient who is on a ventilator.
- Demonstrate the following procedures:
  - Procedure 87 Checking Capillary Refill
  - Procedure 88 Using a Pulse Oximeter
  - Procedure 89 Collecting a Sputum Specimen

VOCABULARY

Learn the meaning and the correct spelling of the following words and phrases:

angina pectoris	congestive heart failure	infarction	peripheral
arteriosclerosis	(CHF)	ischemia	phlebitis
ascites	continuous positive	laryngectomee	pneumonia
asthma	airway pressure	laryngectomy	pulse oximetry
atherosclerosis	(CPAP)	myocardial infarction	respiratory care
bronchitis	dyscrasias	(MI)	practitioner
cannula	dyspnea	nasal cannula	(RCP)
capillary refill	emphysema	nebulizer	sputum
cardiac decompensation	heart block	orthopnea	stoma
chest tubes	high Fowler's position	orthopneic position	tracheostomy
chronic obstructive	humidifier	oxygen concentrator	tripod position
pulmonary disease	hypertrophy	oxygen mask	upper respiratory
(COPD)	hypoxemia	oxygenation	infection (URI)
compensates	incentive spirometer	pacemaker	varicose veins

INTRODUCTION

Life cannot be maintained without oxygen, and carbon dioxide must be eliminated from the body. Diseases of the respiratory tract that interfere with this vital exchange of gases bring acute distress. The need for oxygen is at the base of Maslow's hierarchy of needs, making it one of the most important needs. Nursing care is directed toward making breathing easier and preventing transmission of infection.

The circulatory system is a transportation system that carries nutrients and oxygen to the cells throughout the body and removes wastes. It is also called the cardiovascular system. This is a closed system, somewhat like a radiator. Diseases of this system interfere with overall body function. Long-standing conditions will also affect the pulmonary system.

The circulatory and respiratory systems work closely together. Because of this, the two systems may be referred to as a single system, called the cardiopulmonary system (*cardio* means heart, and *pulmonary* refers to the lungs).

Clinical Information ALERT

The lungs are the only organs of the body that float in water. Humans breathe 20 times per minute, more than 10 million times per year, and about 700 million times in a lifetime. The lungs contain almost 1,500 miles of airways and more than 300 million alveoli. The average person breathes in 13 pints of air each minute. ■

Clinical Information ALERT

The heart is about the same size as your fist. It beats about 100,800 times each day. The most powerful chamber is the left ventricle. The pressure exerted by this chamber will squirt a stream of blood approximately 10 yards. There are approximately 60,000 miles of blood vessels in the human body, the equivalent of approximately 2.5 times around the world. A single drop of blood contains about 5 million red blood cells. It takes about a minute for a blood cell to travel throughout the body. ■

Clinical Information ALERT

Patients with some types of heart disease will have a fever. This is an inflammatory response to heart cell damage after conditions such as a heart attack or acute infection of the heart. ■

AGING CHANGES TO THE CARDIOVASCULAR SYSTEM

- The heart rate slows, causing a slower pulse and less efficient circulation.
- Blood vessels lose elasticity and develop calcium deposits, resulting in narrowing.
- Blood pressure increases because of changes to the walls of the blood vessels.
- It takes longer for the heart rate to return to normal after exercise.
- Veins become enlarged, causing the blood vessels near the surface of the skin to become more prominent.

DISORDERS OF THE CIRCULATORY SYSTEM

Common disorders of the circulatory system include:
- Diseases of the heart and blood vessels
- Blood **dyscrasias** (abnormalities); these can also involve the bone, bone marrow, liver, or spleen

Peripheral Vascular Diseases

The blood vessels that serve the outer parts of the body, particularly those of the hands and feet, are referred to as **peripheral** (toward the outer part) blood vessels. Diseases of these vessels affect the parts of the body through which the vessels pass. The health of these vessels also influences heart function.

Protecting the feet Patients with impaired circulation are at great risk of ulceration, gangrene (Figure 36-1), and amputation due to pressure on or injuries to the feet and ankles. A small injury or ulcer can lead to major complications. Be sure all pressure is relieved from the feet when the patient is in bed.

Nursing assistant responsibilities include:
- Protecting the feet from injury.
- Checking the feet daily for irritation or injury.
- Making sure the patient wears socks with shoes that fit correctly.

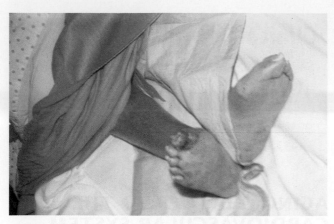

FIGURE 36-1 Both feet are edemetous, the left more than the right. The right big toe is gangrenous, and the doctors considered a below-the-knee amputation, believing that the lower leg and foot could not be saved. However, the patient responded to treatment; the right great toe eventually was amputated, but the foot and lower leg were saved. *(Photo courtesy of Barbara Acello)*

Clinical Information ALERT

Edema (Figure 36-2) develops when the heart cannot pump blood efficiently. Extra fluid has nowhere to go, so it enters the tissues in lower parts of the body. To check for edema, gently press two fingers into the skin and release immediately. If marks from the fingers remain, the person has pitting edema. Table 36-1 provides an overview of pitting edema, which is a potentially serious problem. Notify the nurse promptly. ■

- Not cutting toenails and not using sharp objects (such as nail files) on the toes.
- Making sure bed linen is not too tight on the feet, and using a bed cradle, if needed.
- Removing support hose regularly and checking the skin.
- Keeping the heels elevated above the surface of the bed.
- Making sure the feet are supported on footrests when the patient is using a wheelchair; avoid dragging them across the floor.

Arteriosclerosis

Arteriosclerosis is a very general term used to describe narrowing of the inside walls of the arteries, which makes

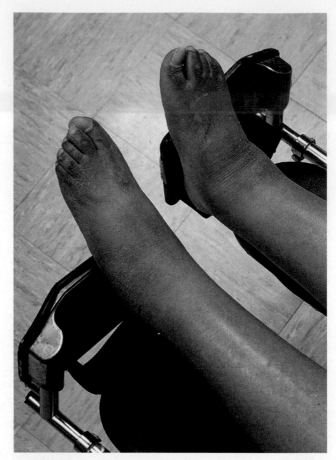

FIGURE 36-2 Persons with heart, circulatory, or kidney problems may develop edema of the lower extremities. (The patient's shoes have been removed so the edema could be pictured. Never get a patient up in a chair without proper foot covering.) *(© Delmar/Cengage Learning)*

TABLE 36-1 ESTIMATING PITTING EDEMA

+1 = slight pitting (about 2 mm depression), barely detectable, no visible distortion, disappears rapidly
+2 = greater depth (approximately 4 mm), no visible distortion of extremity, disappears in 10 to15 seconds
+3 = visible change in limb contour, definite pit (approximately 6 mm) that persists for more than 1 minute
+4 = grossly distorted limb, very deep pit (approximately 8 mm) lasting 2–5 minutes

them rigid and thick. The lay term for this condition is "hardening of the arteries." This describes the loss of elasticity that occurs with the arteriosclerosis process. Because the arteries have become narrower, adequate blood flow cannot pass through the vessel walls to nourish the body. High blood pressure is common because the heart has to work harder to force blood through the narrow, rigid vessels. Persons with this condition are at high risk of stroke and heart attack.

Atherosclerosis

Atherosclerosis is very similar to arteriosclerosis, and the two terms are often used interchangeably, but they are not the same thing. Atherosclerosis is the most common form of vascular disease, in which lipids (fats) consisting

of cholesterol are deposited on the walls of arteries. In later stages, calcium deposits, immune cells, and connective tissue also accumulate. This causes rough areas to form on the inner walls of the arteries. The deposits narrow the vessels. They grow progressively larger until blood flow is blocked (Figure 36-3). Blood clots form on the rough area, then break off and travel through the body, eventually blocking a blood vessel. The narrowing of blood vessels can lead to other serious complications in many parts of the body (Figure 36-4), such as myocardial infarction, stroke (cerebrovascular accident or CVA), and gangrene.

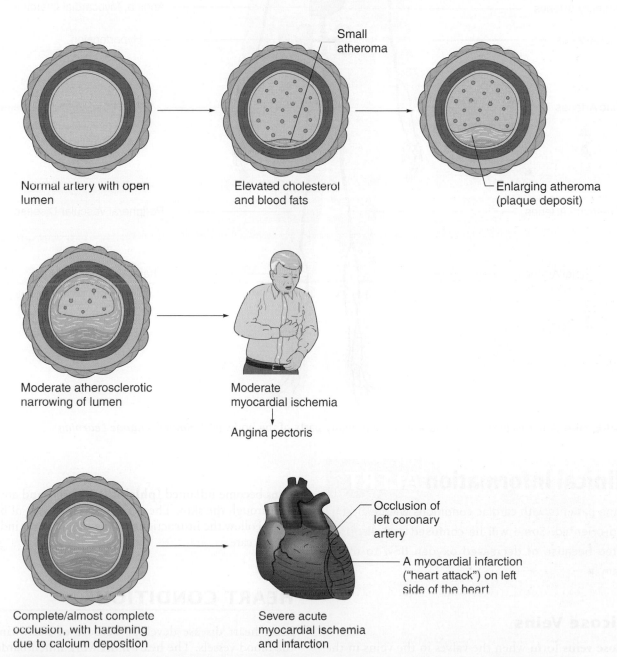

Normal artery with open lumen

Elevated cholesterol and blood fats

Small atheroma

Enlarging atheroma (plaque deposit)

Moderate atherosclerotic narrowing of lumen

Moderate myocardial ischemia

Angina pectoris

Complete/almost complete occlusion, with hardening due to calcium deposition

Severe acute myocardial ischemia and infarction

Occlusion of left coronary artery

A myocardial infarction ("heart attack") on left side of the heart

FIGURE 36-3 Cross-sections through a coronary artery undergoing atherosclerotic changes. (© Delmar/ Cengage Learning)

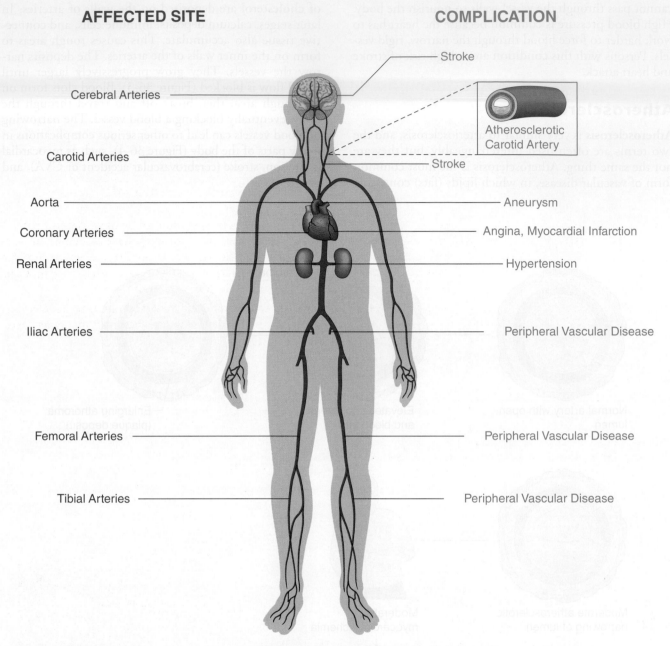

AFFECTED SITE   **COMPLICATION**

Stroke

Cerebral Arteries

Atherosclerotic
Carotid Artery

Carotid Arteries — Stroke

Aorta — Aneurysm

Coronary Arteries — Angina, Myocardial Infarction

Renal Arteries — Hypertension

Iliac Arteries — Peripheral Vascular Disease

Femoral Arteries — Peripheral Vascular Disease

Tibial Arteries — Peripheral Vascular Disease

FIGURE 36-4 Atherosclerosis can cause disease in many parts of the body. (© *Delmar/Cengage Learning*)

Clinical Information ALERT

Some patients with cardiac conditions will be alert and oriented. Some will be confused and disoriented because of decreased oxygen flow to the brain. ∎

Varicose Veins

Varicose veins form when the valves in the veins in the legs become weakened (Figure 36-5). When this occurs, blood does not flow through the veins as it should. The

veins become inflamed (**phlebitis**), enlarge, and are visible through the skin. The person is at high risk of blood clots. Follow the instructions on the care plan for individualized care.

HEART CONDITIONS

Most heart disease develops because of narrowing of the blood vessels. The heart must work much harder to pump blood around the body through these narrow vessels.

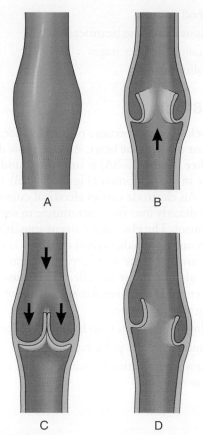

FIGURE 36-5 Veins contain valves to prevent the backward flow of blood. A. External view of the vein shows wider area of valve. B. Internal view with the valve open as blood flows through. C. Internal view with the valve closed. D. Vein with weakened valve that causes a varicose vein. (© Delmar/Cengage Learning)

Clinical Information ALERT

Poor circulation is common in persons with cardiovascular disorders. This causes reduced blood flow to all parts of the body. Pain is a common sign of reduced blood flow, which in this case is called **ischemia**. Chest pain is caused by ischemia of the heart muscle. Pain in the legs from lack of oxygen to the leg muscles is also common. ■

Angina Pectoris

Angina pectoris is known as cardiac "pain of effort" or "pain of exertion." The coronary arteries, which nourish the heart, often are the site of atherosclerotic changes. When a person has an angina attack, the vessels cannot meet the heart's demand for oxygen. Signs and symptoms differ with each person, but the symptoms are usually consistent each time the individual experiences an attack. Signs and symptoms of angina pectoris that you should report include:

- Pain when exercising or under stress. The pain is dull, with increasing intensity. It is usually under the sternum, and may radiate to the neck and left arm.
- Pale or flushed face.
- Perspiration.

Myocardial Infarction (Heart Attack)

An acute **myocardial infarction** (MI) occurs when the coronary arteries, which nourish the heart, are blocked. Part of the heart muscle supplied by these vessels becomes ischemic (loses its blood supply). Unless circulation is restored quickly, the cells die (**infarction**). If too much tissue dies, the person cannot survive. The signs and symptoms of a heart attack include:

- Pain—resembles severe indigestion in some people. It is often described as "crushing" chest pain that radiates to the jaw and left arm (Figure 36-6).
- Nausea and vomiting.
- Irregular pulse and respiration.
- Perspiration (*diaphoresis*).
- Feelings of anxiety and weakness.
- Indications of shock, which include drop in blood pressure and pallor.
- Shortness of breath.
- Syncope (fainting).
- Restlessness.
- Cyanosis or gray skin color.

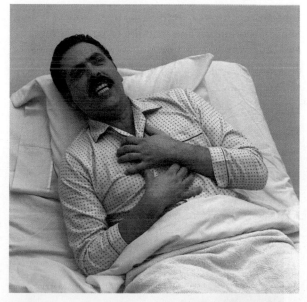

FIGURE 36-6 The patient having a heart attack usually experiences crushing chest pain that is described as "the worst pain I've had in my life," or "It feels like an elephant is standing on my chest." (© Delmar/Cengage Learning)

Always take complaints of chest pain seriously. Have the patient stop activity immediately and assume a comfortable position. Stay with the patient and call for assistance.

Congestive Heart Failure

Like any other muscle, the heart will enlarge and tire if it has to work against increasing pressure. When blood vessels narrowed by atherosclerosis increase the resistance to blood flow, it is more difficult to maintain the circulation. The heart does not pump well enough to meet the body's demands. At first, the heart enlarges (**hypertrophy**) and makes up (**compensates**) for the additional workload. However, eventually it reaches a point when it can no longer compensate. Heart failure follows.

This form of heart disease is known as **congestive heart failure (CHF)** or **cardiac decompensation**. The condition got its name because of *failure* of the *heart* to pump efficiently, which results in *congestion* of the lungs. The signs and symptoms are the result of the heart being unable to pump the blood with sufficient force. The person with CHF may experience:

- Hemoptysis (spitting up blood)
- Cough
- Dyspnea (difficulty breathing)
- **Orthopnea** (difficulty in breathing unless sitting upright)
- **Ascites** (fluid collecting in the abdomen)
- Neck vein swelling
- Fatiguing easily
- Hypoxemia
- Confusion
- Edema
- Shortness of breath and inability to lie flat at night
- Congestion and fluid accumulation in the lungs
- Cyanosis
- Rapid, irregular pulse
- Pulse deficit (see Unit 19) (Figure 36-7)

- High blood pressure
- Palpitations (galloping heartbeat)
- Kidney failure, in later stages
- Liver malfunction

Heart Block

Heart block develops because of interference in the electrical current through the heart. An electronic device called a **pacemaker** (Figure 36-8A) is implanted under the chest muscles or in the abdomen (Figure 36-8B) to treat this condition. An electrode carries electrical current from the pacemaker directly into the heart muscle to replace the lost natural control. The electrical current signals the heart to contract. Some pacemakers send messages only if normal messages carried by the conduction system are delayed. This type of pacemaker is called a *demand pacemaker*. Other pacemakers send regular signals to keep the heart contracting at a preset rate.

When caring for a patient who has a pacemaker:

- Count and record the pulse rate
- Report any irregularities or changes below the present rate

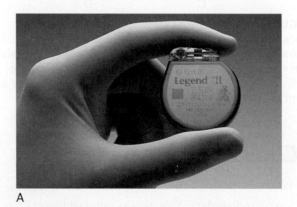

A

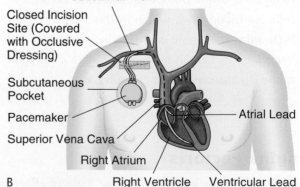

Subclavian Vein
Closed Incision Site (Covered with Occlusive Dressing)
Subcutaneous Pocket
Pacemaker
Superior Vena Cava
Right Atrium
Atrial Lead
Right Ventricle   Ventricular Lead

B

FIGURE 36-8 The electronic pacemaker sends electrical impulses to the heart muscle, causing it to contract. A. A typical pacemaker. B. The pacemaker is inserted under the skin with the electrode placed inside the heart, resting on the heart muscle. *(Photo courtesy of Medtronic, Inc.)*

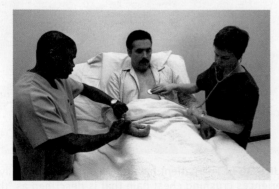

FIGURE 36-7 Ineffective heart contractions may cause a pulse deficit. *(© Delmar/Cengage Learning)*

- Report any discoloration over the implant site
- Report hiccupping, because this may indicate problems
- Keep the patient away from microwave ovens and cellular phones, because they may disrupt the function of the pacemaker

As you can see, each cardiopulmonary disorder has a set of signs and symptoms suggesting complications. Although these are similar, they are not identical. Table 36-2 provides an overview of cardiopulmonary signs and symptoms that warrant prompt reporting.

RESPIRATORY CONDITIONS

Patients with respiratory disorders have many needs that require highly skilled care. The **respiratory care practitioner (RCP)** is a licensed professional who specializes in the care of patients with disorders of the circulatory and respiratory systems, and sleep disorders that affect the patient's breathing.

Patients at Risk of Poor Oxygenation

Hypoxemia is a condition in which there is insufficient oxygen in the blood. Most people with disorders of the respiratory and cardiac systems are at high risk for this condition. However, hypoxemia can develop as a complication of many conditions. This makes it very challenging to identify, because most of these patients are on medical and surgical units, in a long-term care facility, or in patient care areas other than a critical care or respiratory area. Patients who are immobile and those on bedrest have an increased risk of hypoxemia. When hypoxemia develops, immobility makes a positive outcome less likely. The reporting guidelines in Tables 36-2 and 36-4 also apply to hypoxemia.

Capillary Refill

Checking capillary refill is a quick, easy, painless test to evaluate how well oxygen is getting to the body tissues. **Capillary refill** shows how well the tissues are being nourished with oxygen (**oxygenation**). In a light-skinned patient, skin should be pink, indicating an adequate supply of oxygen. In a dark-skinned patient, you must look at the nail beds, oral mucous membranes, and lips to determine how well the person is using oxygen. If any of these areas are cyanotic, the patient most likely has a problem with oxygen delivery, due to lack of oxygen in the blood or poor circulation.

The capillary refill test helps identify problems with oxygenation. Although capillary refill varies somewhat with age, skin color should return to normal within 2 to

TABLE 36-2 SIGNS AND SYMPTOMS OF CARDIOPULMONARY DISORDERS THAT SHOULD BE REPORTED TO THE NURSE IMMEDIATELY

- Abnormal pulse below 60 or above 100
- Pulse irregular, weak, or bounding
- Blood pressure below 100/60 or above 140/90
- Unable to hear blood pressure or palpate pulse
- Pain over center, left, or right chest
- Chest pain that radiates to shoulder, neck, jaw, or arm
- Headache, dizziness, weakness, paralysis, vomiting
- Cold, blue, or gray appearance
- Cold, blue, numb, painful feet or hands
- Coughing (dry or moist/productive)
- Retractions
- Blue color of lips or nail beds, mucous membranes
- Feeling faint or lightheaded, losing consciousness
- Capillary refill > 3 seconds
- Pulse oximeter value < 95

Also review the respiratory symptoms in Table 36-4. Because these systems are closely related, both may be symptomatic at the same time.

3 seconds in all patients. The color should be restored to the nail bed in the length of time it takes to say the words *capillary refill*. (Refer to Procedure 87.) You can check capillary refill any time you suspect a problem. If the capillary refill time is greater than 3 seconds, inform the nurse.

The Pulse Oximeter

Pulse oximetry is another simple, painless test to determine how well oxygen is being carried in the body. Hemoglobin is the part of the blood that carries oxygen to the cells. The pulse oximeter measures how full the hemoglobin molecules are with oxygen (Figure 36-10A), and converts the oxygen in the blood to a percentage. The measurement may be continuous or intermittent. The pulse oximeter is attached to the patient's skin with a sensor (Figure 36-10B). The pulse oximeter will identify critical changes in the patient's oxygen levels before other signs are apparent, making it a valuable tool. The patient's outcome is usually better when early treatment is provided.

Before applying a pulse oximeter, document the liter flow of supplemental oxygen, if used. Check the skin under the sensor every few hours. Never use an adult sensor on an infant or child. The meanings of pulse oximeter values are listed in Table 36-3.

PROCEDURE

87

CHECKING CAPILLARY REFILL

1. Carry out initial procedure actions.

2. Inspect the nails, noting the color.

3. Press the nail for a few seconds, until the skin underneath blanches, or turns white (Figure 36-9A).

4. Release the nail and evaluate the time it takes for the skin to return to its normal color. With normal oxygenation, this will occur within 2 to 3 seconds (Figure 36-9B).

5. Carry out ending procedure actions.

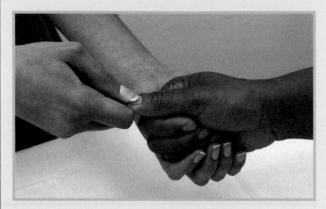

FIGURE 36-9A Inspect the color of the patient's hand, then pinch the thumb. (© *Delmar/Cengage Learning*)

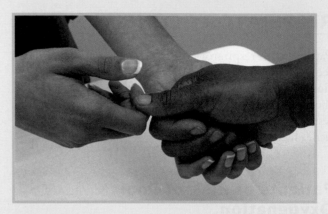

FIGURE 36-9B Observe the color again after releasing the thumb. (© *Delmar/Cengage Learning*)

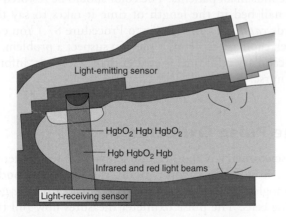

FIGURE 36-10A The pulse oximeter uses light to measure the amount of oxygen in the arterial blood. (© *Delmar/Cengage Learning*)

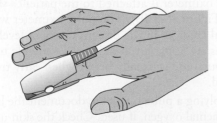

FIGURE 36-10B Clip the sensor to the finger. Rotate it every 2 hours or more often to prevent pressure-related problems. (© *Delmar/Cengage Learning*)

TABLE 36-3 MEANINGS AND INTERPRETATION OF PULSE OXIMETER VALUES

Pulse Oximeter Reading	Interpretation
95% to 100%	Normal
90% to 94% (or 3% to 4% less than usual value)	Potential problem. Have the patient take a deep breath and recheck the value. Inform the nurse of the results.
Inform the nurse promptly of the following values:	
86% to 89%	Suggests complications, impending hypoxemia
85%	Inadequate oxygen for body function, condition worsening, potential impending crisis
Below 70%	Life-threatening

Safety ALERT

Always monitor the patient, not the equipment. For example, the pulse oximeter alarm sounds and the oxygen saturation value reads 63%, suggesting that the patient is in serious distress. However, he is visiting with his family, smiling and talking. His color is good, nail beds and mucous membranes are pink, and capillary refill time is less than 2 seconds. You are having an equipment problem, not a patient problem. This example shows that although monitoring devices are good adjuncts to patient evaluation, the human component is more important. If you cannot identify and correct the problem, ask the nurse or respiratory professional to help. Although your findings suggest an equipment problem, inform the nurse of the situation and your evaluation of the patient. ■

Upper Respiratory Infections

An **upper respiratory infection (URI)** follows invasion of the upper respiratory organs by microbes. The upper respiratory organs include the nose, sinuses, and throat. A common cold, which is caused by a virus, is an example of a URI. It is one of the most ordinary illnesses found in people. Symptoms include:

- Elevated temperature (fever)
- Runny nose
- Watery eyes

This usually self-limiting disease is best treated by:

- Use of a drug to reduce fever, such as acetaminophen
- Rest
- Increased fluid intake

Patients with respiratory infections should be taught to:

- Cover the nose and mouth with a tissue when coughing or sneezing
- Dispose of soiled tissues by placing them in a plastic or paper bag to be burned

PROCEDURE

USING A PULSE OXIMETER

1. Carry out initial procedure actions.

2. Assemble equipment:
   - Pulse oximeter unit
   - Sensor appropriate to the site
   - Adhesive tape, if needed, to secure the sensor

3. Select and apply the sensor. If the sensor has position markings, align them opposite each other to ensure an accurate reading.

4. Fasten the sensor securely (Figure 36-11A), or the reading will not be accurate. Use a self-adhesive sensor, if this is your facility policy (Figure 36-11B). Make sure the sensor is not wrapped so tightly with tape that it restricts blood flow.

5. Attach the sensor to the patient cable on the pulse oximeter.

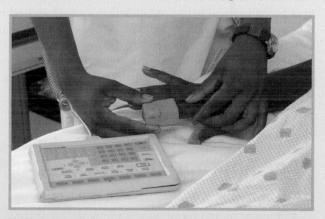

FIGURE 36-11A Firmly attach the sensor to the finger. (© Delmar/Cengage Learning)

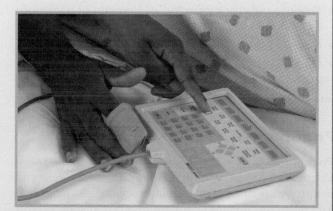

FIGURE 36-11B The self-adhesive finger sensor. (© Delmar/Cengage Learning)

continues

PROCEDURE 88 CONTINUED

6. Turn the unit on. You will hear a beep with each pulse beat. Adjust the volume as desired. Some units also use light bars to measure pulse strength (Figure 36-11C). Note the percentage of oxygen saturation.

7. Monitor the patient's pulse rate, if the unit provides this reading. Compare with the patient's actual pulse to make sure the unit is picking up each beat.

8. Monitor the patient's respirations and general appearance. Check capillary refill time. Inform the nurse and document according to facility policy. If the patient's general condition changes at any time, notify the nurse.

9. Carry out ending procedure actions.

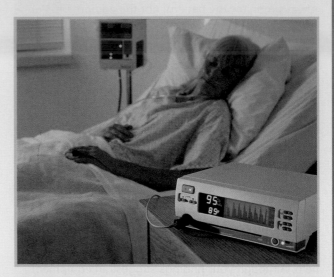

FIGURE 36-11C Turn the unit on and adjust the volume and other controls. (© *Delmar/Cengage Learning*)

• Turn the face away from others when coughing or sneezing

• Wash hands after handling soiled tissues

You have learned that respiratory infections are spread by the airborne and droplet methods of transmission. Secretions containing pathogens make their way to the environment where you pick them up on your hands. Good handwashing is the best method of preventing infection, including respiratory infection. For further information, review the CDC recommendations for respiratory hygiene in Unit 13.

You must take special note of and report the following:

• **Dyspnea** (difficult breathing)

• Changes in rate and rhythm of respiration

• Presence and character, color, and amount of respiratory secretions

• Cough

• Changes in skin color, such as pallor or cyanosis

URIs sometimes move down into the chest and develop into bronchitis or even pneumonia.

Pneumonia

Pneumonia is a serious inflammation of the lungs. It can be caused by a variety of infectious organisms. Signs and symptoms are usually fever, chills, a productive cough, and pain when breathing. The patient may take shallow breaths to relieve pain. This leads to worsening of congestion. The sputum may be rust colored. The patient may become cyanotic.

Chronic Obstructive Pulmonary Disease

Chronic obstructive pulmonary disease (COPD) is also called *chronic obstructive lung disease (COLD)*. This term refers to multiple conditions that cause irreversible blockage or obstruction of the respiratory system. Common conditions are emphysema, asthma, and chronic bronchitis.

Asthma is caused by narrowing and clogging of the bronchi, the small tubes that carry air into and out of the lungs. The bronchi normally narrow during the night, in everyone. This increases resistance to air flow. People who do not have asthma probably will not notice the change. However, in asthmatics the change may be enough to bring on an asthma attack, whether the person is awake or asleep. A person having an asthma attack has labored breathing and frequent coughing. An attack may result when the person contacts an allergen. Respiratory infections can also cause an asthma attack.

Age-Appropriate Care ALERT

The incidence of asthma in children is increasing. Asthma accounts for at least 14 million lost school days annually. ∎

Chronic Bronchitis

Chronic **bronchitis** is prolonged inflammation of the bronchi due to infection or irritants. Signs and symptoms include:

- Swollen and red bronchial tissues, resulting in narrowed bronchial passageways
- Persistent cough
- Sputum production
- Respiratory distress

Emphysema

Emphysema develops after chronic obstruction of the air flow to the alveoli. The air sacs enlarge and lose their elasticity and ability to recoil. The person can bring air into the lungs, but it becomes difficult to expel the air. As a result, there is less and less room for air to reenter, and the person becomes very short of breath.

Nursing Assistant Care of Patients with Respiratory Disorders

- Check vital signs, capillary refill, and pulse oximeter as ordered.
- Monitor the frequency and type of cough (productive or nonproductive).
- Note the color, consistency, and amount of sputum.
- Position the person in semi-Fowler's position to facilitate breathing.
- Place necessary items, such as tissues and the wastebasket, within reach.
- Encourage fluids, to loosen secretions and replace fluids lost through fever and rapid respirations.
- Monitor intake and output.
- Assist with deep breathing and coughing every 2 hours.
- Plan for and encourage rest periods before meals, before activities of daily living, and exercise.
- Prioritize necessary tasks and eliminate nonessential tasks, to conserve energy.
- Assist with range-of-motion exercises 3 times a day.

Surgical Conditions

Most respiratory problems are not treated with surgery. However, several problems require surgical correction to ensure uninterrupted air flow.

Tracheostomy A **tracheostomy** may be temporary or permanent. An incision is made in the neck for air to enter. The external opening on the skin surface is the **stoma**. A plastic or metal tube is inserted through the stoma to keep it open (maintain patency). This tube is the **cannula**. An outer and inner cannula are used. Several types of outer cannulae are available. The most common has an inflatable

cuff (Figure 36-12A). It seals or reduces the air flow to the nose and throat, so virtually all breathing is done through the tracheostomy. The parts of the tracheostomy apparatus are shown in Figure 36-12B.

Cancer of the larynx A **laryngectomy** is surgical removal of the larynx. This is done as a treatment for cancer of the larynx. The airway is separated from the mouth, nose, and esophagus. The patient breathes through an artificial opening in the neck and trachea. A person who has had this surgery may be called a **laryngectomee**. When the larynx is removed, there is no longer a connection between the upper and lower airways (Figure 36-13).

The laryngectomy may look like a regular tracheostomy, but it is very different. You must know the type of device each patient has. When a patient has a tracheostomy, the passageway from the mouth and nose through the trachea remains intact. The patient continues to be able to smell odors, blow the nose, and drink liquid through a straw.

A patient who has had a laryngectomy has had the larynx (voice box) removed. The upper airway is no longer connected to the trachea. The patient can no longer talk and

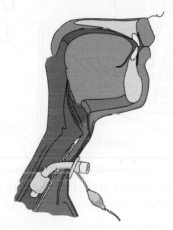

FIGURE 36-12A A tracheostomy with the cuff inflated. (© Delmar/Cengage Learning)

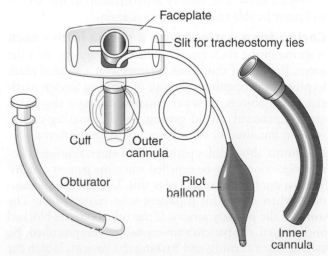

Faceplate
Slit for tracheostomy ties
Cuff
Outer cannula
Obturator
Pilot balloon
Inner cannula

FIGURE 36-12B Parts for the tracheostomy. (© Delmar/Cengage Learning)

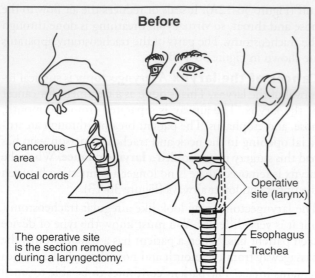

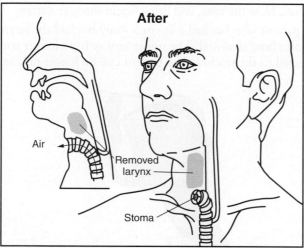

FIGURE 36-13 The anatomy of the face and neck before and after laryngectomy surgery. *(© Delmar/Cengage Learning)*

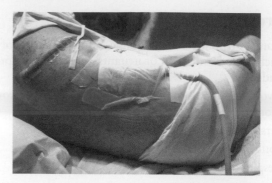

FIGURE 36-14 The chest tube is securely covered with dressings. *(© Delmar/Cengage Learning)*

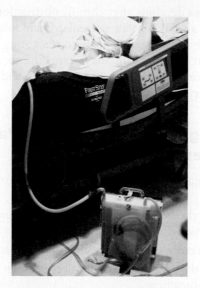

FIGURE 36-15 Make sure the tubing is not obstructed, and that the bottle is lower than the patient's heart. *(© Delmar/Cengage Learning)*

must use other forms of communication. The patient cannot smell, blow the nose, whistle, gargle, or drink liquid through a straw. The surgery is permanent, so the patient will never be able to do these things again.

Caring for a patient with a stoma in the neck

A stoma in the neck creates a direct passageway into the lungs. Because of this, some patients wear a surgical mask to protect the opening. The risk of inhaling foreign particles, small objects, or water (such as during a shower) is greatly increased. Avoid getting powder, shaving cream, cologne, lint, dust, or other items near or in the stoma.

The stoma also enables pathogens to enter, causing infection. Secretions may be expelled when the patient coughs. The patient has no control over this. Use standard precautions when caring for a patient who has a stoma. The stoma is the primary airway. If the tube becomes blocked or dislodged, the patient's airway will be compromised. Be careful when turning and bathing the patient. Watch for cyanosis, changes in color of the nail beds or mucous membranes, or respiratory distress.

Chest tubes Chest tubes (Figure 36-14) are sterile, plastic tubes that are inserted through the skin of the chest and into the space between the covering of the lung and the membrane lining the chest wall. Chest tubes are used to treat an air leak or to drain fluid from the area surrounding the lungs. The chest tube is attached to a drain (Figure 36-15). Make sure that nothing pulls on the tube. Position the drainage system upright, below the level of the heart. Never disconnect any part of the system.

Observations to make and report for patients with respiratory disorders are listed in Table 36-4.

SPECIAL THERAPIES RELATED TO RESPIRATORY ILLNESS

Nursing assistants aid patient breathing by proper positioning and by helping provide moisture and oxygen. You will also be responsible for making observations and reporting to the nurse, as outlined in Table 36-5.

TABLE 36-4 OBSERVATIONS OF PATIENTS WITH RESPIRATORY DISORDERS

- Respiratory rate below 12 or above 20
- Irregular respirations
- Noisy, labored respirations
- Dyspnea
- Shortness of breath
- Gasping for breath
- Cheyne-Stokes respirations
- Wheezing
- Coughing (dry or moist/productive)
- Retractions
- Blue color of lips or nail beds, mucous membranes
- Capillary refill > 3 seconds
- Pulse oximeter value < 95

TABLE 36-5 SIGNS AND SYMPTOMS OF INADEQUATE BREATHING TO REPORT TO THE NURSE IMMEDIATELY

- Movement in the chest is absent, minimal, or irregular.
- Breathing movement appears to be in the abdomen, not the lungs.
- Air movement cannot be detected by listening and feeling for breath sounds on your cheek and ear.
- Respiratory rate is too slow or rapid; there is a marked change in rate.
- Respirations are irregular, gasping, very deep, or shallow; there is a marked change in rhythm.
- Patient has dyspnea (difficult breathing).
- Patient expels respiratory secretions (note character, color, and amount).
- Patient's skin, lips, tongue, ear lobes, mucous membranes, or nail beds are pale, blue, or gray.
- Patient is unable to speak at all, or cannot speak in sentences because of shortness of breath.
- Respirations are noisy.
- Nasal flaring is present during inspiration.
- The muscles below the ribs and/or above the clavicles retract inward during respiration.
- Cough is present. Note whether the cough is *productive* (expelling secretions) or *nonproductive* (patient is not coughing anything up).

Oxygen Therapy

Many patients with respiratory problems will be using oxygen. Oxygen must be ordered by the physician. Review the oxygen precautions and safety information in Unit 14.

Oxygen may be delivered to the patient by several different methods. The same basic care is required for each method, with modifications.

- *Nasal cannula:* Delivery of oxygen by **nasal cannula** (Figure 36-16) is the most common method. A strap around the patient's head holds the cannula in place.
- *Mask:* The **oxygen mask** is held in place by straps around the head. Several different masks are used, depending on the patient's needs (Figure 36-17A). A special mask fits over a stoma (Figure 36-17B).

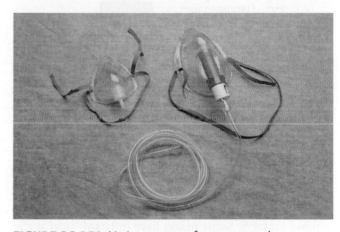

FIGURE 36-16 Oxygen being administered by nasal cannula. (© Delmar/Cengage Learning)

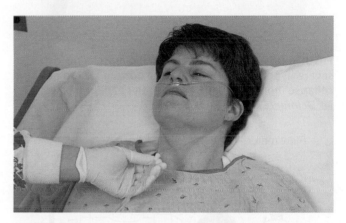

FIGURE 36-17A Various types of oxygen masks. (© Delmar/Cengage Learning)

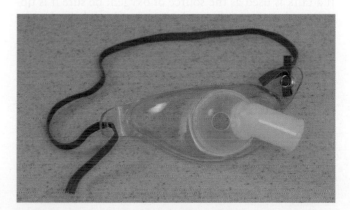

FIGURE 36-17B An adult tracheostomy mask. (© Delmar/Cengage Learning)

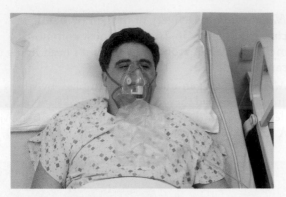

FIGURE 36-17C The nonrebreathing mask is used for severe hypoxemia. The bag at the bottom should not collapse more than halfway when the patient inhales. *(© Delmar/Cengage Learning)*

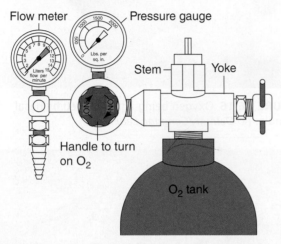

FIGURE 36-18 The flow meter shows the amount of oxygen being delivered. The pressure gauge shows the amount of oxygen remaining in the tank. *(© Delmar/ Cengage Learning)*

An oxygen mask is necessary when high liter flows of oxygen are ordered. A mask is never used with liter flows under 5. Some masks have inflatable bags at the bottom (Figure 36-17C). If this is the case, the bag should be inflated at all times.

If a tank is used as the source of oxygen, be sure it is upright and secure on the carrier, in a stand, or chained to the wall. Check the gauge each time you are in the room (Figure 36-18).

Humidifiers

In some facilities, a **humidifier** (Figure 36-19) is used if the flow of oxygen exceeds 5 liters. Humidification is not necessary with liter flows below 5. Some facilities do not use humidifiers at all.

Oxygen Concentrators

Room air is approximately 21% oxygen. An **oxygen concentrator** (Figure 36-20) removes gases other than

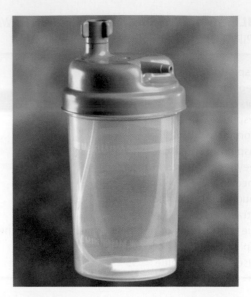

FIGURE 36-19 A humidifier. *(Courtesy of Hudson RCI, Temecula, CA, USA)*

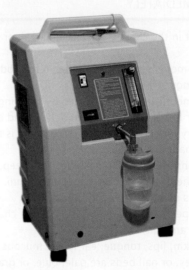

FIGURE 36-20 The oxygen concentrator delivers low liter flows. Although the concentrator pictured has a humidifier attached, humidification is not necessary at low liter flows. *(Courtesy of Hudson RCI, Temecula, CA, USA)*

oxygen, which concentrates the oxygen in the unit. The air delivered to the patient through a cannula is more than 90% oxygen. The flow rate is usually 2 liters per minute (L/min). A concentrator should not be used in emergencies or when high liter flows are necessary.

Liquid Oxygen

Oxygen also comes as a liquid in a canister (Figure 36-21). One advantage is that large amounts of liquid oxygen can be stored in small containers. The canister delivers higher oxygen concentrations than a concentrator, it is quieter, and does not require electricity to operate.

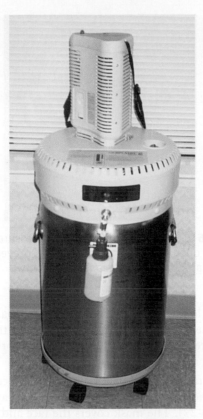

FIGURE 36-21 The liquid oxygen canister. The portable tank on top is filled from the large tank, then detached. There are special environmental requirements for filling the small tank, and this must not be done in a patient care area. (© Delmar/Cengage Learning)

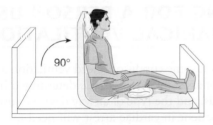

FIGURE 36-22 The patient is in the high Fowler's position. (© Delmar/Cengage Learning)

Respiratory Positions

Positioning to permit expansion of the lungs and a straightened airway is helpful to patients with respiratory distress.

High Fowler's position In the **high Fowler's position**, the patient is sitting up with the backrest elevated (Figure 36-22).

Orthopneic position The **orthopneic position** (Figure 36-23) may be used as an alternative to the high Fowler's position. The patient sits as upright as possible and leans slightly forward, supporting herself with the forearms. This makes the thorax larger during inspiration, enabling the patient to inhale more air.

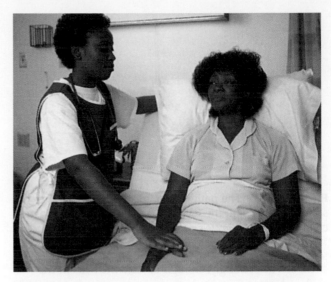

FIGURE 36-23 The patient in the orthopneic position sits straight up, supported on the arms. (© Delmar/Cengage Learning)

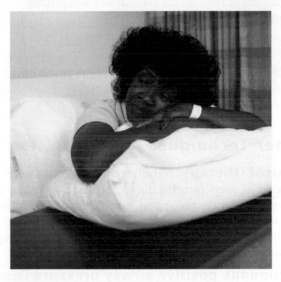

FIGURE 36-24 The tripod position enlarges the chest cavity, making breathing easier. (© Delmar/Cengage Learning)

The **tripod position** (Figure 36-24) is another alternative to improve ventilation.

Incentive Spirometer

The physician may write orders for use of an **incentive spirometer** (Figure 36-25) to help the patient's lungs expand fully and prevent complications. It is often ordered after surgery.

This procedure may be carried out with the patient in bed, with person sitting as upright as possible.

- The patient is instructed how to use the incentive spirometer by the RCP or nurse.
- The patient exhales normally and then, with the lips placed tightly around the mouthpiece, inhales through

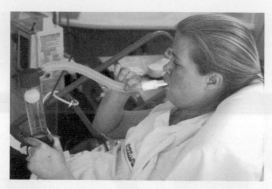

FIGURE 36-25 The patient inhales into the incentive spirometer, raising the level of the ball inside the plastic chamber. *(© Delmar/Cengage Learning)*

the mouth strongly, enough to raise the balls in the chambers.

- The patient holds the deep breath as long as possible (or as ordered), which keeps the balls suspended.
- The patient removes the mouthpiece and exhales normally.
- The exercise is repeated as many times as is ordered.

Tips: The incentive spirometer is usually left at the bedside. Prompt the patient to use it throughout the day by taking four to five slow, deep breaths using the spirometer, or as ordered.

Other Techniques

Aerosol therapy Nebulizers deliver moisture or medication deep into the lungs. Drugs that dilate the bronchi are often prescribed. Small-volume nebulizers (Figure 36-26) turn liquid medicine into a mist that can be breathed in by the patient. Encourage the patient to cough up loose secretions after the treatment.

Continuous positive airway pressure Persons with *sleep apnea* stop breathing periodically while they sleep. This is usually caused when the tongue blocks the airway during sleep, when the muscles relax. Persons with sleep apnea may stop breathing hundreds of times a night,

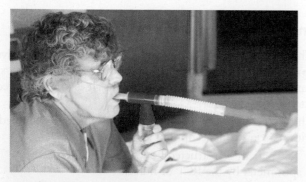

FIGURE 36-26 A hand-held, small-volume nebulizer. *(© Delmar/Cengage Learning)*

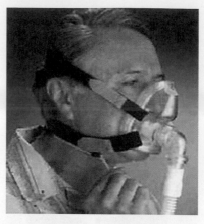

FIGURE 36-27 The CPAP mask applies pressure to keep the airway open while the patient sleeps, preventing sleep apnea. *(Courtesy of Medline Industries)*

then snore loudly when they start to breathe again. This interrupts their sleep, causing them to feel very tired during the day. Treatment consists of use of a mask that applies pressure to the airway, keeping it open.

The mask treatment is called **CPAP** (pronounced see-pap) which stands for **continuous positive airway pressure** (Figure 36-27). The mask covers the face and is held securely in place with a head strap. Tubing connects the mask to a device (sometimes called a blower) that creates low levels of pressure. The amount of pressure is ordered by the physician.

CARING FOR A PERSON USING MECHANICAL VENTILATION

Patients with some conditions need ventilation assistance. The type of assistance necessary is determined by the patient's needs, and the type of airway device in use. For example, a patient in cardiac arrest will need management different from a patient who is being ventilated during transport from one location to another. The RN and RCP will provide specific directions.

Most patients who require continuous mechanical ventilation have a tube called an *endotracheal tube* inserted into the airway (Figure 36-28). Because of the position of the tube, the patient will be unable to speak. The endotracheal tube is used in conjunction with a *ventilator*, a positive pressure device that forces air into the lungs. The RCP and RN will care for the ventilator, and will suction through the endotracheal tube to remove secretions, if needed. These patients need a great deal of nursing assistant care, comfort measures, and reassurance. The patient may be restrained to prevent him or her from removing the endotracheal tube. A patient who is restrained will need total nursing care, including turning and repositioning, and restraint care and observation. The care plan or critical pathway will provide instructions. The RN will guide you if you have

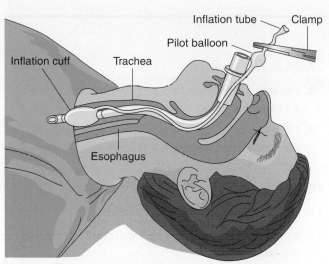

FIGURE 36-28 A properly placed endotracheal tube is connected to a ventilator, which provides positive pressure respirations. The tube is inserted between the vocal cords, so the patient will be unable to speak with it in place. (© Delmar/Cengage Learning)

questions. In general, care for a patient who is mechanically ventilated involves:

- Monitoring the patient frequently and anticipating his or her needs.
- Keeping the head of the bed elevated in the semi-Fowler's or Fowler's position, as directed. Remember that this increases the risk of pressure ulcers on the torso, coccyx, and buttocks.
- Keeping the patient's head turned to the side if an oral or nasal airway is used; turning the head helps prevent aspiration.
- Providing oral and nasal care as directed.
- Keeping the lips and mucous membranes moist.

- Repositioning the patient every 2 hours, or more often, if indicated.
- Monitoring restraints, if used, and releasing restraints according to facility policy.
- Monitoring the bony prominences for signs of redness, irritation, or breakdown.
- Monitoring the tube insertion site for signs of redness, irritation, or breakdown.
- Monitoring the vital signs, capillary refill, and pulse oximeter values, and reporting abnormalities to the RN immediately.
- Monitoring for signs of respiratory distress, and reporting to the RN immediately.
- Reassuring the patient and family.
- Developing a means for communicating with the patient, such as using a magic slate or by writing.

COLLECTING A SPUTUM SPECIMEN

Sputum is a secretion from the mucous membranes lining the trachea and lungs. A sputum specimen may be collected to help diagnose problems in the respiratory tract. Although the specimen is collected by the patient, you must provide the collection container, and give very specific instructions. The patient must understand that the fluid collected must be from the lungs, and not saliva from the mouth.

A sputum specimen is best collected early in the morning, if possible. Instruct the patient to avoid using mouthwash or toothpaste before obtaining the specimen. Assist the patient into a sitting position when he or she produces the specimen. If possible, obtain 5 to 15 mL of fluid. Once obtained, transport the specimen to the laboratory immediately.

PROCEDURE

89

COLLECTING A SPUTUM SPECIMEN

1. Carry out initial procedure actions.

2. Assemble equipment:
   - Disposable gloves
   - Sterile sputum collection container
   - Glass of water
   - Properly completed label
   - Tissues
   - Emesis basin
   - Biohazard specimen transport bag
   - Laboratory requisition

3. Wash your hands and put on disposable gloves.

4. Ask the patient to rinse the mouth with water and spit into the emesis basin.

continues

PROCEDURE 89 CONTINUED

5. Ask the patient to breathe deeply and then cough to bring up sputum. The patient spits the sputum into the container.

   a. Have the patient shield the mouth with a tissue while coughing.

   b. Collect 1 to 2 tablespoons of sputum unless otherwise ordered.

   c. Do not contaminate the outside of the container.

   d. Instruct the patient not to touch the inside of the container or lid.

6. Remove your gloves and discard them according to facility policy.

7. Wash your hands.

8. Cover the specimen container tightly and attach a completed label.

9. Place the specimen container in a biohazard transport bag and attach a laboratory requisition.

10. Assist with mouth care, if needed.

11. Carry out ending procedure actions.

12. Follow facility policy for transporting specimen to the laboratory.

REVIEW

A. Multiple Choice

Select the one best answer for each of the following.

1. When your patient is receiving oxygen, you should
   a. monitor intake and output.
   b. know the ordered rate.
   c. check the flow rate once each shift.
   d. check the flow rate every 3 hours.

2. When a patient receives oxygen through a concentrator,
   a. pull the mask straps until they are very tight.
   b. a cannula delivers the air.
   c. make sure the mask covers only the mouth.
   d. a high liter flow is used.

3. You suspect that the patient needs immediate attention for a possible heart attack because the patient
   a. has chest pain.
   b. complains of not feeling well.
   c. has ankle edema.
   d. has pink nail beds.

4. An oxygen concentrator
   a. has an inflatable bag at the bottom.
   b. delivers high oxygen flows.
   c. should not be used in an emergency.
   d. should always be used with a mask.

5. The capillary refill test
   a. is used to monitor cyanosis.
   b. checks the heart rate.
   c. measures the strength of the heart.
   d. is used to check for hypoxemia.

6. Angina pectoris is
   a. common in heart attack.
   b. a sign of heart failure.
   c. pain of exertion.
   d. a symptom of heart block.

7. When a patient is short of breath, this position may help make breathing easier.
   a. High Fowler's
   b. Sims'
   c. Lithotomy
   d. Supine

8. A sputum specimen
   a. should be collected at bedtime.
   b. analyzes mucus from the lungs.
   c. is used to diagnose leukemia.
   d. must be collected by an RN.

9. The pulse oximeter
   a. must be used continuously.
   b. counts the pulse rate.
   c. analyzes pulse rhythm.
   d. measures oxygen in the blood.

10. A normal capillary refill value is
   a. less than 6 seconds.
   b. more than 4 seconds.
   c. less than 3 seconds.
   d. more than 10 seconds.

B. Nursing Assistant Challenge

Mrs. Harvey has had asthma all her life. She is sensitive to many allergens. She is admitted to your facility for em-physema. She is receiving respiratory assistance with an oxygen concentrator. Answer the following questions related to her care.

11. The oxygen flow rate of the concentrator is usually set at _____.

   (10 L/min)   (2 L/min)

12. Smoking in the same room _____ permitted.

   (is)   (is not)

13. The flow rate of oxygen _____ be changed by the nursing assistant.

   (may)   (may not)

UNIT 37

Caring for Patients with Disorders of the Musculoskeletal and Nervous Systems

OBJECTIVES

After completing this unit, you will be able to:
- Spell and define terms.
- Identify aging changes of the musculoskeletal system and nervous system.
- Describe some common conditions of the musculoskeletal system and nervous system.
- Describe nursing assistant actions and observations related to the care of patients with conditions and diseases of the musculoskeletal system and nervous system.
- Demonstrate the following procedures:
  - Procedure 90 Assisting with Continuous Passive Motion
  - Procedure 91 Performing Range-of-Motion Exercises (Passive)

VOCABULARY

Learn the meaning and the correct spelling of the following words and phrases:

abduction pillow
absence seizure
amputation
amyotrophic lateral
  sclerosis (ALS)
aphasia
arthritis
atrophy
aura
autonomic dysreflexia
brain attack
bursitis
cerebrovascular accident
  (CVA)
chorea
closed (simple) fracture
compartment syndrome
complete fracture
compound (open) fracture
continuous passive
  motion (CPM)

convulsion
countertraction
degenerative joint
  disease (DJD)
ecchymosis
epilepsy
exacerbation
fibromyalgia (FM)
flaccid paralysis
fracture
generalized tonic-clonic
  seizure
gout
grand mal seizure
hemiparesis
hemiplegia
Huntington's disease
  (HD)
incomplete fracture
intention tremor
intracranial pressure

Lhermitte's sign
meningitis
multiple sclerosis (MS)
nystagmus
open (compound)
  fracture
open reduction/internal
  fixation (ORIF)
osteoarthritic joint
  disease (OJD)
osteoporosis
paralysis
paraplegia
Parkinson's disease
passive range of motion
  (PROM)
pathologic fracture
petit mal seizure
phantom pain
post polio syndrome
  (PPS)

quadriplegia
range-of-motion (ROM)
  exercises
remission
rheumatoid arthritis
  (RA)
simple (closed) fracture
spastic paralysis
spica cast
status epilepticus
stroke
tetraplegia
total hip arthroplasty
  (THA)
transient ischemic attack
  (TIA)
tremor
vascular
vertigo

MUSCULOSKELETAL SYSTEM INTRODUCTION

The bony frame of the body is called the *skeleton*. Tissue that is made up of fibers that contract and relax or cells that produce movement are called *muscles*. Together, the skeleton and muscles form the musculoskeletal system. This system functions to:

- Give shape and form to the body
- Protect and support organs and body parts
- Permit movement
- Produce some blood cells
- Store calcium and phosphorus

When muscles, bones, or joints have been injured, a long period of rest and inactivity may be required. During this time, other parts of the body need regular exercise. Bones that are not used lose calcium and become less functional.

AGING CHANGES TO THE MUSCULOSKELETAL SYSTEM

Aging changes in the musculoskeletal system include:

- Decreased strength, endurance, muscle tone, and reaction time caused by loss of elasticity of muscles and decrease in size of muscle mass.
- Bones lose minerals, become brittle and break more easily.
- The spine is less stable, less flexible, and more easily injured.

Clinical Information ALERT

Approximately 40% of your body weight consists of muscles. Muscles usually work in pairs. This is the reason they can move in different or opposite directions. Muscles are attached to the bones. When the muscles contract, the bones act as levers and cause the body parts to move. You use 17 muscles to smile, and 43 to frown. Scientists estimate that the eye muscles move more than 100,000 times a day! The largest muscle in your body is the gluteus maximus. This is the muscle that you sit on. The femur bone in the upper leg is the longest bone in the body. The smallest bone is in the inner ear. A giraffe has the same number of neck bones as a human. ∎

TABLE 37-1 SIGNS AND SYMPTOMS OF MUSCULOSKELETAL DISORDERS THAT SHOULD BE REPORTED TO THE NURSE IMMEDIATELY

- Pain
- Deformity
- Edema
- Immobility
- Inability to move arms and legs
- Inability to move one or more joints
- Limited/abnormal range of motion
- Shortening and external rotation of one leg in patient with a history of fall
- Sudden onset of falls, difficulty balancing
- Jerking, tremors, shaky movements, muscle spasms
- Weakness
- Sensory changes
- Changes in the ability to sit, stand, move, or walk
- Pain upon movement
- Change in color or appearance of an affected extremity
- Loss of pulse distal to an injury

- Posture may become slumped over because of weakness in back muscles.
- Deterioration in the joints resulting in limited movement, stiffness, and pain.

Signs and symptoms of musculoskeletal disorders to report to the nurse are listed in Table 37-1.

COMMON CONDITIONS OF THE MUSCULOSKELETAL SYSTEM

Many conditions can affect the musculoskeletal system. When one structure is diseased or injured, the surrounding tissues are often involved.

Bursitis

Bursae are small sacs of fluid around joints that reduce friction during movement. The joint is painful if the bursae are inflamed. This condition is known as **bursitis**.

Arthritis

Arthritis (Figure 37-1) is inflammation of the joints. The most common forms of chronic arthritis are:

- **Rheumatoid arthritis (RA)**, which affects the lining of joints and can affect other body systems. It is a condition of **exacerbations**, or times in which the condition seems to worsen, and **remissions**, when the disease appears stable. RA reduces joint function and causes deformities that are severe and disabling.

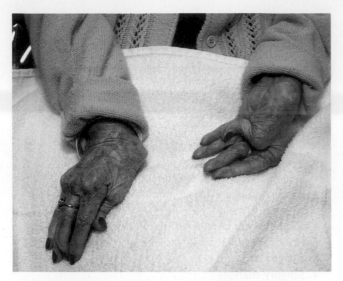

FIGURE 37-1 These deformities, caused by rheumatoid arthritis, make hand movement difficult and painful. *(© Delmar/Cengage Learning)*

- **Osteoarthritic joint disease (OJD)** or **degenerative joint disease (DJD)**, which affects the ends of the bones that form joints. The bones rub together, causing pain and deformity. The weight-bearing joints are usually affected.
- **Gout** (gouty arthritis), which is caused by increased uric acid in the blood. The uric acid crystallizes in the joints, and is very painful. Gout can lead to complete disability, hypertension, and chronic renal disease.

Osteoporosis

Osteoporosis is a metabolic disorder in which bones become porous and spongy (Figure 37-2). Affected bones are

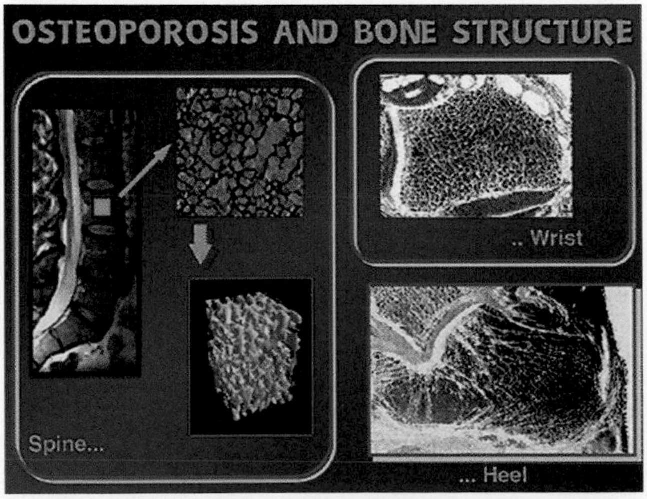

FIGURE 37-2 Bone loss from osteoporosis causes painful, disabling fractures. About 40% of women and 13% of men will suffer a bone fracture due to osteoporosis in their lifetime. *(Courtesy of Sharmila Majumdar, PhD, Professor, University of California, San Francisco)*

at very high risk of fracture. The cause of osteoporosis is unknown, but is believed to result from years of inadequate calcium intake.

The first sign of osteoporosis may be a fracture. Commonly, the patient moves and hears a "pop" or snapping sound in a bone. The patient who is walking may suddenly fall. In this case, the fall is the *result* of the fracture; in most falls, the opposite is true. After the initial incident, the area is very painful, particularly upon movement. Sometimes the onset of osteoporosis begins with a curvature of the spine and loss of height. The back progressively weakens, straining the neck, hips, and low back. Spontaneous fractures may occur during movement or as a result of a minor injury.

Fibromyalgia

Fibromyalgia (FM) is a chronic pain syndrome for which there is no known cause or cure. It affects more women than men. To be diagnosed with this condition, the person must have pain both above and below the waist and on both sides of the body. He or she must have pain in at least 11 of the 18 body sites shown in Figure 37-3.

Fibromyalgia complicates treatment for many other medical problems because of the pain and difficulty in assuming some positions for examination and treatment.

Caring for Patients with Chronic Musculoskeletal Disorders

Arthritis, osteoporosis, and fibromyalgia can cause mild discomfort to severe deformities and disability. Patients are at high risk of contractures (Figure 37-4). If you are assigned to provide range-of-motion exercises for patients with these conditions, follow the care plan, go slowly, and be gentle. Avoid moving joints past the point

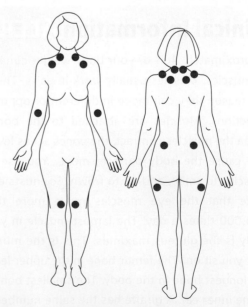

FIGURE 37-3 The patient must have pain at 11 of 18 specific areas of the body for a diagnosis of fibromyalgia. *(© Delmar/Cengage Learning)*

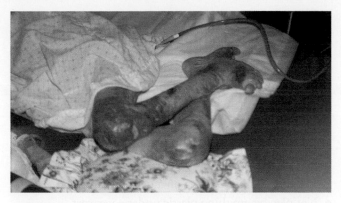

FIGURE 37-4 This patient has many problems with her legs, including injuries, arthritic deformities, and contractures. (© Delmar/Cengage Learning)

of pain or resistance. Be especially mindful of the care plan instructions for patients with osteoporosis.

Use a transfer belt or mechanical lift for transfers. Try to use sheets or turning devices when the patient is in bed. Avoid pulling on the patient's body. Make sure you have enough help if you will be moving or positioning the patient.

FRACTURES

A **fracture** is a break in the continuity of a bone. Falls are the most common cause. Fractures (Figure 37-5) are classified by type of break and whether the skin is broken.

- A **complete fracture** is a break across the entire cross-section of the bone. The bone may be displaced or improperly aligned.
- An **incomplete fracture** involves only part of the cross-section of bone.
- In a **closed** or **simple fracture**, the skin is not broken.
- An **open** or **compound fracture** occurs when the skin over the fracture is broken. The bone may or may not protrude.
- A **pathologic fracture** is a fracture in a diseased bone.

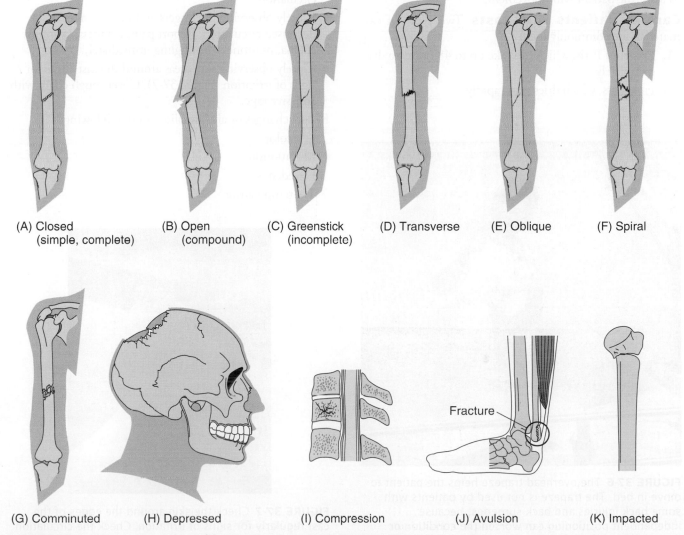

(A) Closed (simple, complete)   (B) Open (compound)   (C) Greenstick (incomplete)   (D) Transverse   (E) Oblique   (F) Spiral

(G) Comminuted   (H) Depressed   (I) Compression   Fracture   (J) Avulsion   (K) Impacted

FIGURE 37-5 Types and patterns of fractures. (© Delmar/Cengage Learning)

Fractures are very painful. Movement is limited, and sometimes the person will be unable to move the injured area at all. The skin surrounding the fracture may appear deformed or have edema. **Ecchymosis**, or bruising, may occur in some parts of the body that are very **vascular** (contain many blood vessels). An ecchymosis the size of a fist over the femur indicates loss of approximately one pint of blood.

Caring for Patients with Fractures

Fractures are treated by immobilizing the injured area until healing takes place. Surgical repair may be necessary, depending on the location and type of injury. Injured bones take from several weeks to several months to heal.

You will assist patients who have fractures with range-of-motion exercises of noninjured extremities. Check with the nurse or care plan for specific instructions. You may also assist the patient with coughing and deep breathing exercises to prevent pneumonia. Encourage fluid intake. The increased fluid liquefies secretions that accumulate in the lungs. A *trapeze* (Figure 37-6) may be attached to the bed to assist the patient with movement.

Care of patients with casts
Two types of cast materials are commonly used:

1. Plaster of Paris, which can take up to 48 hours to dry completely
2. Fiberglass, which dries very rapidly

Cast material is wet when it is applied. During the drying period, the cast gives off heat. Special care for the newly casted patient includes:

- Supporting the cast and body in good alignment with pillows covered by cloth pillowcases, and keeping the cast uncovered, if possible.
- Elevating the casted extremity on a pillow. When positioning a patient who has a leg cast, elevate the foot higher than the hip. For an arm cast, keep the fingers higher than the elbow.
- Avoiding resting the cast on a hard or flat surface.
- Not placing anything plastic under a wet cast.
- Turning the patient frequently to permit air circulation to all parts of the cast. Use the palm of your hand, not your fingers, to move a wet cast.
- Covering the cast loosely with a sheet, if needed for warmth. The greatest amount of heat loss occurs from the head. Covering the upper body and back and top of the head with a blanket may help keep the patient warm.
- Checking the skin distal to the cast for signs of poor circulation.
- Closely observing the fingers and toes for signs of decreased circulation. Report pain, coldness, cyanosis, edema, numbness, or tingling immediately.
- Closely observing skin areas around the cast edges for signs of irritation (Figure 37-7). Cover rough edges with adhesive tape.

Report changes or abnormalities of the following:

C = color
M = motion
E = edema
T = temperature

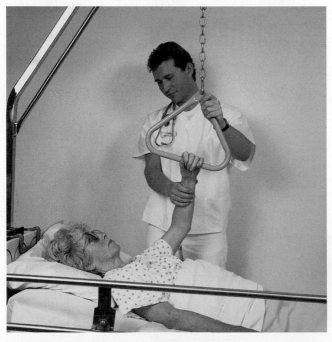

FIGURE 37-6 The overhead trapeze helps the patient to move in bed. The trapeze is not used by patients with some back injuries and back surgeries, because independent positioning can worsen the condition or cause further injuries. (© Delmar/Cengage Learning)

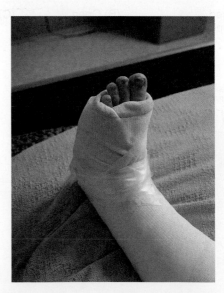

FIGURE 37-7 Check the skin around the edges of the cast regularly for signs of irritation. Check the circulation in the toes. (© Delmar/Cengage Learning)

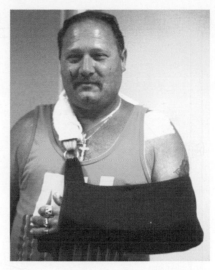

FIGURE 37-9 A sling may be ordered to elevate the hand and wrist. *(© Delmar/Cengage Learning)*

Age-Appropriate Care ALERT

A **spica cast** (Figure 37-8) may be used as a treatment for infants and small children who have fractures or have had surgical procedures. Having a body cast is difficult for children of this age, who are usually active. When caring for a child in a body cast:

- Turn the child to the noncasted side. Turning to the casted side may crack the cast.
- Support the cast when moving the child. Avoid pulling the bar between the legs.
- Protect cast edges near the genitals with plastic to help prevent soiling during toileting.
- Monitor for signs and symptoms of pain if the child is too young to communicate. ∎

A sling (Figure 37-9) may be used to elevate an arm cast when the patient is out of bed. A wheelchair with an elevated leg rest is used for patients who have leg casts. A pillow may be placed on the leg rest, for support and to prevent the casted leg from falling off the elevated leg rest. Cover the cast with plastic during bathing. Keep small objects from getting inside the cast. The patient may complain of an itching sensation under the cast. Discourage him or her from placing objects down the cast to scratch. Report complaints of itching to the nurse.

Care of patients in traction Traction pulls two body areas slightly apart to relieve pressure, relax muscles, and maintain alignment. Two types of traction are used:

- Skin traction, in which traction is applied to the skin (Figure 37-10).
- Skeletal traction (Figure 37-11), which uses tongs or pins placed into bones. Weights are attached to the tongs or pins. Skeletal traction is always continuous. Do not lift or remove the weights.

Traction is applied by attaching weights to the body above or below the injured area. The patient's body weight serves as **countertraction** by pulling in the opposite direction.

GUIDELINES *for*

Caring for Patients in Traction

- Review the correct placement of straps and weights with the nurse. Get instructions for moving the patient in bed.
- Do not permit the weights to swing, drop, or rest on any surface. Avoid releasing the weights.
- Keep the patient in good alignment in the center of the bed. Keep the head of the bed low. Position the patient so the feet do not rest against the end of the bed.
- Check under straps and belts for areas of pressure or irritation.
- Make sure straps and belts are smooth, straight, and properly secured.
- Keep bed covers off ropes and pulleys.

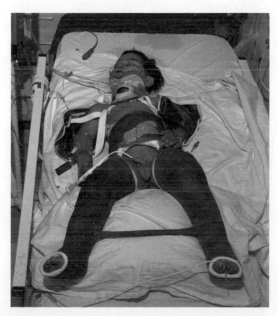

FIGURE 37-8 The spica cast is a full body cast that is commonly used to treat hip fracture and after hip surgery in children. *(© Delmar/Cengage Learning)*

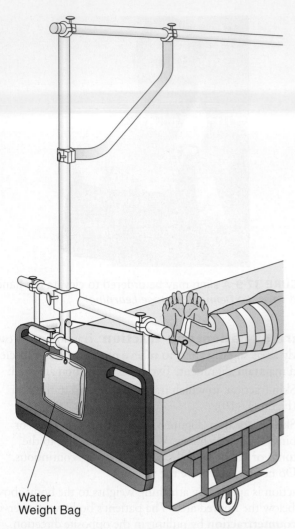

FIGURE 37-10 Buck's traction is a type of skin traction that may be used for a hip fracture. It may be used to stabilize the bone before surgery, or until the fracture heals in patients who are not candidates for surgery. (© Delmar/Cengage Learning)

Water
Weight Bag

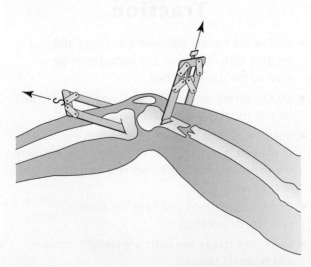

FIGURE 37-11 Skeletal traction immobilizes a body part by attaching weights directly to the patient's bones with pins, screws, wires, or tongs. (© Delmar/Cengage Learning)

Fractured Hip

Hip fractures are the most common type of fracture in older patients. Falls are the usual cause. The term *hip fracture* really is not accurate. A "hip" fracture can occur anywhere in the upper third or head of the femur. It is not limited to the hip joint.

Open reduction/internal fixation The most common treatment for a fractured hip is a surgical procedure called **open reduction/internal fixation (ORIF)**. The surgeon makes an incision, aligns the bone, then inserts a nail, pin, or rod to hold the bone ends in place.

Total hip arthroplasty Total hip arthroplasty **(THA)**, or insertion of a hip prosthesis, is a common procedure. The surgery is done to replace a painful hip joint that has degenerated due to arthritis, and as a treatment for hip fractures that cannot be repaired by other methods.

In a THA, the hip joint is surgically removed and a metal or synthetic ball and socket are inserted (Figure 37-12). While the area is healing, the patient must avoid certain body positions to prevent damage to the new joint. Follow the care plan.

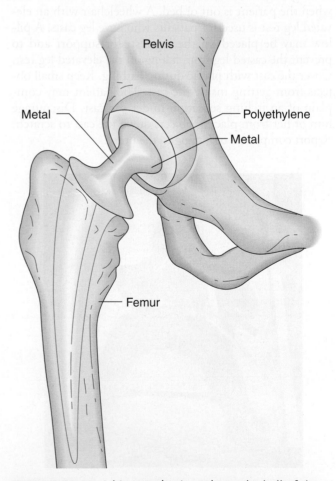

Pelvis

Metal

Polyethylene

Metal

Femur

FIGURE 37-12 A hip prosthesis replaces the ball of the femur and the socket when the patient has a total hip arthroplasty. (© Delmar/Cengage Learning)

GUIDELINES *for*

Caring for the Patient Who Has Had Hip Surgery

After hip surgery, the following general procedures are commonly ordered:

- A trapeze is attached to the bed. Teach the patient to avoid pressing down on the foot of the affected leg when using the trapeze.
- Apply anti-embolism stockings (Unit 29), as ordered.
- Provide a fracture bedpan for elimination, if needed.
- Avoid elevating the head of the bed more than 45° without a specific order.
- Position the **abduction pillow** to keep the legs apart (Figure 37-13) when turning, and when the patient is positioned on the back or sides. Some physicians also want the pillow used when the patient is sitting in a chair. Support the leg when moving the patient.
- Keep the affected leg in good alignment, without internal or external rotation. Avoid flexion of the hip and knee, keep the knees lower than the hips when sitting, and never cross the legs.
- Avoid rolling the affected leg toward the other leg during turning.
- Support the affected leg when moving the patient to the side of the bed.
- Remind the patient to avoid crossing the legs.
- Instruct the patient to:
  - Avoid sleeping on the stomach or operative side.
  - Avoid crossing the legs, as this may cause hip dislocation.
  - Avoid sitting on low chairs or couches. Position these patients only in chairs with arms and ensure that the knees remain lower than the hips.
  - Avoid leaning forward while sitting, and avoid picking up items from the floor or bending to put on shoes and socks.

- - Avoid flexing the hips more than 80° or rotating the foot and leg inward.
  - Avoid raising the knee higher than the hip on the operative side.
  - Keep the legs at least 3 to 6 inches apart when sitting, or use the abduction pillow.
  - Avoid stretching the affected hip back.
  - Avoid kneeling on one knee.
  - Avoid turning the foot outward on the affected side.
  - Avoid twisting the body away from the affected hip.
  - Avoid standing with the toes pointed outward. Keep the toes of the affected leg pointed forward when standing, sitting, or walking.
  - Avoid swinging the affected leg outward away from the body.
  - Avoid assuming a straddling position.
- Follow the care plan instructions for full and partial weight bearing, activity, and use of a walker or other ambulation device.

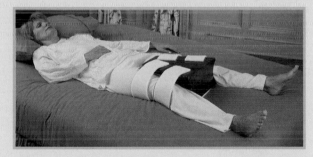

FIGURE 37-13 An abduction pillow is commonly used after hip surgery to keep the legs from crossing over at the ankles or adducting. *(Courtesy of OrthoRehab, Inc.)*

Difficult SITUATIONS

A patient who has had hip surgery will probably wear anti-embolism hosiery and use an incentive spirometer. The patient is at high risk for pressure ulcers, particularly on the heels. The skin on the heels is very thin, so breakdown can develop rapidly. ■

Continuous Passive Motion

Continuous passive motion (CPM) therapy (Figure 37-14) may be ordered following orthopedic procedures. CPM therapy prevents pain and stiffness by providing passive exercise that is effortless for the patient. The machine moves the affected joint through the range of motion.

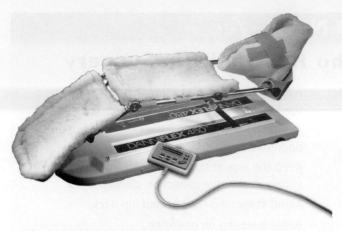

FIGURE 37-14 The CPM machine performs passive range-of-motion exercises on the affected joint without straining the patient's muscles. *(Courtesy of OrthoRehab, Inc.)*

COMPARTMENT SYNDROME

Compartment syndrome occurs when pressure within the muscles increases, blocking the flow of blood and oxygen. Bleeding or swelling take place in the muscle tissue, and the syndrome develops over time. If the swelling is not relieved, pressure will exceed the blood pressure, causing the capillaries to collapse. Blood flow to the muscles and nerves then stops. If it is not restored promptly, tissue death begins. Notify the nurse immediately if a patient has signs or symptoms of this condition.

The most common symptom of acute compartment syndrome is severe pain, especially when the muscle is moved. The pain may seem out of proportion to the injury.

PROCEDURE

 90

ASSISTING WITH CONTINUOUS PASSIVE MOTION

 Note: Be sure this is a nursing assistant procedure at your facility.

Note: These instructions are generic and are not device-specific. The person setting up the device should be trained in use of the specific device, and have an operating manual for that device.

1. Carry out initial procedure actions.

2. Gather equipment:
   - CPM unit
   - Soft goods kit, if available
   - Sheepskin foot pad (if soft goods kit not available)
   - Tibia/femur sling
   - Hip pad
   - Velcro fasteners

3. Check the unit for safety and stability. Make sure that the attachments are tight, the frame is stable, and the electric controls work. Have the nurse adjust the settings according to the physician's orders.

4. Raise the side rail on the side of the bed where you will be placing the unit.

5. Position the CPM unit on the bed and secure the attachment (depending on the type of device being used).

6. Fasten the foot pad to the foot plate with a Velcro fastener.

7. Attach the tibia/femur sling (wide section toward the footrest). Fasten the Velcro closures under the sling.

8. Apply the hip pad to the hinge area of the adjustment bar. Position the femur sling straps over the hinges, then fasten underneath with Velcro.

9. Lengthen or shorten the frame to fit the CPM machine to the patient's leg length.

10. Align the knee joint with the corresponding hinge on the unit (Figure 37-15A).

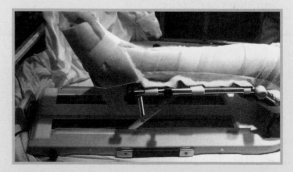

FIGURE 37-15A Position the leg straight, with the toes upright. Line the knee up with the marking at the hinge. *(© Delmar/Cengage Learning)*

PROCEDURE 90 CONTINUED

11. Center the leg on the unit. Avoid pressure on the side and middle of the knee joint.

12. Make adjustments to the foot pad so the foot is well supported (Figure 37-15B). Secure the Velcro straps across the thigh and top of foot (Figure 37-15C).

13. When the leg is in the proper position, give the patient the control (Figure 37-15D). Instruct the patient to start the unit.

14. Stay with the patient for two full cycles to be sure that she tolerates the procedure.

15. Return to check on the patient frequently when the unit is in use.

16. Carry out ending procedure actions.

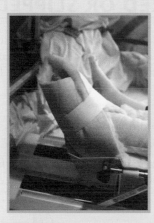

FIGURE 37-15B Make sure the foot is comfortable and well supported. Add padding if needed for patient comfort. (© Delmar/Cengage Learning)

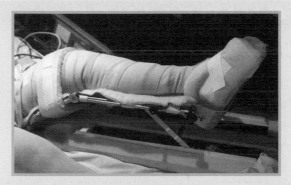

FIGURE 37-15C Secure the straps across the leg and foot. Make sure the strap is not too tight. (© Delmar/Cengage Learning)

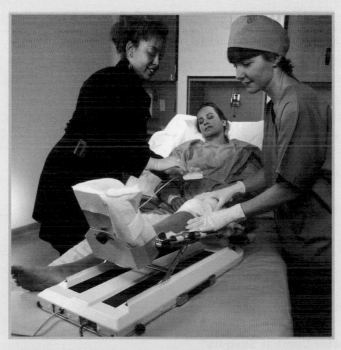

FIGURE 37-15D Show the patient how to turn the unit on, then give her the switch. Stay in the room until the machine goes through at least two cycles if the patient is using the unit for the first time. (Courtesy of OrthoRehab, Inc.)

Age-Appropriate Care ALERT

The most common location of compartment syndrome in adults is the tibia. The most common location of compartment syndrome in children is the humerus. ∎

GUIDELINES *for*

Caring for Patients after Spinal Surgeries

- Monitor vital signs and provide routine postoperative care.
- Keep the spine in good alignment.
- Logroll the patient when turning (Unit 15).
- Monitor the dressing for bleeding and clear fluid leakage.
- Offer the fracture bedpan for elimination if needed.
- Inform the nurse if the patient is unable to void or voids less than 240 mL in 8 hours.

Caring for Patients after Cervical (Neck) Surgery

- Do not remove the cervical collar.
- Keep the head straight in midline position; avoid turning the head toward the sides.
- Support the head, neck, and upper shoulders when repositioning or moving from lying to sitting to standing position, and when getting into and out of a chair.
- Observe for and report complications on one side of the body:
  - Abnormal drooping of the eyelid
  - Constricted pupil
  - Eye that appears to be sinking into the orbit
  - Lack of perspiration on one side of the face

Caring for Patients after Lumbar Surgery

- Turn every 2 hours or more often.
- Advise the patient to call for help with moving; the patient should avoid turning himself or herself.

You may make the following observations:

- The color of the extremity may appear pale, cyanotic, or red
- The skin of an extremity with no cast may feel warm to the touch
- The fingers or toes of a casted extremity may feel cool to the touch
- Edema (swelling)
- Loss of pulse in the extremity (a late sign)

RUPTURED OR SLIPPED DISC

If a disc bulges or slips out of place, pressure is placed on the spinal nerves (Figure 37-16). The parts of the body affected depend on which disc is injured. The person may experience:

- Pain
- Numbness and tingling
- Weakness of one or more muscles

If conservative attempts to relieve pressure fail, surgery may be needed to relieve pressure on the spinal cord.

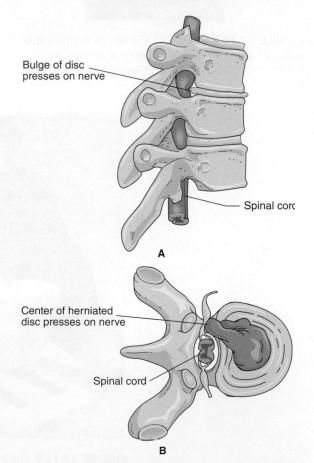

Bulge of disc presses on nerve

Spinal cord

A

Center of herniated disc presses on nerve

Spinal cord

B

FIGURE 37-16 A. Uneven pressure causes the disc to bulge, putting pressure on the nerve root (slipped disc). B. A herniated (ruptured) disc applies pressure on the nerve root as the gel-like center oozes backward. *(© Delmar/Cengage Learning)*

LOWER EXTREMITY AMPUTATION

You may care for patients who have had one or both legs surgically removed (amputated). **Amputation** (Figure 37-17) may be necessary because of circulatory problems, gangrene, or an accidental injury. **Phantom pain** is common after the removal of a limb. The person may feel pain or tingling where the limb used to be. These feelings may persist for months. The pain is real, although it is difficult to explain.

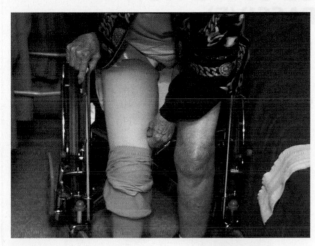

FIGURE 37-17 Some patients are admitted to learn how to apply and use a prosthesis following an amputation. *(© Delmar/Cengage Learning)*

GUIDELINES *for*

Caring for a Patient Who Has Had a Lower Extremity Amputation

When positioning a patient with a leg amputation:

- Avoid abduction and flexion of the hip—without the weight of the lower leg, the affected hip will contract quickly if positioned in flexion. Avoid elevating the head of the bed for prolonged periods, because this position also promotes hip flexion.
- Avoid flexion of the knee if the person has a below-the-knee amputation (BKA).
- Position the leg flat on the bed. Avoid placing pillows under an amputated extremity.
- Keep the legs in a position of adduction. Do not place pillows between the legs. A trochanter roll is helpful.
- Position the patient in the prone position twice a day, if permitted.

RANGE OF MOTION

Patients who are bedfast are not as active, so joints may not move through the normal range of motion daily. Weakness and muscle wasting from lack of use is called **atrophy**. Over time, muscles become rigid. Contractures and deformities develop when the patient is immobile. *Contractures* are disfigurements caused by muscle shortening. They make caring for the patient more difficult. There is a direct relationship between contractures and pressure ulcers.

To prevent complications, patients' joints must be moved regularly. If the patient cannot move independently, you will be responsible for exercising the joints. This includes patients

GUIDELINES *for*

Assisting Patients with Range-of-Motion Exercises

- Check the care plan or ask the nurse for specific guidelines and limitations.
- Help the patient relax during exercise.
- Encourage the patient to assist, if able, but keep your hands in position to provide support.
- Make sure you have enough space for full movement of the extremities.
- Expose only the part of the body you are exercising.
- Support each joint by placing one hand above and one hand below the joint.
- Slowly move each joint through the normal range of movement, stopping briefly after each motion.
- Work from the top of the body to the bottom, performing each motion three to five times, or as ordered.
- In some facilities, the neck is not exercised without a physician's order. Follow your facility policy.
- Never push the patient past the point of pain or joint resistance. Stop the exercise and inform the nurse if the patient complains of pain.
- Be alert for changes in the patient's condition during the activity. If you feel that the activity is harming the patient, stop.
- Use the session as quality time to communicate with the patient.
- Consider doing the exercise in the bathtub or whirlpool if the patient is stiff or combative. Check with the nurse.

with no potential for rehabilitation. Like pressure ulcers, contractures are much easier to prevent than to reverse. Active **range-of-motion (ROM) exercises** are done by the patient during activities of daily living. **Passive** **range-of-motion (PROM)** exercises are done for patients when independent movement is impossible. Passive range-of-motion exercises maintain movement and prevent deformities. They do *not* strengthen the muscles.

PROCEDURE

91

PERFORMING RANGE-OF-MOTION EXERCISES (PASSIVE)

Note: This procedure may be carried out as an independent procedure or as part of the bath. Repeat each action three to five times, or as directed.

1. Carry out initial procedure actions.

2. Assemble equipment:
   - Bath blanket

3. Position the patient on his back close to you.

4. Adjust the bath blanket to keep the patient covered as much as possible.

5. Supporting the elbow and wrist, exercise the shoulder joint nearest you as follows:

   a. Bring the entire arm out at a right angle to the body (horizontal abduction) (Figure 37-18A).

   b. Return the arm to a position parallel to the body (horizontal adduction).

6. a. With the arm parallel to the body, roll the entire arm toward the body (internal rotation of shoulder).

   b. Maintaining the parallel position, roll the entire arm away from the body (external rotation of shoulder).

7. With the shoulder in abduction, flex the elbow and raise the entire arm over the head (shoulder flexion) (Figure 37-18B).

8. With the arm parallel to the body (palm up—supination), flex and extend the elbow (Figures 37–18C and 37–18D).

9. Flex and extend the wrist (Figure 37-18E). Flex and extend each finger joint (Figure 37-18F).

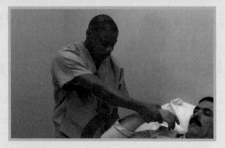

FIGURE 37-18B Shoulder flexion. With the shoulder in abduction, flex the elbow and raise the entire arm over the head. (© Delmar/Cengage Learning)

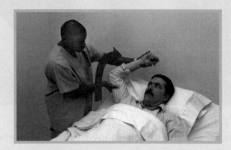

FIGURE 37-18C Flex the lower arm toward the upper arm. (© Delmar/Cengage Learning)

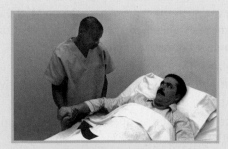

FIGURE 37-18A Shoulder abduction and adduction. Support the arm at the elbow and wrist, then bring the entire arm out at a right angle from the body. (© Delmar/Cengage Learning)

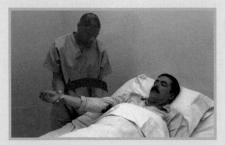

FIGURE 37-18D Elbow extension and flexion. Support the upper arm and wrist, then straighten the elbow. (© Delmar/Cengage Learning)

PROCEDURE 91 CONTINUED

10. Move each finger, in turn, away from the middle finger (abduction) (Figure 37-18G) and toward the middle finger (adduction) (Figure 37-18H).

11. Abduct the thumb by moving it toward the extended fingers (Figure 37-18I).

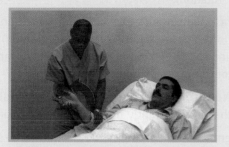

FIGURE 37-18E Wrist extension and flexion. While supporting the arm above the wrist and hand, straighten the wrist. *(© Delmar/Cengage Learning)*

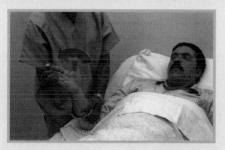

FIGURE 37-18F Finger extension. Slip your fingers over the patient's flexed fingers, then straighten the fingers. *(© Delmar/Cengage Learning)*

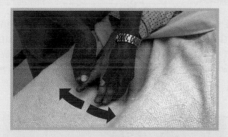

FIGURE 37-18G Abduction of the fingers. *(© Delmar/ Cengage Learning)*

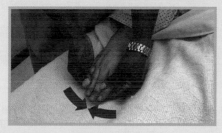

FIGURE 37-18H Adduction of the fingers. *(© Delmar/ Cengage Learning)*

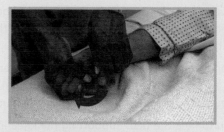

FIGURE 37-18I Abduction and adduction of the thumb and fingers. While supporting the hand, draw the thumb toward and away from the extended fingers. *(© Delmar/Cengage Learning)*

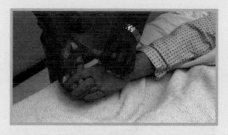

FIGURE 37-18J Thumb opposition. While supporting the hand, touch each finger with the thumb. *(© Delmar/Cengage Learning)*

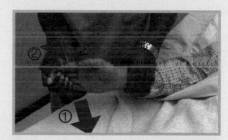

FIGURE 37-18K Wrist inversion (supination) and eversion (pronation). Grasp the patient's wrist with one hand. Grasp the patient's hand with your other hand. Bring the wrist toward the body, then away from the body. *(© Delmar/ Cengage Learning)*

12. Touch the thumb to the base of the little finger, then to each fingertip (opposition) (Figure 37-18J).

13. Turn the hand palm down (pronation), then palm up (supination).

14. Grasp the patient's wrist with one hand and the patient's hand with the other. Bring the wrist toward the body (inversion) and then away from the body (eversion) (Figure 37-18K).

15. Point the hand in supination toward the thumb side (radial deviation), then toward the little-finger side (ulnar deviation).

continues

PROCEDURE **91** CONTINUED

16. Cover the patient's upper extremities and body. Expose only the leg being exercised. Face the foot of the bed.

17. Supporting the knee and ankle, move the entire leg away from the body center (abduction) (Figure 37-18L) and toward the body (adduction).

18. Turn to face the bed. Supporting the knee in bent position (flexion), raise the knee toward the pelvis (hip flexion) (Figure 37-18M). Straighten the knee (extension) (Figure 37-18N), as you lower the leg to the bed.

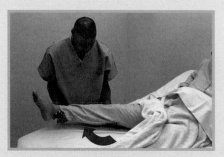

FIGURE 37-18L Abduction of the hip. While supporting the patient's knee and ankle, move the entire leg away from the center of the body. (© Delmar/Cengage Learning)

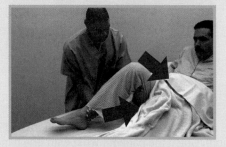

FIGURE 37-18M Hip and knee flexion. While supporting the leg, return toward the center of the body. (© Delmar/Cengage Learning)

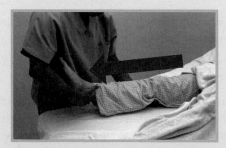

FIGURE 37-18N Knee extension. While supporting the knee and ankle, straighten the leg. (© Delmar/Cengage Learning)

19. a. Supporting the leg at the knee and ankle, roll the leg in a circular fashion away from the body (lateral hip rotation).

 b. Continuing to support the leg, roll the leg in the same fashion toward the body (medial hip rotation).

20. Grasp the patient's toes and support the ankle. Bring toes toward the knee (dorsiflexion) (Figure 37-18O). Then point the toes toward the foot of the bed (plantar flexion) (Figure 37-18P).

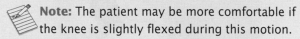 **Note:** The patient may be more comfortable if the knee is slightly flexed during this motion.

21. Gently turn the patient's foot inward (inversion) (Figure 37-18Q) and outward (eversion).

22. Place your fingers over the patient's toes. Bend the toes (flexion) and straighten them (extension).

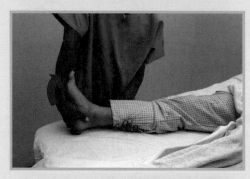

FIGURE 37-18O Ankle flexion. Grasp the patient's heel with one hand, using your upper arm to support the foot. Dorsiflex the ankle by bringing the toes and foot toward the knee. (© Delmar/Cengage Learning)

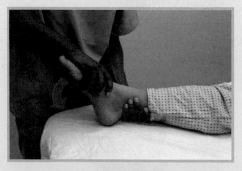

FIGURE 37-18P Plantar flex the ankle by drawing the foot into a downward position. (© Delmar/Cengage Learning)

PROCEDURE 91 CONTINUED

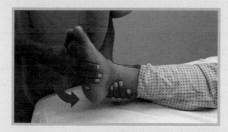

FIGURE 37-18Q Foot inversion. Grasp the patient's foot and gently turn it inward. *(© Delmar/Cengage Learning)*

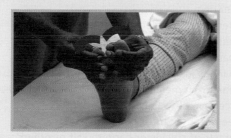

FIGURE 37-18R Toe abduction. Move each toe away from the second toe one at a time. *(© Delmar/Cengage Learning)*

23. Move each toe away from the second toe (abduction) (Figure 37-18R) and then toward the second toe (adduction) (Figure 37-18S).

24. Cover the leg with the bath blanket. Raise the side rail and move to the opposite side of the bed.

25. Move the patient close to you and repeat steps 5 through 23.

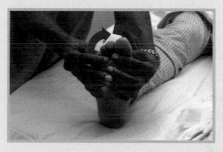

FIGURE 37-18S Toe adduction. Move each toe toward the second toe one at a time. *(© Delmar/Cengage Learning)*

You will find additional information in Unit 42 about emergency care of persons with injuries of the musculoskeletal system.

NERVOUS SYSTEM INTRODUCTION

The nervous system controls all body activities. Some parts are responsible for normal day-to-day functions. Other parts act only in emergencies. Still others control voluntary activities. Neurological conditions require highly specialized nursing care.

Clinical Information ALERT

There are 31 pairs of spinal nerves and 12 pairs of cranial nerves. One nerve can send up to 1,000 impulses per second. A nerve impulse travels at 224 miles per hour. One square inch of skin on the back of the hand has 12,000 nerve endings. Your skin contains 45 miles of nerves. There are 30 times more pain receptors than cold sensors. ∎

AGING CHANGES TO THE NERVOUS SYSTEM

Aging changes to the nervous system include:

- Increased length of time for tasks involving speed, balance, coordination, and fine motor activities, such as those involving the fingers.
- Problems with balance and coordination, as a result of deterioration to the nerve terminals that provide information to the brain on the movement and position of the body.
- Decrease in or loss of ability to feel pressure and temperature, resulting in higher potential for injury.
- Decrease in blood flow to the brain. This may result in mental confusion and memory loss.

COMMON CONDITIONS OF THE NERVOUS SYSTEM

When one or more functions of the nervous system are injured or affected by disease, the person has a neurologic deficit. Conditions ranging from paralysis (loss of voluntary motor control) to Alzheimer's disease (Unit 31) are the result of nervous system problems. Another common condition is **convulsions** (seizures). Most convulsions consist of a series of uncontrolled muscular contractions that may be violent.

Disorders of the nervous system affect other body systems. Care is often complex, and the services of many professionals are needed to return the patient to an optimal level of function.

Head Injuries

The structures within the skull normally exert a certain amount of pressure, called **intracranial pressure**. The pressure is due to a combination of nerve tissue, CSF, and blood flowing through the vessels. Changes to the brain resulting from trauma or medical problems have the potential to increase the pressure within the brain. Increased intracranial pressure must be identified and managed promptly.

Signs and symptoms Indications of increased intracranial pressure are:
- Alteration in pupil size and response to light
- Headache
- Vomiting
- Loss of consciousness and sensation
- Paralysis—loss of voluntary motor control
- Convulsions (seizures)—uncontrolled muscular contractions that are often violent

Nursing care Patients with head injuries or increased intracranial pressure require close observation and skilled nursing care. Notify the nurse promptly if you identify changes in the patient's physical condition, response, or behavior, such as those listed in Table 37-2.

Once medically stable, the patient with a neurologic disorder will require extensive rehabilitation. He or she will continue to be at high risk for complications. The nursing measures first established in the critical care unit must be maintained throughout this extended period. These include:

- Aggressive pressure ulcer and contracture prevention, including regular turning and positioning, provision of range-of-motion exercises, and careful skin monitoring.
- Reporting of early signs of infection.
- Monitoring of elimination. Loss of muscle tone and inactivity may lead to constipation and impaction.
- Checking and management of drainage tubes.
- Monitoring for changes in mood and providing emotional support.
- Careful monitoring of vital signs.

Refer to Unit 42 for information about the emergency care of persons with head injuries and other neurologic conditions.

TABLE 37-2 CHANGES IN MENTAL STATUS TO MAKE AND REPORT TO THE NURSE IMMEDIATELY

- Decreasing level of consciousness—this is the most important indication of a worsening condition
- Change in awareness or alertness
- Sudden onset of mental confusion
- Changes in mood, behavior, or emotional status
- Change in orientation to time, place, and person
- Change in reaction to pain and stimuli
- Abnormal vital signs
- Incontinence (new onset)
- Uncontrolled body movements
- Disorientation
- Dizziness
- Vomiting
- Alterations in speech
- Change in ability to follow directions
- Change in communication
- Changes in ability to respond verbally or nonverbally
- Changes in memory
- Excessive drowsiness
- Sleepiness for no apparent reason
- Threats of suicide or harm to self or others

Transient Ischemic Attack

Transient ischemic attack (TIA) is a temporary interruption of the blood flow to part of the brain. The person may experience:
- Weakness or paralysis of any extremity or the face
- Vision problems
- Difficulty speaking and swallowing

These signs and symptoms come on quickly and may last for up to 24 hours. The effects are not permanent, but the person is at risk for stroke in the future.

Stroke

A **stroke** (Figure 37-19) is also called a **cerebrovascular accident (CVA)** or **brain attack**. It affects the vascular system (blood vessels) and the nervous system. A stroke on one side of the brain results in signs and symptoms on the opposite side of the body. Symptoms vary depending on the extent of damage to the brain. Having weakness (**hemiparesis**) or paralysis (**hemiplegia**) on one side of the body is common (Figure 37-20). **Aphasia**, or loss of ability to express or understand speech, is also common. The person may have difficulty expressing thoughts coherently, which is frustrating and frightening.

Recovery from a stroke is also very frustrating for the patient. Remember two things:

1. The patient has enough frustration for both of you, so be careful not to let yours show. The last thing the patient needs is your silent reinforcement of his helplessness.

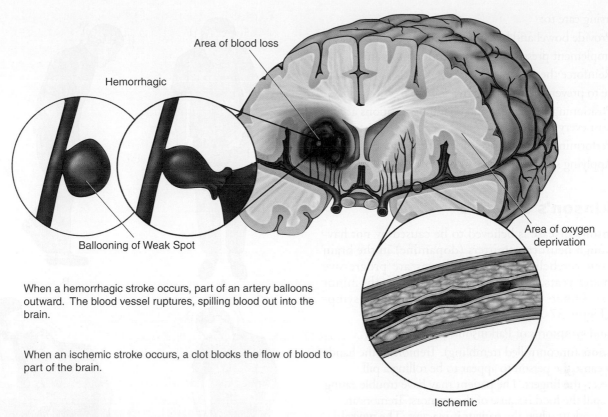

When a hemorrhagic stroke occurs, part of an artery balloons outward. The blood vessel ruptures, spilling blood out into the brain.

When an ischemic stroke occurs, a clot blocks the flow of blood to part of the brain.

FIGURE 37-19 Thrombotic strokes occur more commonly in older adults, and hemorrhagic strokes are more common in younger persons. "Clotbuster" drugs may be given to treat a thrombotic stroke if the condition is identified and treated rapidly, usually within 3 hours of the onset of symptoms. No comparable drugs are available to treat hemorrhagic stroke, and the prognosis is not as good. (© *Delmar/Cengage Learning*)

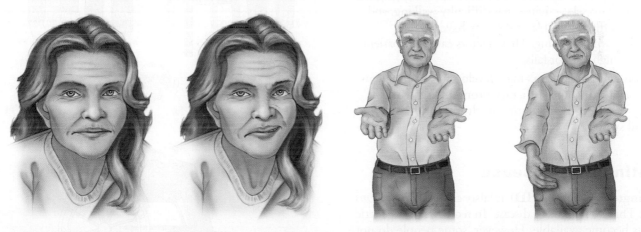

FIGURE 37-20 Compare the right and left sides of the person's body. Weakness or paralysis occurs on the face, arm, and leg on the opposite side in which the stroke occurred. (© *Delmar/Cengage Learning*)

2. The degree and speed of recovery are often related to the patience and encouragement of the caregivers with whom the patient has close contact.

Other interventions during recovery include:

- Physical therapy to increase independent mobility, such as getting to the side of the bed, standing at the bedside, transferring from bed to chair, and ambulation.

- Occupational therapy to regain the ability to perform the activities of daily living, such as bathing, grooming, dressing, and eating, with little or no assistance.

- Speech therapy to regain the ability to communicate and address swallowing problems.

- Nursing care to:
  - Provide bowel and bladder management programs
  - Implement pressure ulcer prevention programs
  - Reinforce the therapy programs
- Care to prevent contractures by:
  - Positioning the patient and changing positions at least every 2 hours
  - Performing passive range-of-motion exercises
  - Applying splints or braces as ordered

Parkinson's Disease

Parkinson's disease is believed to be caused by not having enough neurotransmitters (dopamine) in the brain stem and cerebellum. The symptoms are progressive over many years. Some people will show only minor changes. Others will have much more obvious symptoms (Figure 37-21).

Signs and symptoms of Parkinson's disease include:

- **Tremors** (uncontrolled trembling). Tremors of the hands may cause the person to appear to be rolling a pill between the fingers. The patient may have trouble eating and spill the food because of the tremors. Tremors are more evident when the patient is inactive. The typical posture of a person with Parkinson's disease is shown in Figure 37-22.
- Muscular rigidity and loss of flexibility. These are cardinal signs of Parkinson's. The facial muscles lose expression. The patient becomes slow, has trouble carrying out voluntary muscle activities, has difficulty walking, and uses a shuffling gait. He or she may have trouble stopping when walking. These factors cause the patient to be at high risk for falls.
- Persons with Parkinson's may develop speech problems, such as slurring and difficulty pronouncing words. They may become incontinent, drool, and have mood swings.

Huntington's Disease

Huntington's disease (HD) is also called *Huntington's chorea.* This is a hereditary disease. In recent years, a genetic test has become available. However, some people do not want to know if they have the gene, because they fear the diagnosis.

Clinical signs of the disease usually begin when the person is the 40s or 50s. However, signs may occur in childhood or young adulthood. The disease is progressive and there is no cure. Disability and death occur within 15 to 20 years. Abnormal movements, called **chorea**, are the primary sign of HD. The movements are subtle early in the course of the illness. The individual will appear anxious or restless. He moves frequently, but may try to disguise the activity with voluntary movements, such as

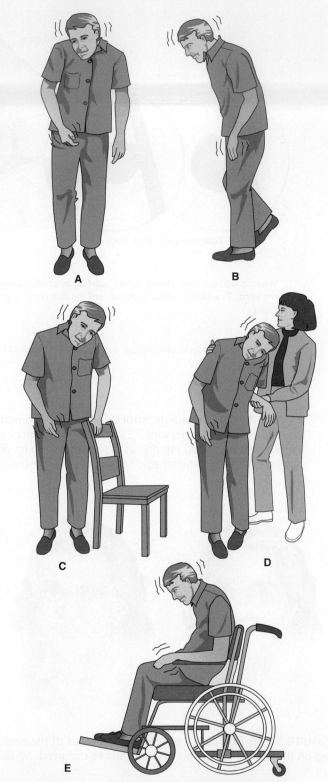

FIGURE 37-21 Progression of Parkinson's disease. A. The person leans slightly forward and develops flexion of an affected arm. B. The person stoops forward and walks with a shuffling gait. C. The person tends to shuffle faster and faster, leaning farther forward until he falls on his face. D. The disease progresses to the point of needing assistance for ambulation. E. The person has profound weakness and severe tremors. Ambulation becomes impossible. (© *Delmar/Cengage Learning*)

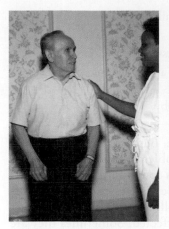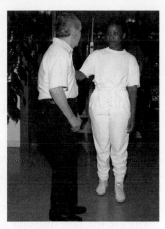

FIGURE 37-22 The typical posture of a person with Parkinson's disease. In addition to the standing posture, note the patient's hands. (© *Delmar/Cengage Learning*)

scratching the head or crossing the legs. The movement increases with stress and attempts to control the motions. As the disease progresses, rapid, jerking choreiform movements involve the entire body. The person will develop a strange, swaying gait in which she extends the hips in an attempt to balance. The person also loses control of the bowel and bladder.

Individuals with HD also develop mental changes. The person becomes nervous, suspicious of others, and irritable. Mood swings are common, as is depression. As the

GUIDELINES *for*

Care of Persons with Parkinson's Disease and Huntington's Disease

- Maintain a consistent routine, avoiding change as much as possible
- Maintain safe ambulation and reduce the risk of falls and other injuries
- Prevent weight loss by replacing calories used by the involuntary movements
- Ensure adequate intake of fluids
- Promote safe swallowing and prevent choking
- Maintain the patient's current abilities
- Keep the patient as independent as possible for as long as possible
- Assist the patient with self-care deficits by completing tasks the patient cannot finish

condition progresses, the individual develops dementia and becomes totally dependent on others.

Multiple Sclerosis

Multiple sclerosis (MS) usually occurs in young adults as a result of the loss of insulation around nerve fibers. However, it can develop in middle age as well. The cause is unknown. This is another condition in which the person will experience remissions and exacerbations. The mind remains alert, but the person experiences gradual nervous system deterioration. Incontinence of bowel and bladder are common. One of the most disabling features of MS is fatigue. The fatigue is very real and is not psychological.

The symptoms are variable and may not be the same for all individuals. Symptoms may include:

- Loss of sensation with regard to temperature, pain, and touch.
- Feelings of numbness and tingling.
- **Vertigo** (a spinning or dizzy sensation).
- **Lhermitte's sign** (a tingling, shock-like sensation that passes down the arms or spine when the neck is flexed).
- Blurred vision, double vision, and **nystagmus** (jerky eye movements).
- Mobility problems, such as pain in the legs.
- Spasticity of muscles.
- **Intention tremor** (a tremor that worsens with voluntary movement).
- **Paraplegia** (paralysis of both legs) and **quadriplegia** (paralysis of all four extremities) in advanced cases. Another term for paralysis of the arms and legs is **tetraplegia**. When a person is paralyzed, voluntary movement, strength, and sensation are limited or absent.
- In severe MS, speech may be slow, with poor articulation. Do not mistake this problem for mental confusion. The patient's mind remains alert.

Nursing care of the patient with multiple sclerosis includes pressure ulcer and contracture prevention. Encourage independence, but help the patient maintain a balanced schedule of rest and activity. Provide emotional support.

Post Polio Syndrome (PPS)

Polio is a very serious neurological disease that has been with us since at least 1350 BC. This disease is caused by a virus that attacks the motor neurons in the spinal cord. There were large annual outbreaks of polio in the United States every summer until 1955, when the first vaccine became available.

Post polio syndrome (PPS) is marked by increased weakness and abnormal muscle fatigue in persons who had polio many years earlier. It is believed to be related to the loss of motor neurons. Most polio survivors have about 10% to 50% as many motor neurons as other people. These neurons have served the person by adapting so they could innervate areas that are five to seven times larger than normal. PPS develops when the neurons being to wear out from years of overuse. As the neurons die, the muscles stop responding.

Signs and symptoms of PPS range from annoying to debilitating. Any new injury strains the remaining neurons, reducing function and increasing pain and fatigue. Signs and symptoms include:

- Fatigue that may be debilitating.
- New joint and muscle pain. Most PPS patients experience pain daily.
- New weakness in muscles affected by polio; formerly unaffected muscles are also affected.
- New dyspnea and other respiratory problems.
- Severe cold intolerance, which causes muscle weakness to worsen, the arms or legs to become pale or cyanotic, and the extremities to feel cold to the touch.
- Muscle spasms and cramps that are sometimes severe and painful.
- Difficulty swallowing.
- Difficulty falling asleep and waking frequently during the night.

PPS patients are much more sensitive to anesthesia than persons who have not had polio. They require less medication and half the anesthesia, yet take twice as long as others to recover from the anesthesia. Because of this, the patient with PPS must be monitored closely after use of anesthesia.

Amyotrophic Lateral Sclerosis

Amyotrophic lateral sclerosis (ALS), also called *Lou Gehrig's disease*, is a disease that causes muscle weakness and paralysis. The cause is unknown. ALS affects the motor nerves that control voluntary movement. It is a progressive condition for which there is no cure. It is almost always fatal.

Signs and symptoms Common signs and symptoms of ALS are:

- Stumbling, tripping, and falling
- Loss of strength and muscle control in hands, arms, and legs

Difficult SITUATIONS

Persons with post polio syndrome are fiercely independent, often to their detriment. Most were taught that part of their recovery includes being "normal." Asking for help may be very difficult for them. ■

- Difficulty speaking and swallowing
- Drooling
- Breathing becoming progressively more difficult
- Muscle cramping, shaking, and twitching, progressing to spasticity
- Muscle weakness and atrophy
- Abnormal reflexes

ALS is not a painful disease, but its effects often cause pain. Despite the many problems, the person's mental acuity is intact. Depression is common. The heart, bowel and bladder control, and sexual function are not affected. The muscles controlling eye and eyelid movement are the last muscles affected. Sometimes they are not affected at all.

Nursing assistant care Most ALS patients are cared for at home. Nursing care is designed to prevent complications of immobility. Allow patients to be in control of daily routines, and respect their intelligence. Adaptive equipment is used to maintain independence for as long as possible. Many ALS patients are not bedridden, despite being paralyzed. Special wheelchairs and ventilators are used so patients can get out of bed.

Care of the patient depends on the stage of the disease at hospital admission. Turn the patient every 2 hours when in bed. Assist with food and fluid intake. Follow the care plan and the nurse's instructions.

Seizure Disorder (Epilepsy)

Seizure disorder (convulsions, **epilepsy**) involves recurrent attacks of disturbed brain function. There are many causes of this condition, which is characterized by various forms of convulsions called *seizures*. Not all seizures are alike. A seizure occurs when one or more of the following is present:

- An altered state of consciousness
- Uncontrolled convulsive movements
- Disturbances of feeling or behavior

Some persons experience an aura just before a seizure occurs. An **aura** involves one of the senses, such as smelling an unusual odor or hearing a sound. The aura is the same each time it is experienced. For some people, the aura serves as a warning that allows the person to get to a safe place. Others may not remember the aura.

There are many different types and categories of seizure activity. The most common are:

- Generalized seizures (Figure 37-23). These include **grand mal seizures**. A newer name is **generalized tonic-clonic seizures**. There is bilateral motor movement and muscular rigidity. Consciousness is lost. The person falls to the floor. The muscles stiffen (tonic phase), then the extremities begin to jerk and twitch (clonic phase). The person may lose bladder control. Consciousness returns slowly. After the seizure, the

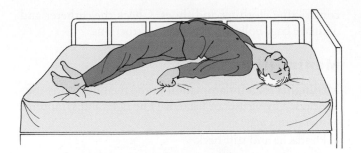

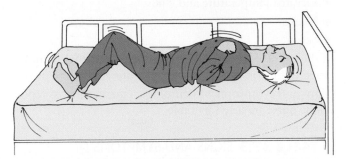

FIGURE 37-23 Generalized tonic-clonic seizures involve the entire body. Side rails should be padded for patients who have seizure disorder. Side rails in this picture are down for clarity only. (© *Delmar/Cengage Learning*)

person may feel tired, or be confused and disoriented. He or she may fall asleep, or gradually become less confused until full consciousness returns.

- **Petit mal seizures**, which are characterized by momentary loss of muscle tone. A more recent name is **absence seizures**. The seizure begins without warning, and consists of a period of unconsciousness, in which the patient blinks or breathes rapidly, stares, or makes chewing movements. The seizure lasts 2 to 10 seconds, then ends abruptly. The person usually resumes normal activity right away. The seizures are mild and may go unnoticed.

- **Status epilepticus** is a seizure that lasts for a long time or repeats without recovery. It is very serious. Death may result if the person is not treated immediately.

Review the information in Unit 42 on caring for a person during and after a seizure.

Spinal Cord Injuries

Injuries to the spinal cord result in loss of function and sensation below the level where the spinal cord was damaged. For example, an injury in the upper neck will cause respiratory depression because the control center is near the upper neck. The person will be unable to move the arms and legs, and lose bowel and bladder control. An injury near the waist also causes loss of bowel and bladder control and inability to move the legs. Patients with spinal cord injuries are at high risk of contractures and pressure ulcers.

Paralysis **Paralysis** is seen in many medical conditions, but is most commonly associated with spinal cord injury. Terms used to describe paralysis are:

- *Paraplegia*—paralysis below the waist and both legs
- *Tetraplegia (quadriplegia)*—paralysis below the neck, both arms, and both legs

Flaccid paralysis involves loss of muscle tone and absence of tendon reflexes. Persons with **spastic paralysis** have no voluntary movement. Their extremities are very jerky (spastic). The person is aware of the movements, but cannot stop them.

The goals of nursing care include:

- Keeping the lungs clear
- Preventing complications of immobility
- Preventing deformities
- Restoring the patient to the highest degree of independence possible
- Enhancing self esteem by encouraging the patient to make choices and direct her own care

Autonomic dysreflexia **Autonomic dysreflexia** (Figure 37-24) is a potentially life-threatening complication of spinal cord injury. It usually occurs in persons with injuries above the mid-thoracic area. Any problem that would normally cause pain below the level of spinal injury triggers this condition. For example:

- Overfull bladder (this is the most common cause)
- Urinary retention, urinary tract infection, or blocked catheter
- Constipation, fecal impaction, or medical problems in the abdomen
- Hemorrhoids
- Pressure ulcers
- Prolonged pressure by an object in the chair, bed, or a shoe; wrinkles in clothing, pressure on skin from tight clothing
- Minor injury, such as a cut, bruise, abrasion, sunburn
- Ingrown toenails

Signs and symptoms of autonomic dysreflexia are:

- Extremely high blood pressure, over 200/100
- Severe headache, stuffy nose

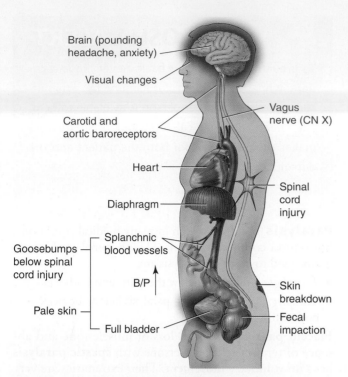

FIGURE 37-24 In autonomic dysreflexia, lower motor neurons sense a painful stimulius and send a signal to the brain. The signal cannot go past the spinal cord injury, so it cannot reach the brain. This triggers hypertension and other signs and symptoms. The body tries to notify the brain of the hypertension, but again the message cannot penetrate the spinal cord injury. This triggers the vagus nerve to slow the heart rate, and the patient develops bradycardia as a result of the body's attempt to normalize internal conditions. (© Delmar/Cengage Learning)

- Red, flushed face, sweating and red blotches on the skin *above* the level of injury
- Cold, clammy skin and goosebumps *below* the level of injury
- Nausea
- Bradycardia (pulse below 60)

If you observe any of these signs and symptoms, notify the nurse immediately. Treatment involves identifying and removing the offending stimulus. Remove tight and constricting clothing and shoes. Check the catheter and drainage bag. Follow the nurses' instructions.

Meningitis

Meningitis is an inflammation of the meninges. It is usually caused by viruses or bacteria. The signs and symptoms of meningitis are:

- Headache and stiff neck
- Elevated temperature and chills
- Nausea
- Seizures

If the cause is bacterial, meningitis is treated with antibiotics. If it is communicable, droplet precautions are used.

Signs and symptoms of neurologic emergencies to report to the nurse are listed in Table 37-3.

TABLE 37-3 SIGNS AND SYMPTOMS OF NEUROLOGIC EMERGENCIES THAT SHOULD BE REPORTED TO THE NURSE IMMEDIATELY

- Change in level of consciousness, orientation, awareness, or alertness
- Feeling faint or lightheaded, losing consciousness
- New onset of inability to recognize familiar persons or objects
- New onset of disorientation (does not know person, place, time)
- Increasing memory or mental confusion, worsening confusion
- Progressive lethargy
- Loss of sensation
- Numbness, tingling
- Change in pupil size; unequal pupils
- Abnormal or involuntary motor function
- Spasticity
- Loss of ability to move a body part
- Incoordination
- Changes in speech
- Changes in ability to swallow
- Drooping of one side of the face
- New onset of weakness or paralysis on one side of the body

REVIEW

A. Multiple Choice

Select the one best answer for each of the following.

1. When assigned to perform ROM, you should
   a. exercise every joint.
   b. exercise joints to the point of pain.
   c. dress the patient in a hospital gown.
   d. perform each exercise 20 times.

2. While a leg cast is drying,
   a. cover it tightly so moisture will not be lost.
   b. support the cast on a hard surface.

   c. cover the bed under the cast with plastic.

   d. use only fingertips to handle the cast.

3. When caring for a patient who is in traction,

   a. maintain proper alignment.

   b. lift the weights rapidly.

   c. allow weights to rest on the floor.

   d. position the patient's feet against the footboard.

4. Your patient has a ruptured disc. You should note and report

   a. crossing of the legs.

   b. ambulation in the room.

   c. numbness and tingling.

   d. complaints of feeling tired.

5. The most common symptom of osteoarthritis is

   a. swollen joints.

   b. pain.

   c. redness.

   d. limited mobility.

6. Gout is caused by

   a. allergies.

   b. hypertension.

   c. an adverse reaction to medication.

   d. elevated uric acid levels in the blood.

7. When positioning a patient who has had hip replacement surgery, you should

   a. elevate the head of the bed at least 60°

   b. cross the legs at the ankles.

   c. avoid elevating the head more than 45°.

   d. position the hips and knees in complete flexion.

8. Compartment syndrome is a

   a. serious surgical emergency.

   b. normal side effect of a fracture.

   c. chronic condition related to arthritis.

   d. complication of spinal cord injury.

9. Position the patient who has had a leg amputation

   a. with both legs in flexion.

   b. with pillows between the legs.

   c. with the head elevated at least 90°.

   d. with the legs in adduction.

10. Patients with which condition are usually very sensitive to anesthesia?

   a. Post polio syndrome

   b. Amyotrophic lateral sclerosis

   c. Huntington's disease

   d. Parkinson's disease

11. Paralysis of all four extremities is

   a. paraplegia.

   b. hemiplegia.

   c. tetraplegia.

   d. hemiparesis.

12. Lhermitte's sign is seen in

   a. hip fracture.

   b. osteoporosis.

   c. multiple sclerosis.

   d. Huntington's disease.

13. Persons with Parkinson's disease generally have

   a. pain.

   b. rigidity.

   c. spasticity.

   d. hearing impairment.

14. Patients with stroke

   a. need proper positioning to prevent contractures.

   b. must be repositioned every 4 hours.

   c. will be unable to speak during the acute phase.

   d. require tube feeding during the acute phase.

15. Multiple sclerosis occurs because

   a. the myelin sheath of the neuron is damaged.

   b. of a hemorrhage in the brain.

   c. the axons and dendrites are dying.

   d. of muscle damage.

16. Patients with multiple sclerosis may experience

   a. hemiplegia.

   b. a shuffling gait and pill-rolling tremors.

   c. loss of sensation to temperature, pain, and touch.

   d. inability to swallow.

17. The person with post polio syndrome experiences

   a. nausea and vomiting.

   b. visual disturbances and facial droop.

   c. cold intolerance and weakness.

   d. hemiplegia.

18. A person who has had a TIA is at risk for

   a. stroke.

   b. heart attack.

   c. paraplegia.

   d. neurologic disorders.

19. Patients with ALS commonly experience

   a. hemiplegia.

   b. muscle weakness and atrophy.

   c. difficulty hearing.

   d. mental confusion.

20. When caring for a patient who has ALS, the nursing assistant should
   a. make decisions for the patient because of mental confusion.
   b. allow the patient to direct care, because mental clarity is unaffected.
   c. keep the patient in bed and as still as possible.
   d. limit fluids to prevent choking and aspiration.

21. Autonomic dysreflexia can be caused by
   a. hunger.
   b. thirst.
   c. overfull bladder.
   d. drowsiness.

22. Autonomic dysreflexia is
   a. a life-threatening condition.
   b. a minor complication of surgery.
   c. very painful.
   d. common in patients with multiple sclerosis.

B. Nursing Assistant Challenge

You are assigned to care for Mr. McGhie, who has had a stroke. You learn from his care plan that he has right hemiplegia and aphasia. Answer the following questions about his care.

23. From this information, you know that which part of Mr. McGhie's brain was affected by the stroke?

24. What does right hemiplegia mean?

25. List two complications of stroke. What can you do to prevent complications?

Caring for Patients with Disorders of the Sensory Organs

OBJECTIVES

After completing this unit, you will be able to:
- Spell and define terms.
- Identify aging changes of the sensory organs.
- Describe common disorders of the sensory organs.
- Describe nursing assistant actions and observations related to the care of patients with disorders of the sensory organs.

- Explain the proper care, handling, and insertion of a hearing aid.
- Demonstrate the following procedures:
  - Procedure 92 Caring for the Eye Socket and Artificial Eye
  - Procedure 93 Applying Warm or Cool Eye Compresses

VOCABULARY

Learn the meaning and the correct spelling of the following words and phrases:

braille	macular degeneration	otitis media	retinal degeneration
cataracts	Ménière's disease	otosclerosis	sign language
glaucoma			

INTRODUCTION

The nervous system is the command center for the body. As a nursing assistant, you will depend on your sensory organs to help you identify problems and changes in patients' conditions. Your nervous system controls sensation by identifying a situation, sending a message to the brain, interpreting the message, then responding appropriately.

INTRODUCTION TO THE SENSORY ORGANS: THE EYES AND EARS

The eyes provide information to the brain, which interprets and acts on it. The eye changes shape and the lens becomes thicker when viewing a close-up object. When viewing something far away, the muscles squeeze the lens, making it thinner and easier to see clearly. The lenses in the eyes do not always focus light properly on the back of the retina. When the eye is too short, the image falls behind the retina. This is called *farsightedness*, because the eyes can focus on items that are far away but not on those that are close up. If the eye is too long, the person can see things nearby but not far away. This is called nearsightedness. The eyes work together, but if a person goes blind in one eye, he or she will lose only about one-fifth of the vision and 100% of the depth perception.

Ear wax is a protective body mechanism that coats the inside of the ear canals. The ear canal also sheds skin cells, which become part of the ear wax. In addition, the wax contains sweat and fatty acids, such as those found in fatty foods. Ear wax protects the inner ears from foreign invaders, such as dust, dirt, and bugs. Persons who live in big cities produce more ear wax than those in rural areas.

Clinical Information ALERT

The eyes do not grow. An infant does not blink at all in the first few months of life. Adults blink every 2 to 10 seconds. Blinking causes the eyes to be closed for approximately one hour each day. Women blink nearly twice as much as men. The corneas obtain oxygen from the air, and are the only part of the body with no blood supply. One in every 12 men is color-blind. Few women are color-blind. ∎

Clinical Information ALERT

Having an insect in the ear is a common problem. People often place cotton swabs and other objects into the ear to remove the insect. This pushes the insect farther back in the ear canal. Pouring mineral oil into the ear will smother the insect. Although uncomfortable, the sensations are less annoying when the insect dies and movement stops. The insect should be professionally removed by a health care provider. ∎

The wax dries up and forms into little balls. The balls move outward and eventually drop out during yawning, chewing, or swallowing. Placing objects into the ears pushes the wax farther back in the ear canal. This can result in reduced hearing acuity or even loss of hearing if the wax is packed against the eardrum.

AGING CHANGES AFFECTING THE EYES AND EARS

The sensory organs need a minimum amount of stimulation before the person notices a sensation. This minimum level of stimulation is the *threshold*. As a person ages, normal body changes increase this threshold. The result is that more sensory input is needed before the person becomes aware of the sensation. Aging changes in hearing and vision changes are the most noticeable. Although some of these can be corrected with aids such as eyeglasses, the improvement may not seem to fully regain the sharpness (*acuity*) of the senses the person remembers from his or her younger years. Aging changes to the sensory organs include:

- Development of cataracts or glaucoma.
- Changes in fluid levels in the eye, which cause some persons to see flashing lights.

- Decreased flexibility of the lens in the eye, which causes visual changes.
- Decreased tear production, which causes discomfort.
- Decreased sensitivity of the cornea; injuries to and foreign bodies in the eye may not be noticed.
- Decrease in the size of the pupils; by age 60, the pupils are about one-third of the size they were at age 20.
- Slower pupil reaction to darkness or bright light. The person may have difficulty adapting to glare and bright light.
- Gradual decline in visual acuity. Almost everyone older than age 55 needs glasses at least part of the time. Most also need bifocals.
- More difficulty distinguishing blues and greens compared with reds and yellows. This problem worsens with age, though all people experience it at some time.
- Decreased muscle movement of the eye, making it difficult to move the eye in all directions. Upward gaze may be limited. The visual field becomes smaller.
- Reduction in peripheral vision.
- Problems with balance and coordination, resulting from deterioration of the nerve terminals that provide information to the brain on the movement and position of the body.
- Thickening of the eardrum, which affects the bones of the inner ear and thus the person's ability to maintain balance.
- Slight decline in hearing, especially of high-frequency sounds. The problem may be worse in persons who were exposed to a lot of noise when they were younger.
- Decline in hearing acuity because of aging changes in the auditory nerve. This problem worsens if aging or disease have reduced the brain's ability to process or translate sounds into useful information.
- Impacted ear wax (more common with advancing age). This problem can be treated, but until the problem is correctly identified, the person may experience difficulty hearing.
- Difficulty hearing or loss of hearing in one or both ears. This may be correctible, depending on the cause. About 30% of adults over the age of 65 have a hearing problem.
- Development of persistent, abnormal ringing, roaring, whistling, hissing, or other annoying ear noise. This condition is called *tinnitus*, and has several causes.

COMMON CONDITIONS OF THE EYE

Cataracts

Cataracts (Figure 38-1) are the leading cause of vision loss in older adults. Because of this, cataract surgery is very common. Cataracts cause the lens to become

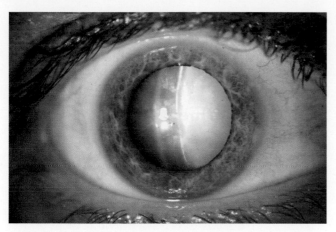

FIGURE 38-1 When the patient develops a cataract, the lens is cloudy instead of transparent. *(Photo courtesy of Linda Jaakobovitch, Cincinnati Eye Institute)*

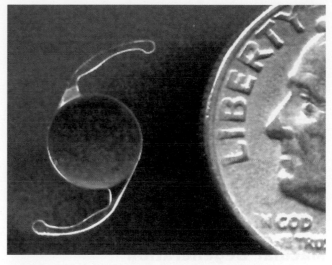

FIGURE 38-2B The lens implant is left in place. The patient cannot feel it after the eye heals. The lens implant is similar to a contact lens and smaller than a dime. *(Photo courtesy of Linda Jaakobovitch, Cincinnati Eye Institute)*

cloudy. The cloudy (opaque) lens blocks light rays so the person cannot see.

Treatment Sight is restored when the lens is removed or replaced, permitting light to enter the eye. Cataract surgery is an outpatient procedure that is comfortable and convenient. The patient is discharged after surgery, or when vital signs are stable. Eye drops are used to numb the eye. The cataract is removed, an artificial lens is implanted (Figures 38-2A and 38-2B), and the incision is naturally sealed. Stitches are not used. Some surgeons apply an eye patch, but most do not.

Lens Implant Surgery for Cataracts

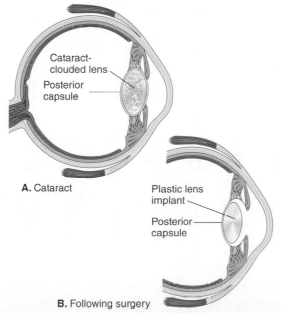

A. Cataract

Cataract-clouded lens

Posterior capsule

Plastic lens implant

Posterior capsule

B. Following surgery

FIGURE 38-2A The lens is removed and the plastic intraocular lens is permanently placed in the eye. *(© Delmar/Cengage Learning)*

Nursing care Nursing care of the patient who has had cataract surgery includes:

- Routine postoperative care and vital sign monitoring.
- Relief of pain, which is usually mild. If the person complains of sharp pain, or decreased vision, promptly notify the nurse.
- Ensuring that all needed items are within reach.
- Avoiding irritation to the surgical site. The patient may complain of itching, or feel as if something (such as an eyelash) is in the eye. Fluid discharge may be present, and the eye may be sensitive to light and touch. Instruct the patient not to rub, scratch, or squeeze the eye.
- Helping the patient to adapt to temporarily blurred vision. This is normal due to the bright lights used in surgery and drops used to dilate the eyes. The problem will resolve on its own very quickly.
- Assisting with initial ambulation, if needed. Most patients are able to walk without help immediately after surgery.

Glaucoma

Glaucoma is a condition of increased pressure within the eye. There are no early signs and symptoms. The person experiences decreased vision and gradual loss of peripheral vision. (In this context, *peripheral* vision means side vision.) Untreated, the pressure in the eye gradually increases, compressing the lens and causing gradual loss of central vision and blindness.

Glaucoma is treated with medications and eye drops that reduce pressure. Surgery may be done to drain fluid and relieve pressure. The person must have regular eye examinations to measure the pressure within the eye. Patients with glaucoma are usually in the hospital for treatment of another condition, but the glaucoma must also be managed. Care of the patient with glaucoma includes:

- Monitoring accurate intake and output if the patient is on intravenous medication to reduce eye pressure
- Checking vital signs every 2 to 4 hours
- Reporting complaints of eye pain promptly to the nurse
- Keeping the patient safe and making sure the call signal and needed items are within reach
- Avoiding strain and exertion that will increase pressure in the eye
- Keeping the patient from stooping or lifting
- Avoiding tight or constrictive clothing, which also increases pressure

Macular Degeneration

Breakdown of the retina, known as **retinal degeneration** or **macular degeneration**, occurs over a period of months or years. The incidence of this condition increases with age. Central vision is progressively lost. Hemorrhages lead to scarring of this area. Early diagnosis and treatment with laser therapy can seal the tiny capillaries to prevent further damage.

Vision Impairment

Cataracts, glaucoma, retinal degeneration, infections, tumors, and other conditions can cause blindness. Persons who are legally blind may still have partial vision. Consider the patient's limitations when giving care. Also consider the patient's attitude to the limitations. Adjustment to blindness is both a physical and an emotional process.

Allow the patient to do as much as possible independently. Many blind people are independent. In fact, most blind people do well once they are oriented to their surroundings.

GUIDELINES *for*

Communicating with Patients Who Have Visual Impairments

Patients who have visual impairments may have problems communicating because they are unable to see the sender or the sender's facial expressions and body language.

- Address the patient by name and then touch lightly on the hand or arm to avoid startling the patient.
- Identify yourself and explain why you are there.
- Be specific when giving information or directions.
- Position yourself so the light is not behind your back while you are speaking.
- Inform the patient when you are leaving the room.
- Offer to read menus, mail, and other printed materials.
- Make sure the telephone is within reach. The patient can count the buttons to make calls.
- Tactfully inform the patient if clothing is soiled, mismatched, or in need of repair.
- Provide radio or television the patient can listen to for information, news, and current events.
- Inform Social Services if the patient requests a talking-book machine.
- Describe the environment so the patient can establish a frame of reference. Avoid moving furnishings or personal item without the patient's consent.

Some patients may read **braille**, a system of raised dots (Figure 38-3). The patient reads the letters and words by moving his or her fingertips over the dots.

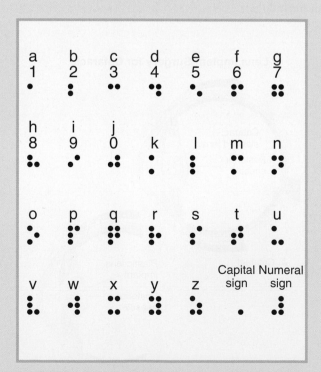

FIGURE 38-3 Many persons with visual impairment use braille. (© *Delmar/Cengage Learning*)

ARTIFICIAL EYE

Situations such as severe injury to the eye or untreatable cancer may require surgical removal of an eye. An eye prosthesis (artificial eye) is usually inserted after the surgery. The care plan will provide information if a patient has an artificial eye.

Some patients remove the artificial eye at night. Others prefer not to remove the eye at all. You may be responsible for removing the eye. If it is to remain out of the socket, store it in a marked cup in contact lens disinfectant solution or sterile saline (Figure 38-4) (see Procedure 92). The socket is usually cleansed and irrigated when the eye is removed. Irrigation of the socket may be a licensed nursing procedure in your facility. Apply the principles of standard precautions when caring for the artificial eye and mucous membranes in the eye socket.

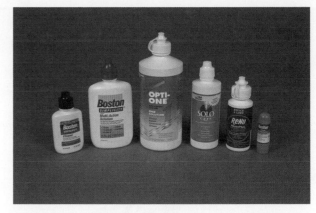

FIGURE 38-4 Many different products and solutions are used to clean, disinfect, and remove protein deposits from the artificial eye. Most of these were developed to be used in the care of contact lenses. They are safe and useful for eye prostheses. The patient must bring the eye in to be polished once or twice a year. (© Delmar/ Cengage Learning)

PROCEDURE

92

CARING FOR THE EYE SOCKET AND ARTIFICIAL EYE

1. Carry out initial procedure actions.

2. Assemble equipment:
   - Eye cup or clean denture cup
   - Prescribed solution
   - Small plastic bag
   - 4 to 6 cotton balls
   - 24 × 4 gauze pads
   - Emesis basin with lukewarm water
   - Disposable gloves
   - Towel

3. Position the patient in the supine position. Drape a towel across the chest.

4. Put on disposable gloves.

5. Moisten cotton balls in lukewarm water in the emesis basin.
   a. Ask the patient to close the eyes.
   b. Wipe the upper lid from the inner corner to the outer edge. Repeat with a clean cotton ball until the area is clean and free of mucus.

6. Discard the used cotton balls in a plastic bag.

7. Place a 4 × 4 gauze pad in the bottom of the eye cup or denture cup.

8. Remove the artificial eye:
   a. Gently pull down the lower eyelid with your thumb (Figure 38-5A). Open the upper lid with your index finger.
   b. Grasp the artificial eye as it comes out of the eye socket and place it on the gauze in the cup.
   c. Some patients use a small suction cup to remove the eye. Gently hold the eye open with

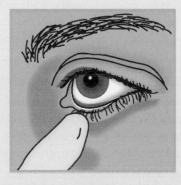

FIGURE 38-5A To loosen the eye, pull the lower lid down, then push back up slightly. (© Delmar/Cengage Learning)

continues

PROCEDURE 92 CONTINUED

the fingers of one hand. Depress the suction cup between your thumb and index finger (Figure 38-5B). Place the suction cup in the center of the artificial eye. Release the pressure so the cup adheres to the eye. Gently pull the eye from the socket (Figure 38-5C).

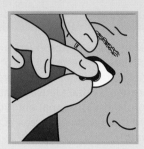

FIGURE 38-5B Squeeze the cup, place it against the eye, then release the suction. (© Delmar/Cengage Learning)

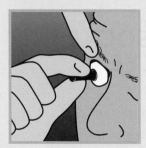

FIGURE 38-5C Pull the eye down gently from the socket. Never try to pull it straight out. (© Delmar/Cengage Learning)

9. Use clean cotton balls moistened with water or solution to clean the empty eye socket. Dry gently with clean, dry cotton balls. Use a new cotton ball for each wipe. Pat the face dry. If the external eyelid has mucus or matter on the surface, wash it gently with warm water and baby shampoo.

10. Carry the cup with the artificial eye to the sink. Fill the sink one-third full with lukewarm water.

11. Wash the eye using lukewarm water or the prescribed solution. Use gauze, if necessary, to loosen and remove any accumulation from the eye. Wipe gently to avoid scratching the eye.

12. Rinse the eye and place it on a dry 4 × 4 gauze pad, or store the eye in sterile water or the prescribed solution, according to the care plan. (Do not dry an artificial eye.)

Inserting an Artificial Eye

13. Carry out initial procedure actions.

14. Put on disposable gloves.

15. Discard the water or solution in the eye cup and rinse the cup.

16. Remove your gloves. Wash your hands. Carry the artificial eye to the bedside.

17. Explain what you are going to do.

18. Insert the artificial eye into the eye socket:

   a. Clean and rinse the artificial eye with the prescribed solution, if you have not already done so. The eye should be moist for insertion. Do not attempt to insert it dry.

   b. Position the notched edge of the eye toward the patient's nose (Figure 38-5D).

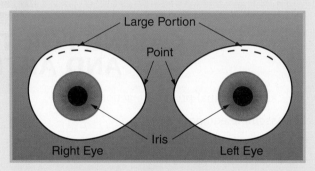

FIGURE 38-5D The notched part of the eye is positioned next to the patient's nose. (© Delmar/Cengage Learning)

   c. Gently open the upper eyelid. Bring the prosthesis up past the lower lid and under the upper lid. Set it flush once it is past the lower lid and touching the upper tissues (Figure 38-5E).

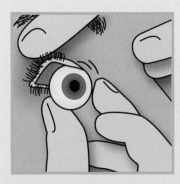

FIGURE 38-5E Gently move the artificial eye up past the lower lid. (© Delmar/Cengage Learning)

PROCEDURE 92 CONTINUED

d. Place your index finger on the prosthesis and slip it up under the upper lid (Figure 38-5F).

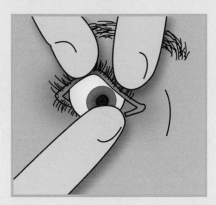

FIGURE 38-5F Using your index finger, push the eye the rest of the way up and under the upper lid. (© Delmar/Cengage Learning) •

e. Release the upper lid.

f. Draw the edge of the lower lid forward, covering the lower edge of the eye. Press down lightly.

19. Carry out ending procedure actions.

Note: Some professionals advise their patients to remove the eye only occasionally, because removing the eye increases the potential for infection. Many people reinsert the prosthesis immediately after cleaning because the socket contracts slightly when the eye is removed. After several hours, insertion becomes more difficult. The person may complain of discomfort when the eye is reinserted. Lack of natural lubrication causes the discomfort. It may take up to several days for the eye to feel comfortable again. Until then, the person may use artificial tears to lubricate the eye. Ask the patient or family caregiver if you have questions about the prosthesis.

WARM AND COOL EYE COMPRESSES

Many elderly patients have dry, itchy eyes. The patient may complain of burning, itching, and excess mucus production. The eyes may appear red, with swollen eyelids. If patient rubs or scratches the eyes, they may become infected. Observe the patient for:

• Redness or drainage
• Scaly, flaky skin or crusts around the eyes
• Edema of the eyelids

Report your observations to the nurse. You may be instructed to apply warm or cool soaks to the eyelids. Apply the principles of standard precautions during this procedure. If an infection is suspected, use separate gloves and equipment for each eye.

PROCEDURE

APPLYING WARM OR COOL EYE COMPRESSES

1. Carry out initial procedure actions.

2. Assemble equipment:
   • Disposable exam gloves
   • Towel
   • Small bottle of sterile saline
   • Small sterile basin
   • Sterile gauze pads
   • Ice, if cool compresses are ordered
   • Plastic bag for used items

3. Position the patient for comfort. The Fowler's or high Fowler's position helps reduce edema. Cover the neck and shoulders with a bath towel.

continues

PROCEDURE **93** CONTINUED

4. Heat the saline under hot water, or soak in a bowl of hot water. The solution should be comfortably warm, not hot. Check the temperature to be sure it is approximately 105°F.

 Note: Never use a microwave oven to heat water for heat treatments.

If cool compresses are ordered, cool the bottle of saline by packing it in ice.

5. Pour the warm or cool solution into the small, sterile basin.

6. Wash your hands, or use alcohol-based cleaner.

7. Apply disposable gloves.

8. Place the gauze pads into the bowl.

9. Remove a gauze pad from the bowl, squeezing out the excess solution.

10. Instruct the patient to close the eyes.

11. Apply one compress to the affected eye (Figure 38-6).

12. Remove a second gauze pad from the bowl, squeezing out the excess solution.

13. Apply the second compress on top of the first.

14. Repeat with the other eye, as directed.

15. If the patient complains that the compress is too hot or cold, remove it immediately.

16. Change the compresses every few minutes for the prescribed length of time. The treatment should not last longer than 15 to 20 minutes. Check the skin under the compress each time you change it.

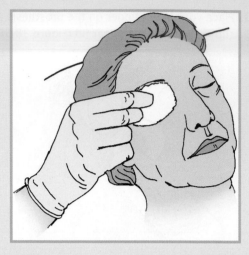

FIGURE 38-6 Instruct the patient to close her eyes. Apply one compress to the affected eye. Follow with a second compress. (© Delmar/Cengage Learning)

17. You may be directed to cover the compress with an ice pack or warm pack. Make a small ice pack by placing ice chips in a sandwich bag or disposable glove. Squeeze the air out of the bag and tie the end. Cover the compress with the pack. Remove it immediately if the patient complains of pain.

18. After 15 to 20 minutes, or as directed, remove the compresses. Discard them in the plastic bag.

19. Use clean gauze pads to gently pat the eye dry. Pat from the inner corner to the outer corner. Use each gauze pad once, then discard in the bag.

20. Carry out ending procedure actions.

COMMON CONDITIONS OF THE EAR

Otitis Media

Otitis media is an infection of the middle ear. Infections of the nose and throat can move along the eustachian tube to the middle ear, causing inflammation. Fluid and pus form within the middle ear, which causes fusion (locking) of the middle ear bones. Increased pressure may cause the eardrum to rupture. This condition is rare in adults, but common in children.

Ménière's Disease

Ménière's disease is a disorder resulting from fluid buildup in the inner ear. It can affect both hearing and balance. It may cause dizziness, vertigo, tinnitus, vomiting, and the sensation of fullness in the ear. Hearing loss may develop in both ears, but one-sided hearing loss is most common.

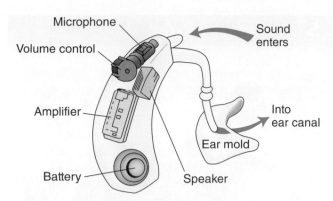

FIGURE 38-7A Parts of a behind-the-ear hearing aid. The ear mold is placed in the ear canal. The rest of the hearing aid is worn outside and over the top of the ear. (© Delmar/Cengage Learning)

Otosclerosis

Otosclerosis is a progressive form of deafness of un known cause. A new, abnormal bone grows in the bony labyrinth, preventing the stapes (one of the small bones)

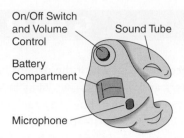

FIGURE 38-7B This hearing aid is worn inside the outer ear canal. (© Delmar/Cengage Learning)

from vibrating properly. Hearing is improved by the use of a hearing aid. Surgery removes the excess bone and replaces it with a prosthesis.

Hearing Impairment

Some people are hard of hearing or completely deaf. They hear less well when tired or ill. A hearing aid (Figures 38-7A and 38-7B) may be helpful. Lip reading or sign language may be used for communication.

GUIDELINES *for*

Communicating with Patients Who Have Hearing Impairments

- Get the patient's attention, and make sure he or she sees you. Touch the patient lightly to indicate that you wish to speak.
- Be sure the patient is wearing his or her hearing aid and that the hearing aid is on.
- If the patient has a "good" ear, stand or sit on that side.
- Do not chew gum, eat, or cover your mouth while talking.
- Face the patient and position your body so your face can be clearly seen (Figure 38-8).
- Reduce outside distractions.
- Start conversations with a key word or phrase to provide clues as to what you are saying.
- Avoid abrupt changes of subject.
- Keep the pitch of your voice low and speak slowly, distinctly, and naturally.
- Form words carefully, use familiar words, and keep sentences short.

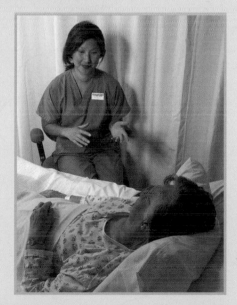

FIGURE 38-8 The light source should be behind the patient so that it lights your face. Make sure the light does not shine directly in the patient's face. (© Delmar/Cengage Learning)

continues

GUIDELINES *continued*

- Pronounce words clearly. If the patient has difficulty with letters and numbers, say: "M as in Mary," "2 as in twins," "B as in boy." Say each number separately: "five six" instead of fifty-six. Remember that *m, n*, and *2, 3, 56, 66*, and *b, c, d, e, t*, and *v* are groups that sound alike.

- Rephrase as needed.

- Avoid shouting, mouthing, exaggerating words, or speaking very slowly.

- Try writing if the patient does not understand.

- Use facial expressions, gestures, and body language to help express your meanings.

- Some patients with hearing impairment use **sign language**.

  - Signing uses hand and finger movements and facial expressions to convey meaning.

  - This skill requires learning and practice (Figure 38-9).

  - There are different forms of sign language, just as there are different spoken languages.

  - There are some basic signs that may be helpful (Figure 38-10).

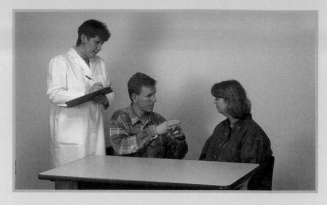

FIGURE 38-9 Learning sign language takes special education and practice with the signs. (© Delmar/ Cengage Learning)

- Some hearing-impaired patients are embarrassed to tell you when they do not understand you.

- Patients who cannot hear may appear confused when they are not.

- Never leave the patient puzzling over what you said and thinking that you do not care. Avoid speaking from another room, while walking away, or with your back turned to the patient.

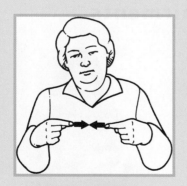

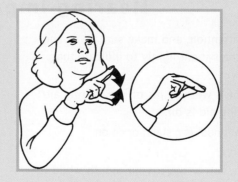

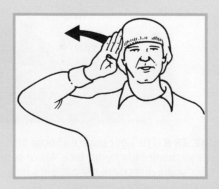

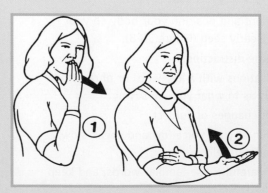

FIGURE 38-10 Basic signs. (© Delmar/Cengage Learning)

GUIDELINES *for*
Caring for a Hearing Aid

- Store hearing aids at room temperature when not being worn. Temperature extremes can damage hearing aids. Their use should be limited in very cold weather.
- Keep hearing aids dry. If an aid accidentally becomes wet, ask the nurse how to dry it. Do not use a hair dryer near the aid. The noise is annoying and the heat will damage the aid.
- Store extra batteries in a cool, dry place. Remove the batteries from the hearing aid at night or open the battery compartment to allow trapped moisture to evaporate.
- Keep hearing aids safe. They break easily if dropped on a hard surface.
- Check bed linen carefully before placing it in the soiled linen hamper. A hearing aid is small, expensive, and easily lost. It will not survive a trip through the washer and dryer!
- Remove the hearing aid when hair spray is being used.

- Turn the hearing aid off before removing it and when it is not in use.
- Wipe in-the-ear aids daily with a dry tissue.
- Be sure the opening of the aid or ear mold is free of wax. In-the-ear types come with a cleaning tool. Use this only if you have been instructed how to use it. Never use a toothpick, paper clip, or other sharp object to clean the hearing aid.
- Insert the hearing aid properly. The shape of the ear may change and the aid may have to be refitted. If the patient complains of pain or the aid is difficult to insert, inform the nurse.
- Shave the patient with an electric razor *before* inserting the hearing aid, or remove it before using the razor. The hearing aid amplifies the noise, making it loud and annoying.

You will find information for troubleshooting hearing aid problems in the Online Companion to this book.

CARING FOR HEARING AIDS

A hearing aid is a delicate and expensive prosthesis that requires safe handling and regular care.

SMELL AND TASTE

A delicious meal or pleasant aroma promotes good social interaction and enjoyment of life. You may have heard the expression, "You eat with your eyes." This means that you are much more likely to select food that is attractive in appearance, because it looks good to you. Your senses of smell and taste are closely related: Most tastes originate with odors, so smell is also closely associated with your appetite. In fact, up to 75% of taste is associated with smell. The sense of smell begins in the nerve receptors high in the nose. Both taste and smell affect the appetite and food likes or dislikes. They also affect overall safety and food enjoyment. Most people can identify hazards, such as natural gas and other noxious gases, spoiled food or beverages, and smoke by using the senses of taste and smell.

Clinical Information ALERT

The human infant can distinguish his or her mother's smell from the scent of other humans. However, adult humans have about 5 million scent receptors in the nose. If your nose is at its best, you can distinguish somewhere between 4,000–10,000 smells. However, humans use only seven primary odors. These are camphoric (mothball smell), musk (perfume smell), rose, peppermint, etheral (dry cleaning fluid smell), pungent (vinegar smell), and putrid (rotten egg smell). ■

AGING CHANGES RELATED TO SMELL AND TASTE

You learned about the papillae (taste buds) on the tongue in Unit 5. Of the five senses, the sense of taste is the weakest. Adults have approximately 9,000 taste buds on the tongue that identify sensations of sweet, salt, bitter, sour, and umami. Other tastes (such as fat) are strong contenders for taste bud recognition, but none have been officially identified and accepted.

Humans also have a total of about 1,000 taste buds on the roof of the mouth and cheeks. Each individual taste bud contains between 10 and 100 taste receptors that send messages to the brain for taste interpretation. Taste buds begin to decrease in number, and lose sensitivity and mass, at about age 40 to 50 in women and age 50 to 60 in men. However, the five distinct taste sensations do not seem to diminish until after age 60, if at all. The cause of aging changes may be hard to identify, because a lifetime of smoking, exposure to environmental pollutants, and some diseases also affect smell and taste. Other changes are:

- Reduced saliva production, which makes swallowing more difficult and digestion less efficient, and may increase dental problems.
- Diminished sense of smell; this usually occurs because of the loss of nerve endings in the nose after age 70.
- Loss of appetite and reduced interest and pleasure in eating as a result of changes to smell and taste. This may lead to weight loss.
- Lack of awareness of unpleasant odors (such as poor personal hygiene), dangerous odors, and odors suggesting pollutants or toxins.
- Loss of enjoyment related to activities and the environment (such as the smell of flowers or freshly cut grass) because of diminished sense of smell.

Observations to make and report related to sensory organs are listed in Table 38-1.

Review the information in Unit 10 about the effects of noise. Review the information in Units 5, 27, and 36 for additional information about sensations of the nose and mouth, and Units 35 and 37 related to other sensory nerves.

SENSE OF TOUCH

The most sensitive areas of the human body are the hands, lips, face, neck, tongue, fingertips, and feet. The least sensitive part of your body is the middle of your back. Each hand contains approximately 17,000 tactile (touch) receptors. Each fingertip contains approximately 100 touch receptors. These receptors send messages to the brain through the spinal cord. The brain interprets the message and causes you to react. Humans have more pain nerve endings than any other type. The pain receptors are also the most important for safety and protection.

TABLE 38-1 OBSERVATIONS TO MAKE AND REPORT RELATED TO SENSORY ORGANS

- Loss of balance or coordination
- Patient withdraws when an area of the body is touched
- Complaints that a body area is painful, burning, numb, tingling, or sensation is absent
- Change in pupil size; unequal pupils
- Abnormal color of sclera (yellow, red)
- Complaints of pain, pressure, or burning in eyes or ears
- Complaints of pain or pressure in ears
- Drainage from eyes or ears
- Ability to hear on one side, but not the other
- Eyelid, corner of the mouth drooping on one side
- Impaired vision
- Frequently rubbing the eyes
- Presence of foreign body in eyes or ears
- Dizziness upon sudden movement of head
- Complaints of ringing in ears
- Complaints of spots or "lightning" in front of eyes
- Eyes appear swollen or inflamed
- Edema around the eye area
- Excessive tear production
- Eyes deviate toward one side
- Eating food on one side of meal tray, but not the other
- Applying excessive condiments (such as salt or sugar) to food
- Dry mucous membranes in mouth
- Difficulty swallowing due to dry mouth and throat
- Mouth breathing
- Dry area between the patient's gums and cheeks (indicates dehydration; this area usually stays moist in mouth breathers)
- Furrows or lines in tongue
- Swollen tongue

About 20 different types of nerve endings send messages to the brain. Of these, the most common are heat, cold, pain, and pressure (touch) receptors. Other common sensations are hard, soft, wet, dry, hot, cold, rough, and smooth. People develop variations of these sensations, such as feelings of warmth, coolness, feeling something that is mushy, or something bumpy. These sensations are very important to your work as a nursing assistant and making observations. Various diseases and injuries can impair the patient's sense of touch, so he or she may interpret various signals differently than you do. Using your sense of touch is essential to reporting both normal and abnormal patient observations.

REVIEW

A. Multiple Choice

Select the one best answer for each of the following.

1. Glaucoma is
   a. a clouding of the lens of the eye.
   b. caused by chemical exposure.
   c. related to retinal degeneration.
   d. caused by very high pressure in the eye.

2. When caring for a person with glaucoma, the nursing assistant should
   a. apply patches to the patient's eyes at bedtime.
   b. perform tasks that would strain or exert the patient.
   c. apply eye drops to the affected eye.
   d. apply cool eye compresses every 2 hours.

3. Cataracts
   a. are a clouding of the lens of the eye.
   b. are caused by increased pressure.
   c. occur when a tear duct is blocked.
   d. must be treated with warm compresses.

4. When caring for an artificial eye, you should
   a. wrap the eye in tissue and store in the drawer.
   b. soak the eye in alcohol after removal.
   c. insert the eye when it is moist.
   d. wash the eye with soap and water.

5. Patients with visual impairment should
   a. stay in their rooms to avoid getting lost.
   b. have identification on their clothing.
   c. learn to use sign language.
   d. be oriented to the environment.

6. When working with a patient who has a hearing impairment, you should
   a. get the patient's attention before speaking.
   b. talk loudly in the patient's good ear.
   c. avoid speaking if possible.
   d. speak very slowly in a high-pitched voice.

7. Aging changes related to saliva production
   a. enhance digestion.
   b. may make swallowing difficult.
   c. protect the tooth enamel.
   d. increase sinus drainage.

8. A condition that results from fluid buildup in the inner ear and affects hearing and balance is
   a. Ménière's disease.
   b. otosclerosis.
   c. macular degeneration.
   d. otitis media.

9. Otitis media involves the
   a. outer ear.
   b. external canal.
   c. middle ear.
   d. inner ear.

10. Otosclerosis is a
    a. common vision impairment.
    b. complication of glaucoma.
    c. type of cancer of the eye.
    d. progressive hearing loss.

B. Nursing Assistant Challenge

You are assigned to care for Dr. Petrick, a professor from the local college who has had an artificial eye for many years. Dr. Petrick is right handed, and just returned from surgery where he had a complex procedure to repair injuries to the right hand. The hand is wrapped with the fingertips exposed. The artificial eye is in a cup of solution in the bedside stand. Answer the following questions related to his care.

11. From this information, you know that Dr. Petrick has an artificial eye. What is the best way to find out who will care for the eye?

12. Should you reinsert the artificial eye as soon as Dr. Petrick returns to the unit?

13. Are gloves necessary when caring for the eye socket?

14. The notched surface of the artificial eye should face the
    a. outside.
    b. inside.
    c. ceiling.
    d. floor.

UNIT 39

Caring for Patients with Disorders of the Endocrine and Reproductive Systems

OBJECTIVES

After completing this unit, you will be able to:

- Spell and define terms.
- Identify aging changes of the endocrine and reproductive systems.
- Recognize the signs and symptoms of hypoglycemia and hyperglycemia.

- Describe nursing assistant actions and observations related to the care of patients with disorders of the endocrine and reproductive systems.
- Perform the following procedures:
  - Procedure 94 Obtaining a Fingerstick Blood Sugar
  - Procedure 95 Giving a Nonsterile Vaginal Douche

VOCABULARY

Learn the meaning and the correct spelling of the following words and phrases:

acetone
Addison's disease
benign prostatic
  hypertrophy (BPH)
brachytherapy
chancre
Cushing's syndrome
diabetes mellitus
douche
fingerstick blood sugar
  (FSBS)

glucose
gonorrhea
herpes simplex II
hyperglycemia
hypersecretion
hyperthyroidism
hypertrophies
hypoglycemia
hyposecretion
hypothyroidism

insulin
insulin-dependent
  diabetes mellitus
  (IDDM)
lancet
metabolism rate
non–insulin-dependent
  diabetes mellitus
  (NIDDM)

prolapsed uterus
prostatectomy
sexually transmitted
  disease (STD)
simple goiter
syphilis
tetany

INTRODUCTION TO THE ENDOCRINE SYSTEM

The nervous system uses electrical messages to control the body. The endocrine system uses chemicals to coordinate, regulate, and control body functions. The endocrine glands send hormones into the bloodstream. From there, they travel throughout the body, causing various activities and changes. The hormones are responsible for helping you feel hunger, thirst, and the need to sleep. Hormones are responsible for growth and development, reproduction, and stress responses. They play an important role in regulating fluid and energy balance in the body.

AGING CHANGES TO THE ENDOCRINE SYSTEM

Changes occur in the way that hormones control body systems. Some tissues become less sensitive to their controlling hormone. The total amount of hormone production may change, but this is highly variable. Blood levels of

Clinical Information ALERT

Laughing lowers the level of stress hormones in the body and strengthens the immune system. In addition, people who laugh a great deal often experience a sense of well-being. Six-year-olds laugh an average of 300 times a day. Adults usually laugh 15 to 100 times a day. ■

some hormones increase, some decrease, and some will be unchanged. Hormones are also broken down more slowly. Aging changes to the endocrine system include:

- Increased blood sugar level caused by delayed release of insulin, a hormone that regulates sugar use in the body
- Lower **metabolism rate**, or slower body function, which reduces the amount of calories needed for the body to function normally

COMMON CONDITIONS OF THE ENDOCRINE SYSTEM

Thyroid Gland Conditions

The thyroid gland may secrete too much or not enough hormones. Either situation is treatable. If not treated, severe illness or death will occur.

Hyperthyroidism Hyperthyroidism, or overactivity of the thyroid gland, results in production of too much thyroxine (**hypersecretion**). The person shows:

- Irritability and restlessness
- Nervousness
- Rapid pulse
- Increased appetite
- Weight loss
- Sensitivity

When caring for these patients, the nursing assistant must be understanding and have patience. Keep the room quiet and cool. This patient will burn extra calories due to increased activity, and is at risk for weight loss and nutritional problems. Meet the patient's increased nutritional needs with foods that the patient likes.

Thyroidectomy It may be necessary to treat hyperthyroidism with surgery. You may be assigned to assist in the postoperative care. Following surgery:

- The patient is placed in a semi-Fowler's position, with neck and shoulders well supported. Remember at all times to support the back of the neck. Hyperextension of the neck may damage the operative site.
- Assist with oxygen, if ordered, using all oxygen precautions.
- Give routine postoperative care.

- Check for and report the following:
  - Any signs of bleeding (this may drain toward the back of the neck). Also check the pillows behind the patient, as well as the dressings.
  - Signs of respiratory distress.
  - Inability of the patient to speak. Initial hoarseness is common, but report any increase.
  - Greatly elevated temperature and pulse, pronounced apprehension, or irritability.
  - Numbness, tingling, or muscular spasm (**tetany**) of the extremities.

Hypothyroidism Hypothyroidism results in an undersecretion of the hormone thyroxine. Recall that iodine is an essential component of thyroxine. A lack of iodine in the diet can result in low thyroxine production.

- The condition is called **simple goiter**.
- The thyroid gland enlarges (**hypertrophies**).
- Secretions produced have low thyroxine content.

Hypothyroidism can usually be successfully managed with thyroxine replacement. Table 39-1 compares signs and symptoms of hyperthyroidism and hypothyroidism.

TABLE 39-1 HYPERTHYROIDISM AND HYPOTHYROIDISM COMPARED

Hyperthyroidism	Hypothyroidism
Increased appetite	Decreased appetite; loss of appetite
Intolerance to heat	Intolerance to cold
Elevated body temperature	Low body temperature
Weight loss despite increased appetite	Weight gain despite loss of appetite
Tachycardia	Bradycardia
Moderate hypertension	Hypotension
Nervousness; insomnia	Lethargy, sleepiness
Flushed, warm, moist skin	Pale, cool, dry skin
Anxiety	Face appears puffy
Tremors	Hair coarse
Irregular or scant menses	Heavy menses
	May be unable to conceive
	Loss of fetus possible

Adrenal Gland Conditions

Adrenal gland secretions regulate:

- Development and maintenance of sexual characteristics
- Carbohydrate, fat, and protein metabolism
- Fluid balance
- Electrolyte levels of sodium and potassium

Hypersecretion results in **Cushing's syndrome**, which is characterized by:

- Weakness due to loss of body protein
- Increased blood sugar levels (hyperglycemia)
- Edema
- Hypertension
- Loss of potassium and retention of sodium
- Masculinization of a female

Therapy is primarily surgical and supportive.

Hyposecretion results in **Addison's disease**, which is characterized by:

- Loss of sodium and retention of potassium
- Abnormally low blood sugar (hypoglycemia)

- Dehydration
- Low stress tolerance

Addison's disease is treated by hormone replacement therapy and techniques to combat dehydration.

Observations to make and report for patients with disorders of the endocrine system are listed in Table 39-2.

Diabetes Mellitus

In the United States, 20.8 million people (7% of the population) had diabetes by 2005. Diabetes occurs in people of all ages and races. The incidence increases with age.

Diabetes mellitus is a chronic disease that results from a deficiency of the hormone **insulin** or a resistance to the effects of insulin. This causes the body to be unable to properly process food into energy. The glucose from the food remains in the blood, resulting in elevated blood sugar. Persistent, elevated blood glucose affects the whole body.

The reason why diabetes develops is not fully understood. Factors that are related to development of diabetes are heredity, obesity, age, diet, and lack of exercise.

TABLE 39-2 OBSERVATIONS TO MAKE AND REPORT ON PATIENTS WITH DISORDERS OF THE ENDOCRINE SYSTEM

- Complaints of feeling very warm or cold, heat or cold intolerance
- Difficulty swallowing
- Insomnia
- Easy excitability, hyperactivity
- Palpitations
- Chest pain
- Flank pain
- Tingling in the arms and legs
- Respiratory difficulty
- Muscle contractions, spasms, spasticity
- Convulsions
- Complaints of gastrointestinal distress
- Nausea and vomiting
- Abdominal cramps
- Diarrhea
- Muscle weakness
- Decreased stress tolerance
- Variation from previous weight (+/−)
- Decreasing urine output
- Imbalance between intake and output
- Fluid retention, with or without swelling
- Edema
- Excessive perspiration
- Craving salt
- Consuming more fluid than usual
- Loss of appetite
- Dark pigmentation of skin or mucous membranes
- Decreased hair growth anywhere on body, hair loss
- Any abnormal vital signs

- Dizziness
- Metallic taste in mouth
- Hunger
- Headache
- Sweating
- Weakness
- Nervousness
- Lethargy
- Fatigue
- Brittle nails
- Depression
- Trembling or shaking
- Unusual clumsiness
- Emotional instability
- Confusion
- Disorientation
- Loss of consciousness
- Visual disturbances, visual changes (such as blurred or double vision)
- Bulging/protruding eyes
- Neck swelling
- Skin excessively oily or dry
- Skin breaks that heal poorly
- Loss of motor function
- Decreased sensitivity to pain or touch in the extremities
- Change in mental and emotional status and demeanor (e.g., dull, apathetic, extremely nervous)
- Change in ability to process information and respond to questions

Clinical Information ALERT

Almost 1 in 20 people worldwide are diabetic. Before developing type 2 diabetes, most people develop a condition called *prediabetes*, in which the blood glucose is elevated, but not high enough to be called diabetes. Damage to the body may occur in this stage. The person may be able to delay or prevent diabetes through diet and exercise. ∎

Disease mechanism In diabetes, the metabolism of fats, carbohydrates, and proteins is unbalanced. Normally, the blood sugar rises when carbohydrates enter the bloodstream. The pancreas responds to an increase in **glucose** by secreting more insulin to reduce the blood sugar. In diabetes, glucose cannot be properly utilized for energy, either because the pancreas does not make enough insulin or because the person's system does not respond properly to the insulin (*insulin resistance*).

Types of diabetes mellitus Diabetes mellitus is typed and named according to the need for insulin. Examples are **insulin-dependent diabetes mellitus (IDDM)** (type 1) and **non–insulin-dependent diabetes (NIDDM)** (type 2). IDDM is more common in children and young adults. NIDDM occurs most often when the body does not properly use insulin. This is the most common form of diabetes. NIDDM is much more stable than IDDM.

Care of the patient with diabetes The goal of care of the patient with diabetes is maintaining a normal blood glucose. This may require lifestyle changes. People with diabetes who are willing to manage the condition can live happily and productively (Figure 39-1).

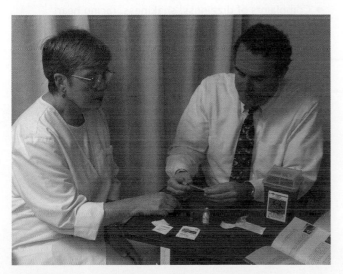

FIGURE 39-1 Patients are taught to manage their diabetes by the nurse. (© *Delmar/Cengage Learning*)

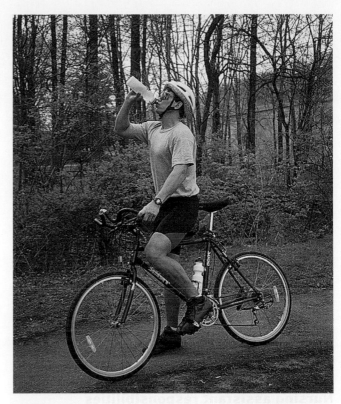

FIGURE 39-2 Exercise and sufficient water intake are important factors in maintaining good health. (© *Delmar/Cengage Learning*)

Diet is an important part of diabetic treatment. Weight reduction is favored, and this alone may be sufficient to bring the condition under control in NIDDM.

Exercise (Figure 39-2) is an important part of the overall treatment. The amount and type of exercise the patient routinely engages in are balanced by the food intake and insulin or hypoglycemic drug requirements.

Hypoglycemia (low blood sugar) Hypoglycemia occurs when the blood glucose level is below normal. It is also called *insulin reaction* or *insulin shock*. Common causes are too much insulin or oral medication, skipping meals, excessive activity, medication problems, vomiting, and diarrhea. The signs and symptoms of hypoglycemia include:

- Complaints of hunger, weakness, dizziness, shakiness
- Skin cold, moist, clammy, pale
- Rapid, shallow respirations
- Nervousness and excitement
- Rapid pulse
- Unconsciousness
- Low blood sugar test results and no sugar in the urine

If the patient is awake and alert, treatment includes intake of orange juice or an easily absorbed carbohydrate. If the patient is unconscious, the nurse may give medication to increase the blood sugar. A glucose paste that can be administered by absorption from the mucous membranes of the mouth is also available.

Hyperglycemia (high blood sugar) Hyperglycemia (diabetic coma):

- Occurs when there is insufficient insulin for metabolic needs
- Develops slowly, usually over a 24-hour period
- May be seen as confusion, drowsiness, or a slow slippage into coma

Hyperglycemia may be brought on by illness such as dehydration, infection, forgotten medication, and intake of too much food. The signs and symptoms of diabetic coma include:

- Early headache, drowsiness, or confusion
- Sweet, fruity odor to the breath
- Deep breathing, labored respirations
- Full, bounding pulse
- Low blood pressure
- Nausea or vomiting
- Flushed, dry, hot skin
- Weakness
- Unconsciousness
- High blood sugar test results and sugar in the urine

Nursing assistant responsibilities

- Know the signs of insulin shock and diabetic coma.
- Be alert for the signs of high or low blood sugar and notify the nurse.
- Know the location of orange juice or other carbohydrates.
- Check the patient's meal tray to be sure the foods are permitted on the diet.

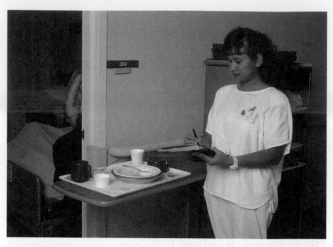

FIGURE 39-3 The amount and type of food consumed by diabetic patients is closely observed and recorded. (© Delmar/Cengage Learning)

- Document food consumption, and report uneaten meals (Figure 39-3).
- Give special attention to care of the diabetic patient's feet. Wash daily, carefully drying between toes. Do not allow moisture to collect between toes. Do not cut the toenails of a patient with diabetes. Do not allow the patient to go barefoot. Be sure shoes and socks fit well and are not too tight.
- Test the blood sugar as ordered and report abnormal values.

Observations of diabetic patients to report to the nurse are listed in Table 39-3.

TABLE 39-3 IMPORTANT OBSERVATIONS OF DIABETIC PATIENTS

- Loss of consciousness or change in mental status
- Inadequate food intake
- Eating food not allowed on diet
- Refusal of meals, supplements, or snacks
- Nausea, vomiting, or diarrhea

- Inadequate fluid intake
- Excessive activity
- Complaints of dizziness, shakiness, racing heart
- Blood sugar values outside of normal range

Signs and Symptoms of Hyperglycemia	Signs and Symptoms of Hypoglycemia
• Nausea, vomiting • Weakness • Headache • Full, bounding pulse • Fruity smell to breath • Hot, dry, flushed skin • Labored respirations • Drowsiness • Mental confusion • Unconsciousness • Sugar in the urine • High blood sugar by fingerstick test	• Complaints of hunger, weakness, dizziness, shakiness • Feeling faint or lightheaded • Skin cold, moist, clammy, pale • Rapid, shallow respirations • Nervousness and excitement • Rapid pulse • Unconsciousness • No sugar in the urine • Low blood sugar by fingerstick test

Blood Glucose Monitoring

The physician will order specific times for blood sugar testing. The nurse administers insulin based on the blood sugar value. Always report the value to the nurse, and document your findings. If the patient is suspected of having complications, the nurse may request a stat blood sugar. This test must be performed immediately.

Fingerstick blood sugar Fingerstick blood sugar (FSBS) testing is done by collecting a sample of capillary blood with a **lancet**, or tiny needle. The blood is transferred to a test strip. If the instructions call for a drop of blood on the reagent pad, avoid smearing the strip against the finger. Some strips can be read visually, by comparing the color on the reagent strip with the key on the bottle (Figure 39-4).

Many newer meters do not use reagent strips. After making the fingerstick, a drop of blood is drawn into a tiny tube, which is inserted into the meter before beginning. An audible beep informs you when the tube has collected enough blood.

Many different blood glucose meters are available. All are accurate and simple to use. Each meter has its own reagent

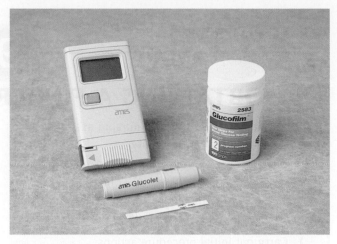

FIGURE 39-5 The reagent strips must be compatible with the glucose meter. (© Delmar/Cengage Learning)

or test strip. For accuracy, make sure the strip is compatible with the meter you are using (Figure 39-5). Do not use strips beyond the expiration date. Follow the directions for the meter and strips you are using.

The normal blood sugar values vary with the health care facility. The normal fasting range is usually between 65 and 120, with the normal value being 70 to 110. Values below 70 suggest hypoglycemia. Fasting values above 110 suggest elevated blood sugar. If the patient is not fasting when the sample is obtained, the value should be 150 or less, if the diabetes is in good control. If the meter displays the word *low* or *high*, the value is below or above the capacity of the meter, which has a wide range. This is a potentially serious problem. Notify the nurse if blood sugar values are outside of the normal range.

Acetone Monitoring

You may be expected to test the patient's urine for acetone. **Acetone** is a substance that accumulates in the body when the blood glucose is out of balance. A simple urine test detects the presence of acetone.

Infection Control ALERT

Several episodes of hepatitis B infection developed as a result of use of a shared glucose meter in a long-term care facility. Other diseases may also be spread in this manner. Bloodborne pathogens are stable on environmental surfaces at room temperature. They are easily passed if improper techniques are used. Disinfect the shared glucose meter and spring-loaded lancet holders after each use. Discard used lancets in the sharps container. ■

Difficult SITUATIONS

Ketone bodies are created when body fat is burned for fuel. The ketone bodies cause a chemical imbalance, upsetting the patient's buffer system. If the blood sugar is over 250 mg/dL, the nurse may request a urine check for ketones. If the patient is very ill, the nurse may request a ketone test even if the blood sugar is not high. ■

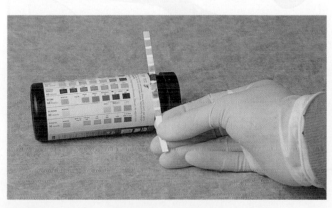

FIGURE 39-4 Multistix are used for many different blood tests. (© Delmar/Cengage Learning)

PROCEDURE

94

OBTAINING A FINGERSTICK BLOOD SUGAR

 Note: Be sure this is a nursing assistant procedure in your facility.

Note: This procedure is generic and applies the principles used for most blood glucose meters. Follow the directions for the meter and strip you are using.

1. Carry out initial procedure actions.

2. Assemble equipment:
   - Disposable exam gloves
   - Alcohol sponge
   - Lancet
   - Blood glucose meter
   - Reagent strip or test strip for the blood glucose meter being used
   - Sharps container
   - Plastic bandage strip
   - Plastic bag for used supplies

3. Wipe the patient's finger with the alcohol sponge. Allow the alcohol to dry.

4. Pierce the side of the middle or ring finger using the lancet (Figure 39-6A).

5. Discard the lancet in the sharps container.

6. Squeeze the sides of the finger gently to obtain a drop of blood.

7. Hold the puncture site directly over the reagent strip, and place a hanging drop of blood onto the reagent pad. If using capillary tube (straw-like) strips, peel the package back to open it. Hold the package firmly with your thumb and forefinger over the test end (patient end) of the strip. Insert the strip into the meter (Figure 39-6B). Remove and discard the package. Hold the strip next to the puncture site to draw blood into the straw (Figure 39-6C).

8. Insert the strip into the meter, if this was not done previously.

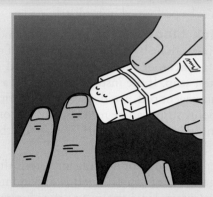

FIGURE 39-6A Pierce the side of the finger with the lancet. (© Delmar/Cengage Learning)

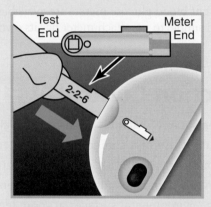

FIGURE 39-6B Insert the strip in the meter. (© Delmar/Cengage Learning)

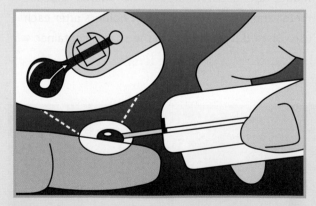

FIGURE 39-6C This strip is like a straw that will draw blood into the base. (© Delmar/Cengage Learning)

PROCEDURE 94 CONTINUED

9. Wipe the patient's finger with the alcohol sponge and allow it to dry. Apply pressure until bleeding stops. Apply a bandage strip, if necessary.

10. When the meter makes an audible beep, the blood sugar value is displayed on the screen (Figure 39-6D). Inform the nurse and document the value.

11. Carry out ending procedure actions.

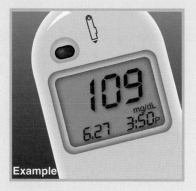

FIGURE 39-6D Read the meter after the designated period of time. (© Delmar/Cengage Learning)

INTRODUCTION TO THE REPRODUCTIVE SYSTEM

The functions of the reproductive system are gender-specific. This system works closely with the endocrine system through the use of hormones to control body function and secondary sex characteristics.

AGING CHANGES IN THE REPRODUCTIVE SYSTEM

The following changes occur with age in the male reproductive system:
- Hormone production decreases, causing decreased size of testes and a lower sperm count.
- More time is needed for an erection to occur.
- The prostate gland may enlarge, causing urinary problems.
- The risk of prostate cancer increases.

The following changes occur with age in the female reproductive system:
- Menstrual periods stop.
- Fewer female hormones are produced, resulting in uncomfortable symptoms and loss of ability to conceive a child.
- The vagina becomes shorter and narrower.
- Vaginal secretions decrease.
- Breast tissue decreases and the muscles supporting the breasts weaken.
- The risk of breast cancer increases.

CONDITIONS OF THE MALE REPRODUCTIVE ORGANS

The male organs are subject to the same kinds of diseases that affect other body parts. A common problem experienced by many men involves the prostate gland.

Prostate Conditions

Benign prostatic **hypertrophy (BPH)** or *hyperplasia* (*prostatic* means "of the prostate gland") (Figure 39-7)

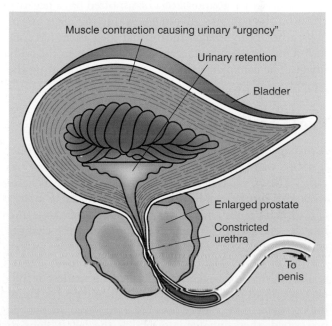

FIGURE 39-7 Cell growth causes the prostate to enlarge, constricting the urethra. The bladder may not empty completely, causing discomfort and increasing the risk of infection. (© Delmar/Cengage Learning)

is an enlargement of the prostate gland. This growth compresses and narrows the urethra, causing urinary retention. Signs and symptoms include difficulty starting the stream of urine or inability to empty the bladder completely.

Prostate cancer is the second leading cause of cancer deaths in males. Prostate cancer usually grows slowly. In the early stages, there may be no symptoms. If identified early, the outcome is usually positive.

Various surgical approaches are used to remove all or part of the prostate gland (**prostatectomy**) to relieve urinary retention. **Brachytherapy** is a form of radiation therapy in which tiny radioactive seeds are implanted inside the prostate gland. This treatment for prostate cancer is very successful and preferred over traditional radiation therapy because it has fewer side effects.

CONDITIONS OF THE FEMALE REPRODUCTIVE ORGANS

Like the male organs, female reproductive organs are subject to disease processes, including tumors and infections.

Tumors of the Breast

Tumors, both benign and malignant, are commonly found in the breasts. Breast cancer is the second most common cancer in women. However, men can also develop breast cancer. The usual treatment is to remove the cancerous area (only), or part or all of the breast and lymph nodes under the arm. Radiation and chemotherapy are also used. Removal of a breast often has a negative effect on the patient's self-image. A nursing diagnosis of "Disturbed Body Image" means that the patient has confusion and problems concerning the changes in the body image. The care plan will list methods of supporting the patient.

Prolapsed Uterus

A **prolapsed uterus** may also be called a *pelvic floor hernia*. It occurs when the uterus slips downward into the vaginal canal. The uterus is held in place by ligaments, which are weakened during childbirth, especially with large infants and difficult labor and delivery. Loss of muscle tone and muscle relaxation, combined with normal aging changes and a reduction of estrogen, are the most common cause of uterine prolapse. Signs and symptoms are pain during sexual activity, low backache, a feeling of heaviness or fullness, feeling as if sitting on a tennis ball, and protrusion of the uterus from the vaginal opening. Kegel exercises may be prescribed; these involve contracting the pelvic floor to strengthen the muscles surrounding the urethra and vagina that support the pelvic structures. Surgery may be necessary in some cases.

SEXUALLY TRANSMITTED DISEASES

Sexually transmitted diseases (STDs) affect both men and women. STDs can be transmitted from contact with mucous membranes, blood, and body fluids (Unit 13). Using standard precautions correctly (Unit 13) will protect the nursing assistant and the patients. Common STDs are HIV and AIDS (Unit 12), gonorrhea, herpes simplex II, and syphilis. Signs and symptoms of sexually transmitted diseases to make and report are listed in Table 39-4.

Gonorrhea

Gonorrhea is caused by a bacterium. Males will have greenish-yellow discharge from the penis within two to five days after contact. Burning upon urination is common. Females may have no signs or symptoms for a long time after infection. Because of this, a woman may spread the disease before she is aware that she is infected.

Syphilis

Syphilis is caused by the *Treponema pallidum* bacterium. The disease affects men and women in the same ways. This infection is treated with antibiotics. If untreated, this disease passes through three stages.

1. First stage—a sore (**chancre**) (Figure 39-8A) develops within 90 days of exposure. The chancre heals without treatment. Because it is not painful, it may go entirely unnoticed.

2. Second stage—may be accompanied by a rash, sore throat, or other mild symptoms suggestive of a viral infection (Figure 39-8B). Again, the signs and symptoms

TABLE 39-4 SIGNS AND SYMPTOMS OF SEXUALLY TRANSMITTED DISEASES TO MAKE AND REPORT

- Vaginal or urethral discharge
- Vaginal pain or burning
- Redness and irritation of genital tissue
- Burning upon urination
- Lower abdominal pain in women
- Testicular pain in men
- Bleeding between menstrual periods
- Painful bowel elimination
- Rectal discharge
- Sore throat
- Skin rash
- Fever
- Painful joints
- Painful lesions on genitalia, throat, or mouth
- Burning or itching of external genitalia
- Warts on genitalia

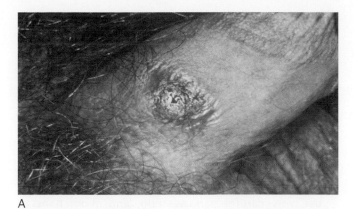

A

FIGURE 39-8A This person contracted an STD through genital to oral contact. *(Courtesy of Centers for Disease Control and Prevention)*

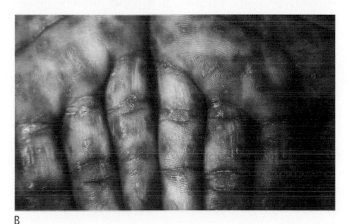

B

FIGURE 39-8B Although less common, lesions on the hands can develop as a result of contact with the genitalia of an infected person. *(Courtesy of Centers for Disease Control and Prevention)*

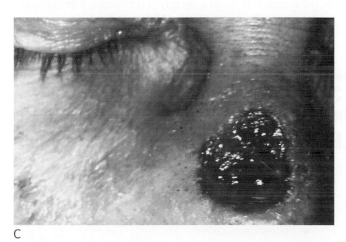

C

FIGURE 39-8C The signs and symptoms of third stage syphilis include loss of coordination, dementia, paralysis, numbness, and gradual blindness. Occasionally, the patient develops a painless, nodular, ulcerative lesion, such as the one pictured. The lesion can occur anywhere on the body. The patient is not contagious in this stage, but the damage is serious enough to cause death. *(Courtesy of Centers for Disease Control and Prevention)*

disappear without treatment. The disease is infectious during the first and second stages and may be transmitted to a sexual partner. By this time, the microorganisms have gained entry into vital organs such as the heart, liver, brain, and spinal cord.

3. Third stage—permanent damage is done to vital organs, though the damage may not become apparent for many years. Patients in this stage are usually cognitively impaired, but there is no way to differentiate cognitive impairment caused by syphilis from impairment due to other causes. Aside from this, the patient usually has no other signs or symptoms, and the diagnosis of tertiary syphylis is usually made after a routine blood test shows an abnormality. Occasionally, the person will develop painless lesions (*gumma*) on various parts of the body (Figure 39-8C). The patient is not infectious in this stage.

You may also wish to review the information in Unit 31 on untreated syphilis.

Herpes

Herpes simplex II (genital herpes) is an infectious disease caused by the herpes simplex virus. It is transmitted primarily through direct sexual contact. The person who has herpes:

- May develop painful, red, blister-like sores on the reproductive organs (Figure 39-9A)

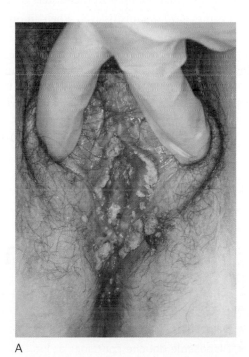

A

FIGURE 39-9A One out of every four women and one out of every five men in the United States have genital herpes. The lesions appear as one or more painful blisters on or around the genitals or rectum. The blisters eventually break, leaving tender ulcers that may take 2 to 4 weeks to heal the first time they appear. Oral herpes can be spread to the genital area just as genital herpes can be spread to the mouth. *(Courtesy of Centers for Disease Control and Prevention)*

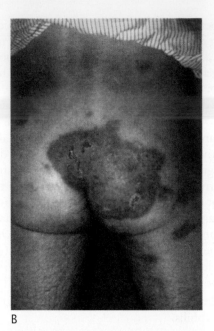

FIGURE 39-9B Chronic herpes in an AIDS patient *(Courtesy of Daniel J. Barbaro, MD, Fort Worth, Texas)*

- Has sores that are associated with a burning sensation
- Usually has sores that heal in about 2 weeks
- Must remember that the fluid in the blisters is infectious
- May transmit (*shed*) organisms even when an outbreak or sore is not present

One in five American adults has genital herpes and may not know it. People with the herpes infection may have only one episode or may have repeated attacks. In many cases, repeated attacks are milder. Individuals who have weakened immune systems often develop chronic cases of herpes (Figure 39-9B). Because herpes is caused by a virus, there is no cure. Oral medications are available to stop the replication of the virus, which makes an outbreak subside more quickly. Topical creams are available to relieve discomfort and reduce the danger of spreading the infection.

VAGINAL DOUCHE

A vaginal **douche** is an irrigation of the vagina with fluid or medication. It is done by physician's order. Use standard precautions when performing this procedure.

PROCEDURE

GIVING A NONSTERILE VAGINAL DOUCHE

1. Carry out initial procedure actions.

2. Assemble equipment:
- Disposable gloves
- Disposable douche container or kit
- Bed protectors
- Toilet tissue
- Bath blanket
- Cotton balls
- Disinfectant
- Cup
- Irrigating standard
- Bedpan and cover
- Plastic bag

3. Pour a small amount of disinfecting solution over the cotton balls in the cup.

PROCEDURE 95 CONTINUED

4. Measure water into the douche container. The water temperature should be about 105°F. Add powder or solution as ordered.

5. Hang the douche bag on the standard. Close the clamp on the tubing. Leave the protector on the sterile tip.

6. Place a bed protector on the chair and assemble equipment where you can reach it. Screen the unit.

7. Elevate the bed to a comfortable working height and put up the side rails on the opposite side of the bed for safety.

8. Wash your hands and put on gloves.

9. Assist the patient into the dorsal recumbent position.

10. Place a bed protector beneath the buttocks.

11. Remove the perineal pad (if used) from front to back and discard it in a plastic bag.

12. Drape the patient with a bath blanket (Figure 39-10). Fanfold top bedding to the foot of the bed.

13. Place a bedpan under the patient and ask her to void. Follow facility policies for emptying the bedpan, if necessary.

14. Cleanse the perineum.

   a. Use one cotton ball with disinfectant for each stroke.

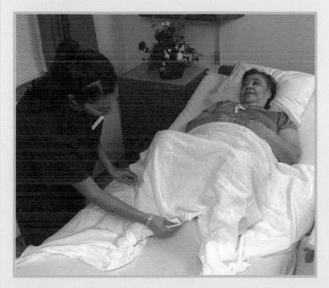

FIGURE 39-10 Drape the patient. (© Delmar/Cengage Learning)

   b. Cleanse from the vulva toward the anus.

   c. Cleanse the labia majora first.

   d. Expose the labia minora with your thumb and forefinger and cleanse.

   e. Give special attention to folds.

   f. Discard used cotton balls in a plastic bag.

15. Replace the bedpan, if necessary. Reposition the patient and readjust the bath blanket. Elevate the head for comfort, if desired.

16. Open the clamp to expel air. Remove the protector from the sterile tip of the disposable douche.

17. Allow a small amount of solution to flow over the inner thigh and then over the vulva. Do not touch the vulva with the nozzle.

18. Allow solution to continue to flow and insert the nozzle slowly and gently into the vagina, with an upward and backward movement, for about 3 inches.

19. Rotate the nozzle from side to side as solution flows.

20. When all solution has been given, remove the nozzle slowly and clamp the tubing.

21. Have the patient sit up on the bedpan to allow all the solution to return.

22. Remove the douche bag from the standard and place it on the bed protector.

23. Dry the perineum with tissue. Discard used tissue in the bedpan.

24. Cover the bedpan and place it on the bed protector on the chair.

25. Have the patient turn on her side. Dry her buttocks with tissue.

26. Place a clean pad over the vulva, if needed. Do not touch the inside of the pad.

27. Remove the bed protector and bath blanket. Replace with top bedding.

28. Note the character and amount of discharge, if any. Discard the contents of the bedpan. Care for equipment. Remove your gloves and discard them properly. Wash your hands.

29. Carry out ending procedure actions.

REVIEW

A. Multiple Choice

Select the one best answer for each of the following.

1. Hypersecretion of the adrenal gland results in
   a. Cushing's disease.
   b. Addison's disease.
   c. elevated blood sugar.
   d. diabetes mellitus.

2. Your patient is an insulin-dependent diabetic. You know that this
   a. is a stable form of the disease.
   b. affects only older persons.
   c. requires oral hypoglycemic drugs.
   d. is a less stable form of the disease.

3. Insulin is an important hormone because it
   a. lowers blood sugar.
   b. raises blood sugar.
   c. stimulates the conversion of glycogen to glucose.
   d. breaks fat down to form glucose.

4. You are to give a nonsterile douche. You will remember to
   a. place the patient in a high Fowler's position.
   b. use a solution with a temperature of about 115°F.
   c. insert the nozzle about 3 inches into the vagina.
   d. rest the nozzle on the side of the vulva.

5. The normal range for fasting blood glucose is
   a. 90 to 170.
   b. 70 to 110.
   c. 30 to 80.
   d. 220 to 400.

6. Brachytherapy is a/an
   a. type of chemotherapy.
   b. implanted medication.
   c. form of radiation.
   d. hormonal implant.

7. Benign prostatic hypertrophy is
   a. a condition that occurs at puberty.
   b. the first sign of cancer.
   c. an enlargement of the prostate.
   d. the second leading cause of death in males.

8. Signs of hypoglycemia include
   a. sweet, fruity odor to the breath.
   b. deep breathing, labored respirations.
   c. flushed, dry, hot skin.
   d. nervousness and excitement.

9. Signs of hyperglycemia include
   a. skin cold, moist, clammy, pale.
   b. full, bounding pulse.
   c. rapid, shallow respirations.
   d. no sugar in urine.

10. When caring for a patient who has an STD, the nursing assistant should
    a. use standard precautions.
    b. avoid touching the patient whenever possible.
    c. practice contact precautions.
    d. wear a gown, gloves, eye shield, and mask.

B. Nursing Assistant Challenge

You are assigned to two patients who both have diabetes. Sally Sakowski is 29 years old and has had diabetes for 10 years. She is considered to be IDDM. Ruth Young is 72 years old and has just been diagnosed with NIDDM. Although these patients both have diabetes, there may be many differences in their signs, symptoms, and problems. Answer the following questions about care of these patients.

11. Of the two types of diabetes, which is the least stable?

12. Ms. Sakowski receives insulin injections. Mrs. Young's diabetes is regulated with an oral medication. Whose blood sugar will be monitored?

13. Hypoglycemia and hyperglycemia may be complications for either patient. List the differences in the signs and symptoms of both complications.

Expanded Role of the Nursing Assistant

UNIT 40
Caring for Obstetrical Patients and Neonates

UNIT 41
Rehabilitation and Restorative Services

UNIT 40

Caring for Obstetrical Patients and Neonates

OBJECTIVES

After completing this unit, you will be able to:
- Spell and define terms.
- Define *doula* and identify the role and responsibilities of the doula as a member of the childbirth team.
- Assist in care of the normal postpartum patient.
- Properly change a perineal pad.
- Recognize reportable observations of patients in the postpartum period.
- Assist in care of the normal newborn.
- Demonstrate three methods of safely holding a baby.
- Describe nursing assistant actions and observations related to the care of the newborn infant.
- List measures to prevent inadvertent switching, misidentification, and abduction of infants.
- Assist in carrying out the discharge procedures for mother and infant.

- Demonstrate the following procedures:
  - Procedure 96   Changing a Diaper
  - Procedure 97   Weighing an Infant
  - Procedure 98   Measuring an Infant
  - Procedure 99   Bathing an Infant
  - Procedure 100 Changing Crib Linens
  - Procedure 101 Changing Crib Linens (Infant in Crib)
  - Procedure 102 Measuring an Infant's Temperature
  - Procedure 103 Determining an Infant's Heart Rate (Pulse)
  - Procedure 104 Counting an Infant's Respiratory Rate
  - Procedure 105 Bottle-Feeding an Infant
  - Procedure 106 Burping an Infant

VOCABULARY

Learn the meaning and the correct spelling of the following words and phrases:

amniotic fluid	fetus	lochia	prenatal
amniotic sac	foreskin	placenta	status
circumcision	involution	postpartum	umbilical cord
doula			

INTRODUCTION

When a baby is ready to be born, it is normally upside down in the mother's uterus with its head toward the birth canal (Figure 40-1). Before the baby is born, it is known as a **fetus**. It is surrounded by a membranous bag called an **amniotic sac**. The fetus floats in a liquid called **amniotic fluid**.

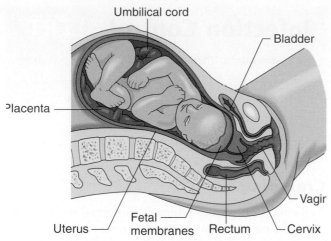

Umbilical cord

Bladder

Placenta

Vagir

Uterus

Fetal membranes

Rectum

Cervix

FIGURE 40-1 The usual position of the fetus at birth. *(© Delmar/Cengage Learning)*

The fetus gets nourishment from the mother through the **umbilical cord**. The umbilical cord is attached to the fetus and the **placenta**. The placenta is attached to the wall of the mother's uterus.

After the baby is born and separated from the umbilical cord, the placenta, amniotic sac, and remaining cord are expelled as the *afterbirth*. After a period of time, the mother's uterus, which was greatly stretched during pregnancy, will return to its normal size and shape.

There are three phases of pregnancy:

1. **Prenatal** (before birth)
2. **Labor and delivery**
3. **Postpartum** (after birth)

THE DOULA

Some patients who come to the hospital in labor may be accompanied by both the spouse and a **doula**. The word *doula* is derived from Greek, and means "woman's servant." Doulas are members of the childbirth team. The doula is not a caregiver. A doula may work for a physician, midwife, or a hospital, or be self-employed. They are responsible for supporting and comforting the mother and enhancing communication between the mother and hospital staff. Two types of doulas assist families during the childbirth process:

1. A *birth doula* provides support and nurture to the mother before, during, and just after childbirth.
2. A *postpartum doula* works with a postpartum family to help them care for and enjoy the infant.

POSTPARTUM CARE

You may assist in caring for the mother during the postpartum period. With other team members, you will assist the mother from the stretcher into bed. A bed protector should be placed under the patient's buttocks. Always wear gloves and follow standard precautions when caring for the postpartum patient. There is a high probability of contact with blood, mucous membranes, urine, and breast milk.

Anesthesia

If an anesthetic was used, follow the procedures for postoperative care of surgical patients (Unit 29).

- Keep the patient flat on her back if spinal anesthesia was used.
- Make sure the patient has a fresh gown and clean bed linen.
- Check vital signs as ordered until the patient is stable, then continue to recheck every 4 hours for 24 hours.
- If the patient complains of being cold, an extra blanket may provide comfort.
- Record the first voiding. Inform the nurse if the patient has not voided by the end of your shift.

Drainage

Carefully check the condition of the perineum and the perineal pad for the amount and color of drainage.

- Always lift the pad away from the body from front to back.
- Red vaginal discharge, called **lochia**, is expected. *Lochia rubra* (Figure 40-2) is the discharge that occurs during the first 3 days after delivery. Report the amount of discharge and any clotting.

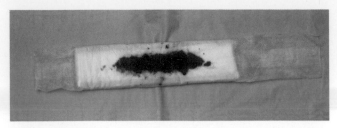

FIGURE 40-2 Moderate lochia is normal during the first few days. (© Delmar/Cengage Learning)

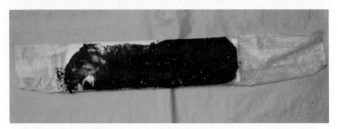

FIGURE 40-3 Heavy lochia must be promptly reported to the nurse. (© Delmar/Cengage Learning)

Clinical Information ALERT

If the patient has been in bed for a long time, lochia pools in the vagina. When the patient stands, she may have very heavy flow. This is normal. Exercising vigorously will also increase the flow. If the flow is heavy, inform the nurse. ■

Clinical Information ALERT

Women who have had a cesarean section usually have less lochia than women who deliver vaginally. This is because the surgeon usually wipes the inside of the uterus, removing blood and loose tissue, before suturing the abdomen closed. ■

Initially, the lochia is bright red and moderate in amount. Report heavy lochia to the nurse (Figure 40-3). Over the next week, the lochia will lessen and become pink to pink-brown in color. A yellowish-white or brown discharge may continue for 1 to 3 weeks after delivery and then stop.

Infection Control ALERT

Peri pads are normally packaged in sterile containers. Teach the mother to handle the pad only by the ends, so that the part that contacts the perineum remains sterile. ■

Cramping

As the uterus begins to return to its normal size (**involution**), the patient may experience strong cramps. Cramping may also be associated with breast feeding. This is normal, but be sure to report any complaints of pain to the nurse, who can administer medication for relief.

Voiding

Encourage the new mother to void within the first 6 to 8 hours after the delivery. Check carefully for signs of urine retention.

Toileting and Perineal Care

The mother may be:
- Provided with a squeezable bottle filled with warm tap water.
- Instructed to rinse the genitals and perineum after voiding or defecating.
- Instructed to gently pat, not wipe, the perineal area with tissue or special medicated pads—once only, from front to back. Discard the tissue in the toilet.
- Taught to wash her hands before applying a fresh perineal pad.
- Taught not to touch the inside of the perineal pad.

If the perineum is very uncomfortable:
- Specially medicated pads may be used for cleansing. The procedure is always the same—front to back and discard.
- Anesthetic sprays may be ordered.
- Ice packs may be used to reduce edema and relieve discomfort.

Breast Care

The breasts should be washed daily with soap and water even if the mother is not breast-feeding. The breasts must be supported continuously by a well-fitted brassiere. Medication to suppress milk production is sometimes ordered.

GUIDELINES *for*

Assisting with Breast-Feeding

A recent trend holds that "the breast is best," and many mothers elect to breast-feed their newborns. Assist the mother by:

- Instructing her to wash the nipples and areolae with clear water on a cotton ball before nursing. She should begin at the nipple, working outward in a circular motion.

- Helping to position the baby. The football hold (Figure 40-4A) or cradle hold (Figure 40-4B) is usually easiest.

- Gently stroking the infant's cheek near the mouth to get the baby to open the mouth and turn toward the breast.

- Instructing the mother to place the nipple and areola into the baby's mouth. The infant should begin to suck and swallow.

- Checking the position of the breast. Advise the mother to press and hold the breast back, if necessary, so it does not obstruct the baby's nose.

- Allowing the baby to nurse for 5 to 7 minutes, if he or she has not stopped by then. If the infant has not stopped nursing, avoid pulling it from the breast. Break the infant's suction by placing a finger into the side of the mouth and moving the breast. Instruct the mother to burp the infant.

- Switching to the other breast after the infant has burped. Help the mother reposition the infant and get the baby started nursing on the opposite breast.

The infant will stop nursing when he or she is full. Have the mother burp the baby again.

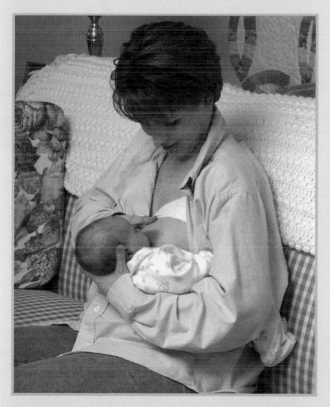

FIGURE 40-4A The football hold is used for nursing and other activities when the baby must be supported well, such as when washing the hair. (© *Delmar/Cengage Learning*)

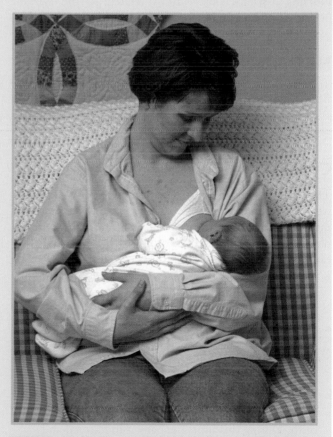

FIGURE 40-4B The cradle hold is also a comfortable position for nursing. (© *Delmar/Cengage Learning*)

TABLE 40-1 OBSERVATIONS OF POSTPARTUM PATIENTS TO MAKE AND REPORT TO THE NURSE IMMEDIATELY

- Uterus that is unusually high or pushed to one side
- Swelling just above the pubis
- Complaints of urgency (the need to void), but with voidings of 200 mL or less
- Signs of possible urine retention
- Inability to void within the first 8 hours postpartum
- Voidings of less than 100 mL
- Temperature of 100.4°F or greater
- Pulse over 100
- Blood pressure of 140/90 or above
- Progressively falling blood pressure
- Signs of inflammation
- Presence of large blood clots
- Foul-smelling lochia
- Saturation of a pad in 15 to 30 minutes
- Bruised appearance of perineum
- Complaints of constipation

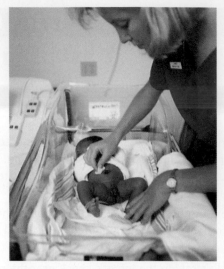

FIGURE 40-5 The cord is carefully cleaned to cause it to dry. *(© Delmar/Cengage Learning)*

Nursing assistant observations related to the care of postpartum patients are listed in Table 40-1.

NEONATAL CARE

After the newborn is admitted to the nursery, some additional procedures are completed. The physician will examine the baby and evaluate his or her **status**.

Care of the Newborn Infant

The baby's vital signs are determined. The infant is weighed and measured. The infant's axillary temperature is monitored and recorded every 30 to 60 minutes until stable, then every 4 hours or according to the nurse's instructions. When the newborn's status becomes stable:

- The baby is given an admission bath using an antiseptic soap. The umbilical cord is carefully cleaned with a solution prescribed by the facility (Figure 40-5).
- The baby must be kept warm because his or her temperature has not yet stabilized. The baby is dressed. Cover the head with a stockinette cap, because much body heat can be lost through this surface.
- The baby is placed in a crib or isolette (Figure 40-6).
- Feeding is not usually started until 4 to 6 hours after birth. During this time, the baby is monitored and observed carefully. After 4 to 6 hours, the baby is either taken to breast-feed or started on feedings of glucose and water. Babies whose mothers are unable to feed them will be fed in the nursery.
- Male babies may be circumcised before discharge. In **circumcision**, the excess tissue (**foreskin**) is cut from the

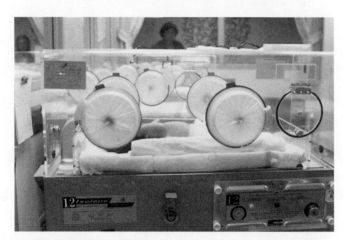

FIGURE 40-6 Some babies are cared for in the controlled environment of the isolette. *(Courtesy of Memorial Medical Center of Long Beach, CA)*

tip of the penis (Figure 40-7). This procedure is usually performed according to the parents' personal choices, as well as cultural, ethnic, and religious traditions.

Handling the Infant

Take care when lifting, carrying, and positioning an infant. Remember to lift the baby by grasping the legs securely with one hand while slipping the other hand under the baby's back to support the head and neck (Figures 40-8A and 40-8B). You may also use the cradle hold or football hold. Back through doorways when carrying a baby. Never turn your back when the infant is on an unprotected surface.

Elimination

The passage of urine and stool in a newborn infant are important observations. A normal newborn will urinate 6 to 10 times a day. Elimination is recorded and the color

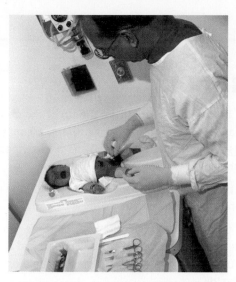

FIGURE 40-7 The infant is circumcised shortly after birth at the parents' request. (© Delmar/Cengage Learning)

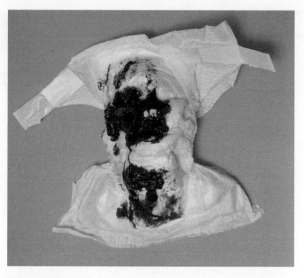

FIGURE 40-9A The first stools are meconium stools. (© Delmar/Cengage Learning)

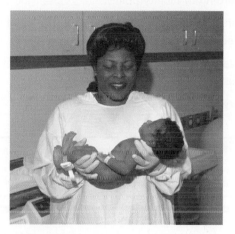

FIGURE 40-8A Always support the infant's bottom and neck. (© Delmar/Cengage Learning)

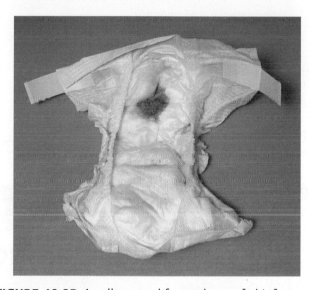

FIGURE 40-9B A yellow stool from a breast-fed infant. (© Delmar/Cengage Learning)

Postcircumcision Care

The circumcision should be checked each time the diaper is changed. Observe the area for bleeding and report anything unusual. The crib identification and nursery record will note the circumcision. Document the first voiding after circumcision.

Weighing the Infant

Routine care includes weighing the infant. This procedure should also be done before feeding.

Tips: Put clean paper on the scale before using it. Balance the scale with the paper in place. Keep your hand on the infant. Work quickly to prevent heat loss in the infant. Disinfect the scale each time it is used, to prevent cross-contamination.

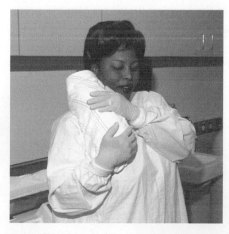

FIGURE 40-8B Shoulder hold. (© Delmar/Cengage Learning)

of stool documented. Stools should change from dark, meconium stools (Figure 40-9A) to brown-yellow, pasty transitional stools, then finally to yellow stools that are slightly loose (Figure 40-9B).

PROCEDURE

96

CHANGING A DIAPER

1. Carry out initial procedure actions.

2. Assemble equipment:
   - Clean diaper
   - Gloves
   - Plastic bag or container for trash
   - Damp washcloths, wipes, or cotton balls for cleansing
   - Mild soap, if used
   - Supplies for cord care and/or circumcision care, according to facility policy

3. Remove the soiled diaper and observe for color, consistency, and quantity.

4. Roll the soiled diaper so the clean side faces out. Put it in the trash or place it out of reach of the infant.

5. Cleanse the diaper area with wipes or a damp washcloth. Clean from the front toward the back

in a female infant, and from the tip of the penis toward the scrotum for a male infant. Cleanse all folds of the groin and anus. Discard the wipes or washcloth.

6. Lift the buttocks with one hand and slide the new, open diaper underneath.

7. Pull the diaper between the legs. Fold the top edge of the diaper down so it is positioned under the umbilical cord. Fasten the tape snugly on each side.

8. Perform cord care with alcohol or antiseptic according to facility policy.

9. Change other clothing, blanket, or crib linen if soiled or wet.

10. Discard the soiled diaper and your gloves, if not done previously.

11. Carry out ending procedure actions.

PROCEDURE

97

WEIGHING AN INFANT

1. Wash your hands.

2. Place exam paper or a receiving blanket on the scale and balance the scale.

3. Check the infant's previous weight, if any.

4. Remove the infant's diaper and shirt.

5. Place the infant on the scale, keeping a hand over the infant to prevent falling (Figure 40-10).

6. Move the bar to the correct weight until the scale balances.

7. Return the infant to the crib. Diaper and dress the infant.

8. Record the infant's weight according to hospital policy.

9. Remove the linen from the scale and place it in a laundry hamper.

10. Return the scale to its proper storage place.

11. Wash your hands.

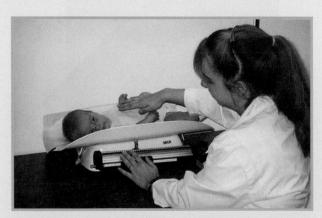

FIGURE 40-10 Maintain light hand contact with the infant while adjusting the weights with the other hand. *(© Delmar/Cengage Learning)*

Measuring Length

Length refers to a measurement taken with the infant in the supine position. Infants move and flex their extremities, so having two people measure is best. Measure the infant twice. The measurements must be within 1/8 inch of each other.

In some facilities, infants are measured by using a calibrated length board with a fixed headrest and movable footrest (similar to the device used for measuring shoe size). This is the most accurate method. In other facilities, the infant is measured using a disposable paper tape measure.

PROCEDURE

98

MEASURING AN INFANT

1. Wash your hands.
2. Assemble equipment:
   - Paper to cover the surface
   - Calibrated length board, if used
   - Paper tape measure, if used
   - Pen and paper
   - Supplies for disinfecting the measuring surface
3. Check the infant's identification band.

Calibrated length board: Complete steps 1 through 3 above.

4. Position the infant on the back in the center of the length board with the head touching the headrest and the buttocks and shoulders flat against the measuring surface.
5. One person gently holds the infant's head in contact with the headpiece. He or she gently cups the infant's ears to be sure the infant's chin is not tucked in against the chest or stretched too far back.
6. The other person aligns the infant, extending both legs. Place one hand gently on the knees to keep the legs in extension with the toes pointing upward.
7. Slide the movable footrest up until it rests firmly against the soles of the infant's feet. Read the measurement and write the value on your note pad.
8. Remove the infant and return him or her to the crib.
9. Discard paper cover and sanitize the board.
10. Document the measurement.
11. Perform your procedure completion actions.

Tape measure method #1: Complete steps 1 through 3 above.

4. One person gently holds the infant's head in contact with a solid surface. This person gently cups the ears to be sure the infant's chin is not tucked in against the chest or stretched too far back.
5. The other person aligns the infant, extending both legs. Place one hand gently on the knees to keep the legs in extension with the toes pointing upward.
6. Using a paper tape measure, measure from the top of the head to the soles of the infant's feet. Read the measurement and write the value on your note pad.
7. Remove the infant and return him or her to the crib.
8. Discard the paper and sanitize the measuring surface.
9. Document the value.
10. Perform your procedure completion actions.

Tape measure method #2: Complete steps 1 through 3 above.

4. Place a piece of exam table paper on a clean surface. Make sure the paper is smooth and wrinkle-free.
5. One person gently holds the infant's head in contact with a solid surface. This person gently cups the infant's ears while holding the head to be sure the infant's chin is not tucked in against the chest or stretched too far back.
6. Make a mark on the paper at the center top of the head.
7. Align the infant, extending both legs. Place one hand gently on the knees to keep the legs in extension with the toes pointing upward.
8. Make a mark on the paper at the bottom of the heels. Repeat to verify accuracy.

continues

PROCEDURE 98 CONTINUED

9. Pick the infant up and return him or her to the crib.

10. Using a paper tape measure, measure the distance between the two marks.

11. Document the value.

12. Discard the paper and sanitize the measuring surface.

13. Perform your procedure completion actions.

Bathing the Infant

The infant may be bathed after the temperature has stabilized. Bathing is done daily, and as needed. The nurse will teach the parents how to bathe the infant.

 Note: Before beginning the bathing procedure, check with the nurse to make sure the infant's temperature is stable enough for bathing. Keep the infant warm throughout the procedure.

Security

All infants must be identified to prevent inadvertent switching, misidentification, and abduction. The nurse

Difficult SITUATIONS

Babies are dressed in a long-sleeved T-shirt, a diaper, and a stockinette cap on the head, then covered with a receiving blanket. Despite these measures, some newborns cannot maintain temperature. Try adding a second long-sleeved T-shirt. Place the baby's legs in the armholes and pull the shirt up to create leggings. ■

PROCEDURE

99

BATHING AN INFANT

1. Carry out initial procedure actions.

2. Assemble equipment:
   - Clean diaper
   - Gloves
   - Washbasin with warm water (98°F to 100°F)
   - Plastic bag or container for trash
   - Washcloths (2–3)
   - Towel
   - Cotton balls
   - Liquid infant cleanser/shampoo
   - Supplies for cord care and/or circumcision care, according to facility policy
   - Blankets
   - Sheet

3. Place the infant in a bassinet with sides. Arrange the supplies within reach.

4. Check the infant's skin for dryness, peeling, or signs of infection. If present, notify the nurse and obtain instructions for care.

5. Check the site of the umbilical cord for redness, drainage, drying, and bleeding. If present, notify the nurse and obtain instructions for care.

6. Remove the infant's clothing. Cover the infant with a blanket for warmth.

7. Moisten a cotton ball with plain water. Cleanse the far eye from inside to outside, in one wipe. Repeat with a new cotton ball for the near eye.

8. Wash the outer ears with plain water and a cotton ball or twisted end of the washcloth.

9. Make a mitt with the washcloth. Wash the face and neck with plain water, with attention to areas behind the ears and creases in the neck.

PROCEDURE 99 CONTINUED

10. Pat the face and neck dry with a towel.

11. Pull the blanket down to expose the upper body.

12. Cleanse the upper body with soap and a washcloth. Rinse soap from the hands quickly, then rinse the rest of the upper body. Pat dry.

13. Cleanse and rinse the area around the umbilicus. Pat dry. Apply alcohol or drying solution used by the facility.

14. Cover the upper body. Pull the blanket up to expose the lower body.

15. Wash the legs and outer buttocks with soap and water. Rinse well and pat dry.

16. Obtain a fresh washcloth.

17. Cleanse the genitalia with plain water.

Female infant:

   a. Spread labia gently. Wash from front to back toward the anus. Turn the washcloth so a separate part is used for each wipe.

   b. Wash the remaining portions of the labia and the folds in the groin.

   c. Rinse and pat dry.

Uncircumcised male infant:

   d. Avoid retracting the foreskin.

   e. Wash from the urethra outward, then scrotum and folds in the groin.

   f. Rinse and pat dry.

Circumcised male infant:

   g. Care for the circumcision according to the nurse's instructions.

   h. Check for bleeding.

   i. Gently cleanse the area with warm water and cotton balls.

   j. Apply petroleum jelly and a gauze dressing, or provide care according to facility policy.

18. Cleanse the anal area with soap. Rinse and pat dry.

19. Diaper the infant.

20. Wrap the infant in the blanket.

21. Pick up the infant, using the football hold. Hold the head over the basin.

22. Wet the scalp well with a washcloth and water.

23. Lather and gently wash the scalp with baby shampoo or gentle cleanser.

24. Rinse the scalp by pouring water from a small cup over the scalp and into the washbasin, or rinse well using a washcloth.

25. Pat dry.

26. Comb the infant's hair. Cover the head.

27. Dress the infant.

28. Replace the damp blanket and sheets.

29. Carry out ending procedure actions.

---

will apply identification bands to the infant's wrist and ankle while in the delivery room. The mother is given a matching wrist band. In some facilities, the father is also given a wrist band. The identification bands must be checked each time the infant is brought to the mother for feeding or rooming-in. Crib cards and other documents are also used for infant identification. Each facility has policies for checking identification. In some, the identification is also checked at the beginning and end of each shift.

Infant Abduction

Unfortunately, a number of infant abductions occur each year. In addition to wearing an identification badge, reinforce your identity and position to the mothers each time

Safety ALERT

Your facility will issue photo identification to all personnel working in the maternity department. Many workers turn the cards around so only the back side shows. This is an unsafe practice that most likely violates hospital policy. Wear the badge on your upper body, with the picture on the front. The mother will be informed to check the worker's identification badge if someone tries to remove the infant from the room. ■

you provide care. The mother will be instructed not to hand the infant over to someone she does not know. Hospitals have various security measures in place to prevent abduction. Some apply magnetic-sensor ankle bands in the delivery room. An alarm will sound if the infant is removed from the unit. A few are using global positioning systems (GPS) for tracking. Some apply a tamper-proof band to the ankle or umbilical cord. If the band is removed or the infant is taken off the unit, doors automatically lock. Infants are transported to other areas of the hospital in a crib (Figure 40-11), never carried. A transport identification card may also be used. Nursing staff must remain with the infant while he or she is off the unit.

Many hospitals have infant abduction drills, similar to fire drills. Take these drills seriously. There is no room for error in responding to an abduction, and the drills help staff react automatically to the emergency, increasing the odds that the infant will be found.

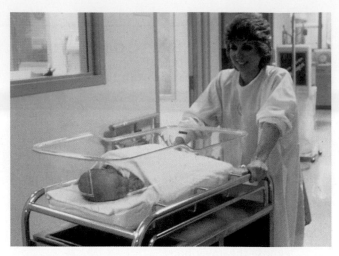

FIGURE 40-11 Babies are transported in their own bassinets, never carried. The nursing assistant wears a cover gown when leaving the department. *(Courtesy of Memorial Medical Center of Long Beach, CA)*

Changing Crib Linen

Newborn infants are placed in a plastic bassinette or a crib. The mattress is covered with a pillowcase. Change the pillowcase after the infant's bath, and as needed. Older infants are placed in a regular crib. Again, the linen is changed after the bath, and as often as needed. Procedures 100 and 101 are used for a regular crib.

PROCEDURE

100
CHANGING CRIB LINENS

1. Wash your hands.

2. Gather supplies:
   - Disposable gloves
   - Sheet (or pillowcase for bassinette)
   - Blanket
   - Shirt
   - Diaper
   - Pad

3. Apply the principles of standard precautions as you would with an adult.

4. After bathing, diaper and dress the infant.

5. Place the infant in a stroller, playpen, or other safe place.

6. Strip the linen from the crib. Wear gloves if linen is soiled. Dispose of soiled or used linen according to facility policy.

7. Remove gloves and discard them according to facility policy. Wash hands.

8. Wash your hands.

9. Place clean linen on the bed and open the sheet, hem side down.

10. Make one side of the crib; miter the corners top and bottom, and tuck in the side (Figure 40-12A).

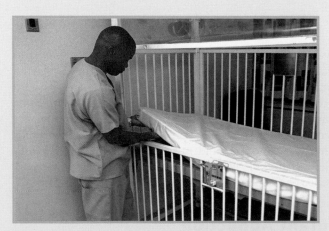

FIGURE 40-12A Make one side of the crib. Miter corners at the top and bottom and tuck under mattress. *(© Delmar/Cengage Learning)*

PROCEDURE 100 CONTINUED

11. Pull down the crib top (Figure 40-12B). Pull up the crib side (Figure 40-12C).

12. Repeat step 10 on the opposite side of the crib.

13. Place a diaper pad on top of the sheet.

14. Place a clean blanket at the bottom of the bed.

15. Arrange bumper pads around the sides of the crib, if used.

16. Wash your hands.

17. Return the infant to the crib, cover with the blanket, and pull the side up.

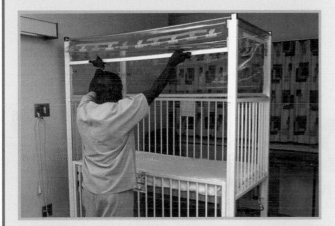

FIGURE 40-12B Pull the crib top down. (© Delmar/Cengage Learning)

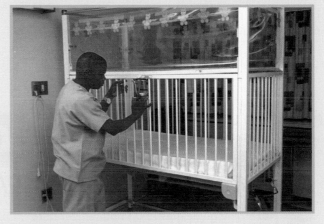

FIGURE 40-12C Pull the side up and check for security. (© Delmar/Cengage Learning)

PROCEDURE

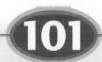

CHANGING CRIB LINENS (INFANT IN CRIB)

1. Wash your hands.

2. Gather supplies:
   - Sheet (or pillowcase for bassinette)
   - Blanket
   - Shirt
   - Diaper
   - Bathing equipment
   - Disposable gloves

3. After bathing, diaper and dress the infant.

4. Pick up the infant and hold him in one arm.

5. With your free hand, strip the old linen off the crib. Wear gloves if linen is soiled.

6. Place the clean linen on the mattress and open the sheet, placing the hem side down. Place the infant on the sheet.

7. Place one hand on the infant and keep it on him at all times.

8. Make one side of the crib. Miter the sheet corners and tuck in the side.

9. Remove your hand from the infant and pull up the crib side.

10. Go around to the other side of the crib.

11. Take down the crib side, place one hand on the infant, and repeat step 8.

12. Place a diaper pad under the infant and cover him with the blanket.

13. Arrange bumper pads around the crib, if used.

14. Pull up the crib side.

15. Wash your hands.

DETERMINING VITAL SIGNS

Measure the infant's vital signs every 4 hours or as ordered after the birth temperature has stabilized. The infant's heart and respiratory rates are normally faster than an adult's. The rates increase if the infant is crying, or has a fever or infection. Take the pulse and respiratory rates when the infant is quiet, either awake or asleep. Count the pulse and respirations for one full minute.

Temperatures on children 5 years of age and under are usually taken rectally or by the temporal artery or tympanic method unless there is a medical reason not to. Axillary temperature can be taken in place of rectal temperature,

but remember that this is the least accurate temperature value. The temporal artery method is the most accurate and desirable method to use.

Difficult SITUATIONS

Take the rectal temperature *last*. Taking the rectal temperature first may cause the infant to cry, which will accelerate the pulse and respirations. ∎

PROCEDURE

MEASURING AN INFANT'S TEMPERATURE

Note: The guidelines for taking temperature vary slightly from state to state, and from one facility to the next. Your instructor will inform you if the sequence you are to use differs from the procedure listed here. Know and follow the required sequence for your facility and state.

Rectal Temperature

1. Carry out initial procedure actions.

2. Assemble equipment:
   - Gloves (standard precautions)
   - Clinical thermometer (glass or digital)
   - Protective sheath (unopened package)
   - Water-soluble lubricant
   - Clean diaper
   - Pad and pencil

3. Inspect the glass thermometer for breaks (if used).

4. Shake down the glass thermometer (if used).

5. Cover the thermometer with a disposable sheath or probe cover, depending on the type of thermometer used.

6. Lubricate the thermometer sheath, if it is not prelubricated.

7. Remove the infant's diaper. Lay the infant on his back on the bed (Figure 40-13A) or on his stomach across your lap (Figure 40-13B).

8. Insert the thermometer 1/2 inch into the child's rectum and hold. Hold the child securely and gently so the child does not move about.

9. Leave the thermometer in place for the required amount of time (3 minutes for a glass thermometer). Follow your facility's policy.

10. Remove the thermometer. Discard the sheath or probe cover.

11. Read the thermometer and write the value on your pad.

12. Apply a clean diaper.

13. Carry out ending procedure actions.

14. Report any unusual variations to the nurse at once.

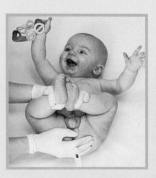
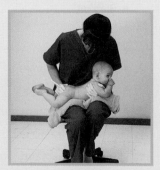

| A | B |

FIGURE 40-13 A. Infant in supine position B. Infant in prone position. (© Delmar/Cengage Learning)

PROCEDURE 102 CONTINUED

Axillary Temperature

1. Carry out initial procedure actions.

2. Assemble equipment:
   - Clinical thermometer (glass or digital)
   - Protective sheath (unopened package)
   - Pad and pencil

3. Inspect the glass thermometer for breaks.

4. Shake down the glass thermometer.

5. Cover the thermometer with a disposable sheath or probe cover, depending on the type of thermometer used.

6. Place the thermometer in the child's armpit.

7. Hold the child's arm close to the chest for the required amount of time (10 minutes for a glass thermometer).

8. Remove the thermometer. Discard the sheath according to facility policy.

9. Read the thermometer and write the value on your pad.

10. Carry out ending procedure actions.

11. Report any unusual variations to the nurse at once.

   Note: If an electronic thermometer is used, follow the manufacturer's directions supplied with the equipment.

Tympanic Temperature

1. Carry out initial procedure actions.

2. Assemble equipment:
   - Tympanic thermometer
   - Protective sheath (unopened package)
   - Pad and pencil

3. Check the lens on the thermometer to make sure it is clean and intact.

4. Set the appropriate mode on the thermometer.

5. Place a clean probe cover on the probe.

6. Position the patient so you will have access to the ear you will be using.

7. If the patient is under age 1, pull the ear straight back, then down. In children over age 1, pull the ear up and back. While gently tugging the ear,

fit the probe snugly into the canal, aiming at the tympanic membrane. Point the probe tip at the midpoint between the eyebrow and sideburn on the opposite side of the face. The probe tip should penetrate at least one-third of the ear canal and form a complete seal.

   Note: Tympanic thermometers measure temperature by aiming an infrared light beam at the tympanic membrane. Light does not go around corners. If the ear canal is not fully straightened when the thermometer is inserted, the value will not be accurate. Because of this, step 7 is very important to the accuracy of this procedure.

8. Press the activation button. Leave the thermometer in place until the display blinks or signals that the temperature is final.

9. Remove the thermometer. Discard the probe cover. Write the value on your pad.

10. Carry out ending procedure actions.

11. Report any unusual variations to the nurse at once.

Temporal Artery Temperature

1. Carry out initial procedure actions.

2. Assemble equipment:
   - Temporal artery thermometer
   - Probe covers, alcohol sponges, or disinfectant wipes

3. Check the lens to make sure it is clean and intact.

4. Apply a clean probe cover, or wipe the probe with alcohol or a disinfectant wipe.

5. Hold the thermometer as you would a pencil or pen. Gently press the probe (head) of the thermometer against the center of the forehead. Push the switch to the "ON" position with your thumb. Keep this button depressed.

6. Slowly move the probe across the forehead to the hair line on one side.

7. Push the hair back with the opposite hand, then lift the probe slightly. Quickly place it down just behind the earlobe. (This is the area in which perfume is normally applied). Release the button and remove the thermometer. Note and remember the value on the digital display until you can write it on your pad. The value should

continues

PROCEDURE 102 CONTINUED

remain on the display for about 30 seconds before disappearing.

8. Discard the disposable probe cover, or wipe with an alcohol or disinfectant wipe.

9. Carry out ending procedure actions.

10. Report any unusual variations to the nurse at once.

Safety ALERT

When taking a rectal temperature, grasp the child's ankles gently, but firmly, with one hand. Cover the penis of a male infant with a diaper. Insert the lubricated thermometer while holding the ankles. Continue to hold the ankles with one hand and the thermometer with the other throughout the procedure. ■

FEEDING

Feeding is important to the infant because it satisfies hunger and sucking needs. Sucking provides the infant with a pleasant sensation, whether she receives food or not. The amount of time an infant needs to suckle will vary with each infant. Provide the infant with the opportunity to suck, even if the infant cannot eat. Wash your hands well before feeding an infant or assisting a mother with breast-feeding.

PROCEDURE

103

DETERMINING AN INFANT'S HEART RATE (PULSE)

With infants and children, the easiest way to find the heart rate is to measure the apical pulse by placing a stethoscope over the heart (Figure 40-14). This should be done when the child is quiet, because stress and crying will result in a reading that is higher than normal.

1. Carry out initial procedure actions.

2. Assemble equipment:
   - Stethoscope
   - Alcohol sponges
   - Pad of paper and pen

3. Clean stethoscope earpieces and diaphragm with an alcohol sponge.

4. Rub the diaphragm so that it will not be cold.

5. Place the stethoscope over the heart and count the number of beats you hear in a minute.

6. Clean the stethoscope earpieces and diaphragm with an alcohol sponge.

7. Write the value on your pad.

8. Carry out ending procedure actions.

9. Report any unusual variations to the nurse at once.

📝 **Note:** The radial pulse can be used for children 6 years of age and over. The procedure used is the same as for adults. Refer to Procedure 30 in Unit 19.

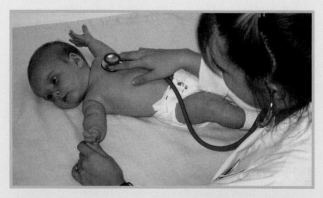

FIGURE 40-14 Measuring the apical pulse. (© Delmar/ Cengage Learning)

PROCEDURE

104

COUNTING AN INFANT'S RESPIRATORY RATE

Infants and toddlers use their abdominal muscles for breathing. To count the respiratory rate for this age group, look at the abdomen and chest and count the respirations for a full minute.

To obtain the respiratory rate for preschoolers and older children, follow Procedure 32 in Unit 19, as for adults, but count the respirations for a full minute.

When feeding an infant:

- Hold the infant unless there is a medical reason not to. Holding the infant during a feeding allows close, physical contact with the person feeding her.
- Infants breathe from the nose. Nasal congestion will cause feeding problems. Inform the nurse if the newborn experiences nasal congestion or has difficulty during feeding.
- If an infant cannot be held, hold the bottle while she eats.
- Never leave an infant in a crib with a bottle propped in the mouth. This is dangerous because the infant could vomit and/or choke.
- Burp the infant during and following feeding.
- If the infant hiccups after feeding, try to get her to swallow a little more formula, or burp the infant to make the hiccups stop.

   Note: If an infant cannot be fed, hold and allow her to suck on a pacifier unless a medical reason prevents removal of the infant from the crib.

Burping

The frequency with which you burp the infant will depend on the infant's age and medical condition. Burping is important because bottle-fed infants swallow a lot of air while sucking. The infant can be burped as frequently as after every half-ounce of formula. Older infants can be burped after 1 to 2 ounces during feeding and at the conclusion of feeding. There are two methods of burping an infant (see Procedure 106).

Breast-Feeding

If the rooming-in or visiting mother is breast-feeding, she should be directed to an area where she can be assured of privacy as well as comfort. As a nursing assistant, you may be responsible for weighing the infant before and after feeding. (See Procedure 96.) When returning the infant to the crib after feeding, place him on his back or side. A rolled blanket can be used to keep him on the side.

Safety ALERT

Shake the bottle slightly to ensure that the formula is mixed well. Remove the plastic cap and place it on its side or with the clean inner side up. (The caps for disposable bottles used in hospitals are very lightweight and may fall over if placed upside down.) Invert the bottle and drop a few drops of formula on your wrist to check the temperature of the formula and patency of the nipple. Formula should drip freely, but not come out in a stream. If the formula runs out in a stream, change the nipple. Elevate the child's head and shoulders slightly during feeding. Keep the nipple filled with formula at all times, to prevent ingestion of air. A steady stream of bubbles should rise in the bottle during feeding. If the infant pushes the nipple out with her tongue, reinsert it. This is a normal reflex and does not mean that the child is full or does not want to eat. ■

Infection Control ALERT

The formula and bottle for bottle-feeding an infant should be sterile. Most facilities use prepared, sterile formula in disposable glass bottles. Avoid touching the nipple or the inside of the cap. Keep the nipple covered until you are ready to begin feeding. Check the expiration date on the bottle to make sure the formula has not expired. ■

PROCEDURE

105

BOTTLE-FEEDING AN INFANT

1. Wash your hands.

2. Gather the infant's formula and diaper pad, washcloth, or bib.

3. Check the infant's identification band.

4. Pick up the infant and hold her in the crook of your arm, with the head slightly raised (Figure 40-15).

5. Sit in a chair or rocker.

6. Place a diaper, washcloth, or bib under the infant's chin, covering the chest.

7. Tip the bottle so the nipple is filled with formula.

8. Stroke the side of the infant's cheek closest to you. The infant will automatically turn toward the side stroked and open her mouth. Place the nipple in the mouth.

9. If the nipple is in the mouth but the infant is not sucking, gently lift up under the infant's chin to close her mouth on the nipple.

10. Hold the bottle so the nipple stays filled with formula while the infant feeds.

11. Feed the infant and burp as needed. (See Procedure 106.)

12. If the infant starts to vomit, remove the bottle and turn the infant to the side, with head lowered, to prevent aspiration. Seek help as needed.

13. After feeding, return the infant to the crib and place her on her back or side.

14. Pull up the crib side.

15. Carry out ending procedure actions.

16. Record the amount of formula the infant took, according to hospital policy.

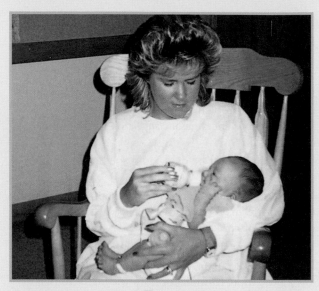

FIGURE 40-15 Hold the infant with the head elevated during bottle-feeding. Keep the nipple filled with fluid to prevent excess air in the stomach, which is painful. (© Delmar/Cengage Learning)

PROCEDURE

106

BURPING AN INFANT

Burping (Method A)

1. Place a diaper or cloth over your shoulder.

2. Lift the infant up to your shoulder, holding the infant close to your chest (Figure 40-16).

3. Holding the infant with one hand, use the other hand to gently rub or pat the infant's back until the infant burps.

Burping (Method B)

1. Place a diaper, cloth, or bib under the infant's chin.

2. Place the child in a sitting or upright position. Put one hand on the infant's chest and chin, supporting the infant's weight (Figure 40-17). With the other hand, gently rub or pat the infant's back until the infant burps.

PROCEDURE 99 CONTINUED

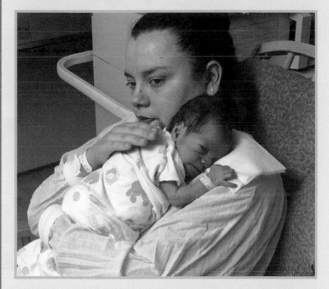

FIGURE 40-16 Burping the infant during and after feeding helps eliminate swallowed air. Gently rub or pat the infant's back. (© Delmar/Cengage Learning)

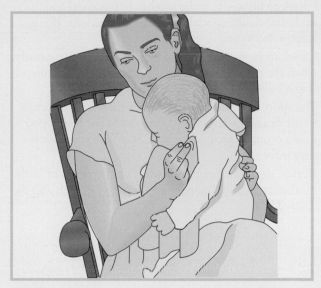

FIGURE 40-17 An alternative method of burping is to sit the infant on your lap with a cloth or bib under the chin. (© Delmar/Cengage Learning)

SUMMARY OF NURSING ASSISTANT RESPONSIBILITIES WHEN CARING FOR INFANTS

- Maintain a safe environment
- Provide information through monitoring of vital signs (temperature, pulse, respiration), weight, length, intake, and output
- Provide routine care such as bathing, feeding, and changing
- Assist with treatments, examinations, and procedures
- Provide warmth, security, and affection

Observations of newborn infants to make and report are listed in Table 40-2.

DISCHARGE

When delivery is uncomplicated, mothers and healthy newborns do not stay in the hospital very long. They are usually able to go home within 2 days. To carry out the discharge procedure:

- Match the baby's identification with the mother's.
- Dress the child in his or her own clothing (Figure 40-18).

TABLE 40-2 OBSERVATIONS OF NEWBORN INFANTS TO MAKE AND REPORT

- Temperature below 97.6°F (36.6°C)
- Temperature above 98.6°F (37.0°C)
- Apical pulse below 110 when infant is at rest (not crying)
- Apical pulse above 160 when infant is at rest (not crying)
- Respiratory rate below 30 when infant is at rest (not crying)
- Respiratory rate above 60 when infant is at rest (not crying)
- Noisy or grunting respirations
- Retractions when breathing (below the sternum, below the ribs, between the ribs, above the sternum, or above the clavicle)
- Systolic blood pressure below 50 mm Hg
- Systolic blood pressure above 80 mm Hg
- Heel stick blood glucose below 40 mg/dL
- Fewer than 6 wet diapers in 24 hours
- Flaring of the nostrils
- Nasal congestion
- Drainage from eyes or ears
- Bleeding from circumcision (more than a small amount)
- Accepting less than 1 ounce of formula every 3 hours

- Wrap the baby in a blanket, using the technique of "papoosing," as shown in Figures 40-19A through 40-19D.
- Check to be sure that the mother has received and understands any special discharge instructions. If not, inform the nurse.
- Check to be sure equipment or needed formula is ready when the parents and newborn are ready to go home (Figure 40-20).
- Transport the mother, carrying her baby, by wheelchair to the discharge area. Make sure the infant is strapped into a properly secured car seat. Stay with them until they leave.
- Record the discharge information on the charts of both mother and child. Include the condition of each and the time of release.

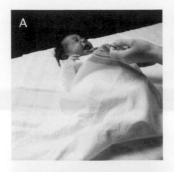
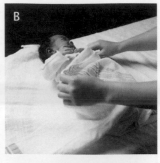
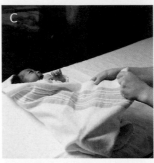
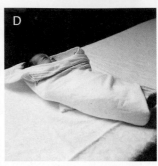

FIGURE 40-19 A. Position the receiving blanket under the infant so the corners are at the head and feet. Bring the bottom corner up over the infant. B. Fold one side corner over the infant. C. Bring the corner from the other side over the infant. D. Tuck the final corner under the infant, who is now ready for discharge. (© Delmar/Cengage Learning)

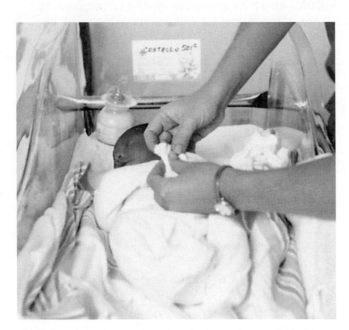

FIGURE 40-18 Dress the infant in his or her own clothing. (© Delmar/Cengage Learning)

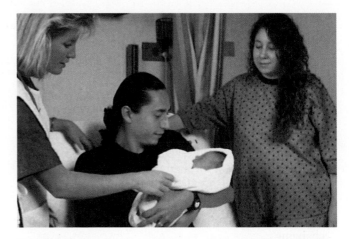

FIGURE 40-20 Parents prepare to leave the hospital with the newborn. (© Delmar/Cengage Learning)

REVIEW

A. Multiple Choice

Select the one best answer for each of the following.

   1. The doula
   a. is a member of the clinical staff.
   b. actively assists with the birth.
   c. supports and comforts the mother.
   d. provides anesthesia, if needed.

2. The usual vaginal discharge after birth is called
  a. lochia.
  b. menses.
  c. vernix.
  d. colostrum.

3. Immediately after birth, you would expect the vaginal drainage to be
  a. brown.
  b. yellow.
  c. yellow-brown.
  d. red.

4. The temperature of a newborn infant is usually
  a. elevated.
  b. stable.
  c. hypothermic.
  d. unstable.

5. The *most* desirable and accurate method of taking the infant's temperature is the
  a. tympanic membrane method.
  b. axillary method.
  c. temporal artery method.
  d. rectal method.

6. The color of the newborn's first stool is expected to be
  a. brown.
  b. black.
  c. yellow.
  d. red.

7. When caring for a new circumcision, you will wash the area, then wipe it with
  a. petroleum jelly.
  b. an alcohol sponge.
  c. disinfectant solution.
  d. povidone iodine.

8. When feeding a newborn infant, the formula and bottle should be
  a. cold.
  b. clean.
  c. hot.
  d. sterile.

9. After feeding the infant, position her in the crib
  a. on her abdomen.
  b. with the head elevated.
  c. on her back or side.
  d. with the feet elevated.

10. Burp the newborn infant after every
  a. half ounce.
  b. 2 ounces.
  c. 3 ounces.
  d. 4 ounces.

B. Nursing Assistant Challenge

You are assisting Mrs. Acuff to the bathroom for the first time since she delivered her first child, a nine-pound infant. Answer the following questions about care of this patient.

11. What will you instruct the patient to do before removing the perineal pad?

12. You must instruct Mrs. Acuff to remove the perineal pad. What will you tell her?

13. Mrs. Acuff starts to flush the toilet before standing up. What will you tell her? Why?

14. What color will you expect the vaginal discharge to be?

Rehabilitation and Restorative Services

OBJECTIVES

After completing this unit, you will be able to:
- Spell and define terms.
- Compare and contrast rehabilitation and restorative nursing care.
- Describe the role of the nursing assistant in rehabilitation and restorative care.
- Describe the principles of rehabilitation.

- List the elements of successful rehabilitation/restorative care.
- List six complications resulting from inactivity.
- Describe four approaches used for restorative programs.
- List guidelines for providing restorative care.
- Describe monitoring of the patient's response to care.

VOCABULARY

Learn the meaning and the correct spelling of the following words and phrases:

activities of daily living (ADLs)	disability	mobility skills	restoration
	geriatric	physiatrist	restorative
adaptive devices	handicap	rehabilitation	self-care deficit

INTRODUCTION TO REHABILITATION AND RESTORATIVE CARE

Rehabilitation and restorative care are provided to improve and maintain the patient's physical abilities. This may include **mobility skills** (Figure 41-1) and the ability to carry out **activities of daily living (ADLs)**. Activities of daily living are the tasks that we learn as children and do throughout life. These tasks include bathing, oral care, hair and nail care, dressing and undressing, eating, toileting, and mobility. Being independent with daily care promotes positive self-esteem.

Rehabilitation is a process in which the person is assisted to reach an optimal level of physical, mental, and emotional health. Rehabilitation and restorative care are similar, but there are some differences. These are compared and contrasted in Table 41-1.

How Rehabilitation and Restorative Nursing are Alike

- Assists patient to attain optimum level of physical, mental, and psychosocial function in light of condition
- Considers how one weak area of function can affect the whole person

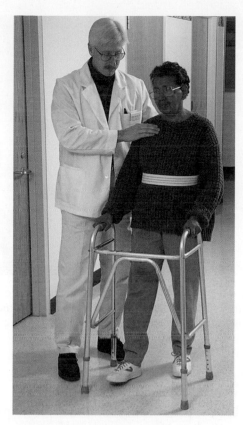

FIGURE 41-1 Rehabilitation and restorative nursing both work on increasing mobility and independence. (© Delmar/Cengage Learning)

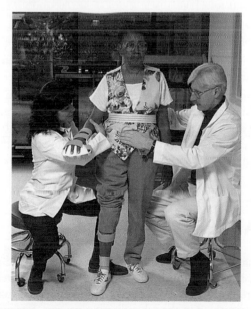

FIGURE 41-2 Rehabilitation is more aggressive and intensive than restorative care. (© Delmar/Cengage Learning)

- Helps patient adapt to limitations imposed by illness or injury
- Helps patient regain lost skills or learn a new way of doing skills lost because of illness or injury
- Requires physician order

TABLE 41-1 COMPARISON OF REHABILITATION AND RESTORATIVE NURSING

Rehabilitation	Restorative Nursing
Aggressive and intensive	Slower pace
Scheduled 1–4 hours a day, 7 days a week	Not scheduled, given 24 hours a day, whenever needed
A separate and distinct service	Approaches integrated into regular nursing care
Goal is to improve	Goal is to maintain; improvement is desirable, but not required
Patient makes rapid, significant progress	Patient may or may not progress, but does not decline
Planned and implemented by therapists	Planned and implemented by nursing
Must have potential for improvement	May participate even if no potential for improvement
Provided in any setting, but not required	Required in long-term care; usually provided in home health care, long-term care facilities, subacute care, and long-term acute care hospitals
Licensed personnel provide most services	Licensed and unlicensed personnel provide services; unlicensed personnel are primary caregivers
Paid by Medicare, Medicaid, private insurance	Inconsistently paid by Medicare and Medicaid in some situations; usually not paid by private insurance

- Requires initial evaluation and periodic re-evaluation (Figure 41-2)
- Must be verified by documentation
- Documentation must be measurable
- Safety an important factor
- Patient teaching is part of program; staff and family teaching may also be done
- May use services of others outside the department
- Assists with activities of daily living
- Works toward goals
- Patient benefits from service

- Provides a necessary service; not given as an activity or to keep the patient occupied
- Prevents complications
- Maintains current abilities
- Improves quality of life

The information in this unit applies to both rehabilitation and restorative care. These services complement each other. They do not compete. A **restorative** program established by the therapist to complement the rehabilitation program reinforces what the therapists are teaching, and the patient masters the skill more quickly. When you follow the program developed by the licensed nurse, you are helping the patient master skills for which nursing is responsible, such as bowel and bladder management. Regardless of whether the service is planned and provided by therapy or nursing, it is a functional service for the patient. For example:

- The speech therapist works with a patient who is recovering from a stroke to communicate the need for basic services that are essential to daily life, such as hunger, thirst, pain, and elimination. The therapist would not work with the patient to teach words that the patient is not likely to use, such as *aardvark* or *kumquat*.
- The physical therapist works with a patient who recently had a hip replacement to relearn safe ambulation. On the nursing unit, personnel follow a safe ambulation program to complement rehabilitation rather than applying restraints to prevent falls.
- A restorative nursing program may establish a goal for a patient to walk 150 feet with a walker, gait belt, and one assistant. The purpose of the program is to walk to the dining room, which is 150 feet from the patient's room. The patient would not walk back and forth in the hallway until the 150-foot goal is reached.

As you can see, both rehabilitation and restorative nursing work with functional skills that the patient needs each day. This process is called **restoration.**

REASONS FOR REHABILITATION/ RESTORATIVE CARE

A person may need rehabilitation because of a **disability.** A disability exists when the person has an impairment that affects the ability to perform an activity that a person of that age would normally be able to do. Adults, for example, are able to dress and undress independently. If a person is unable to do this because of a disease or injury, a disability exists. A disability may be temporary or permanent. Impairments or disabilities result from trauma or disease. Disorders of the musculoskeletal system, such as amputation (Figure 41-3) of an extremity or arthritis, may require rehabilitation.

A **handicap** exists if the disability limits or prevents the person from fulfilling a role that is normal for that person.

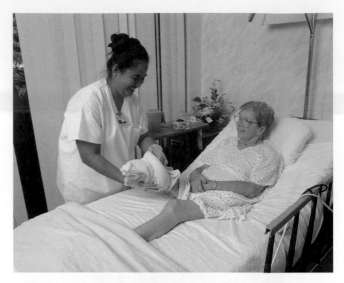

FIGURE 41-3 Patients who have had an amputation often benefit from intensive rehabilitation and a companion restorative nursing program. (© *Delmar/Cengage Learning*)

This might include such functions as holding a job, managing a household, and raising a family.

If a disability is permanent, such as tetraplegia (paralysis from the neck down) from a spinal cord injury, it is unrealistic to expect that rehabilitation will enable the patient to walk again. In these situations, the goals will be to teach the patient to:

- Adapt to the present circumstances.
- Use adaptive devices to increase independence.
- Learn new ways of doing routine tasks, such as dressing or bathing.
- Become as independent as possible in light of the disability. Patients with severely limiting conditions, such as tetraplegia, are taught to assume responsibility for personal well-being, including verbally directing caregivers to accomplish the results the patient wants.

THE INTERDISCIPLINARY HEALTH CARE TEAM

Physicians who specialize in rehabilitation are called **physiatrists.** Nurses and nursing assistants who work in rehabilitation receive specialized education. Many other disciplines may be involved in the rehabilitation process. For instance, a person who has had a stroke may receive:

- Physical therapy to learn how to walk again
- Occupational therapy to relearn the activities of daily living
- Speech therapy to learn new communication or swallowing methods
- Nursing services for bowel and bladder management, prevention of pressure ulcers, and other complications

- Dietitian services to help the patient learn to manage new dietary restrictions for a low-sodium diet (to reduce blood pressure), and to plan and prepare meals
- Psychological support to adapt to the sudden changes brought about by the stroke
- Social services to plan for the impending discharge

All disciplines work together with the patient and family to solve problems and plan care. There are many subspecialties in rehabilitation. Health care professionals may choose to work in **geriatric** (care of the elderly) or pediatric rehabilitation. Others may specialize in the care of patients with strokes, spinal cord injuries, brain injuries, amputations, burns, or arthritis.

THE ROLE OF THE NURSING ASSISTANT

The nursing assistant who works in the rehabilitation and restorative nursing unit will assist the nurses with:

- Procedures to prevent complications
- Mobility skills (transfers and ambulation)
- Bathing and personal care procedures
- Bowel and bladder management programs
- Maintaining the patient's nutritional status
- Programs to increase the patient's independence

PRINCIPLES OF REHABILITATION

Four principles form the foundation of successful rehabilitation or restorative care.

1. *Treatment begins as soon as possible.*

   This means that services begin as soon as the patient's condition is stable. For example, if a patient has had a stroke, passive exercises and positioning techniques are initiated in the critical care unit to prevent contractures, pressure ulcers, and other complications that would prohibit or delay rehabilitation.

2. *Stress the person's ability, not the disability.*

   Workers must think in terms of what the patient can do, not what he or she cannot do. The patient's strengths are used to help in adapting to limitations. A *strength* refers to anything the patient can do. Perhaps a patient whose dominant hand is paralyzed cannot use that hand to feed himself—but instead of having nursing staff feed him, he can be taught to use the other, stronger hand. Use the restorative philosophy when communicating with patients. Avoid statements such as, "You *can't* use your right hand." Instead, say, "You *can* use your left hand." Allow the patient to struggle a little, but avoid letting him progress to the point of frustration before you step in to assist.

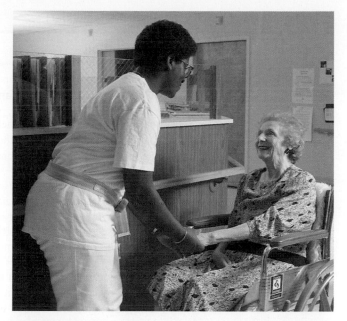

FIGURE 41-4 The patient's mental and emotional state are as important as her physical condition. (© *Delmar/Cengage Learning*)

3. *Activity strengthens and inactivity weakens.*

   Complications result from physical and mental inactivity. These can cause further disability or even be life-threatening. A rehabilitation or restorative plan of care always includes approaches and goals for physical and mental activity.

4. *Treat the whole person.*

   When we give care to patients, we are concerned with the whole person (Figure 41-4). We must also work with the patients' families. They directly influence the emotional and mental health of the patients.

Keys to success in rehabilitation and restorative nursing programs are:

- Teamwork. All staff cooperate with each other and other departments involved in care of the patient.
- Use of the care plan. All staff are familiar with the patient's problems, goals, and approaches.
- Consistency of care. All staff use the same approaches (as listed on the care plan) when caring for the patient.
- Continuity of care. There is a smooth progression and flow between caregivers and between shifts.
- Good communication among all caregivers, the patient, and interested family members.

COMPLICATIONS FROM INACTIVITY

People with disabilities may be unable to move about at will. The inactivity or immobility can result in numerous complications affecting body systems, as shown in Table 41-2.

TABLE 41-2 COMPLICATIONS OF IMMOBILITY

System	Complication
Integumentary	Pressure ulcers may develop in a short time from lack of oxygen to the tissues. Pressure ulcers may worsen quickly and be difficult or impossible to reverse.
Muscular	Weakness and atrophy from lack of use. Contractures (Figure 41-5) develop because of the patient's position, freezing the muscle in a permanent state of flexion. Contractures are painful and difficult or impossible to reverse.
Skeletal	Calcium drains from the bones when they are inactive. This contributes to fractures, lack of healing, osteoporosis, and other complications.
Respiratory	Fluid and secretions collect in the lungs. The patient has more difficulty expanding the lungs, increasing the risk of pneumonia and other lung infections.
Circulatory	Blood clots caused by pooling of blood and pressure on the legs (Figure 41-6). Edema may be caused by lack of movement. The heart must work harder to pump blood through the body. Changes in the blood vessels may cause dizziness and fainting when the patient is placed in the upright position.
Genitourinary	The extra calcium in the system from the bones promotes the development of kidney stones. Retention of urine is common, and is often caused by the patient's position in bed. Overflow of a full bladder leads to incontinence. The patient is at high risk of urinary tract infection.
Gastrointestinal	Indigestion and heartburn may result if the patient is not positioned properly for meals. Loss of appetite may occur from lack of activity, illness, and boredom. Constipation and fecal impaction result from immobility.
Nervous	Weakness and limited mobility. Insomnia may result from sleeping too much during the day, then being unable to sleep at night.
Mental changes	Irritability, boredom, lethargy, and depression result from the patient's frustration and feelings of helplessness. Lack of social contact and sensory stimulation result in disorientation (Figure 41-7).

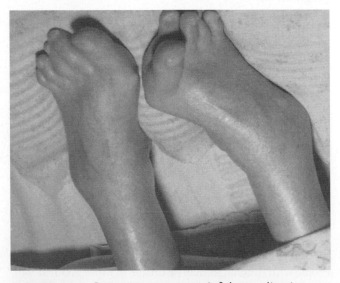

FIGURE 41-5 Contractures are a painful complication of immobility. This patient has foot drop, a serious contracture of the feet. (© Delmar/Cengage Learning)

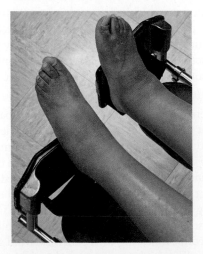

FIGURE 41-6 Patients with heart, circulatory, or kidney problems may develop edema of the lower extremities. (The patient's shoes have been removed so the edema could be pictured. Never get a patient up in a chair without proper foot covering.) (© Delmar/Cengage Learning)

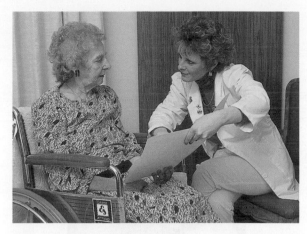

FIGURE 41-7 Immobility and lack of sensory stimulation often result in disorientation of elderly persons. (© Delmar/Cengage Learning)

ACTIVITIES OF DAILY LIVING

One purpose of restorative care is to increase the person's physical abilities. Healthy adults do ADLs automatically. If a person cannot complete any or all of the ADLs, a **self-care deficit** exists. Deficits are caused by problems that limit the ability to do self care, such as decreased strength, lack of endurance, or disorientation.

Patients with self-care deficits are evaluated by therapists and nurses. The results of the evaluations will determine whether the patient's functional (physical) abilities can be increased. In other words, can the interdisciplinary team help this patient to relearn an activity of daily living? This is discussed with the patient and the family (Figure 41-8).

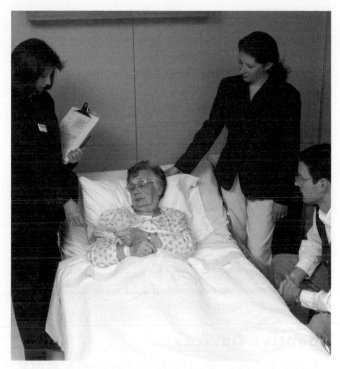

FIGURE 41-8 Members of the interdisciplinary team evaluate the patient to determine whether she will benefit from a restoration or rehabilitation program. Part of the evaluation involves meeting with the patient and her family to learn what their goals are. (© Delmar/Cengage Learning)

Clinical Information ALERT

Elderly and chronically ill patients usually lose independence by degrees. Loss of independence as a result of trauma can be devastating for the patient. Imagine being normal one minute, then having an auto accident that leaves you completely paralyzed. This type of injury immediately changes the lives of the patient and her entire family. Some patients will regain all or part of their independence, but most have to cope with the loss and adjust activities and routines to disability. Because their bodies now work differently, they must learn to do things differently. This is also difficult and frustrating. Being completely unable to perform ADLs is even more frustrating. Despite the best medical and rehabilitative care, an unfortunate few will be physically dependent on others for the rest of their lives. One important goal of rehabilitation and restorative nursing is to promote mental and emotional independence, so the patient can direct his or her care. ■

Clinical Information ALERT

We normally think of the grieving process in relation to death and dying. However, the process applies to any major loss. Patients and families experience the grieving process because of disability and loss of independence. The stage of grieving often affects rehabilitation and safety. Some health care workers label patients as "difficult" or "trying" when in fact they are grieving. Avoid stereotyping and labeling patients. Recognize the stages of the grieving process and use the skills you learned in Unit 33 to support the patient. ■

Restorative Programs

If the patient has the potential to relearn an ADL and is motivated to try, a restorative program is planned. These programs are sometimes called *retraining programs* or *ADL programs*.

Approaches Used in Restorative Programs

The approaches to use will be listed on the care plan. It is important that the same approach be used consistently.

- *Setup.* Patients with self-care deficits are not able to set up or prepare for activities of daily living. You may need to provide the setup (Figure 41-9).
- *Verbal cues.* The care provider uses short, simple phrases to prompt the patient. Example: Give the patient a prepared washcloth and then say, "Please wash your face" (Figure 41-10).
- *Hand-over-hand techniques.* Example for eating program: Place a glass in the patient's hand. Place your hand over the patient's hand. Guide the glass to the patient's mouth (Figure 41-11).
- *Demonstration.* Act out what you want the patient to do. Example: Before giving the patient a toothbrush, make the motions of brushing your teeth with the toothbrush (Figure 41-12).

Adaptive Devices

Adaptive devices are sometimes used to simplify an ADL. **Adaptive devices** are ordinary items that have been modified for use by patients with various types of problems. A person with a disability may be unable to perform certain ADLs. Adding a device that changes the way the task is done may enable the person to perform it independently. The person is taught to use the device for everyday tasks

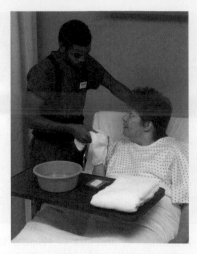

FIGURE 41-10 The nursing assistant uses verbal cues to assist the patient with ADLs. *(© Delmar/Cengage Learning)*

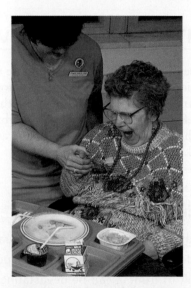

FIGURE 41-11 Hand-over-hand technique is another approach that helps patients relearn essential skills. *(© Delmar/Cengage Learning)*

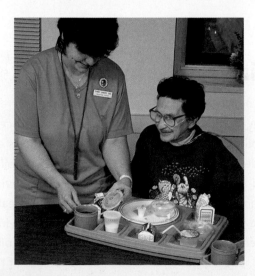

FIGURE 41-9 This patient is able to feed herself if the nursing assistant sets up the tray. *(© Delmar/Cengage Learning)*

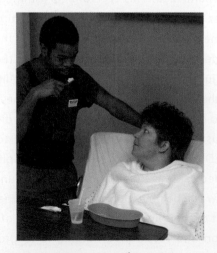

FIGURE 41-12 Demonstrating the activity is a good way to help the patient understand the directions. *(© Delmar/Cengage Learning)*

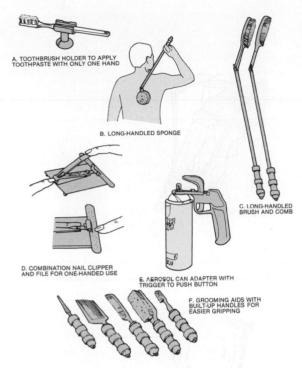

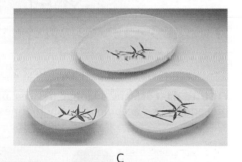

A. TOOTHBRUSH HOLDER TO APPLY TOOTHPASTE WITH ONLY ONE HAND

B. LONG-HANDLED SPONGE

C. LONG-HANDLED BRUSH AND COMB

D. COMBINATION NAIL CLIPPER AND FILE FOR ONE-HANDED USE

E. AEROSOL CAN ADAPTER WITH TRIGGER TO PUSH BUTTON

F. GROOMING AIDS WITH BUILT-UP HANDLES FOR EASIER GRIPPING

FIGURE 41-13 These devices enable the patient to be independent with grooming and personal hygiene. *(© Delmar/Cengage Learning)*

(Figure 41-13). Your role as a nursing assistant is to make sure the device is clean, available, and used by the patient. You may need to work on the skill with the patient while she is learning to use the device. The care plan will provide instructions on the types of devices the patient uses.

Adaptive devices for eating The most common adaptive devices are used to enable patients to feed themselves. Many individual devices are available to meet patients' needs. The most common devices are adaptive silverware (Figures 41-14A and 41-14B), plates and plate guards (Figure 41-14C), and cups (Figure 41-14D). Other items, such as a straw holder (Figure 41-14E), may also be necessary.

Adaptive devices for dressing Dressing aids are also commonly used (Figures 41-15). These devices make it easier for patients to dress themselves. Using these adaptive devices may appear awkward to you, but being able to dress independently is important to a patient's self-esteem.

Adaptive devices for grooming and hygiene Being able to bathe and groom oneself are important skills. Everyone has a personal hygienic routine. Grooming and hygiene are very private activities. Using adaptive devices (Figure 41-16) permits the patient to perform these skills and increases self-esteem and comfort.

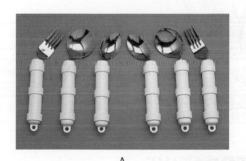

A

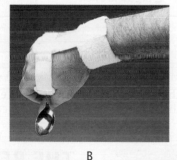

B

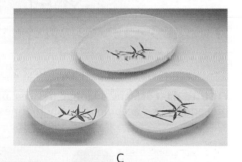

C

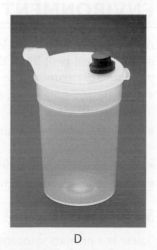

D

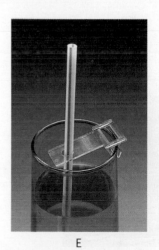

E

FIGURE 41-14 A. Many types of adaptive utensils are available to meet individual needs and enable patients to feed themselves. B. The wrist cuff enables the patient to hold silverware and eat independently. C. Adaptive plates and bowls have raised edges so patients can scoop food easily. D. An adaptive cup. E. The straw holder centers the straw and holds it in place. *(Courtesy of Maddak, Inc.)*

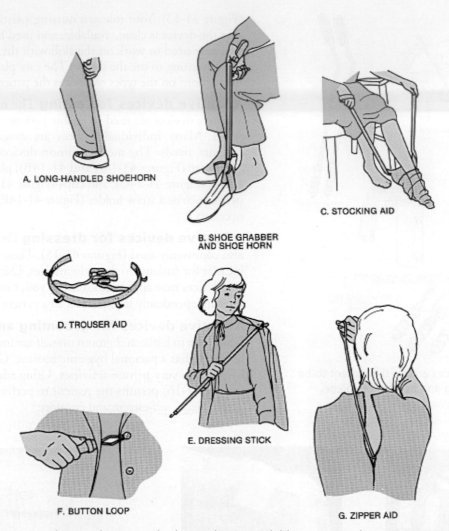

A. LONG-HANDLED SHOEHORN

B. SHOE GRABBER AND SHOE HORN

C. STOCKING AID

D. TROUSER AID

E. DRESSING STICK

F. BUTTON LOOP

G. ZIPPER AID

FIGURE 41-15 Many adaptive devices and other tools are available to ensure that patients are able to perform self-care procedures and accomplish daily routines at the highest level of independence possible. (© Delmar/Cengage Learning)

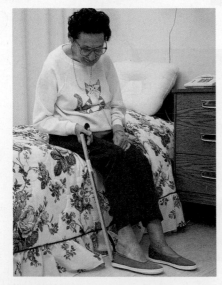

FIGURE 41-16 The patient learned how to use this device by working with the occupational therapist. Now she uses it independently to put her shoes on each day. (© Delmar/Cengage Learning)

THE RESTORATIVE ENVIRONMENT

All patients benefit from living in an environment that promotes quality of life. The interdisciplinary team helps promote this environment.

- Give the patient a sense of control and opportunities to make decisions.
- Remember that mental and physical activity are essential to well-being.
- Provide cues for orientation.
- Create an environment that is safe, serene, and colorful.

Safety Concerns

Safety is a primary concern when there is a loss of function. If a patient's condition changes, evaluate his or her awareness. If the level of consciousness or mental status has changed, report to your supervisor. Changes in consciousness and mental status may indicate serious problems. Other important observations that should be reported are:

- Whether the patient is aware of the change
- Whether the patient denies that there has been a change
- Whether the patient asks for assistance when needed
- The patient's desire to remain independent despite the increased safety risk
- Any falls that you know of
- Changes in vision
- Changes in bowel and bladder control
- The patient's ability to ambulate
- Problems with standing, balance, or coordination

If you observe any of these changes, notify your supervisor immediately. A licensed health care professional will assess the patient. He or she makes other team members aware of the changes. They will reevaluate the care plan and write new approaches, if necessary. The restorative program will be designed with the changes in mind. The overall goal is keeping the patient safe.

If the patient has been on bedrest for a long time, he or she must gradually increase activity. Inactivity and bedrest cause changes in blood pressure and balance. Your supervisor will develop a schedule to gradually increase the length of time that the patient will be up.

GUIDELINES *for*

Restorative Care

- Become familiar with the patient's condition.
- Provide restorative care at the usual time of day for the activity.
  - Make sure that the treatment area is ready, equipment is gathered, and the patient's physical needs are met before beginning.
- Follow the instructions on the care plan. Check frequently for changes to the plan.
- Provide privacy. The patient will make mistakes and become frustrated. Avoid embarrassing the patient in front of others.
- Eliminate as many distractions as possible.
- Apply orthotic and prosthetic devices as ordered. These will be listed on the care plan. Orthotic devices improve function and prevent deformities. Prosthetic devices are replacements for body parts, such as the eye, breast, hand, leg, or foot.
- Modify the environment to promote independence, if necessary.
- Practice good body mechanics for yourself and the patient.
- Practice safety, and teach the patient safety measures.
- Remember that all ADLs have many steps. If the patient cannot complete one step, he or she will not be able to complete the activity.
- Treat the patient with dignity.
- Be positive and encouraging. Stress what the patient can do.
- Give the patient as much control as possible by allowing him or her to make choices and decisions.

- Allow enough time for the activity. Be patient and avoid rushing the patient.
- Work on one step at a time. When the patient masters one step, move to the next.
  - Remember that the patient's progress may be inconsistent from one day to the next.
- Provide frequent, positive feedback during the procedure.
- Be patient.
- Provide simple, clear directions. Keep directions as clear and simple as possible. If the patient does not understand, demonstrate.
- Give verbal cues, whenever necessary, to describe what you want the patient to do.
- If the patient does not respond to verbal cues, use hand-over-hand technique. Place your hand on top of the patient's hand and guide him or her to begin the activity. If the patient does not respond, replace your hand and guide the patient through the activity.
- Allow the patient to do as much self-care as possible. Show the patient that you are confident in his or her ability.
- Use adaptive devices, if necessary.
- If the patient cannot complete an ADL, praise his or her accomplishment. Complete the task without comment or complaint.
- Report your observations to your supervisor. Notify the proper person if you feel that the patient's condition requires evaluation.
- Document care immediately after providing it. Never document in advance.

MONITORING THE PATIENT'S RESPONSE TO CARE

You must observe how the restorative program affects the patient. This is particularly true in the early stages of an illness. The patient may become easily frustrated. Allow the patient to struggle a little. Intervene before the patient reaches the point of frustration. Remind him or her that learning takes time. Practice empathy. Tell the patient you understand how frustrated he or she feels. Be aware of the patient's fears. A fear of falling or spilling may prevent the patient from participating in an activity or attempting to do a task.

Early in the restorative program, the patient may have an unexpected physical response. You have learned that even a short period of bedrest has a negative effect on the body. Any physical activity may cause a change in the physical condition. Monitor for signs of fatigue. Be alert for changes, and report them to your supervisor. A good practice is to take the patient's pulse before beginning, then perform the activity. Monitor the pulse every five minutes during the activity. Normally, the pulse increases slightly with activity. Assuming the pulse is under 100 during the activity, continue. If the rate is more than 100, or if the patient develops other problems, such as pain, shortness of breath, nausea, or perspiration, stop the activity. If the patient is standing, assist him or her to sit down. Notify your supervisor or a nurse immediately. Pull the call signal, or send someone else to get help. Do not leave the patient alone. After you complete the activity, check the pulse again. It should return to within 10 beats of the resting pulse rate within 5 minutes.

Precautions and Special Situations

Patients with certain conditions require special care and handling. Avoid exercising extremities that have fractures or dislocations. The bones of patients with osteoporosis or bone cancer break easily. Osteoporosis is a condition in which bone mass decreases, leading to fractures with little or no trauma. Check with your supervisor and the care plan before continuing. Notify a nurse if the patient has a wound, red, or open area on the joint you are exercising. Inquire if exercise will be harmful before continuing. If a patient is combative or resists care, explain why it is important. Try to coax him or her into participating. Try singing a song with the patient for distraction. Avoid forcing a patient to accept care. Notify your supervisor if the patient continues to refuse.

REVIEW

A. Multiple Choice

Select the one best answer for each of the following.

1. A patient with a permanent disability is
   a. taught to adapt to the present circumstances.
   b. not a good candidate for rehabilitation.
   c. given much sympathy.
   d. encouraged to be helpless.

2. Disabilities may result from
   a. too much exercise.
   b. getting inadequate sleep.
   c. spinal cord injury.
   d. not drinking enough water.

3. A patient who is unable to communicate verbally will be treated by a
   a. physical therapist.
   b. occupational therapist.
   c. nursing assistant.
   d. speech language pathologist.

4. Physical inactivity is *most likely* to cause
   a. pressure ulcers.
   b. dehydration.
   c. pain.
   d. infection.

5. Adaptive devices are
   a. inappropriate for patients receiving rehabilitation.
   b. used by nursing assistants to feed patients.
   c. ordinary items modified for use by patients who have self-care deficits.
   d. used only by occupational therapists.

6. Placing your hand over the patient's hand to guide an action is
   a. giving verbal cues.
   b. demonstration.
   c. hand-over-hand technique.
   d. setting up.

7. When providing restorative care, the nursing assistant should
   a. stress what the patient can do. ✓
   b. treat only signs related to the diagnosis.
   c. begin treatment after the patient's recovery.
   d. encourage the patient to rest.

8. If a person cannot complete one or more ADLs, he or she has a/an
   a. readiness for enhanced self-care.
   b. activity impairment.
   c. risk for compromised ADLs.
   d. self-care deficit. ✗

9. ADLs are
   a. things you buy at the store.
   b. actions during life.
   c. all done in life.
   d. activities of daily living.

10. Restorative nursing care is designed to
    a. be given only by licensed personnel.
    b. require the skills of a therapist.
    c. maintain or improve patients' conditions.
    d. promote dependence in ADLs.

B. Nursing Assistant Challenge

You are working as a nursing assistant in the rehabilitation unit of a subacute care section of a skilled nursing facility. Think about what you have learned in this unit and answer the following questions.

11. What types of patients will you see?

12. What kinds of disabilities will the patients have?

13. List some causes of self-care deficits.

14. What kinds of problems can limit a person's ability to do self-care?

15. What are the differences between rehabilitation and restorative care?

Response to Basic Emergencies

UNIT 42

Response to Basic Emergencies

OBJECTIVES

After completing this unit, you will be able to:

- Spell and define terms.
- Recognize emergency situations that require urgent care.
- Evaluate situations and determine the actions to be taken.
- List and describe the 11 standardized codes.
- Describe how to maintain the patient's airway and breathing.
- Recognize the need for CPR.
- List the benefits of early defibrillation.
- Identify the signs, symptoms, and treatment of common emergency situations.
- Demonstrate the following procedures:
  - Procedure 107 Head-Tilt, Chin-Lift Maneuver
  - Procedure 108 Jaw-Thrust Maneuver

- Procedure 109 Mask-to-Mouth Ventilation
- Procedure 110 Positioning the Patient in the Recovery Position
- Procedure 111 Heimlich Maneuver—Abdominal Thrusts
- Procedure 112 Assisting the Adult Who Has an Obstructed Airway and Becomes Unconscious
- Procedure 113 Obstructed Airway: Infant
- Procedure 114 Assisting a Child Who Has a Foreign Body Airway Obstruction

VOCABULARY

Learn the meaning and the correct spelling of the following words and phrases:

adjunctive devices	defibrillation	head-tilt, chin-lift	respiratory arrest
automatic external	dislocation	maneuver	respiratory failure
defibrillator (AED)	emergency	Heimlich maneuver	shock
cardiac arrest	emergency care	hemorrhage	sprain
cardiopulmonary	Emergency Medical	jaw-thrust maneuver	strain
resuscitation	Services (EMS)	pocket mask	ventilation
(CPR)	first aid	recovery position	victim

DEALING WITH EMERGENCIES

An **emergency** is an unexpected situation that requires immediate action. In a true emergency, prompt action is needed to prevent complications and to save the life of the **victim** (person needing help). Nursing assistants must recognize common emergencies and take immediate, decisive action. The guidelines in this chapter are basic actions to remember for any emergency.

GUIDELINES *for*

Responding to an Emergency

- Always remember the priorities of any emergency as the ABCs:
  - **A**irway: obstructed or unobstructed?
  - **B**reathing: is the victim able to breathe?
  - **C**irculation: is the heart beating, is there bleeding?
- Stay calm. Nothing is accomplished and more problems will result if the people at the scene of the emergency become upset. If you are calm, you will be a calming influence on the victim.
- Know how to summon immediate help. Stay with the victim and call out for help. If you are out in the community, tell the closest person to call. **Emergency Medical Services (EMS)**.
- Do not move the victim unless he or she is in danger.
- Stay with the victim until the person in charge gives you permission to leave.
- Know your limitations. Provide care for which you have been trained and are qualified to give.
- Know the code names for various emergencies in your facility.
- Know the procedures for activating the Emergency Medical Services (EMS) system (Figure 42-1). In most areas, you will dial 9-1-1 (Figure 42-2).
- Keep the victim warm. Cover with blankets.
- Do not give the victim any fluids or food.
- If the victim starts to vomit, turn the head to one side to avoid aspiration.
- If the victim is conscious, reassure him or her.
- Protect the victim's privacy. Keep other people away from the scene unless they are qualified to assist.
- Apply standard precautions to prevent exposure to blood, body fluids, mucous membranes, and nonintact skin during the emergency.

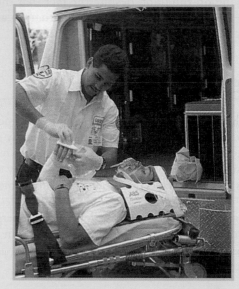

FIGURE 42-1 Know the procedure for activating the EMS system in your community. (© *Delmar/Cengage Learning*)

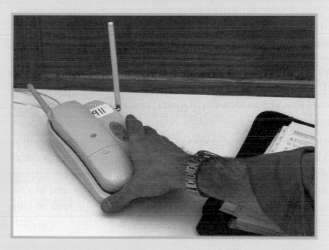

FIGURE 42-2 9-1-1 is the universal telephone number for obtaining professional help in an emergency in the United States. (© *Delmar/Cengage Learning*)

BEING PREPARED

While working in the hospital or long-term care facility, you are always close to professional medical help. When you witness an accident away from the medical facility, professional help is not always readily available. Whatever course of action you choose, the victim should not be further endangered.

First Aid

First aid includes immediate care for victims of illness or injury. This care is especially important if medical help is delayed or is not available.

Evaluating the Situation

At the scene of an accident, evaluate the situation and identify the injuries. Quickly note the number of victims, their injuries, and any dangerous factors at the scene.

In the medical facility, unless there is a fire, you usually will be dealing with a single victim. You will be able to focus on the needs of that individual. For example, you might enter a patient's room and find the patient lying on the floor, despite the fact that the bed side rails are up. Quickly evaluate the situation as you signal for help.

CODE EMERGENCIES

Most health care facilities call the various types of emergencies *codes*. They have code designations for many situations. The most common of these is a cardiac arrest. In 1999, three employees of a hospital were killed by an intruder. As a result, a trade association met with its member facilities to establish standardized emergency codes. The California Hospital Association adopted the emergency code words listed in Table 42-1. Many facilities in other states also adopted the code words. As a result, they are being used throughout the country.

Assisting with a Code

Your responsibilities in a code are determined by the facility. Many facilities have unannounced "mock code" practices. For example, personnel respond to a cardiac arrest code and find that a manikin is being used. However, the code is conducted as if it were a real patient. This provides everyone with an opportunity to practice their skills, learn their responsibilities, and become comfortable with and proficient in providing lifesaving care.

Always follow the directions of the nurse in an emergency. A code is a very busy time, and many tasks must be accomplished in a rapid, orderly manner. Accuracy is very important. Become familiar with your responsibilities so that you are confident in your ability to perform your best in this highly critical situation.

TABLE 42-1 STANDARDIZED CODE WORDS

- Code Red: Fire
- Code Blue: Medical emergency—adult
- Code White: Medical emergency—pediatric
- Code Pink: Infant abduction
- Code Purple: Child abduction
- Code Yellow: Bomb threat
- Code Gray: Combative person
- Code Silver: Person with a weapon and/or hostage situation
- Code Orange: Hazardous material spill/release
- Code Triage Internal: An internal disaster
- Code Triage External: An external disaster

EMERGENCY CARE

Emergency care is care that must be given right away to prevent loss of life.

- Whether you are out in the community or in the health care facility, ask someone nearby to summon help.
- Do not leave people who need urgent care to get help yourself. (Exception—CPR)
- As help is on the way, check, in the following order, for the victim's:
  - Degree of responsiveness
  - Airway/breathing capability
  - Presence and rate of heartbeat
  - Signs of bleeding
  - Signs of shock
- Do not move the victim if you do not have to.
- Do not allow the victim to get up and walk around.
- Check for other injuries.

Maintaining the Patient's Breathing

The normal respiratory rate is determined by age. **Respiratory failure** occurs when breathing is insufficient to sustain life. **Respiratory arrest** occurs when breathing stops. It is caused by many conditions, including heart attack and stroke. Follow the criteria in Table 42-2 to determine if the patient's breathing is adequate. Stay with the patient and use the call signal or telephone to request assistance. Report problems to the nurse immediately.

Opening the Airway

If you discover that a patient is in respiratory failure or respiratory arrest, remain in the room and call for help. Open the patient's airway. The most common cause of airway obstruction is the tongue falling back into the throat. Opening the airway lifts the tongue from the back of the throat, making breathing easier. This procedure, as well as some other procedures in this unit, is most effective when the

TABLE 42-2 MONITORING FOR BREATHING ADEQUACY

- The patient can talk, and respirations are between 12 and 20.
- The rhythm is regular.
- The patient's color is normal, with no cyanosis or gray coloration.
- The chest expands equally with each inspiration.
- Listen and feel for breath sounds on your cheek and ear by kneeling next to the patient's nose and mouth, if necessary. The sounds should be quiet and normal.

patient is lying in the supine position. Always remove the pillow. Position the patient on the back before beginning.

Because of the nature of the situation, you may not have time to wash your hands or perform other initial procedure actions. Immediately after the patient is safe, wash your hands well. Avoid contact with secretions if you are not wearing gloves or other protective equipment. Obtain protective apparel as soon as you can safely do so.

The **head-tilt, chin-lift maneuver** (Procedure 107) is the most common method of opening the airway. If the victim has a neck injury, do not perform this procedure. Instead, use the jaw-thrust maneuver.

The **jaw-thrust maneuver** (Procedure 108) is used to open the airway of persons with known or suspected neck injuries, and for those whose airways cannot be opened using the head-tilt, chin-lift method.

PROCEDURE

HEAD-TILT, CHIN-LIFT MANEUVER

1. Place one hand on the victim's forehead. Place the fingers of the opposite hand below the center of the jaw bone, directly under the chin.

2. Tilt the victim's head back gently.

3. With your fingertips, lift the lower jaw forward (Figure 42-3).

4. Keep the victim's mouth open.

5. As soon as the patient is safe, and the nurse or other professionals have assumed responsibility for care, wash your hands well.

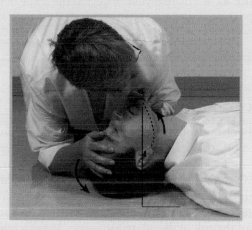

FIGURE 42-3 Use the head-tilt, chin-lift technique to open the airway unless head injury is suspected. (© Delmar/Cengage Learning)

PROCEDURE

JAW-THRUST MANEUVER

1. Move the patient into the supine position as a single unit. Avoid twisting the neck, back, or spine during movement.

2. Pull the head of the bed away from the wall.

3. Position yourself above the patient's head.

4. Position your elbows on the mattress.

5. Using your forearms, stabilize the sides of the patient's head to prevent movement.

6. Place one hand on each side of the lower jaw, just below the ears (Figure 42-4).

continues

PROCEDURE 108 CONTINUED

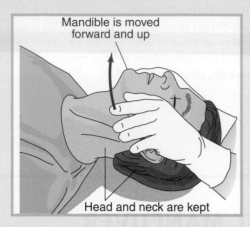

Mandible is moved forward and up

Head and neck are kept

FIGURE 42-4 Position your fingers at the angle of the jaw, pushing it upward and forward. (© Delmar/Cengage Learning)

7. Use the tips of your index fingers to push the lower jaw forward.

8. Keep the patient's mouth open. If necessary, pull the chin forward. Avoid inserting your fingers into the mouth.

9. If the patient cannot maintain this position, maintain the airway manually, by holding your hands in place, if necessary.

10. As soon as the patient is safe, and the nurse or other professionals have assumed responsibility for care, wash your hands well.

Mask-to-Mouth Resuscitation

When a person stops breathing, his respirations must be sustained by artificial means to prevent brain damage and other complications. If you have taken a CPR class, you may have learned mouth-to-mouth **ventilation**. This is a technique of breathing for the victim. Most health care facilities discourage staff from using this method on patients because of the risk of disease transmission. Various **adjunctive devices** are used instead. An airway adjunct is a secondary device used to maintain respirations. This is done by a trained and qualified health care professional.

Mask-to-mouth ventilation is performed using a **pocket mask** (Figure 42-5). This is a temporary measure until more advanced airway support becomes available. The mask has a special valve that prevents the patient's exhaled air and secretions from entering the caregiver's mouth. (Refer to Procedure 109.)

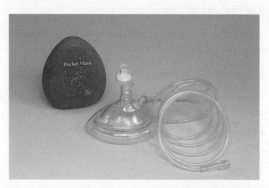

FIGURE 42-5 A pocket mask is a simple, efficient device that provides a one-way barrier if mouth-to-mouth (mask) ventilation is necessary. Supplemental oxygen may be added by connecting the tubing to the male adapter on the mask. However, do not delay resuscitation if oxygen is not available. (© Delmar/Cengage Learning)

PROCEDURE

MASK-TO-MOUTH VENTILATION

1. Supplies needed:
   - Disposable exam gloves
   - Pocket mask with anti-reflux (one-way) valve

2. Pull the head of the bed away from the wall.

3. Apply gloves.

4. Open the patient's airway using the head-tilt, chin-lift method or the jaw-thrust maneuver.

5. Position yourself at the patient's head.

PROCEDURE 109 CONTINUED

6. Position the mask on the patient's face, with the small end over the bridge of the nose and the wide end on the patient's chin. Center the ventilation port over the patient's mouth.

7. Seal the mask by positioning your thumbs on the top of the mask and fingers at the sides. Hold the airway in the open position.

8. Take a normal breath, then seal your mouth over the ventilation port, exhaling into the mask. The ventilation should take 1 second in adults. During the ventilation, look at the patient's chest. It should rise as you blow air in. If it does not, reposition the airway and try again.

Note: Remember to take a normal breath, not a deep breath, to avoid overinflating the patient's lungs or filling the stomach with air.

9. Remove your mouth from the mask and allow the patient to exhale passively. Continue to breathe into the mask once every 5 to 6 seconds.

Age-Appropriate Care ALERT

Turn the pocket mask upside down if the victim of respiratory arrest is an infant or child. ∎

Cardiac Arrest

When respiratory arrest occurs, the person stops breathing but still has a heartbeat. The heart will stop unless the problem is not reversed quickly. **Cardiac arrest** is the term used when the heart has stopped beating and respirations have ceased. When this occurs, blood and oxygen are not circulated to the rest of the body. The person is clinically dead.

Permanent damage to the brain occurs within 4 to 6 minutes. Signs of cardiac arrest are:

- No response from the victim
- No breathing can be detected
- No pulse

Cardiopulmonary resuscitation (CPR) is a procedure used to maintain circulation until the EMS (or a facility code team) can respond. *You must never perform CPR unless you have completed an approved course.* The American Heart Association and the American Red Cross both offer such courses. The information in this book is not intended to take the place of an approved course. Use these guidelines as a quick reference or refresher.

In the health care facility, you must know whether CPR is to be initiated. A patient with an advance directive may not wish to be resuscitated if cardiac arrest occurs. In this situation, the patient will have a "do not resuscitate" (DNR) or "no code" order (Figure 42-6). (See Unit 33.) If there is no DNR order, full life support measures are given for cardiac arrest. For additional information, refer to the Online Companion for your book.

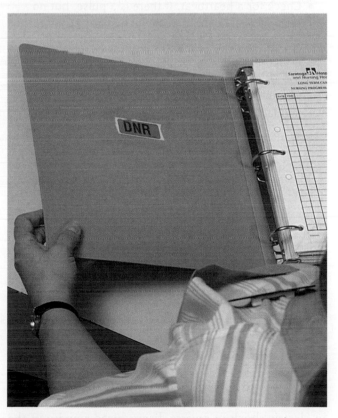

FIGURE 42-6 A DNR on the patient's chart means the patient does not wish to be resuscitated in the event of cardiac arrest. A physician's order is needed to place a patient on DNR status. (© *Delmar/Cengage Learning*)

GUIDELINES *for*

Performing CPR

 Note: Perform CPR *only* if you have completed an approved course, taught by an approved instructor.

- Follow standard precautions if at all possible. Wear gloves and use a barrier device. If the victim is bleeding, a gown, mask, and eye protection may also be necessary. In a health care facility, these items should be readily available.

- Careful evaluation is required before CPR is administered.

Adult Victim

- Call for help, or have another person call the EMS system.

- For CPR to be effective, the victim must be lying on his back on a hard surface.

- Make sure the victim's airway is open. Look, listen, and feel for breathing.

- If the victim is not breathing, ventilate 2 times, taking 1 second for each ventilation.

- Check for a heartbeat. If there is a pulse, but no respirations, continue with ventilations at the rate of 1 every 6 to 8 seconds.

- If there is no pulse, begin chest compressions at the ratio of 30 compressions to 2 ventilations. Compressions should be smooth, rhythmic, hard, and fast. Make sure hand placement on the sternum

is correct, and compress the victim's chest straight down $1\frac{1}{2}$ to 2 inches.

- With 2 rescuers, one rescuer does chest compressions and the other checks for pulse and breathing and gives ventilations. The ratio remains 30 compressions to 2 ventilations.

- Two rescuers may switch positions and roles about every 2 minutes; try to complete the switch in 5 seconds or less.

Infant Victim

- The compression-to-ventilation ratio is the same as for adults: 30 compressions to 2 ventilations.

- If there are 2 rescuers, use a 15:2 ratio of compressions to breaths.

- Breaths are given with the rescuer's mouth covering the infant's nose *and* mouth.

- Breaths must be gentle because of an infant's small size; do not overinflate the lungs.

- Use your fingers to give chest compressions. Compress about $\frac{1}{3}$ to $\frac{1}{2}$ the depth of the chest. Do not compress over the xiphoid process.

For additional information, refer to the Online Companion for your book.

THE RECOVERY POSITION

If the victim is unresponsive, but is breathing and has a pulse, she should be positioned in the **recovery position** after the emergency is over, to prevent complications. The recovery position is a modified lateral position (Figure 42-7).

EARLY DEFIBRILLATION

Public access to defibrillation has proven to be highly successful. **Defibrillation** is a method of treatment that uses an electric shock to reverse disorganized activity in the heart during cardiac arrest. Early defibrillation has proven to be critical to survival in a victim with cardiac arrest. In health care facilities, the goal is to defibrillate within 3 minutes.

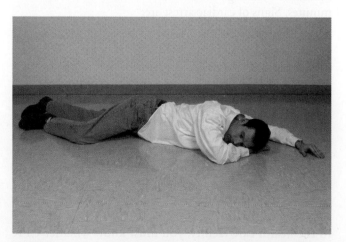

FIGURE 42-7 If the victim is breathing but not conscious, place him in the recovery position. (© *Delmar/Cengage Learning*)

PROCEDURE

110

POSITIONING THE PATIENT IN THE RECOVERY POSITION

1. Kneel beside the patient and straighten his legs.

2. Place the arm nearest you above the patient's head, with the palm up and the elbow bent slightly.

3. Position his opposite arm across his chest.

4. Place your lower hand on the patient's thigh on the far side of the body. Pull the thigh up slightly, closer to the center of the patient's body.

5. Place your upper hand on the patient's shoulder on the opposite side of the body.

6. With one hand on the thigh and the other on the shoulder, roll the patient onto his side, facing you.

7. Move the patient's upper hand close to the cheek, bending the elbow. This hand should be close to the face, but not under the body. Adjust the upper body so that the hip and knee are at right angles.

8. Tilt the patient's head back slightly to keep the airway open. Now place his upper hand, palm facing down, under the cheek to maintain the head position.

9. Continue to monitor the patient closely for adequate breathing.

Automatic external defibrillators (AEDs) are computerized devices that are simple to operate. The AED is used *only* when a person is unresponsive, not breathing, and pulseless. When the device is attached to the victim's chest, the unit determines if an electrical shock is necessary. Several different models are available, and the operating instructions are slightly different for each. The four basic steps to using an AED are:

1. Turn the power to the unit on.

2. Apply the electrode pads to the victim's chest.

3. All rescuers stand back to allow the machine to analyze the heart rhythm.

4. All rescuers continue to stand back; the operator of the unit presses the shock button and/or follows the unit's instructions, which are usually audible through a voice-synthesized message.

CHOKING

A person chokes when the throat is occluded (closed up or blocked) and air cannot get into the airway. In this situation, you must take quick, decisive action. The airway can be blocked by the tongue, food, dentures, or other foreign body in the back of the throat. Tilting the head back may open the airway by pulling the tongue forward.

• If the person can speak and is coughing vigorously, do not intervene. Stay close by and encourage coughing.

• A complete blockage is signaled by the person being unable to speak, high-pitched sounds on inhalation, and grasping the throat in the universal distress signal (Figure 42-8).

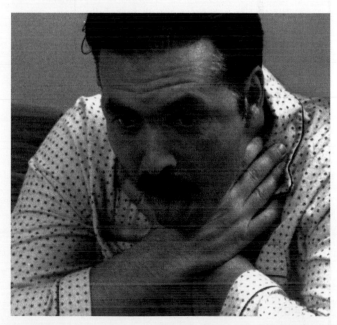

FIGURE 42-8 The universal distress signal for choking is one or both hands about the throat. (© *Delmar/Cengage Learning*)

PROCEDURE

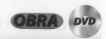

HEIMLICH MANEUVER—ABDOMINAL THRUSTS

1. Ask the person if he is choking.

2. If the person starts to cough, wait.

3. If the person cannot speak, cough, or breathe, but is conscious, apply abdominal thrusts (**Heimlich maneuver**) until the foreign body is expelled.

   a. Stand behind the victim and wrap your arms around the waist.

   b. Clench your fist, keeping the thumb straight (Figure 42-9A).

   c. Place your fist, thumb side in, against the victim's abdomen slightly above the navel and below the tip of the xiphoid process.

   d. Grasp your clenched fist with your opposite hand (Figure 42-9B).

   e. Avoid pressing on the patient's ribs with your forearms.

   f. Thrust forcefully with the thumb side of your fist against the midline of the victim's abdomen, slightly above the navel, inward and upward (Figure 42-9C). Be sure you are below the tip of the sternum (xiphoid process). Deliver each thrust with the intention of freeing the obstruction.

4. Keep thrusting if the object is not dislodged. If the victim begins to cough forcefully, wait.

5. Activate the EMS system.

6. Continue the Heimlich maneuver until the obstruction is expelled or the victim becomes unconscious. If the victim becomes unconscious,

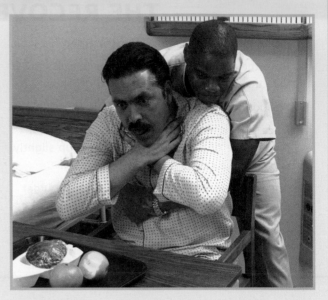

FIGURE 42-9B Grasp the clenched fist with your opposite hand. Avoid pressing against the ribs with your forearms. *(© Delmar/Cengage Learning)*

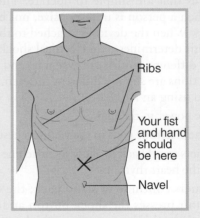

FIGURE 42-9C Thrust forcefully, inward and upward, with the thumb side of your fist just above the navel. *(© Delmar/Cengage Learning)*

place the victim in supine position. Proceed with Procedure 112.

Alternative Action: Chest thrusts are used when pressure to the abdomen would be harmful or impossible. Chest thrusts are used if the choking person is in late pregnancy or if the victim is so large

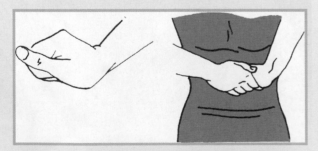

FIGURE 42-9A Clench your fist, keeping the thumb straight. *(© Delmar/Cengage Learning)*

PROCEDURE 111 CONTINUED

you are unable to get your arms around him. Follow steps 1 and 2, then stand behind the victim, place your arms directly under the victim's armpits, and around the chest. Place the thumb side of your fist in the middle of the breastbone (avoid ribs and xiphoid process). Grab your fist with your other hand and perform thrusts until the foreign body is expelled or the victim becomes unconscious.

PROCEDURE

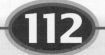

ASSISTING THE ADULT WHO HAS AN OBSTRUCTED AIRWAY AND BECOMES UNCONSCIOUS

1. Activate the EMS system.
2. Apply gloves.
3. Turn the victim on her back.
4. Begin CPR. Use a pocket mask for ventilation.

5. Each time you open the airway, look for a foreign body in the victim's mouth. If you see a foreign body, avoid pushing it farther down into the throat.
6. Continue CPR until the object is expelled, further help arrives, or you are exhausted and unable to continue.

CPR AND OBSTRUCTED AIRWAY PROCEDURES FOR INFANTS AND CHILDREN

The following procedures for infants and children are only guidelines for emergency treatment of an obstructed airway. You *must* successfully complete an approved course before you perform these procedures.

When determining which procedure to use, consider the age and size of the child:

- Newborn—birth to approximately 1 month of age
- Infant—from birth to approximately 1 year of age
- Child—from approximately 1 to 8 years of age

If the child is more than 8 years old, adult CPR and obstructed airway procedures are used.

PROCEDURE

OBSTRUCTED AIRWAY: INFANT

Perform this procedure only if the airway of the infant is completely obstructed and someone has witnessed or strongly suspects that there is a foreign body obstruction.

1. Determine whether there is airway obstruction by observing breathing difficulties, weak or absent cry, or ineffective cough.

2. Supporting the infant's head and neck with one hand, position the infant face down with the head lower than the trunk, over one arm (support your arm on your thigh). Deliver up to 5 back blows (Figure 42-10A).

3. Supporting the infant on your arm, turn the infant face up and deliver up to 5 chest thrusts in the

continues

PROCEDURE 113 CONTINUED

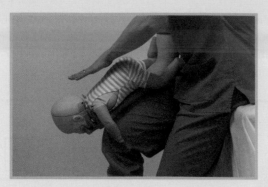

FIGURE 42-10A Position the infant face down, with face lower than trunk. Deliver up to 5 back blows. (© Delmar/Cengage Learning)

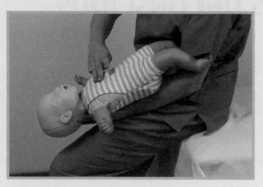

FIGURE 42-10B Turn the infant face up and deliver up to 5 chest thrusts. (© Delmar/Cengage Learning)

midsternal region (Figure 42-10B). Do chest thrusts at a rate of 1 per second.

4. Repeat steps 2 and 3 until the foreign body is expelled or the infant becomes unconscious.

If the Infant Becomes Unconscious

5. Call out for help. If someone responds, have that person call the EMS system. Place the infant on her back.

6. Open the airway with the head-tilt, chin-lift method and try to give rescue breaths.

7. If the chest does not rise with each breath, reposition the infant's head and try again. If you see a foreign body in the mouth, remove it. Take care to avoid pushing it farther down into the throat. Do not perform a finger sweep or attempt to remove an object you cannot see.

8. Check the brachial pulse. If the pulse is absent, begin CPR. Continue until further help arrives, you are exhausted and unable to continue, or the infant has respirations and a pulse above 60.

PROCEDURE

114

ASSISTING A CHILD WHO HAS A FOREIGN BODY AIRWAY OBSTRUCTION

Conscious Child

1. Ask "Are you choking?"

2. Give abdominal thrusts, using the same hand placement as you would for an adult, slightly above the navel and well below the xiphoid process.

3. Repeat thrusts until the foreign body is removed or the victim becomes unconscious.

If the Child Becomes Unconscious

4. If another person is present, have that person activate the EMS system.

5. Open the airway and try to do rescue breathing. If still obstructed, reposition the child's head and try to do rescue breathing again. If you see a foreign body in the mouth, remove it. Take care to avoid

PROCEDURE 114 CONTINUED

pushing it farther down into the throat. Do not perform a finger sweep or attempt to remove an object you cannot see.

6. Check the carotid pulse. If the pulse is absent, begin CPR.

7. If the airway obstruction is not relieved after about one minute, activate the EMS system, if this has not been done.

8. Continue until further help arrives, you are exhausted and unable to continue, or the child has respirations and a pulse.

OTHER EMERGENCIES

For some of the emergencies described here, a patient at home or in a long-term care facility may need to be transported to a hospital emergency room. If the victim is outside of the hospital, be sure that you know:

- Initial emergency actions to perform
- How and when to notify the EMS system
- How and when to notify the nurse

Bleeding

Heavy bleeding and blood loss can be life-threatening. Apply gloves and follow standard precautions if you care for a patient with external bleeding. Internal bleeding is not visible, and is shown when the signs of shock become apparent (described in the next section). Take the following steps to prevent additional loss:

- Identify the area that is bleeding.
- Have the patient apply continuous pressure over the bleeding area, if able.

GUIDELINES *for*

Non-Cardiac Facility Emergencies

- Anticipate and prevent emergencies whenever possible. Think safety when you enter and leave a room.
- If you discover a patient who is ill or injured, stay with the patient and call for help.
- Know facility procedures, phone numbers, and code words for reporting emergencies.
- Do not move a patient who has fallen to the floor, unless the patient is in immediate danger, until the nurse checks the patient and gives permission for the move.
- Stay calm and do not panic. Reassure the patient.
- While you wait for help to arrive, start emergency measures that you are permitted to do.
- Do not give the patient anything to eat or drink.
- Know the location of emergency equipment and supplies on your unit.

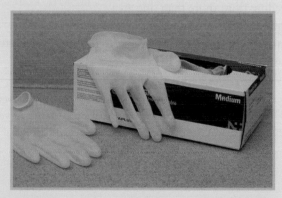

FIGURE 42-11 Know where protective equipment is kept and apply the principles of standard precautions when giving emergency care. (© *Delmar/Cengage Learning*)

- Many emergencies involve bleeding. Always remember and apply the principles of standard precautions (Figure 42-11).
- Once the nurse arrives, do as he or she directs.

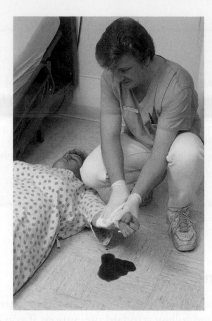

FIGURE 42-12 Apply firm hand pressure over the bleeding area with a pad and your gloved hand. (© Delmar/Cengage Learning)

- If the patient is not able, apply continuous, direct pressure over the bleeding area with a pad and your gloved hand (Figure 42-12).
- Call for help.
- If seepage occurs, increase the padding and pressure. Do not remove the original pads.
- Elevate the wounded area above the level of the heart, but do not release pressure.
- Support the elevated area.
- Use binding to hold the padded pressure if there is bleeding from more than one area.
- Apply pressure over the appropriate pulse point to control **hemorrhage** (heavy bleeding) if direct pressure is ineffective (Figure 42-13).
- Keep the victim warm and quiet until help arrives.

Note: Persons who are bleeding are often very frightened. Their anxiety contributes to the development of shock. Continuous reassurance is essential.

Safety ALERT

Do not be distracted by copious bleeding in an unconscious person. Always check the adequacy of the patient's airway first. If airway, breathing, and circulation are adequate, quickly apply gloves and take measures to stop the bleeding. ∎

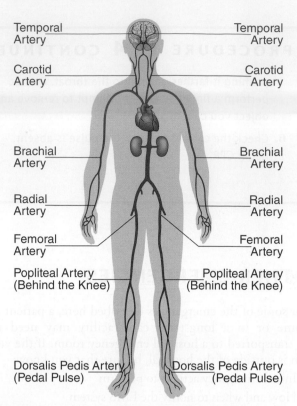

FIGURE 42-13 Pressure on the pulse points is effective for slowing or stopping bleeding. (© Delmar/Cengage Learning)

Shock

Shock is defined as a disturbance of the oxygen supply to the tissues and return of blood to the heart. It can follow any severe injury, hemorrhage, and many medical conditions. Early signs and symptoms of shock include:

- Pale, cold skin that is moist or clammy to the touch
- Complaints of weakness
- Weak, rapid pulse
- Rapid and irregular breathing
- Restlessness, anxiety, and thirst
- Perspiration

Care for the patient according to the guidelines listed under fainting (following). Unless shock is controlled, death can occur. Until help arrives, your care can make the difference between life and death.

Fainting

When the blood supply to the brain is reduced for a short time, the person loses consciousness. This is called *fainting* (*syncope*). Fainting is usually a temporary condition (Figure 42-14). It is corrected as soon as blood flow to the brain is restored.

Unfortunately, when consciousness is lost, the patient is likely to fall and injuries can occur. Ease the patient to the

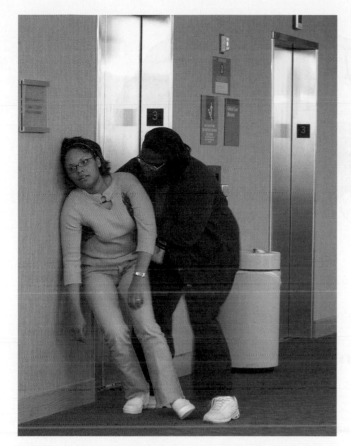

FIGURE 42-14 Fainting occurs when blood flow to the head is suddenly and temporarily decreased. *(© Delmar/Cengage Learning)*

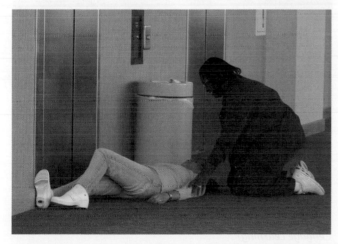

FIGURE 42-15 Do not try to hold the victim up. Ease her to the floor, making sure the airway is open. Stay with the victim and call for help. *(© Delmar/Cengage Learning)*

floor to prevent injury (Figure 42-15). Assist patients who are *feeling* faint to a safe position.

The patient who is sitting and feels faint should be encouraged to lower her head between the knees. To provide

assistance to a patient who is fainting or in whom shock is suspected, the nursing assistant should:

- Help the patient assume a protected position, sitting or lying down
- Loosen tight clothing
- Position the victim's head lower than the heart
- Allow the patient to rest for at least 10 minutes
- Maintain normal body temperature
- Call for additional help
- Monitor pulse, respirations, and blood pressure
- Do not give the patient anything to eat or drink

Heart Attack

Heart attacks can occur in any age group, but the high-risk group includes those who have high blood pressure, smoke, and have a history of heart disease. Signs and symptoms of heart attack include:

- Crushing pain that can radiate to the jaw and arms, or heaviness in chest
- Perspiration; skin cold and clammy
- Nausea and vomiting
- Pale to grayish color of the face
- Difficulty breathing or absence of breathing
- Loss of consciousness
- Irregular pulse or loss of pulse
- Low blood pressure in later stages

Stroke

A *brain attack* (cerebral vascular accident or CVA), also called a *stroke*, occurs when there is interference with normal blood circulation to the brain. It usually is caused by a clot that has lodged in a cerebral vessel or by a blood vessel that has ruptured (Figure 42-16).

The person with a brain attack usually develops weakness or paralysis on one side of the body. He or she may become unresponsive or have a seizure. First aid includes:

- Maintaining an airway (Figure 42-17)
- Providing mask-to-mouth breathing as needed
- Administering CPR, if needed
- Positioning the victim on the side so fluids will drain from the mouth
- Maintaining normal body temperature
- Keeping the victim quiet until help arrives

Seizures

Seizures or convulsions are sometimes seen when there is a head injury, drug overdose, and many other medical conditions. Seizures (Unit 37) do not always follow the same pattern. Their range may be:

- A momentary loss of contact with the environment, in which the person seems to stare blankly.

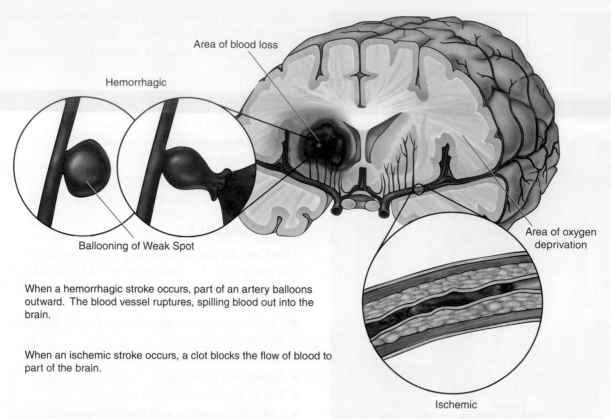

When a hemorrhagic stroke occurs, part of an artery balloons outward. The blood vessel ruptures, spilling blood out into the brain.

When an ischemic stroke occurs, a clot blocks the flow of blood to part of the brain.

FIGURE 42-16 A stroke occurs when blood flow within the brain is interrupted as a result of a blood clot or rupture of a blood vessel. (© Delmar/Cengage Learning)

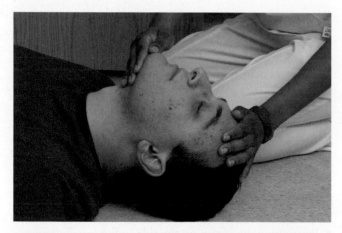

FIGURE 42-17 Maintain the airway by holding it open manually, if necessary. (© Delmar/Cengage Learning)

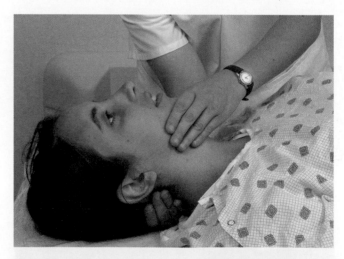

FIGURE 42-18 Protect the patient's head. (© Delmar/Cengage Learning)

- A generalized tonic-clonic seizure, in which consciousness is lost, the person becomes rigid and falls, and the person loses bowel and bladder control.

If you witness a seizure, take the following steps:

- Wear gloves and apply standard precautions.
- Do not restrain the victim's movements.
- Protect the victim from injury.

- Loosen clothing around the neck.
- Maintain an airway by positioning. Do not try to put anything in the victim's mouth.
- Protect the victim's head (Figure 42-18).
- Observe the seizure.

After seizure activity stops:

- Turn the victim to the side so fluid or vomitus can drain.

- Give mask-to-mouth resuscitation if breathing is not resumed immediately.
- Allow the victim to rest undisturbed.
- Stay with the victim but summon medical assistance.
- Report and record seizure activity: time, length of seizure, body parts or activity involved.

Vomiting and Aspiration

Food and air are both taken into the body through the mouth. The passageway by which food and air enter is shared. Occasionally a patient aspirates, which is potentially serious. This occurs when food, water, vomitus, or other objects accidentally go down the trachea and into the lungs. Signs and symptoms of aspiration include choking on food or an object, coughing, cyanosis, and vomiting.

If a patient has aspirated anything:

- Stay with the patient and call for help.
- Use standard precautions and select personal protective equipment appropriate to the procedure.
- Do not give the patient any liquids.
- Keep the patient's head elevated (Figure 42-19).
- Turn the patient's body to the side if she is vomiting while lying down. If turning the patient's body is not possible, turn the head to the side.
- Provide an emesis basin if the patient is vomiting (Figure 42-20).
- If the patient begins choking and an airway obstruction occurs, follow the procedure for clearing an obstructed airway.
- After the episode, assist the patient with mouth care (Figure 42-21).
- Make observations and report to the nurse:
- Observe any vomitus for color, odor, presence of undigested food, blood, or coffee-ground appearance. Save the emesis for the nurse to inspect.

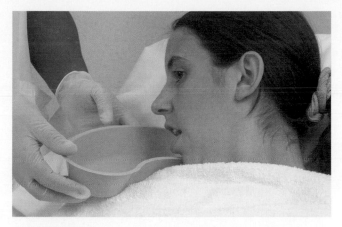

FIGURE 42-20 Provide an emesis basin and assist the patient as necessary. *(© Delmar/Cengage Learning)*

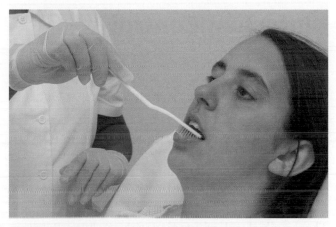

FIGURE 42-21 Provide or assist with oral care when the patient has finished vomiting. *(© Delmar/Cengage Learning)*

- Measure or estimate the amount of vomitus or blood, and record on the intake and output record.

Electric Shock

Severe burns and cardiac and respiratory arrest can result from electric shock. You must protect yourself as you try to rescue the victim. Rescue steps include:

- Turn off the electricity at the source, such as at a fuse box, before touching the victim, if possible.
- If the source of electricity cannot be controlled, try to move the victim away with some nonconductive material, such as a wooden broom handle.
- Once free of the electrical source, check the victim for breathing and pulse.
- Summon medical help.
- Administer CPR, if necessary (Figure 42-22).
- Once breathing and heart function are restored, check for burns and other injuries. Keep the victim lying down and comfortable.
- Give first aid for burns or other injuries.

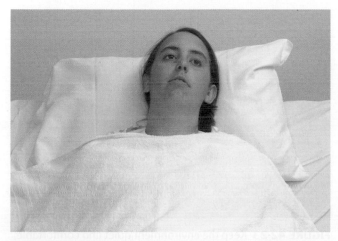

FIGURE 42-19 Elevate the head of the bed. *© Delmar/Cengage Learning.*

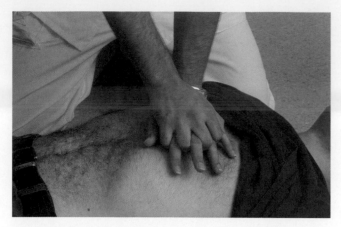

FIGURE 42-22 Perform CPR, if necessary. (© Delmar/ Cengage Learning)

Infection Control ALERT

Cool a burn with cold water. Avoid using ice, which will damage sensitive tissue. Never break blisters on a burn. Cover them loosely with material that will not stick to the tissue. ■

Burns

Burns may be caused by heat, chemicals, or radiation. There is a high risk of infection with any burn. Burns are classified as partial thickness or full thickness, depending on the degree of injury.

Follow these steps for emergency treatment of burns:

1. Call the nurse immediately.
2. If the patient's clothing is on fire, use a coat or blanket to smother the flames.
3. Cool water may be applied to lower skin temperature and to stop further tissue damage.

Orthopedic Injuries

Orthopedic injuries include injuries to bones, joints, muscles, and ligaments.

- A *fracture* is a break in a bone.
- A **sprain** is an injury to a ligament caused by sudden overstretching.
- A **strain** is excessive stretching of a muscle that results in pain and swelling of the muscle. A **dislocation** occurs in a joint when one bone is displaced from another bone.

If you suspect that a patient has suffered a sprain, strain, dislocation, or fracture:

- Stay with the patient.
- Immobilize the injured extremity.

- Do not attempt to move the patient.
- Call the nurse immediately.
- If the patient is on the floor and a fracture is suspected, avoid moving her until after the nurse assesses her and informs you what action to take.
- Monitor the patient's vital signs as instructed.

Head Injury

A patient with a known or suspected head injury always requires close observation and monitoring. Bleeding inside the skull commonly occurs when the head strikes a broad, hard object, such as the floor. Some serious complications of head injuries may not be apparent until 72 hours (or more) after a head injury. This is particularly true in elderly persons.

Signs and symptoms of a possible head injury include:

- Change in the patient's level of alertness or consciousness
- Change in orientation (ability to recognize time, place, person)
- Memory loss
- Unequal pupils
- Visual disturbances
- Blood or clear fluid leaking from ears or nose
- No response to verbal stimulation
- Headache
- Nausea and/or vomiting

If you think a patient has suffered a head injury:

- Stay with the patient and call for help.
- Keep the environment quiet and calm.
- Do not give the patient anything to drink.
- Reassure and orient the person.
- Elevate the head on a pillow (Figure 42-23).
- Do not move the patient if he is on the floor.
- Monitor vital signs regularly after the injury, as instructed.

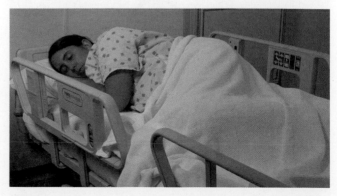

FIGURE 42-23 Keep the environment quiet and comfortable; elevate the patient's head slightly on a pillow. (© Delmar/Cengage Learning)

Accidental Poisoning

If you suspect that a poisoning has happened:
- Call the nurse immediately.
- Try to determine what the patient has taken and save the container.

- The nurse may administer a substance that will cause vomiting. (Not all substances can be safely removed by vomiting.) Follow the nurse's instructions.

GUIDELINES *for*

Action in an Emergency

In the health care facility:
- Stay with the patient and signal for help.
- Have the patient stop any activity and assume a comfortable position.
- Help keep the patient calm.
- Elevate the head of the bed to assist breathing.

If the patient is unconscious:
- Check for breathing and heartbeat.
- If necessary, institute CPR.

In the community, and if the victim is conscious, proceed as follows.
1. Evaluate the situation.
2. Activate the EMS.
3. Have the victim sit and assume a comfortable position. Loosen tight clothing.

4. Provide fresh air but keep the victim comfortably warm.
5. Monitor pulse and respirations and be prepared to initiate CPR.

In the community, if the victim is unconscious, follow steps 1 and 2. Then:
3. Check for breathing and heartbeat.
4. If heartbeat is present but breathing has ceased, open the airway and institute mask-to-mouth resuscitation.
5. If breathing and heartbeat have ceased (cardiac and respiratory arrest), perform CPR until a professional takes charge.

REVIEW

A. Multiple Choice

Select the one best answer for each of the following.

1. An organization that offers instruction in CPR is the
   a. American Emergency Association.
   b. American Association of Nurses.
   c. Association for Resuscitation.
   d. American Heart Association.

2. First aid is care given
   a. for nausea and vomiting.
   b. only upon a physician's order.
   c. if medical help is delayed.
   d. for cough, cold, or sore throat.

3. Which of the following is a life-threatening situation requiring intervention? A person who
   a. broke a finger.
   b. fell and bruised a knee.
   c. is in shock.
   d. is coughing.

4. The first step you should take when arriving on the scene of an accident is to
   a. stop a passerby.
   b. evaluate the situation.
   c. move the victims to one side.
   d. help the victims get up and walk.

5. To assist a person who has fainted,
   a. help the person to walk to circulate the blood.
   b. cover the person with several blankets.
   c. loosen tight clothing.
   d. position the person's head higher than the heart.

6. To assist the person who is experiencing a seizure, you should
   a. keep the person as active as possible.
   b. restrain the person's movements.

c. keep the head straight.

d. protect the person from injury.

7. You suspect that a patient is in shock because the

a. blood pressure is elevated.

b. face is flushed.

c. skin is cold and clammy.

d. pulse is full and bounding.

8. Overstretching of a ligament can result in a

a. fracture.

b. sprain.

c. strain.

d. dislocation.

9. For one-person CPR, the ratio of chest compressions to ventilations is

a. 30 compressions to 2 ventilations.

b. 5 compressions to 1 ventilation.

c. 15 compressions to 2 ventilations.

d. 30 compressions to 1 ventilation.

10. If a victim of cardiac arrest resumes breathing but is unconscious, you should position the victim

a. in recovery position.

b. on his back.

c. on his abdomen.

d. in a chair.

11. The first action to take when an adult is choking and is conscious is to tell the victim what you are going to do. Then

a. slap the person on the back.

b. give abdominal thrusts.

c. begin artificial respirations.

d. begin chest compressions.

12. The first priority in an emergency is

a. airway.

b. bleeding.

c. circulation.

d. level of consciousness.

13. When a person suffers cardiac arrest,

a. the heart has stopped beating.

b. the respirations are less than 12 per minute.

c. biological death has occurred.

d. unconsciousness occurs in about 4 minutes.

14. In the health care facility, you would initiate CPR for cardiac arrest unless

a. the patient has a DNR order.

b. you think the patient would not want to be revived.

c. the patient is very old.

d. the death is unexpected.

15. If you are working in a patient's home and CPR is initiated, you must

a. call the EMS system yourself if you are alone.

b. drive the patient to the closest hospital.

c. do CPR for 20 minutes, then call the EMS system.

d. go next door to have the neighbor call the EMS system.

16. The procedure to clear an obstructed airway on a conscious infant is to position the infant and

a. deliver 5 abdominal thrusts followed by 5 back blows.

b. deliver 5 back blows followed by 5 chest thrusts.

c. perform a blind finger sweep.

d. perform 2 ventilations followed by 5 compressions.

17. When performing single-rescuer CPR on an infant, the procedure is

a. done with 5 back blows and 5 chest thrusts.

b. done only with 2 rescuers.

c. done with a ratio of 1 ventilation to 5 chest compressions.

d. done with a ratio of 2 ventilations to 30 chest compressions.

18. Vomiting may be treated as an emergency because of the risk of

a. airflow.

b. aspiration.

c. hemorrhage.

d. cardiac arrest.

19. The preferred treatment for external bleeding is to apply

a. continuous, direct pressure.

b. a tourniquet.

c. pressure to pulse points.

d. a heat pack.

B. Nursing Assistant Challenge

You and a friend are driving home from work. A car immediately ahead of you goes through a stop sign and is hit on the passenger side by a car going through the intersection. You and your friend park your car to see if your help is needed in this emergency. The people in the other car are conscious, alert, and deny having any injuries. The passenger in the car that ran the stop sign is unconscious and begins to vomit. You see blood coming from the person's right arm. The driver is conscious but dazed and seems to be disoriented. List, in sequence, the actions you will take.

90-90-90 position   a method of positioning the patient in good posture with the feet at a 90° angle to the lower legs, the lower legs at a 90° angle to the thigh, and the thighs at a 90° angle to the torso.

AII (A2) room   an isolation room with an anteroom and negative-pressure ventilation that may be used for patients in airborne precautions.

abbreviation   shortened form of a word or phrase.

abdominal distention   a condition in which the abdomen is bloated and enlarged.

abduction   movement away from midline or center.

abduction pillow   pillow used to maintain separation between the legs of a patient who has had hip surgery.

ablutions   the practice of removing sins and diseases and cleansing negative energy from body, mind, and spirit through ritual washing.

abrasion   injury that results from scraping the skin.

abscess   a collection of pus in the tissue, usually in a confined space; abscesses can occur anywhere in the body.

absence seizure   another name for a petit mal seizure.

abuse   improper treatment or misuse.

accelerated   increased or faster.

acceptance   coming to terms with a situation and awaiting the outcome calmly; final stage of dying, which some people, but not all, reach.

acetone   colorless liquid produced during the metabolism of fats because glucose cannot be oxidized in the blood; has a sweet, fruity odor; appears in blood and urine of persons with diabetes.

acquired immune deficiency syndrome (AIDS)   a progressive disease of the immune system caused by the human immunodeficiency virus; initially an extremely high mortality rate was the norm for the disease, but now combination drug therapy can slow the disease process and lengthen life expectancy of those infected with HIV.

activities of daily living (ADLs)   the activities necessary to fulfill basic human needs.

acute exacerbation   an increase in the severity of signs and symptoms of a chronic disease.

acute illness or disease   illness that comes on suddenly; requires intensive, immediate treatment.

adaptation   adjustment.

adaptive device   item altered to make it easier to use by those with functional deficits to perform any activity of daily living.

Addison's disease   disease caused by underfunctioning of the adrenal glands.

adduction   movement toward midline or center.

adjunctive devices   secondary devices used to maintain the airway and respirations.

ADLs   See **activities of daily living**

admission   procedure carried out when a patient first arrives at a facility.

adolescence   the period of human life from 14 years to 20 years of age.

adrenal glands   endocrine glands that secrete hormones, including epinephrine; one is located on the top of each kidney.

advance directive   document signed before the diagnosis of a terminal illness, when the individual is still in good health, indicating the person's wishes regarding care during dying.

advocate   a person who speaks on behalf of the patient.

AED   See **automatic external defibrillator**

affective disorders   a group of mental disorders characterized by a disturbance in mood. They may also be called *mood disorders*, and are usually marked by a profound and persistent sadness.

agitation   mental state characterized by irregular and erratic behavior.

aiding and abetting   not reporting dishonest acts that are observed.

AIDS   See **acquired immune deficiency syndrome**

airborne precautions   procedures used to prevent the spread of airborne pathogens.

airborne transmission   method of spreading disease by breathing tiny pathogens that remain suspended in the air for long periods of time.

alcoholism   a dependency on alcohol.

alignment   See **body alignment**

ALS   See **amyotrophic lateral sclerosis**

alternative   choice; option.

alveoli   tiny air sacs that make up most of the lungs.

Alzheimer's disease   neurological condition in which there is a gradual loss of cerebral functioning.

AM care   care given in the early morning when the patient first awakens.

ambulate   to walk.

ambulation   the process of walking.

amino acids   basic components of proteins.

amniotic fluid   fluid in which the fetus floats in the mother's womb.

amniotic sac   sac enclosing the fetus and amniotic fluid.

amputation   removal of a limb or other body appendage.

amyotrophic lateral sclerosis (ALS)   a progressive neuromuscular disease that causes muscle weakness and paralysis.

analgesic   pain-relieving medication.

anatomic position   standing erect, facing observer, feet flat on floor and slightly separated, arms at sides, palms forward.

anatomy   study of the structure of the human body.

aneroid gauge   device for measuring and registering blood pressure.

anesthesia   loss of feeling or sensation.

anger   feeling of hostility, rage.

angina pectoris   acute pain in the chest caused by interference with the supply of oxygen to the heart.

anorexia nervosa   an eating disorder in which the patient has a disturbed body image; despite appearing skeletal, he or she views the body as being fat.

anterior   in anatomy, in front of the coronal or ventral plane.

anteroom   a small room just inside the entrance to the isolation room; usually has a sink and containers for trash disposal.

antibodies   proteins produced in the body in response to invasion by a foreign agent (antigen); react specifically with the foreign agent.

anticoagulant   medication that thins the blood and increases the risk of bleeding.

anti-embolism hose   elasticized stockings used to support the leg blood vessels.

antigen   marker on cells that identifies a cell as self or nonself; antigens on foreign substances that enter the body, such as pathogens, stimulate the production of antibodies by the body.

anxiety   fear, apprehension, or sense of impending danger that is often marked by vague physical symptoms, such as tension, restlessness, and rapid heart rate.

anxiety disorder   one of a group of recognized mental illnesses involving anxiety reactions in response to stress.

aphasia   language impairment; loss of ability to comprehend normally.

apical pulse   pulse rate taken by placing a stethoscope over the tip of the heart.

apnea   period of no respiration.

appliance   device used with colostomy or ileostomy to collect drainage from a stoma.

approaches   actions used by the health care team to help resolve a patient's problems; steps taken to reach a goal.

arteriosclerosis   a narrowing of the inside walls of the arteries, causing them to become thick and rigid and restricting blood flow through the vessels.

arthritis   joint inflammation.

ascites   fluid accumulation in the abdomen.

asepsis   without infection.

aspiration   a very serious condition in which food, water, gastric contents, or other materials enter the trachea and lungs. It is usually accidental, such as when the patient "swallows down the wrong tube" or accidentally inhales food or fluids. If you suspect that a patient has aspirated, inform the nurse promptly.

assault   attempt or threat to do violence to another.

assessment   act of evaluating.

assignment   specific list of duties; tells you which patients you will care for during your shift and the specific procedures to be performed.

assistive devices   equipment used to help people be more effective in their physical activity.

asthma   chronic respiratory disease characterized by bronchospasms and excessive mucus production.

atelectasis   decreased or absent air in all or part of a lung, resulting in loss of lung volume and inability to expand the lung fully.

atherosclerosis   the most common form of vascular disease in which lipids (fats) are deposited on the walls of arteries, causing the lumen to gradually narrow and close.

atrium   one of the two upper chambers of the heart.

atrophy   shrinking or wasting away of tissues.

attitude   an external expression of inner feelings about oneself or others.

aura   peculiar sensation preceding the appearance of more definite symptoms in a convulsion or seizure.

auscultatory gap   sound fadeout for 1–15 mm Hg (mercury) pressure, after which sound begins again; sometimes mistaken for the diastolic pressure.

autoclave   machine that sterilizes articles.

automatic external defibrillator (AED)   computerized device that uses an electric shock to reverse disorganized activity in the heart during cardiac arrest.

autonomic dysreflexia   potentially life-threatening complication of spinal cord injury; indicates uncontrolled sympathetic nervous system activity.

axilla   armpit.

axon   extension of neuron that conducts nerve impulses away from the cell body.

bacterium (plural bacteria)   a form of simple microbe.

bag bath   *See* **waterless bathing**

balance bar   section of an upright scale that holds the weights used to determine a patient's weight.

bandages   fabric, gauze, net, or elasticized material used to cover dressings and keep them securely in place.

bargaining   stage of the grieving process in which the individual seeks to make a deal or form a pact that will delay death.

bariatrics   a relatively new field of medicine that focuses on the treatment and control of obesity and diseases associated with obesity.

baseline   measurement of patient's vital signs or other body functions upon admission; future measurements are compared to these initial measurements to track the patient's progress.

baseline assessment   initial observations of the patient and his or her condition.

battery   an unlawful attack upon or touching of another person.

bedbugs   parasites that are difficult to eliminate and have been found throughout the world; they are active mainly at night, seeking a blood meal from a human or animal host.

benign prostatic hypertrophy (BPH) (also called benign prostatic hyperplasia)   noncancerous enlargement of the prostate gland.

bile   substance produced by the liver that prepares fats for digestion.

binders   fabric or elastic wraps that encircle the abdomen; may be used to hold dressings in place or support a surgical site.

biohazard   waste items or laboratory specimens or materials, and their containers contaminated by body fluids; these have the potential to transmit disease. Discarded items must be labeled. Special precautions are taken to handle and contain this waste.

bioterrorism   the use of biological agents, such as pathogenic organisms or agricultural pests, for terrorist purposes.

bipolar affective disorder   a mood disorder in which the person has marked mood swings beyond what most people experience (also called *manic depression* or *bipolar depression*).

bisexuality   having sexual interest in both genders.

blood pressure   pressure of blood exerted against vascular walls.

BMI   *See* **body mass index**

body alignment position of a human body in which the body can properly function.

body language use of facial expression, body positions, and vocal inflections to convey a message.

body mass index (BMI) a mathematical calculation used to determine whether a person is at a healthy, normal weight, is overweight, or is obese. The BMI measures body weight relative to a person's height by dividing a person's weight (in kilograms) by his or her height (in meters, squared).

borderline personality disorder (BPD) a condition in which the patient feels very unstable. He or she may be impulsive, prone to self-injurious behavior, and fear abandonment.

box (square) corner one type of corner used in the making of a hospital bed.

BPD *See* **borderline personality disorder**

BPH *See* **benign prostatic hypertrophy**

brachial artery main artery of the arm.

brachytherapy a form of radiation therapy in which tiny radioactive seeds or pellets are implanted directly inside the prostate gland or tumor site.

bradycardia unusually slow heartbeat.

braille method of communication used by persons with visual impairments, who use fingertips to feel a series of raised dots representing letters and numbers.

brain attack interference with the supply of blood to the brain; also known as *stroke* or *cerebral vascular accident.*

brain stem base of the brain; enlarged extension of the spinal cord, located in the cranium; includes medulla oblongata, diencephalon, pons, and midbrain.

bridging supporting the body on either side of an affected area to relieve pressure on the area.

bronchi tubal structures connecting the trachea to the lungs.

bronchioles smaller subdivisions or branches at end of the bronchi, located in the lungs.

bronchitis inflammation of the bronchi.

bulimia nervosa a condition in which patients usually binge-eat in huge amounts, then vomit (*purge*) to undo the binge. The binge eating causes feelings of guilt, depression, and self-condemnation.

burn traumatic injury to the skin and underlying tissues caused by heat, chemicals, or electricity. Burns are a very painful injury with a high risk of complications. Extensive treatment is often required.

burnout loss of enthusiasm for and interest in an activity.

bursae small sacs of fluid found around joints.

bursitis condition in which the bursae become inflamed and the joint becomes very painful.

cannula an indwelling tube inserted through a stoma (or into the skin) to maintain patency.

capillary hairlike blood vessel; link between arterioles and venules.

capillary refill quick and painless method of checking a patient's peripheral circulation and oxygenation status; done by pressing on a fingernail and noting the time needed for skin color to return to normal when pressure is released.

carbohydrates energy foods; used by the body to produce heat and energy for work.

carbon dioxide (CO_2) gas that is a waste product in cellular metabolism.

cardiac arrest sudden and often unexpected stoppage of effective heart action.

cardiac cycle all (mechanical and electrical) events that occur between one heart contraction and the next.

cardiac decompensation another name for congestive heart failure.

cardiac muscle muscle that forms the heart wall.

cardiopulmonary resuscitation (CPR) emergency medical procedure undertaken to restart and sustain heart and respiratory functions.

care plan nursing plan for care of a resident in a long-term care facility.

care plan conference meeting of members of an interdisciplinary health care team to develop approaches and a plan of care.

caries tooth decay or cavities.

carrier person who hosts infectious organisms without having symptoms of disease. This person can give the disease to others. He or she may not know of the infection.

cataract opacity of the lens of the eye, resulting in loss of vision.

catastrophic reaction severe and unpredictable violent behavior of a person with dementia.

catheter tube for evacuating or injecting fluids.

causative agent etiology (cause) of a specific disease process.

cell basic unit in the organization of living substances.

cellulose basic substance of all plant foods, which can supply the body with roughage.

Celsius scale centigrade scale for measuring temperature.

centimeter (cm) one-hundredth of a meter.

central venous catheter (CVC) tube inserted into a large vein in the area of the clavicle.

cerebellum portion of the brain lying beneath the occipital lobe; coordinates muscular activities and balance.

cerebrospinal fluid (CSF) water cushion protecting the brain and spinal cord from shock.

cerebrovascular accident (CVA) more commonly called *brain attack* or *stroke*; disorder of the blood vessels of the brain resulting in impaired cerebral circulation and often causing motor and cognitive deficits.

cerebrum largest part of the brain, consisting of two hemispheres separated by a deep longitudinal fissure; controls all mental activities.

chain of infection process of events involved in the transmission and development of an infectious disease.

chancre shallow, craterlike lesion; primary lesion of syphilis.

charting entering information (documentation) in a patient's medical record (chart).

chemical burn injury (burn) caused by exposure to chemicals that damage the skin and mucous membranes.

chemical restraint use of medications to control behavior.

chest tubes sterile, clear plastic tubes that are inserted through the skin of the chest, between the ribs, and into the space between the lung and chest wall; used after surgery to drain bloody fluid from the chest and allow air to escape if there is a small leak of air at the suture line after lung surgery.

Cheyne-Stokes respirations periods of apnea alternating with periods of dyspnea.

CHF *See* **congestive heart failure**

cholecystectomy   surgical removal of a diseased gallbladder and stones.

cholecystitis   inflammation of the gallbladder.

cholelithiasis   formation of stones in the gallbladder.

chorea   abnormal, spastic movements that are the primary sign of Huntington's disease.

chronic disease or illness   incurable illness or disease, but treatable; requires ongoing care.

chronic obstructive pulmonary disease (COPD)   any condition, such as emphysema or bronchitis, that interferes with normal respiration over a long period of time.

circumcision   removal of the end of the prepuce by a circular incision.

citation   written notice that informs a facility of violations of government or accrediting agency rules.

clear liquid diet   diet of water and high-carbohydrate fluids given every 2 to 4 hours.

client   person receiving care; depending on the health care setting, also known as *patient* or *resident.*

Clients' Rights   document spelling out rights of persons receiving home health care.

clinical thermometer   instrument used to measure body temperature.

clitoris   small, cylindrical mass of erotic tissue; part of the external female reproductive organs analogous to the penis in the male.

closed bed   bed with sheets and spread positioned to the head of the bed; unoccupied.

closed (simple) fracture   fracture that does not produce an open wound in the skin and in which bones remain in proper alignment.

cochlea   spiral-shaped organ in the inner ear that receives and interprets sounds.

coercion   forcing a patient to do something against his or her wishes.

cognitive impairment   changes in mental function caused by injury or disease. Persons with this condition may have a deficit in intellect, memory, or attention, causing difficulty with learning, processing, and remembering. Their ability to plan and carry out activities of daily living is usually reduced.

coitus   sexual intercourse; copulation.

colostomy   artificial opening in the abdomen for the purpose of evacuation of feces.

combining form   word part that can be used with other word parts to form a variety of new words.

comfort   a state of well-being in which the patient is calm and relaxed, and is not in pain or upset.

communicable disease   disease caused by pathogenic organism; can be transmitted from person to person, either directly or indirectly.

communication   exchange of messages.

community   people who live in a common area and share common health needs.

comorbidities   diseases and medical conditions that are either caused by or contributed to by morbid obesity or another medical problem.

compartment syndrome   a painful condition that occurs when pressure within the muscles builds up, preventing blood and oxygen from reaching muscles and nerves; a very serious complication that may develop following an injury or surgical procedure.

compensate   to seek a substitute for something unattainable or unacceptable.

complete fracture   a break across the entire cross-section of the bone.

complication   situation that makes the original medical condition more serious.

compound (open) fracture   fracture in which part of the broken bone protrudes through the skin.

compulsion   a purposeful, repetitive behavior that is done many times each day and is problematic enough to cause distress, be time-consuming, or interfere with the person's normal routine, occupation, social activities, or relationships.

concurrent cleaning   daily, routine cleaning of the patient unit.

condom catheter   latex sheath that fits over the penis; used for urinary drainage when connected to a urinary collection bag.

confidential   keeping what is said or written to oneself; private; not shared.

congestive heart failure (CHF)   condition resulting from cardiac output inadequate for physiological needs, with shortness of breath, edema, and abnormal retention of sodium and water in body tissues.

conjunctiva   mucous membrane that lines the eyelids and covers the eye.

constipation   difficulty in defecating.

constrict   become smaller.

contact precautions   practices used to prevent spread of disease by direct or indirect contact.

contact transmission   spread of disease by direct or indirect contact with infected person or contaminated objects.

contagious   communicable or easily spread.

contaminated   unclean; impure; soiled with microbes.

continuous passive motion (CPM)   a therapy that prevents stiffness and improves circulation by delivering a form of passive range-of-motion exercise so that the joint is moved without the patient's muscles being used.

continuous positive airway pressure (CPAP)   oxygen therapy in which a mask is placed on the patient's face, then connected to a device that creates low levels of pressure.

continuum   continuous related series of events or actions.

contracture   permanent shortening or contraction of a muscle due to immobility spasm, or paralysis.

contraindication   situation in which a treatment or action is inappropriate.

contusion   mechanical injury (usually caused by a blow) resulting in hemorrhage beneath the unbroken skin.

convulsion   a seizure or change in electrical brain function.

COPD   *See* **chronic obstructive pulmonary disease**

coping   handling or dealing with stress.

cornea   transparent portion of the eye through which light passes.

corporal punishment   use of painful treatment to change or correct behavior.

cortex   outer portion of a kidney.

countertraction   providing opposing balance to traction; used in reduction of fractures.

Cowper's glands   pair of small glands that open into the urethra at the base of the penis; part of the male reproductive system.

CPAP *See* **continuous positive airway pressure**

CPM *See* **continuous passive motion**

CPR *See* **cardiopulmonary resuscitation**

critical list list that patients are placed on when they are dangerously or terminally ill.

critical (clinical) pathways written documents that detail the expected course of treatment and expected outcomes for a DRG.

cross-training education in many different skills across (health care) disciplines.

CSF *See* **cerebrospinal fluid**

culture views and traditions of a particular group.

Cushing's syndrome condition that results from an excess level of adrenal cortex hormones.

cuticle base of the fingernail.

CV catheter *See* **central venous catheter**

CVA *See* **cerebrovascular accident**

cyanosis dusky, bluish discoloration of skin, lips, and nails caused by inadequate oxygen.

cystitis inflammation of the urinary bladder.

dangling sitting up with legs hanging over the edge of the bed.

DD *See* **developmental disability**

deep vein thrombosis (DVT) blood clot that commonly occurs in the femoral vein, the large blood vessel in the groin.

defamation something harmful to the good name or reputation of another person; slander.

defecation bowel movement that expels feces.

defense mechanism psychological reaction or technique for protection against a stressful environmental situation or anxiety.

defibrillation using an electric shock to reverse disorganized activity in the heart during cardiac arrest.

degenerative joint disease (DJD) deterioration of the tissues of the joints.

dehydration excessive water loss.

delegation transfer of the responsibility for the completion of a procedure or nursing activity from a nurse to another person.

delirium acute, reversible mental confusion due to illness and medical problems.

delirium tremens (DTs) part of a serious withdrawal syndrome seen in persons who stop drinking alcohol following continuous and heavy consumption; signs and symptoms commonly begin 48 to 96 hours after taking the last drink.

dementia progressive mental deterioration due to organic brain disease.

dendrite branch of a neuron that conducts impulses toward the cell body.

denial unconscious defense mechanism in which an occurrence or observation is refused recognition as reality in order to avoid anxiety or pain; also, the first stage of grief.

dentures artificial teeth.

depression morbid sadness or melancholy.

dermis layer of tissue that lies under the epidermis.

development gradual growth.

developmental disability (DD) a condition that first occurs in the developmental period, or before the age of 22. Some individuals are born with the condition, whereas others acquire the disability as a result of trauma or medical problems during childhood.

diabetes mellitus disorder of carbohydrate metabolism.

dialysis movement of dissolved materials through a semipermeable membrane, passing from an area of higher concentration to an area of lower concentration; means of cleansing waste or toxic materials from the body.

diaphoresis profuse sweating.

diarrhea a condition in which the patient has multiple, watery stools.

diastole period during which the heart muscle relaxes and the chamber fills with blood.

diastolic pressure blood pressure during period of cardiac ventricular relaxation.

digestion process of converting food into a form that can be used by the body.

digital thermometer hand-held, battery-operated device that registers temperature and displays reading as numbers.

dilate to open, enlarge, or expand.

dirty anything that has potentially been exposed to pathogens.

disability persistent physical or mental deficit or handicap.

discharge procedure carried out as a patient leaves the facility.

disease definite, marked process of illness having characteristic symptoms.

disinfection process of eliminating pathogens from equipment and instruments.

dislocation displacement of the ends of a joint.

disorientation loss of recognition of time, place, or people.

disposable not reusable after one use.

disruption separation of wound edges.

distal farthest away from a central point, such as point of attachment of muscles.

distention the state of being stretched out (distended).

diuresis increase in output of fluids by the kidneys.

diverticulitis inflammation of diverticula.

DJD *See* **degenerative joint disease**

DNR (do not resuscitate) order used when cardiac and respiratory arrest occur in a patient who is not to be revived; issued according to the patient's wishes expressed in an advance directive.

document legal record; recording observations and data about a patient's condition.

dorsal posterior or back.

douche irrigation of the vaginal canal with medicated or normal saline solution.

doula person who accompanies the mother during the childbirth process; he or she is responsible for supporting and comforting the mother and enhancing communication between the mother and medical professionals.

drainage systematic withdrawal of fluids and discharges from wounds, sores, or body cavities.

draw sheet sheet folded under the patient, extending from above the shoulder to below the hips.

dressings gauze, film, or other synthetic substances that cover a wound, ulcer, or injury.

droplet precautions procedures used to prevent spread of disease by droplets in air.

droplet transmission   a method of spreading infection by inhaling pathogens from the droplets of a patient's respiratory secretions. The droplets are believed to stay within 3 feet of the source patient. This is an area of ongoing research.

DTs   *See* **delirium tremens**

durable power of attorney for health care   document stating that a person appointed by the patient can make health care decisions when the patient is unable to do so for himself or herself.

DVT   *See* **deep vein thrombosis**

dyscrasia   abnormality or disorder of the body.

dysphagia   difficulty swallowing food and liquids.

dyspnea   difficult or labored breathing.

dysuria   painful voiding.

eating disorders   a group of disorders characterized by disturbances in appetite or food intake.

EBP   *See* **evidence-based practice**

ecchymosis   bruising.

edema   excessive accumulation of fluid in the tissues.

ejaculatory duct   part of the male reproductive system extending down from the seminal vesicles to the urethra.

elasticity   ability to stretch.

electric bed   bed operated by electricity.

electrical burn   injury (burn) caused by contact with electricity and lightning. Typically deep; the electricity charts an unpredictable path through the body, causing major damage along the pathway from entrance to exit.

electronic thermometer   battery-operated clinical thermometer that uses a probe and records the temperature on a viewing screen in a few seconds.

eloping   wandering away from the health care facility.

embolus   mass of undissolved material carried in the bloodstream; frequently causes obstruction of a vessel.

emergency   situation requiring immediate attention or medical treatment.

emergency care   medical treatment and nursing care provided to emergency patients.

Emergency Medical Services (EMS)   treatment and care provided by specially trained health care personnel during emergencies.

emesis   vomiting.

empathy   understanding how someone else feels.

emphysema   chronic obstructive pulmonary disease in which the alveolar walls are destroyed.

EMS   *See* **Emergency Medical Services**

enabler   a device that empowers patients and assists them to function at their highest possible level.

enabling   reacting to a patient in a manner that shields the patient from experiencing the full impact or consequences of his or her actions or behavior.

endocrine gland   gland that secretes hormonal substances directly into the bloodstream; ductless gland.

enema   injection of water and/or medications into the rectum and colon; commonly used to help the bowels eliminate feces.

enteral feeding   giving nutrition through a tube inserted into the digestive tract.

environmental safety   adaptation of the environment to prevent incidents and injuries.

epidermis   top layer of skin.

epididymis   elongated, cordlike structure along the posterior border of the testes, in the ducts of which sperm is stored.

epilepsy   A disorder in which temporary abnormal activity occurs in brain cells, causing mild, episodic loss of attention, sleepiness, convulsions with loss of consciousness, and various other symptoms.

ergonomics   process of adapting the environment and using techniques and equipment to prevent worker injuries.

erythrocyte   red blood cell.

eschar   a thick crust or slough covering a wound caused by the death of cells. The word *necrosis* may also be used to describe this condition.

essential nutrients   foods required for normal growth and development and to maintain health.

ethical standards   guides to moral behavior.

ethnic   relating to customs, languages, and traditions of specific groups of people.

ethnicity   special groupings within a race.

etiology   cause of a disease.

eustachian tube   auditory tube; leads from the middle ear to the pharynx.

evaluation   judgment.

evidence-based practice (EBP)   a means of decision making based on the strength of the evidence. Using EBP ensures that patient care practices are scientifically sound.

exacerbation   worsening of a chronic medical condition.

excoriation   superficial injury, such as that produced by scratching the skin.

excrete   to eliminate wastes from body.

expiration   exhalation.

exposure incident   an occurrence during which there is possible personal contact with infectious material.

extension   movement by which the two ends of any jointed part are drawn away from each other.

face shield   type of personal protective equipment; protects mucous membranes of eyes, nose, and mouth from pathogens.

facility (health care)   an agency that provides health care.

Fahrenheit scale   system used in the United States to express temperature.

fallopian tube   tubes that serve as a pathway between the ovary and uterus. Fertilization takes place here.

false imprisonment   unlawfully restraining another.

fat   nutrient used to store energy.

fecal impaction   the most serious form of constipation, in which stool is retained in the rectum, where water is absorbed. Over time, the stool becomes hard and dry, and the patient is unable to pass it.

fecal material   another term for feces, stool, or solid body waste (bowel movement or BM). Normally brown, but color can be affected by certain foods, medications, and diseases. A BM is normally soft and formed.

feedback   confirmation that a message was received as intended.

fibromyalgia (FM)   a common pain syndrome for which there is no known cause.

fingerstick blood sugar (FSBS)   a method of checking blood sugar by collecting a sample of capillary blood with a lancet.

first aid emergency care and treatment of an injured person before complete medical and surgical care can be secured.

flaccid paralysis loss of muscle tone and absence of tendon reflexes.

flagged marked in a special way to attract attention.

flatus gas or air in the stomach or intestines; air or gas expelled through the anus.

flexion decreasing the angle between two bones.

flora normal population of organisms found in a given area.

flow sheet clinical record of ongoing patient care and progress.

fluid balance balance between fluid intake and fluid output.

Foley catheter indwelling catheter placed in the urinary bladder to remove urine continuously.

fomite any object contaminated with germs and thus able to transmit disease.

foot drop a neurological problem that causes the foot to point downward.

footboard appliance placed at the foot of the bed so the feet rest firmly against it and are kept at right angles to the legs.

force fluids notation meaning that the patient must be encouraged to take as much fluid as possible.

foreskin prepuce; loose tissue covering the penis and clitoris.

Fowler's position position in which the patient lies on the back with backrest elevated 45 to 60°.

fracture break in the continuity of bone.

friction rubbing of the skin against another surface, such as bed linen.

FSBS *See* **fingerstick blood sugar**

full liquid diet diet consisting of all types of fluids.

full weight-bearing able to stand on both legs.

fungus (plural fungi) class of organisms to which molds and yeasts belong.

gait manner of walking.

gait belt belt placed around the patient's waist to assist in ambulation.

gait training teaching the patient to walk.

gastrostomy feeding nutrition given through a tube inserted into the stomach through the abdominal wall.

gatch bed bed fitted with a jointed backrest and knee rest; patient can be raised to a sitting position and kept in that position by manually adjusting the bed.

general anesthetic medication that induces a state of unconsciousness and reduces or eliminates ability to feel pain.

generalized throughout the entire body.

generalized tonic-clonic seizure another name for grand mal seizure.

genitalia external reproductive organs.

geriatric relating to age or the elderly.

glaucoma a condition in which the pressure within the eye is increased. Untreated, it will lead to blindness.

glucagon hormone produced by pancreas that increases blood sugar level.

glucose simple sugar; also called *dextrose*.

goal an outcome resulting from implementation of a care plan.

goggles type of personal protective equipment used with standard precautions to protect the eyes.

gonads reproductive organs; ovaries and testes.

gonorrhea sexually transmitted disease that causes an acute inflammation.

gout a metabolic disease that results in increased uric acid deposits in the joints, causing pain.

graduate container marked for milliliters, used to measure liquids.

grand mal seizure major epileptic seizure attended by loss of consciousness and convulsive movements.

grievance situation in which a consumer feels there are grounds for complaint.

growth physical changes that take place in body during development.

guarding an unconscious, protective action, position, or movement to shield a painful or injured area of the body.

halitosis bad breath.

handicap inability of person to fulfill a normal role due to disability.

hand-off communication essential communication that must occur when patient care is transferred from one worker or department to another worker or department.

HD *See* **Huntington's disease**

head lice parasites that live in the hair and scalp and feed on blood; spread primarily by direct contact with an infected person.

head-tilt, chin-lift maneuver a procedure used to open a patient's airway if no neck injury is suspected; pressure is placed on the forehead while the jaw is lifted up.

health state of physical, mental, and social well being.

health care consumer person requiring health care services.

Health Insurance Portability and Accountability Act (HIPAA) a law passed in 1996 that protects privacy, confidentiality, and medical records and other individually identifiable patient information.

heart block condition in which conduction of electrical impulses from atrium to ventricles is impaired and pumping action of heart is slowed down (change in rhythm of heart).

Heimlich maneuver procedure that uses abdominal thrusts to relieve obstruction in the trachea.

hematoma a localized mass of blood that is confined to one area.

hematuria blood in the urine.

hemiparesis weakness on one side of the body; usually the result of a stroke.

hemiplegia paralysis on one side of the body.

hemorrhage heavy bleeding.

HEPA *See* **high efficiency particulate air filter mask**

hepatitis inflammation of the liver.

hernia protrusion or projection of a stomach or organ through the wall or cavity that normally contains it.

herpes simplex II the virus that causes genital herpes.

heterosexuality sexual attraction between persons of opposite genders.

high efficiency particulate air (HEPA) filter mask a mask used by health care workers that prevents the spread of airborne infection.

high Fowler's position position in which the head of the bed is elevated to 90°, with the patient sitting upright.

HIPAA *See* **Health Insurance Portability and Accountability Act**

HIV *See* **human immunodeficiency virus**

home health assistant nursing assistant who practices under supervision in a client's home.

homemaker aide person hired to perform light housekeeping tasks in a client's home.

homemaker assistant person who provides home management help to a client in the client's home.

homosexuality sexual attraction between persons of the same gender.

hormone secretion of endocrine gland; chemical messenger carried to other parts of the body where it alters activity.

hospice special facility or arrangement to provide care of terminally ill persons.

hospice care health care for persons who are dying.

hospital facility for care of the acutely ill or injured.

host animal or plant that harbors another organism. *See also* **susceptible host**

human immunodeficiency virus (HIV) virus that causes acquired immune deficiency syndrome (AIDS).

humidifier a water bottle that moistens oxygen for comfort and prevents drying of the mucous membranes in the nose, mouth, and lungs; used when oxygen is administered at flow rates of 5 liters a minute or more.

Huntington's disease (HD) (also called *Huntington's chorea*) a hereditary disease that usually begins when an individual is in the 40s or 50s, although some may be younger. The disease is progressive, and is marked by involuntary, spastic movements called *chorea*; the condition progresses until the person is totally dependent, with cognitive decline or dementia.

hydronephrosis condition resulting from too much fluid on the kidney.

hyperalimentation technique in which high-density nutrients are introduced into a large vein.

hyperglycemia excessive level of sugar in the blood.

hypersecretion excessive secretion.

hypertension high blood pressure.

hyperthyroidism excessive functioning of the thyroid gland.

hypertrophy increase in the size of an organ or structure that does not involve tumor formation.

hypoglycemia abnormally low level of sugar in the blood.

hyposecretion less than normal production of secretions.

hypotension low blood pressure.

hypothermia-hyperthermia blanket a fluid-filled blanket, the temperature of which can be raised or lowered.

hypothyroidism condition due to deficiency of thyroid secretion, resulting in a lower basal metabolism.

hypoxemia a condition in which there is insufficient oxygen in the blood.

hypoxia lack of adequate oxygen supply.

IBW *See* **ideal body weight**

IDDM *See* **insulin-dependent diabetes mellitus**

ideal body weight (IBW) a mathematical formula and concept developed from life insurance statistics related to life span or longevity and health.

ileostomy incision in the ileum.

immunity ability to fight off infectious disease; state of being protected from a disease.

immunization medication that makes a person more resistant to an infectious agent.

impaction *See* **fecal impaction**

implementation putting into effect.

incentive spirometer apparatus used to encourage better ventilation.

incident an occurrence or event that interrupts normal procedures or causes a crisis.

incident report summary of information about an incident.

incomplete fracture a partial break in a bone.

increment specific amount; in measurement, the amount from one marking to the next.

indwelling catheter Foley catheter that remains in the patient's bladder to drain urine.

infarction death of tissue.

infection invasion and multiplication of any organism and the damage this causes in the body.

infectious capable of transmitting disease.

inferior below another part.

inflammation a localized protective reaction of tissue to irritation, injury, or infection; characterized by pain, redness, swelling, and sometimes loss of function.

informed consent permission given after full disclosure of the facts.

insertion distal point of attachment of skeletal muscle.

inspiration drawing of air into the lungs; inhalation.

insulin active antidiabetic hormone that lowers blood sugar secreted by the islets of Langerhans in the pancreas.

insulin-dependent diabetes mellitus (IDDM) form of diabetes mellitus that requires insulin administration as part of the therapy.

intake and output (I&O) recording of the amount of fluid ingested and the amount of fluid expelled by a patient.

integument the skin.

intention tremor involuntary movement of muscles (particularly hands) that increases when the patient attempts to use the muscles.

interdisciplinary health care team group of professionals from different health care disciplines who each contribute their expertise to the care of a single patient.

interpersonal relationships how people interact with each other.

interpreter a communication professional who mediates between speakers of different languages.

intervention actions that influence the eventual outcome of a situation.

intimacy feelings of closeness and familiarity.

intracranial pressure pressure exerted within the cranium.

intravenous (IV) infusion nourishment given through a sterile tube into a vein.

invasion of privacy taking liberties with the person or personal rights of another.

invasive characterized by invading (penetrating into) tissue or spreading in the body.

inversion turning inward.

involuntary muscle muscle not under conscious control, mainly smooth muscle.

involuntary seclusion separation of patient from other patients and people, against the patient's will.

involution return of the uterus to its normal size after delivery of a baby.

I&O   *See* **intake and output**

iris   colored portion of the eye.

ischemia   having inadequate blood flow to an area.

islets of Langerhans   cells in the pancreas that produce insulin.

isolation   place where a patient with easily transmitted infection or disease is separated from others.

isolation technique   special procedures carried out to prevent the spread of infectious organisms from an infected person.

isolation unit   used for patients with communicable illness, for protection of other patients, staff, and visitors.

IV   intravenous.

jaundice   a yellow color of the skin and sclera.

jaw-thrust maneuver   a method of opening the airway of patients with known or suspected neck injuries; involves pushing the jaw forward and upward.

jejunostomy tube (J-tube)   a long, small-bore tube that is threaded through the GI tract until the tip reaches the small intestine. These tubes may be placed through the nose (nasojejunostomy), or surgically through an incision in the abdominal skin. Used for providing enteral nutrition for patients who do not have a stomach and those in whom recurrent formula aspiration is a problem.

Joint Commission   an organization that inspects and accredits health care agencies that meet high quality standards.

Kardex   type of file in which nursing care plans are kept.

kidney   glandular, bean-shaped organ, purplish-brown, situated in back of the abdominal cavity, one on each side of the spinal column; excretes waste matter in the form of urine.

kilogram (kg)   metric unit of weight measurement, equal to 1,000 grams or 2.2 pounds.

labia majora   two large, hair-covered, liplike structures that are part of the vulva.

labia minora   two hairless, liplike structures found beneath the labia majora.

laceration   accidental break in skin, an injury.

lacrimal gland   produces tears.

lancet   a tiny needle.

laryngectomee   a person who has had a laryngectomy (voice box removal); the patient breathes through an artificial opening in the neck and trachea.

laryngectomy   surgical removal of the larynx. The airway is separated from the mouth, nose, and esophagus; there is no longer a connection between the upper and lower airways.

larynx   organ located at upper end of trachea; part of airway and organ of voice (voice box).

lateral   away from the midline.

lateral transfer   *See* **sitting transfer**

legal standards   guides to lawful behavior.

lesions   abnormal changes in tissue formation.

leukocyte   white blood cell.

Lhermitte's sign   sharp, electrical-type sensation felt down spine when head is flexed; found in patients with multiple sclerosis.

liable   legally responsible.

libel   any written defamatory statement.

licensed practical nurse (LPN); licensed vocational nurse (LVN)   graduate of a certificate nursing program, who must pass a state exam before being permitted to practice nursing.

life-sustaining treatment   treatment given to a critically ill or injured patient to maintain life and prevent death.

ligament   band of fibrous tissue that holds joints together.

lithotripsy   procedure that uses sound waves to crush kidney stones.

living will   document describing the wishes of a terminally ill person, relating to health care.

local anesthetics   drugs that induce loss of feeling in a specific area of the body.

lochia   discharge from the uterus of blood, mucus, and tissue during the puerperal period.

long-term acute care hospital (LTACH)   hospital in which a lengthy stay is anticipated; the patients accepted have medically complex problems but have a good chance of improvement.

low bed   bed in which the frame is 4 to 6 inches from the floor to the top of the frame deck; reduces the risk of injury if the patient falls from the bed.

LPN   *See* **licensed practical nurse**

LTACH   *See* **long-term acute care hospital**

LVN   *See* **licensed vocational nurse**

lymph   fluid found in lymphatic vessels.

lymphatic vessel   vessel that conveys electrolytes, water, and proteins.

macular degeneration   vision impairment due to damage to the macula located at the back of the eye, generally related to aging.

Magnet Program for Excellence in Nursing Services   a voluntary program that recognizes hospitals for nursing excellence.

maladaptive behavior   actions and responses that disrupt the person's ability to function smoothly within the family, environment, or community.

malpractice   improper, negligent, or unethical conduct that results in harm, injury, or loss to a patient.

managed care   method of paying for health care, used by insurance companies to provide efficient services at the lowest cost.

manual patient handling   moving a patient by hand or bodily force, including pushing, pulling, carrying, holding, or supporting the patient or a body part.

masturbation   sexually stimulating self.

Material Safety Data Sheet (MSDS)   information provided by a manufacturer about a hazardous product; includes health hazards, safe use guidelines, and emergency procedures for chemical exposure.

mechanical lift   a manually operated hydraulic lift, electrically (or battery-) operated lift, or a ceiling-mounted lift. Used to transfer dependent or heavy patients from one surface to another.

mechanical soft diet   a diet that includes ground meats; served to patients with no teeth, or those with serious dental problems.

mechanically altered diet   diet in which the consistency and texture of food are modified, making the food easier to chew and swallow.

medial   close to the midline of the body or structure.

medical asepsis   procedures followed to keep germs from being spread from one person to another.

medical chart   patient record containing all information about that patient.

medical diagnosis   name of disease; determination made by a physician.

medulla   forms part of the brain stem; also, the middle area of the kidney.

Meniere's disease   a disorder affecting hearing and balance that results from fluid buildup in the inner ear. Other signs and symptoms include dizziness, vertigo, tinnitus, vomiting, a sensation of fullness in the ear(s), and hearing loss in one or both ears.

meninges   three-layered serous membranes covering the brain and spinal cord.

meningitis   inflammation of the meninges.

mental abuse   causing a patient to feel afraid by teasing, threatening to withhold care or harm the patient, demeaning the patient, or using pet names such as "honey" and "dear."

mental illness   behavioral maladaptations.

mental retardation (MR)   a condition in which a person has lower-than-average intelligence. This condition causes the person to have limited ability to learn and social immaturity. Persons with this condition may be unable to care for themselves or live independently.

message   the information the sender wants to communicate.

metabolism rate   body function; speed with which the body processes the calories needed for the body to function.

methicillin-resistant *Staphylococcus aureus* **(MRSA)** bacteria resistant to most antibiotics.

method of transmission   See mode of transmission

MI   *See* **myocardial infarction**

microbe   *See* **microorganism**

microorganism   tiny organism that can be seen only with a microscope, particularly bacteria.

mineral   inorganic chemical compound found in nature; many minerals are important in building body tissues and regulating body fluids.

mite   microscopic organism that cannot be seen with the naked eye.

mitered corner   one type of corner used in making a facility bed.

mobility   ability to move or to be moved easily from place to place.

mobility skills   ability to move about in bed, out of bed, and walking.

mode of transmission   manner in which a pathogen moves from one place to another.

modified Trendelenburg position   position in which the head of the bed is lowered 20° to 30°.

mold   organism in fungus family.

Montgomery straps   long strips of adhesive attached to the skin on either side of a wound, then tied to hold a dressing in place.

morbid obesity   being 100 pounds or more over ideal body weight, or having a BMI of 40 or higher; this condition usually qualifies for surgical treatment.

mores   customs of ethnic groups.

moribund   dying.

MR   *See* **mental retardation**

MRSA   *See* **methicillin-resistant** *Staphylococcus aureus*

MS   *See* **multiple sclerosis**

MSDS   *See* **Material Safety Data Sheet**

multiple sclerosis (MS)   disease characterized by hardened patches scattered throughout the brain and spinal cord that interfere with the nerves in those areas.

myocardial infarction (MI)   formation of an infarct in the heart muscle due to interruption of the blood supply to the area; heart muscle in the infarcted area actually dies.

myocardium   heart muscle.

N95 respirator   mask with small, tightly woven pores that protects the wearer from airborne infection.

NATCEP   *See* **Nurse Aide Training and Competency Evaluation Program**

nasal cannula   tubing inserted into nostrils to administer oxygen.

nasogastric feeding (NG feeding)   nourishment given through a tube inserted through the nose into the stomach.

National Institute of Occupational Safety and Health (NIOSH)   federal agency responsible for conducting research and making recommendations for the prevention of work-related disease and injury.

nebulizer   device used to apply a liquid in the form of a fine spray or mist; may be used to administer medication.

necrosis   tissue death.

negative air pressure room   a room with a special ventilation system in which the room air is drawn upward into the ventilation system and is either specially filtered or exhausted directly to the outside of the building.

neglect   failing to provide services to patients to prevent physical harm or mental anguish.

negligence   failure to exercise the degree of care considered reasonable under the circumstances, resulting in an unintended injury to a patient. Negligence is carelessness that may be caused by hurrying or not focusing on the task at hand.

neonate   a newborn.

nephritis   inflammation of the kidney.

nephron   microscopic kidney unit that produces urine.

nerve   bundle of nerve processes (axons and dendrites) that are held together by connective tissue.

neuron   cell of the nervous system.

neurotransmitter   chemical compound that transmits a nervous impulse across cells at a synapse.

NG   *See* **nasogastric feeding**

NIDDM   *See* **non–insulin-dependent diabetes mellitus**

NIOSH   *See* **National Institute of Occupational Safety and Health**

nits   tiny, oval-shaped eggs of head lice; are yellow-white and adhere to the hair. They look like dandruff, but are firmly attached to the hair and are very difficult to remove.

no-code order   an order not to resuscitate a patient.

non–insulin-dependent diabetes mellitus (NIDDM) diabetes controlled by diet and sometimes oral medication, for which insulin is not needed.

noninvasive   remaining localized and not spreading; not penetrating.

nonpathogen   microorganism that does not produce disease.

nonverbal communication   communication transmitted without spoken words, such as by facial expression and body language.

nonweight-bearing   unable to stand or walk on one or both legs.

nosocomial   pertaining to or originating in a facility.

nourishments   substantial food items given to patients to increase nutrient intake; often planned and ordered by the facility dietitian.

NPO   nothing by mouth.

Nurse Aide Training and Competency Evaluation Program (NATCEP)   training program culminating in a test taken by the nursing assistant which, when passed successfully, entitles the nursing assistant to certification.

nurse practice act   a legal document from a state board of nursing (or a piece of legislation passed by a state legislature) that describes the nursing scope of practice in that state. Facilities use these acts as a guide to develop job descriptions and determine which skills nursing assistants can perform in the facility.

nurse's notes   section of medical record in which nursing staff records procedures, medications, and observations.

nursing assistant   person who provides personal care and assists with ADLs under nursing supervision.

nursing diagnosis   statement of a patient's problems leading to nursing interventions.

nursing process   framework for nursing action.

nursing team   members of the nursing staff who provide patient care.

nutrient   nourishing substance or food.

nutrition   process by which the body uses food for growth and repair and to maintain health.

nystagmus   constant involuntary movement of the eyeball.

obesity   being overweight by 20% to 30% of the ideal body weight. Being overweight or obese increases the risk for many health conditions, including diabetes, heart disease, and stroke.

objective observation   observation made through the senses of the observer.

OBRA   *See* **Omnibus Budget Reconciliation Act**

observation   noticing something.

obsession   an idea, impulse, or thought (which usually does not make sense) but recurs frequently. The person cannot suppress or eliminate it.

obsessive-compulsive disorder (OCD)   an anxiety disorder in which the patient has recurrent obsessions, frequent thoughts, ideas, impulses, or compulsions, resulting in repeated ritualistic activity over which the patient has no control.

obstetric   relating to pregnancy and childbirth.

occupational exposure   coming into contact with infectious materials during the performance of a person's job.

Occupational Safety and Health Administration (OSHA)   federal agency that makes and enforces regulations to protect workers.

OCD   *See* **obsessive-compulsive disorder**

OJD   *See* **osteoarthritic joint disease**

oliguria   decreased urine production.

Omnibus Budget Reconciliation Act (OBRA)   law that regulates the education and certification of nursing assistants in acute care and long-term care facilities.

open bed   bed with top bedding fanfolded to bottom, ready for occupancy.

open (compound) fracture   fracture in which part of the broken bone protrudes through the skin.

open reduction/internal fixation (ORIF)   surgical procedure to reduce a fractured bone. The skin is opened and the fracture is realigned and held in place by screws, plates, and pins.

operative   in the operating room.

OPIM   *See* **other potentially infectious material**

oral hygiene   care of the mouth and teeth.

oral report   verbal report.

organ   any part of the body that carries out a specific function or functions, such as the heart.

organism   any living thing, plant, or animal.

organizational chart   guide for communication; spells out lines of authority.

ORIF   *See* **open reduction/internal fixation**

orifices   body openings.

origin   proximal point of attachment to skeletal muscle.

orthopnea   need to sit upright in order to breathe without difficulty.

orthopneic position   a position in which the patient must sit up to breathe comfortably. The patient sits as upright as possible and leans slightly forward, supporting herself with the forearms.

orthotic devices (orthoses)   devices that restore or improve function and prevent deformity.

OSHA   *See* **Occupational Safety and Health Administration**

ossicles   any small bones, such as one of the three bones in the ear.

osteoarthritic joint disease (OJD)   degenerative disease of joints.

osteoporosis   a metabolic disorder of the bones in which bone mass is lost, causing them to become porous and spongy; affected bones are at very high risk for fracture.

ostomy   suffix meaning "to create a new opening"; for example, colostomy.

other potentially infectious material (OPIM)   material or equipment that could be a source of disease-producing organisms.

otitis media   inflamed condition of the middle part of the ear.

otosclerosis   formation of bone in the inner ear that causes the ossicles to become fixed.

ovaries (singular ovary)   endocrine glands located in the female pelvis; female gonads.

overweight   a condition in which a person weighs more than he or she should, according to standards set according to the person's height and bone (frame) size.

oviduct   *See* **fallopian tube**

ovulation   process during which an ovum is released; occurs about once each month in the human female.

ovum   female reproductive cell; an egg.

oxygen (O₂)   gas that is essential to cellular metabolism and life.

oxygen concentrator   device that removes impurities from room air and concentrates oxygen to be delivered to a patient.

oxygen mask   device to administer oxygen through nose and mouth; placed over patient's face.

oxygenation   movement of oxygen from the lungs into the blood, which carries the oxygen to body cells.

pacemaker   artificial device placed in the body to regulate the heartbeat.

PACU   *See* **post anesthesia care unit**

pain   a state of discomfort; a warning signal that something is wrong.

pallor   paleness; less color than normal.

panic disorder   a condition characterized by unexpected, chronic *panic attacks* (bouts of overwhelming fear). The person usually feels that he is in danger, but there is no specific cause for the fear. The person may be so fearful that she is unable to function.

panniculus   the fatty apron of abdominal skin seen in most bariatric patients.

pannus   a large, hanging flap of skin; usually seen in the abdomen of a person who has recently lost a significant amount of weight.

PAR   *See* **post-anesthesia recovery**

paralysis   loss or impairment of the ability to move parts of the body.

paraphrasing   providing communication feedback by restating one's understanding of what was said.

paraplegia   paralysis of the lower portion of the body and of both legs.

parasite   organism that lives within, upon, or at the expense of another organism known as the *host*.

parathyroid glands   two pairs of endocrine glands situated on the posterior of the thyroid gland; produce the hormone parathormone.

Parkinson's disease   neurological disorder due to deficiency of dopamine, a neurotransmitter; progressive disease characterized by stiffness of muscles and tremors.

partial weight-bearing   unable to bear full weight on one or both legs.

PASS   acronym for fire extinguisher use meaning: *P*ull the pin; *A*im the nozzle; *S*queeze the handle; *S*weep back and forth.

passive range of motion (PROM)   exercises performed for the patient by the nursing assistant when independent movement is not possible. Maintains movement and prevents deformities, but does not strengthen muscles.

pathogen   microorganism or other agent capable of producing a disease.

pathologic fracture   fracture in a diseased bone that occurs as a result of osteoporosis, a tumor, or cancer.

patient   person who needs care; *see also* **resident** and **client**.

patient-focused care   attention given to mental, physical, and emotional aspects of a person's being.

Patients' Bill of Rights   document developed by the American Hospital Association that describes the basic rights to which each patient is entitled.

pediatric   patient from birth to 18 years of age.

PEG   *See* **percutaneous endoscopic gastrostomy**

pelvis   lower portion of the trunk of the body; basin-shaped area bounded by the hip bones, the sacrum, and the coccyx.

penis   male organ of copulation and urinary elimination.

percutaneous endoscopic gastrostomy (PEG)   a gastrostomy tube that is surgically placed by a physician by threading the tube through the mouth, then out an incision in the abdominal wall over the stomach.

perineal care   cleansing of genital and rectal areas.

perineum   in the male, the area between the anus and the scrotum; in the female, the area between the anus and the vagina.

perioperative   occurring in association with an operative procedure.

peripheral   pertaining to the outside or outer part.

peripheral intravenous central catheter (PICC)   intravenous line inserted into a vein in the arm and threaded through to a larger vein.

peristalsis   progressive, wavelike movement that occurs involuntarily in hollow tubes of the body, especially the alimentary canal.

peritoneal dialysis   removal of liquid waste by washing chemicals through the abdominal cavity.

personal protective equipment (PPE)   equipment such as waterproof gowns, masks, gloves, goggles, and other equipment needed to protect a person from infectious material.

personal space   physical closeness that a person is comfortable with during interactions with others.

personality   sum of the behavior, attitudes, and character traits of an individual.

petit mal seizure   type of epileptic attack that is generally short and mild in nature; "absence" attack.

PFR95 respirator   mask with very tiny pores that prevents the wearer from breathing in infectious airborne microorganisms.

phantom pain   pain experienced in a body part that has been removed from the body, as if the part were still attached.

pharynx   muscular, membranous tube between the mouth and esophagus; throat.

phlebitis   inflammation of a vein.

phobia   an unfounded, recurring fear that causes the person to feel panic.

physiatrist   medical doctor specializing in rehabilitation.

physical abuse   mistreatment by hitting or other physical contact.

physical restraint   device used to prevent a patient from moving about or having access to his or her own body.

physiology   the science that deals with the functioning of living organisms.

PICC   *See* **peripheral intravenous central catheter**

pineal body   pea-sized endocrine gland located in the brain.

pituitary gland   "master" endocrine gland located in brain at base of skull (attached to hypothalamus); produces hormones that regulate growth and reproduction.

pivot   to twist or turn in a swiveling motion.

placenta   organ that develops during pregnancy and is attached to the wall of the mother's uterus; supplies the fetus with nutrients and oxygen.

planning   establishing possible solutions for a patient's problems (as determined by nursing diagnoses).

plasma   liquid portion of blood.

pleura   membranes that surround the lungs.

PM care   care given to prepare a patient for sleep.

pneumonia   inflammation and infection of the lungs.

pocket mask   a barrier device used for providing "mouth-to-mouth resuscitation" that prevents the patient's exhaled air and secretions from entering the caregiver's mouth.

port   opening.

portal of entry   area of body through which microbes enter and cause disease.

portal of exit   area of body through which disease-producing organisms leave the body.

post polio syndrome (PPS)   a neurologic disorder marked by increased weakness and/or abnormal muscle fatigue in persons who had paralytic polio many years earlier.

post anesthesia care unit (PACU) room where patients receive immediate care following surgery.

post-anesthesia recovery (PAR) area where patients are monitored until they are stable enough to leave the surgical department.

posterior back or dorsal.

postmortem after death.

postmortem care care given to the body after death.

postoperative after surgery.

postpartum after parturition; after birth.

posttraumatic stress disorder (PTSD) the development of unusual symptoms, such as nightmares or flashbacks, after a psychologically traumatic event.

postural support device used as an enabler that maintains body position and alignment.

pound (lb) unit of measurement of weight, equivalent to 16 ounces or 453.6 grams.

PPE *See* **personal protective equipment**

PPS *See* **post polio syndrome**

preadolescence years between the ages of 12 and 14.

predisposing factor condition that contributes to the development of disease.

prefix word part that is placed before a word root that changes or modifies the meaning of the word root.

prenatal before birth; care of the mother during pregnancy.

preoperative period before surgery.

pressure ulcer ulceration due to ischemia; pressure sore.

private room room in a health care facility that contains only one patient at a time.

probe as used in this text, a long, slender part of an instrument; that portion of the electronic or tympanic thermometer placed into the patient.

procedure the practices and processes used when following facility policies in patient care. A procedure prioritizes and orders your responsibilities when doing the task.

professional boundaries limits on how a health care worker interacts with patients.

prognosis probable outcome of a disease or injury.

prolapsed uterus *See* **uterine prolapse**

PROM *See* **passive range of motion**

prone position in which the patient is on the abdomen, spine straight, legs extended, and arms flexed on either side of the head.

prostate gland gland of male reproductive system that surrounds the neck of the urinary bladder and the beginning of the urethra.

prostatectomy removal of all or part of the prostate gland.

prosthesis artificial substitute for a missing body part, such as dentures, hand, leg.

protein basic material of every body cell; an essential nutrient.

protocol standards of procedure and care developed for preparation of a patient for diagnostic tests.

protozoa (singular protozoon) simple one-celled organisms that live on living matter.

proximal closest to the point of attachment.

psychiatric relating to mental illness.

PTSD *See* **posttraumatic stress disorder**

pubic relating to or near the pubis.

pulmonary embolism blood clot in the lungs.

pulse wave of blood pressure exerted against the walls of the arteries in response to ventricular contraction.

pulse deficit difference between contractions of the heart and pulse expansions of the radial artery.

pulse oximetry procedure for measuring level of oxygen in arterial blood.

pulse pressure difference between the systolic and diastolic pressures.

pupil circular opening in the center of the iris; regulates light entering the eye.

pureed diet diet in which foods are blended with gravy or liquid until they are the consistency of pudding.

push fluids to encourage a patient to drink additional fluids.

QA *See* **quality assurance**

quadrant one of the four imaginary sections of the surface of the abdomen.

quadriplegia *See* **tetraplegia**

quality assurance (QA) an internal review done by facility staff to identify problems and find solutions for improvement.

RA *See* **rheumatoid arthritis**

race classification of people according to shared physical characteristics.

RACE acronym relating to fire emergency procedure, meaning: *R*emove patient from danger; *A*ctivate alarm; *C*ontain fire; *E*xtinguish fire.

radial pulse pulse that can be measured by palpating the radial artery.

range-of-motion (ROM) exercises series of exercises specifically designed to move each joint through its full range.

rash change in the skin affecting color, appearance, temperature, or texture. The rash may be localized or generalized, and cause itching, burning, pain and swelling.

rate valuation based on comparison with a standard.

RCP *See* **respiratory care practitioner**

reality orientation techniques used to help a patient remain oriented to environment, time, and self.

receiver person for whom a communication is intended.

recovery position a modified lateral position used when the patient is recovering from certain emergencies, such as unconsciousness.

recovery room location where surgical patients are taken after surgery; they return to their rooms when their conditions stabilize.

rectal prolapse a condition that occurs when a large portion of the rectum protrudes from the body.

reflex activity performed without conscious thought.

registered nurse (RN) specially educated person who is licensed to plan and direct the nursing care of patients.

rehabilitation process of assisting an ill or injured person to attain an optimal level of well-being and function.

reminiscing thinking and talking about the past.

remission times in which a chronic disease appears stable.

renal calculi kidney stones.

renal colic spasm in an area near the kidney, accompanied by pain.

renal failure inability of the kidneys to maintain fluid and electrolyte balance, excrete waste products, and regulate essential body functions.

GLOSSARY

reservoir   storage area; biologically, an animal or source that maintains infectious organisms that periodically can be spread to others.

resident   person being cared for in a long-term care facility; *see also* **client** and **patient**.

Residents' Rights   document that spells out rights of residents receiving care in long-term care facilities.

respiration   process of taking oxygen into the body and expelling carbon dioxide.

respiratory arrest   cessation of breathing.

respiratory care practitioner (RCP)   a licensed professional who specializes in care of patients with disorders of the cardiopulmonary system, respirations, and sleep disorders that affect the patient's breathing.

respiratory failure   a condition that occurs when breathing is insufficient to sustain life.

rest   state of comfort, calmness, and relaxation.

restoration   basic nursing care measures designed to maintain or improve a patient's function and assist the patient to return to self-care.

restorative   returning to preexisting level or status.

retention   inability to excrete urine that has been produced.

retention catheter   catheter that is kept in the body rather than being removed after use; usually has a balloon that is inflated after the catheter is introduced into the bladder.

retinal degeneration   breakdown and functional loss of the nervous layer of the eye.

rheumatoid arthritis (RA)   autoimmune response that results in inflammation of the joints.

rhythm   the repeat interval of measured time or movement.

rigor mortis   rigidity of skeletal muscles, developing 6 to 10 hours after death.

risk factor   condition indicating that a problem may develop, causing the patient's health to worsen.

ritual   ceremonial acts that reinforce faith.

RN   *See* **registered nurse**

ROM   *See* **range-of-motion exercises**

rotation   act of turning about the axis of the center of a body, as in rotation of a joint.

rubra   redness; flushing of the skin.

Sacrament of the Sick   last rites given by clergy to a person who is terminally ill (dying).

SAD   *See* **seasonal affective disorder**

SARS   *See* **severe acute respiratory syndrome**

scabies   a parasitic disease of the skin that causes a rash and severe itching.

schizoaffective disorder   a condition that is believed to be a combination of schizophrenia and a mood disorder. This chronic, disabling mental illness has symptoms of schizophrenia, alternating with times when the patient also has symptoms of major depression or a manic episode.

scope of practice   extent or range of permissible activities.

seasonal affective disorder (SAD)   a depression that recurs each year at the same time, usually starting in fall or winter and ending in spring or early summer. The cause is not known, but it is believed to be related to lack of exposure to sunlight or abnormal melatonin levels.

self-care deficit   inability to perform an activity of daily living.

self-esteem   feeling of confidence about oneself.

self-identity   personal knowledge of who one is; personal view of self.

semicircular canal   three tubes in the inner ear containing fluid; the function is concerned with balance and detecting motion.

semi-Fowler's position   position in which the patient is on the back with knees slightly flexed, and the head of the bed is elevated 30° to 45°.

seminal vesicles   tissues in the male that store sperm and contribute nutrients to the seminal fluid.

semiprivate room   room in a health care facility that is shared by two patients.

semiprone   patient is positioned between the side and the abdomen.

semisupine   patient is positioned between the side and the back.

sender   the person who originates a communication.

senile purpura   dark purple bruises on the forearms and back of hands, common in elderly individuals.

sensitivity   ability to be aware of and appreciate personal characteristics of others; state of acute or abnormal response to stimuli or allergens.

sequential compression therapy   postoperative procedure in which pneumatic boots are applied to massage the legs using a milking, wavelike motion. Prevents blood clots.

severe acute respiratory syndrome (SARS)   a serious, highly infectious viral respiratory illness caused by a coronavirus.

sexual abuse   use of physical means or verbal threats to force a person to perform sexual acts.

sexual harassment   unwelcome sexual advances, requests for sexual favors, and other verbal or physical conduct of a sexual nature. The action may be physical, verbal, or nonverbal.

sexuality   maleness or femaleness of an individual.

sexually transmitted disease (STD)   disease that is passed from one individual to another through sexual contact.

sharps   needles, knife blades, etc.; items that can cut or puncture skin.

shearing   force on skin over bone when the skin remains at the point of contact while the bone moves; causes damage to skin.

shift report   information about patients passed from outgoing shift to oncoming shift.

shock   condition in which there is a disruption of circulation that results in dangerously low blood pressure and an upset of all bodily functions.

side rails   sliding metal bars that may be pulled up on each side of the bed to prevent the patient from falling out of bed.

sign   any objective evidence of an abnormal nature in the body or its organs.

sign language   communication for persons with hearing impairment; uses gestures and signs made with the fingers and hands.

simple (closed) fracture   fracture that does not produce an open wound in the skin and in which bones remain in proper alignment.

simple goiter   condition that causes hypothyroidism, in which the thyroid gland enlarges and undersecretes thyroxine.

Sims' position   position in which the patient is on the left side with left leg extended and right leg flexed; left arm is extended and brought behind the back; right arm is flexed and brought forward.

singultus   hiccup.

sitting (lateral) transfer   moving a patient from one surface to another with the patient sitting.

skilled care facility   long-term care facility. Skilled nursing facilities provide the most intensive level of care on the residential care continuum. Residents of these facilities have complex medical care and rehabilitation demands. Some are chronically ill and can no longer live independently.

skin tear   shallow injuries in which the epidermis is ripped or torn.

slander   false oral statement that injures the reputation of another person.

sleep   a period of continuous or intermittent unconsciousness in which physical movements are decreased.

sliding board   a plastic or wooden board that is about 2 feet long with a slippery surface. Used for a sitting, *lateral* transfer.

soft diet   intake consisting of low-residue, mildly flavored, easily digested foods.

source   person who has an infection that can be spread to others.

spastic paralysis   paralysis in which there is no voluntary movement. The extremities move in an involuntary pattern, similar to muscle spasms. The patient is aware of the movements, but cannot stop or control them.

sperm   male reproductive cell.

sphygmomanometer   instrument for determining arterial pressures; blood pressure gauge.

spica cast   body cast.

spinal anesthesia   technique of providing anesthesia by introducing drugs into the spinal canal.

spirituality   feeling of wholeness resulting from filling the human need to feel connected to the world and to a power greater than oneself.

splint   type of orthosis used to maintain position and prevent contractures of an extremity.

spores   microscopic reproductive bodies that spread infection and are very difficult to eliminate. They can survive in a dormant form until conditions are ideal for reproduction. The spores then multiply and continue to spread infection.

sprain   injury to ligament, resulting in pain and swelling.

sputum   matter brought up from the lungs; phlegm.

square corner   *See* **box corner**

stable   health condition is steady, predictable, without complications.

staff development   process used to educate staff in health care facilities.

standard   a basis for comparison; a reference point against which performance can be evaluated.

standard precautions   practices used in health care facilities to prevent the spread of infection via blood, body fluids, secretions, excretions, mucous membranes, and nonintact skin.

standing transfer   patient is moved from one surface to another while standing.

status   condition or state of health.

status epilepticus   a seizure that lasts for a long time, or repeats without recovery; a very serious medical emergency.

STD   *See* **sexually transmitted disease**

stereotype   rigid beliefs based on generalizations.

sterile   absence of all microorganisms; incapable of reproducing sexually.

sterilization   process that renders an individual incapable of reproduction; process of cleaning equipment to remove all microbes and make equipment sterile.

stertorous   snoring-type respirations.

stethoscope   instrument used in auscultation to make audible the sounds produced in the body.

stimulus   anything that provokes a response in a cell, tissue, or other structure.

stoma   artificial, mouthlike opening.

stool   another name for feces.

strain   injury to a muscle, resulting in pain.

stressors   situations, feelings, or conditions that cause a person to be anxious about his or her well-being.

stroke   cerebrovascular accident or brain attack; damage to the blood vessels of the brain.

subcutaneous tissue   connective tissue located under the dermis; attaches skin to muscle.

subjective observation   idea based on perceptions made only by the individual involved.

substance abuse   a disorder characterized by the use of one or more substances (such as alcohol or drugs) that alter mood or behavior, resulting in impairment.

suffix   word part added to the end of a word root that changes or modifies the meaning of the word root.

suicide   self-destruction; killing oneself.

suicide precautions   checks and practices a facility follows if a patient states that he or she no longer wishes to live and intends to harm himself or herself. May involve modifying the physical environment and securing the assistance of mental health professionals. The facility maintains these procedures until the patient is discharged or believed to be out of danger.

sundowning   behavior in which a patient becomes more agitated and disoriented during the evening hours.

superior   toward the head; upward.

supine position   lying with the face upward.

supplement   to add; also, the substance added.

supportive care   care given to a dying patient that avoids prolonging life but provides comfort measures only.

supportive device   used to help maintain a patient's body in a specific position.

suppository   medication used to help the bowels eliminate feces.

suprapubic catheter   a urinary catheter that is inserted surgically through the abdominal wall directly into the bladder.

surgical bed   bed prepared for a patient returning from surgery.

surgical mask   mask worn by health care workers during surgery, sterile procedures, standard precautions, and work in a droplet precautions room.

survey   a review and evaluation to ensure that the facility maintains acceptable standards of practice and quality of care.

surveyor   a representative of a private or governmental agency who reviews facility policies, procedures, and practices for quality of care.

susceptible host   a person who cannot resist the pathogen and will become ill from entry of the pathogen into the body. *See also* **host**

symbols   signs, pictures, or other characters used to communicate.

symmetry matching or correspondence in size, form, and arrangement.

symptom any perceptible change in the body or its function that indicates disease or the phases of disease.

synapse space between the axon of one nerve cell and the dendrites of others.

syphilis infectious, chronic, venereal disease characterized by lesions that may involve any organ or tissue; usually exhibits cutaneous manifestations; relapses are frequent; may exist asymptomatically for years.

system group of organs organized to perform a specific body function or functions; for example, the respiratory system.

systole contraction or period of contraction of cardiac muscle.

systolic pressure blood pressure exerted by the ventricles during the heart's contraction phase.

tachycardia unusually rapid heartbeat.

tachypnea pattern of rapid, shallow respirations.

tasks accomplishments throughout life that lead to healthy participation in society; work to be done.

TAT *See* **temporal artery thermometer**

TED hose support hose; anti-embolism stockings.

temporal artery thermometer (TAT) battery-operated thermometer that measures the temperature of the skin surface over the temporal artery.

tendon fibrous band of connective tissue that attaches skeletal muscle to bone.

terminal final; life-ending stage.

testes male gonads; reproductive glands located in the scrotal sac.

testosterone hormone produced by the testes.

tetany nervous condition characterized by intermittent toxic spasms that are usually paroxysmal and involve the extremities.

tetraplegia paralysis of the arms, legs, and trunk below the level of spinal cord injury.

THA *See* **total hip arthroplasty**

theft taking anything that does not belong to you; stealing.

therapeutic diet treatment through specifically planned nutrition.

therapy treatment designated to eliminate disease or other bodily disorder.

thermal burn injury (burn) caused by heat, fire, or flame.

thrombocyte blood platelet that is formed in the bone marrow and is important in blood clotting.

thrombophlebitis development of venous thrombi in the presence of inflammatory changes in the vessel wall.

thyroid gland endocrine gland situated in base of neck; has two lobes, one on either side of trachea; produces hormones thyrocalcitonin and thyroxine.

TIA *See* **transient ischemic attack**

tissue collection of specialized cells that perform a particular function; piece of paper used for cleansing (for example, toilet tissue, facial tissue).

toddler stage of childhood from 1 to 3 years of age.

toe pleat an extra space made by folding the top linen over 2 to 3 inches at the end of the bed to keep the linen from pulling the feet downward. This is more comfortable for the patient and reduces the risk of contractures, such as foot drop.

total hip arthroplasty (THA) surgical replacement of hip joint with a prosthesis.

total parenteral nutrition (TPN) also called *hyperalimentation*. A nutritionally complete IV solution containing proteins, carbohydrates, and fats; given to a patient who cannot digest food normally and whose bowel needs complete rest.

TPN *See* **total parenteral nutrition**

trachea windpipe.

tracheostomy opening made into anterior trachea.

transfer procedure followed when changing a patient's location.

transfer belt gait belt used to assist and support patients during ambulation.

transgender person whose personal feelings about gender identity do not match the anatomical sex he or she was born with, causing the individual to feel as if he or she was born with a physical body of the wrong gender.

transient ischemic attack (TIA) temporary reduction of flow of blood to the brain.

transmission transfer from one place or person to another.

transmission-based precautions isolation practices that prevent the spread of infection by interrupting the way in which the disease is spread.

tremor involuntary trembling.

tripod position a sitting position that makes the thorax larger on inspiration, enabling the patient to inhale more air.

trochanter roll rolled sheet or bath blanket placed under the patient extending from waist to mid-thigh; positioned against the hip to prevent lateral hip rotation.

tuberculosis disease condition occurring when tuberculosis bacteria enter the body and damage tissue.

tuberculosis infection condition in which tuberculosis bacteria enter the body but are walled off and contained and do not cause disease.

turning (moving) sheet *See* **draw sheet**

tympanic membrane membrane serving as the lateral wall of the tympanic cavity and separating it from the external acoustic meatus (outer ear).

tympanic thermometer device used to measure temperature at the tympanic membrane in the ear.

ulcer open sore caused by inadequate blood supply and broken skin.

ulcerative colitis inflammation of the colon resulting in the formation of ulcers.

ultraviolet germicidal irradiation (UVGI) special lights used to irradiate an isolation room to eliminate pathogens.

umbilical cord attachment connecting the fetus with the placenta. It is severed artificially at the birth of the child.

umbilicus depressed scar marking the site of entry of the umbilical cord in the fetus.

upper respiratory infection (URI) infection involving the organs of the upper respiratory tract.

ureter narrow tube that conducts urine from the kidney to the urinary bladder.

urethra mucus-lined tube conveying urine from the urinary bladder to the exterior of the body; in the male, the urethra also conveys the semen.

urgency need to urinate.

URI *See* **upper respiratory infection**

urinalysis laboratory analysis of urine.

urinary bladder receptacle for urine before it is voided.

urinary incontinence inability to control urination.

urinary meatus external opening to urethra.

uterine prolapse a condition that results from weakening of the ligaments, causing the uterus to slip downward into the vaginal canal.

uterus organ of gestation; womb.

UVGI *See* **ultraviolet germicidal irradiation**

vaccine artificial or weakened antigens that help the body develop antibodies to prevent infectious disease.

vagina tube that extends from the vulva to the uterine cervix; female organ of copulation that receives the penis during sexual intercourse.

validation therapy techniques used to help individuals feel good about themselves.

vancomycin-resistant enterococci (VRE) type of bacteria resistant to most antibiotics.

varicose vein enlarged vein in the leg due to an impaired valve in the vein.

vas deferens tube that carries sperm from the epididymis to the junction of the seminal vesicle; ductus deferens.

vascular an area of the body that contains many blood vessels and bleeds readily.

vector carrier, such as an arthropod, that transmits disease.

ventilation process of breathing in oxygen and breathing out carbon dioxide; also, a means of breathing for another person.

ventral front; anterior.

ventricle small cavity or chamber, as in the brain or heart.

verbal abuse use of speech to humiliate, threaten, or cause fear or anxiety in another person.

verbal communication transmitting messages using words.

vertigo sensation of rotation or movement of or about the person.

victim someone who is injured unexpectedly, as in an accident.

virus tiny living organisms by which some infectious diseases are transmitted.

visceral muscle muscle that operates without conscious control.

vital signs measurements of temperature, pulse, respiration, and blood pressure.

vitamin general term for various, unrelated organic substances, found in many foods in small amounts, that are necessary for normal metabolic function of the body.

vocal cords tissue that stretches across the larynx and produces vocal sounds.

void to release urine from the bladder.

volume capacity or size of an object or of an area; measure of the quantity of a substance.

VRE *See* **vancomycin-resistant enterococci**

vulva external female genitalia.

ward multiple-bed room, usually with 3 or 4 beds.

waterless bathing procedure in which a bed bath is given using a package of premoistened, disposable washcloths.

weight-bearing able to stand on one or both legs.

word root word form with a basic meaning; used in forming new words by combining it with prefixes or suffixes.

work practice controls specific procedures implemented to prevent the spread of infections.

workplace violence any physical assault, threatening behavior, or verbal abuse occurring in the workplace.

yeast one type of fungus.

INDEX

Note: Page numbers followed by f refer to Figures; page numbers followed by t refer to Tables

IMPORTANT! READ CAREFULLY: This End User License Agreement ("Agreement") sets forth the conditions by which Cengage Learning will make electronic access to the Cengage Learning-owned licensed content and associated media, software, documentation, printed materials, and electronic documentation contained in this package and/or made available to you via this product (the "Licensed Content"), available to you (the "End User"). BY CLICKING THE "I ACCEPT" BUTTON AND/OR OPENING THIS PACKAGE, YOU ACKNOWLEDGE THAT YOU HAVE READ ALL OF THE TERMS AND CONDITIONS, AND THAT YOU AGREE TO BE BOUND BY ITS TERMS, CONDITIONS, AND ALL APPLICABLE LAWS AND REGULATIONS GOVERNING THE USE OF THE LICENSED CONTENT.

1.0 SCOPE OF LICENSE

1.1 <u>Licensed Content</u>. The Licensed Content may contain portions of modifiable content ("Modifiable Content") and content which may not be modified or otherwise altered by the End User ("Non-Modifiable Content"). For purposes of this Agreement, Modifiable Content and Non-Modifiable Content may be collectively referred to herein as the "Licensed Content." All Licensed Content shall be considered Non-Modifiable Content, unless such Licensed Content is presented to the End User in a modifiable format and it is clearly indicated that modification of the Licensed Content is permitted.

1.2 Subject to the End User's compliance with the terms and conditions of this Agreement, Cengage Learning hereby grants the End User, a nontransferable, nonexclusive, limited right to access and view a single copy of the Licensed Content on a single personal computer system for noncommercial, internal, personal use only. The End User shall not (i) reproduce, copy, modify (except in the case of Modifiable Content), distribute, display, transfer, sublicense, prepare derivative work(s) based on, sell, exchange, barter or transfer, rent, lease, loan, resell, or in any other manner exploit the Licensed Content; (ii) remove, obscure, or alter any notice of Cengage Learning's intellectual property rights present on or in the Licensed Content, including, but not limited to, copyright, trademark, and/or patent notices; or (iii) disassemble, decompile, translate, reverse engineer, or otherwise reduce the Licensed Content.

2.0 TERMINATION

2.1 Cengage Learning may at any time (without prejudice to its other rights or remedies) immediately terminate this Agreement and/or suspend access to some or all of the Licensed Content, in the event that the End User does not comply with any of the terms and conditions of this Agreement. In the event of such termination by Cengage Learning, the End User shall immediately return any and all copies of the Licensed Content to Cengage Learning.

3.0 PROPRIETARY RIGHTS

3.1 The End User acknowledges that Cengage Learning owns all rights, title and interest, including, but not limited to all copyright rights therein, in and to the Licensed Content, and that the End User shall not take any action inconsistent with such ownership. The Licensed Content is protected by U.S., Canadian and other applicable copyright laws and by international treaties, including the Berne Convention and the Universal Copyright Convention. Nothing contained in this Agreement shall be construed as granting the End User any ownership rights in or to the Licensed Content.

3.2 Cengage Learning reserves the right at any time to withdraw from the Licensed Content any item or part of an item for which it no longer retains the right to publish, or which it has reasonable grounds to believe infringes copyright or is defamatory, unlawful, or otherwise objectionable.

4.0 PROTECTION AND SECURITY

4.1 The End User shall use its best efforts and take all reasonable steps to safeguard its copy of the Licensed Content to ensure that no unauthorized reproduction, publication, disclosure, modification, or distribution of the Licensed Content, in whole or in part, is made. To the extent that the End User becomes aware of any such unauthorized use of the Licensed Content, the End User shall immediately notify Cengage Learning. Notification of such violations may be made by sending an e-mail to infringement @ Cengage.com.

5.0 MISUSE OF THE LICENSED PRODUCT

5.1 In the event that the End User uses the Licensed Content in violation of this Agreement, Cengage Learning shall have the option of electing liquidated damages, which shall include all profits generated by the End User's use of the Licensed Content plus interest computed at the maximum rate permitted by law and all legal fees and other expenses incurred by Cengage Learning in enforcing its rights, plus penalties.

6.0 FEDERAL GOVERNMENT CLIENTS

6.1 Except as expressly authorized by Cengage Learning, Federal Government clients obtain only the rights specified in this Agreement and no other rights. The Government acknowledges that (i) all software and related documentation incorporated in the Licensed Content is existing commercial computer software within the meaning of FAR 27.405(b)(2); and (2) all other data delivered in whatever form, is limited rights data within the meaning of FAR 27.401. The restrictions in this section are acceptable as consistent with the Government's need for software and other data under this Agreement.

7.0 DISCLAIMER OF WARRANTIES AND LIABILITIES

7.1 Although Cengage Learning believes the Licensed Content to be reliable, Cengage Learning does not guarantee or warrant (i) any information or materials contained in or produced by the Licensed Content, (ii) the accuracy, completeness or reliability of the Licensed Content, or (iii) that the Licensed Content is free from errors or other material defects. THE LICENSED PRODUCT IS PROVIDED "AS IS," WITHOUT ANY WARRANTY OF ANY KIND AND CENGAGE LEARNING DISCLAIMS ANY AND ALL WARRANTIES, EXPRESSED OR IMPLIED, INCLUDING, WITHOUT LIMITATION, WARRANTIES OF MERCHANTABILITY OR FITNESS FOR A PARTICULAR PURPOSE. IN NO EVENT SHALL CENGAGE LEARNING BE LIABLE FOR: INDIRECT, SPECIAL, PUNITIVE OR CONSEQUENTIAL DAMAGES INCLUDING FOR LOST PROFITS, LOST DATA, OR OTHERWISE. IN NO EVENT SHALL CENGAGE LEARNING'S AGGREGATE LIABILITY HEREUNDER, WHETHER ARISING IN CONTRACT, TORT, STRICT LIABILITY OR OTHERWISE, EXCEED THE AMOUNT OF FEES PAID BY THE END USER HEREUNDER FOR THE LICENSE OF THE LICENSED CONTENT.

8.0 GENERAL

8.1 Entire Agreement. This Agreement shall constitute the entire Agreement between the Parties and supercedes all prior Agreements and understandings oral or written relating to the subject matter hereof.

8.2 Enhancements/Modifications of Licensed Content. From time to time, and in Cengage Learning's sole discretion, Cengage Learning may advise the End User of updates, upgrades, enhancements and/or improvements to the Licensed Content, and may permit the End User to access and use, subject to the terms and conditions of this Agreement, such modifications, upon payment of prices as may be established by Cengage Learning.

8.3 No Export. The End User shall use the Licensed Content solely in the United States and shall not transfer or export, directly or indirectly, the Licensed Content outside the United States.

8.4 Severability. If any provision of this Agreement is invalid, illegal, or unenforceable under any applicable statute or rule of law, the provision shall be deemed omitted to the extent that it is invalid, illegal, or unenforceable. In such a case, the remainder of the Agreement shall be construed in a manner as to give greatest effect to the original intention of the parties hereto.

8.5 Waiver. The waiver of any right or failure of either party to exercise in any respect any right provided in this Agreement in any instance shall not be deemed to be a waiver of such right in the future or a waiver of any other right under this Agreement.

8.6 Choice of Law/Venue. This Agreement shall be interpreted, construed, and governed by and in accordance with the laws of the State of New York, applicable to contracts executed and to be wholly preformed therein, without regard to its principles governing conflicts of law. Each party agrees that any proceeding arising out of or relating to this Agreement or the breach or threatened breach of this Agreement may be commenced and prosecuted in a court in the State and County of New York. Each party consents and submits to the nonexclusive personal jurisdiction of any court in the State and County of New York in respect of any such proceeding.

8.7 Acknowledgment. By opening this package and/or by accessing the Licensed Content on this Web site, THE END USER ACKNOWLEDGES THAT IT HAS READ THIS AGREEMENT, UNDERSTANDS IT, AND AGREES TO BE BOUND BY ITS TERMS AND CONDITIONS. IF YOU DO NOT ACCEPT THESE TERMS AND CONDITIONS, YOU MUST NOT ACCESS THE LICENSED CONTENT AND RETURN THE LICENSED PRODUCT TO CENGAGE LEARNING (WITHIN 30 CALENDAR DAYS OF THE END USER'S PURCHASE) WITH PROOF OF PAYMENT ACCEPTABLE TO CENGAGE LEARNING, FOR A CREDIT OR A REFUND. Should the End User have any questions/comments regarding this Agreement, please contact Cengage Learning at Delmar.help@cengage.com.

StudyWare™ to Accompany Nursing Assistant: A Nursing Process Approach – Basics

Minimum System Requirements

- Operating systems: Microsoft Windows XP w/SP 2, Windows Vista w/ SP 1
- Processor: Minimum required by Operating System
- Memory: Minimum required by Operating System
- Hard Drive Space: 225 MB
- Screen resolution: 800 × 600 pixels
- CD-ROM drive
- Sound card & listening device required for audio features
- Flash Player 9. The Adobe Flash Player is free, and can be downloaded from http://www.adobe.com/products/flashplayer/

Setup Instructions

1. Insert disc into CD-ROM drive. The StudyWare™ installation program should start automatically. If it does not, go to step 2.
2. From My Computer, double-click the icon for the CD drive.
3. Double-click the *setup.exe* file to start the program.

Technical Support

Telephone: 1-800-648-7450

8:30 A.M.–6:30 P.M. Eastern Time

E-mail: delmar.help@cengage.com

StudyWare™ is a trademark used herein under license.

Microsoft® and Windows® are registered trademarks of the Microsoft Corporation.

Pentium® is a registered trademark of the Intel Corporation.